# Diseases of the Ocular Fundus

Commissioning Editor: Paul Fam
Project Development Manager: Belinda Kuhn
Project Manager: Susan Stuart
Illustration Manager: Mick Ruddy
Design Manager: Jayne Jones
Illustrator: Paul Pernson

# Diseases of the Ocular Fundus

**Jack J Kanski** MD, MS, FRCS, FRCOphth
Honorary Consultant Ophthalmic Surgeon
Prince Charles Eye Unit
King Edward VII Hospital
Windsor, UK

**Stanislaw A Milewski** MD, MA, FACS
Clinical Professor of Ophthalmology
University of Connecticut, USA

**Bertil E Damato** PhD FRCS FRCOphth
Professor of Ophthalmology
Director Ocular Oncology Service
The Royal Liverpool University Hospital
Liverpool, UK

**Vaughan Tanner** BSc, MBBS, FRCOphth
Consultant Ophthalmic Surgeon
Prince Charles Eye Unit
Windsor and Royal Berkshire Hospital
Reading, UK

**Photographers**
Irina Gout
Anne Bolton
Matthew J Koyama
Richard Baseler
Peter Fontaine
James Gendron
Bogdan Stoj

**Artists**
T R Tarrant
Jenni Miller

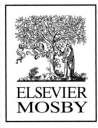

ELSEVIER
MOSBY

Edinburgh   London   New York   Oxford   Philadelphia   St Louis   Sydney   Toronto   2005

**ELSEVIER**
**MOSBY**

MOSBY An imprint of Elsevier Limited

First published 2005

ISBN 0 7234 3370 4

**British Library Cataloguing in Publication Data**
A catalogue record for this book is available from the British Library

**Library of Congress Cataloging in Publication Data**
A catalog record for this book is available from the Library of Congress

**Notice**
Medical knowledge is constantly changing. Standard safety precautions must be followed, but as new research and clinical experience broaden our knowledge, changes in treatment and drug therapy may become necessary or appropriate. Readers are advised to check the most current product information provided by the manufacturer of each drug to be administered to verify the recommended dose, the method and duration of administration, and contraindications. It is the responsibility of the practitioner, relying on experience and knowledge of the patient, to determine dosages and the best treatment for each individual patient. Neither the Publisher nor the author assumes any liability for any injury and/or damage to persons or property arising from this publication.
The Publisher

The
Publisher's
policy is to use
**paper manufactured**
**from sustainable forests**

Printed in China

# Preface

Despite great advances in medicine, diseases of the ocular fundus remain a common cause of severe visual impairment. The purpose of this book is to present an up-to-date, systematic and practical overview of fundus disease. The presentation is intentionally pragmatic in order to attempt to contain a large amount of material within a reasonably sized book.

*Diseases of the Ocular Fundus* is primarily intended for general ophthalmologists, those in training as well as optometrists. The further reading section is not meant to be comprehensive. We have mainly included recent papers and only older publications that have special merit.

JK
SM
BD
VT
2004

# Acknowledgements

We are very grateful to Brad Bowling and Carlos Pavesio for reviewing the manuscript and providing much useful advice.

We would also like to acknowledge and thank the many medical photographic departments as well as the following colleagues for supplying us with additional material without which this book could not have been written: Peter J Hudson, Jerry Neuwirth, Michael S Ruddat, Marion Joseph Stoj and Andrew J Packer.

# Contents

Contents

# Chapter **1**

# EXAMINATION AND INVESTIGATION

## Slit-lamp Biomicroscopy

### SLIT-LAMP INDIRECT OPHTHALMOSCOPY

This examination utilises high-power convex lenses designed to obtain a wide field of view of the fundus (Fig. 1.1); the image is vertically inverted and laterally reversed. The technique is as follows:

- Adjust the slit beam to a width about one-quarter of its full round diameter.
- Set the illumination angle coaxial with the slit-lamp viewing system.
- Set the magnification and light intensity at their lowest settings.
- Focus on the cornea and centre the light beam to pass directly through the patient's pupil.
- Hold the lens directly in front of the cornea just clearing the lashes so that the light beam passes through its centre.
- Examine the fundus by moving the joystick and vertical adjustment mechanism of the slit lamp whilst keeping the lens still.
- Reduce reflections by tilting or angling the light beam.
- Increase the width of the beam to obtain a larger field of view.
- Increase the magnification to show greater detail as necessary.
- To view the peripheral retina, the patient should be instructed to direct their gaze accordingly.

### GOLDMANN THREE-MIRROR EXAMINATION

1. **The Goldmann three-mirror contact lens** consists of four parts; a central part and three mirrors set at different angles. It is important to be familiar with each part of the lens as follows (Fig. 1.2):

   - The central part provides a 30° upright view of the posterior pole.
   - The equatorial mirror (largest and oblong-shaped) enables visualisation from 30° to the equator.

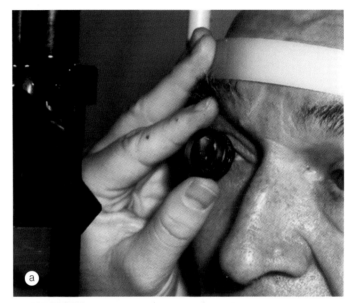

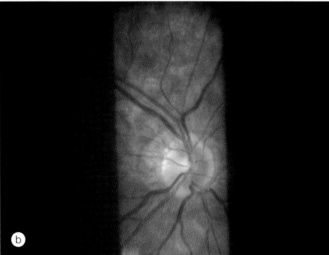

**Figure 1.1 (a)** Indirect slit-lamp biomicroscopy; **(b)** fundus view. (Courtesy of B. Tompkins)

   - The peripheral mirror (intermediate in size and square-shaped) enables visualisation between the equator and the ora serrata.
   - The gonioscopy mirror (smallest and dome-shaped) may be used for visualising the extreme retinal periphery and pars plana. It is therefore apparent that the smaller the mirror, the more peripheral the view obtained.

1

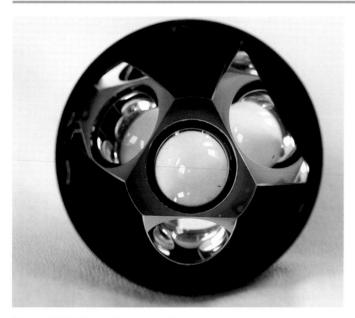

**Figure 1.2** Goldmann three-mirror lens

## 2. Mirror positioning

- The mirror should be positioned opposite the area of the fundus to be examined; to examine the 12 o'clock position, the mirror should be positioned at 6 o'clock.
- When viewing the vertical meridian, the image is upside down but not laterally reversed, as with indirect ophthalmoscopy, so that lesions located to the left of 12 o'clock in the retina will also appear in the mirror on the left-hand side (Fig. 1.3).
- When viewing the horizontal meridian, the image is laterally reversed.

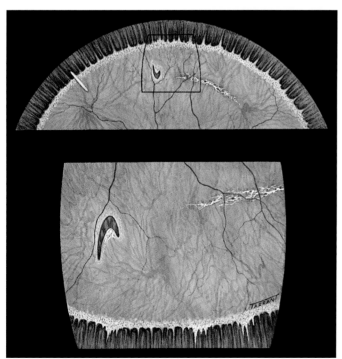

**Figure 1.3 (Top)** U-tear left of 12 o'clock and an island of lattice degeneration right of 12 o'clock; **(bottom)** the same lesions seen with the triple mirror positioned at 6 o'clock

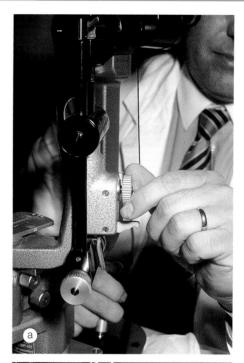

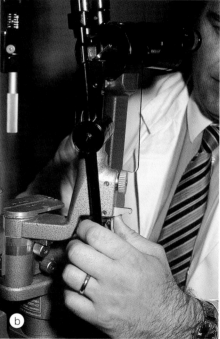

**Figure 1.4 (a)** Unlocking the screw; **(b)** tilting of the illumination column

## 3. Technique

- Dilate the pupils.
- Unlock the locking screw (Fig. 1.4a) to allow tilting of the illumination column (Fig. 1.4b).
- Instruct the patient to keep both eyes open at all times and not to move the head backward when the lens is being inserted.
- Instil topical anaesthetic drops.
- Insert coupling fluid (high-viscosity methylcellulose or equivalent) into the cup of the contact lens but do not overfill; it should be no more than half full.

- Ask the patient to look up, insert the inferior rim of the lens into the lower fornix (Fig. 1.5) and press it quickly against the cornea so that the coupling fluid has no time to escape (Fig. 1.6).
- Ask the patient to look straight ahead and wipe away any excess coupling fluid with a soft tissue.
- The illumination column should always be tilted except when viewing the 12 o'clock position in the fundus (i.e. with the mirror at 6 o'clock).
- When viewing horizontal meridians (i.e. 3 and 9 o'clock positions in the fundus), the column should be kept central.
- When viewing the vertical meridians (i.e. 6 and 12 o'clock positions), the column can be positioned left or right of centre (Fig. 1.7).
- When viewing oblique meridians (i.e. 1.30 and 7.30 o'clock), keep the column right of centre, and vice versa when viewing the 10.30 and 4.30 o'clock positions.
- When viewing different positions of the peripheral retina, rotate the axis of the beam so that it is always at right angles to the mirror.

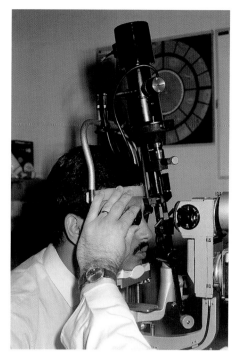

**Figure 1.7** Illumination column tilted and positioned right of centre to view the oblique meridians at 1.30 and 7.30 o'clock

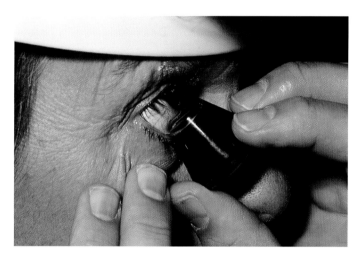

**Figure 1.5** Insertion of the triple-mirror lens into the lower fornix with the patient looking up

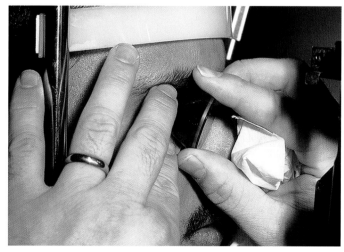

**Figure 1.6** Triple-mirror in position

- To visualise the entire fundus, rotate the lens for 360° using first the equatorial mirror and then the peripheral mirrors.
- To obtain a more peripheral view of the retina, tilt the lens to the opposite side, asking the patient to move the eyes to the same side. For example, to obtain a more peripheral view of 12 o'clock (with mirrors at 6 o'clock), tilt the lens down and ask the patient to look up.
- Examine the vitreous cavity with the central lens using both a horizontal and a vertical slit beam.
- Examine the posterior pole.

## INTERPRETATION OF SIGNS

- The normal vitreous in a young individual appears homogeneous with the same density throughout. Swift ocular movements produce undulating folds in the gel and a few small opacities may be seen.
- The central vitreous cavity contains optically empty spaces (lacunae). The condensed lining of a large cavity may be mistaken for a detached posterior hyaloid surface (pseudo-posterior vitreous detachment [pseudo-PVD]).
- In eyes with PVD, the detached posterior hyaloid surface (Fig. 1.8) can usually be traced to its insertion in to the vitreous base above.
- A Weiss ring (Fig. 1.9) is an annular opacity represent-ing a ring of glial tissue detached from the margin of the optic disc; it is virtually pathognomonic of PVD.
- 'Tobacco dust', consisting of retinal pigment epithelial (RPE) cells and macrophages, in the retrolental space (Fig. 1.10), in a patient complaining of sudden onset of flashing

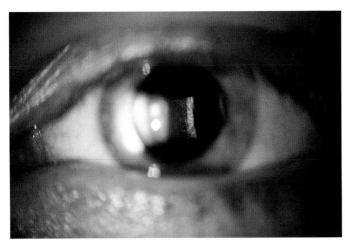

**Figure 1.8** Posterior hyaloid face in an eye with posterior vitreous detachment

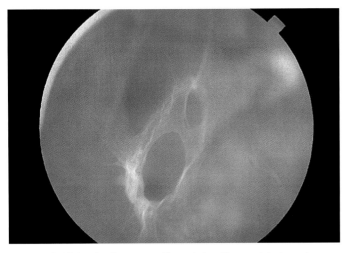

**Figure 1.9** Weiss ring in an eye with posterior vitreous detachment

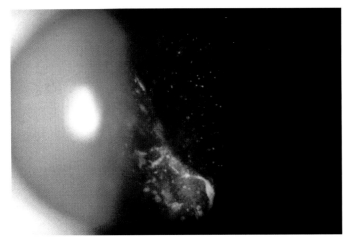

**Figure 1.10** 'Tobacco dust' in the anterior vitreous in an eye with a retinal tear

lights and floaters is strongly suggestive of the presence of a retinal tear. A careful examination of the peripheral retina, particularly superiorly, is mandatory.

● Traces of blood in the vitreous will often appear as numerous small opacities within the anteriorly displaced gel or in the retrohyaloid space.

# Indirect Ophthalmoscopy

## CONDENSING LENSES

Condensing lenses of various powers and diameters are available for indirect ophthalmoscopy. The higher the power, the lower the magnification, the shorter the working distance but the greater the field of view. The following lenses are currently available (Fig. 1.11):

● 15D (magnifies ×4; field about 40°) is used for examination of the posterior pole.
● 20D (magnifies ×3; field about 45°) is the most commonly used for general examination of the fundus.
● 25D (magnifies ×2.5; field is about 50°).
● 30D (magnifies ×2; field is 60°) has a shorter working distance and is useful when examining patients with small pupils.
● 40D (magnifies ×1; field is about 65°) is used mainly to examine small children.
● Panretinal 2.2 (magnifies ×3; field is about 55°).

## TECHNIQUE

● Dilate both pupils well with 1% tropicamide and, if necessary, phenylephrine 10% so that they will not constrict when exposed to a bright light during examination.
● The patient should be in the supine position, with one pillow, on a bed (Fig. 1.12), reclining chair or couch and not sitting upright in a chair (Fig. 1.13).
● Darken the examination room.
● Set the eyepieces at the correct interpupillary distance and align the beam so that it is located in the centre of the viewing frame.
● Instruct the patient to keep both eyes open at all times.
● Take the lens into one hand with the flat surface facing the patient and throughout the examination try to keep it parallel to the patient's iris plane.
● If necessary, gently separate the patient's eyelids with the fingers.
● Find the red reflex and begin at a low-to-medium light intensity.

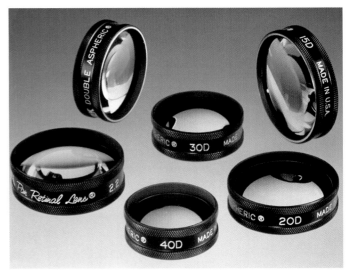

**Figure 1.11** Condensing lenses used for indirect ophthalmoscopy

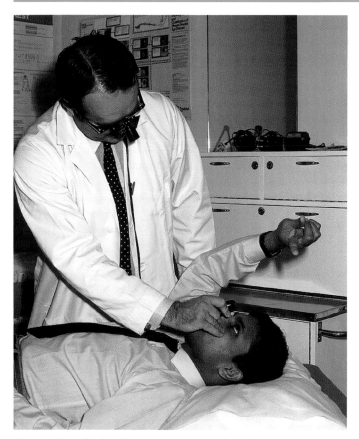

**Figure 1.12** Indirect ophthalmoscopy – correct position

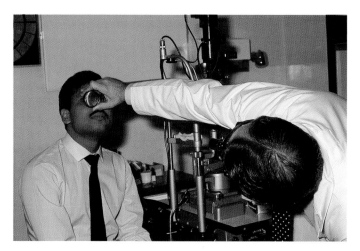

**Figure 1.13** Indirect ophthalmoscopy – incorrect position

- In order to enable the patient to get used to the light, he or she should be asked to look up and the superior peripheral fundus should be examined first.
- Avoid the tendency to move towards the patient if you are having difficulty visualising the fundus.
- Be prepared to move around the patient and stand opposite the clock hour position to be examined. For example, when viewing the 9 o'clock meridian, stand to the patient's left.
- Ask the patient to move the eyes and head into optimal positions for examination. For example, when examining the extreme retinal periphery, ask the patient to look away from you.

## SCLERAL INDENTATION

1. **Purposes.** Scleral indentation should be attempted only after the art of indirect ophthalmoscopy has been mastered. Its main function is to enhance visualisation of the peripheral retina anterior to the equator (Fig. 1.14); it also permits a kinetic evaluation of the retina.

2. **Technique**

- Take the indenter into one hand.
- To view the ora serrata at 12 o'clock, first ask the patient to look down and then apply the scleral indenter to the outside of the upper eyelid at the margin of the tarsal plate (Fig. 1.15a).
- With the indenter in place, ask the patient to look up; at the same time, advance the indenter into the anterior orbit parallel with the globe (Fig. 1.15b).
- Align your eyes with the condensing lens and indenter and then exert gentle pressure and observe the mound created by the indentation in the fundus (Fig. 1.16). The indenter should be kept tangential to the globe at all times, as perpendicular indentation will cause pain.
- Move the indenter to an adjacent part of the fundus, making sure that your eyes, the condensing lens, the fundus image and the indenter are all in a straight line.
- The entire fundus can usually be examined while indenting through the eyelids. Occasionally, in patients with very tight eyelids, indentation directly over the conjunctiva may be necessary to examine the 3 and 9 o'clock positions. If this is done gently, a topical anaesthetic may not be required.

## FUNDUS DRAWING

1. **Technique.** The image seen with the indirect ophthalmoscope is vertically inverted and laterally reversed. This phenomenon can be used to your advantage when drawing the fundus if the top of the chart is placed towards the patient's feet (i.e. upside down). In this way, the inverted position of the chart in relation to the patient's eye corresponds to the image of the fundus obtained by the observer. For example, a U-tear at 11 o'clock in the patient's right eye will correspond to the 11 o'clock position on the chart;

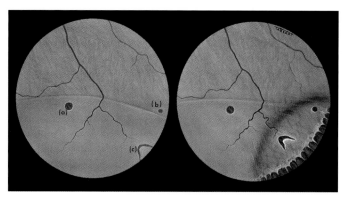

**Figure 1.14** Appearance of retinal breaks in detached retina.
**(Left)** Without scleral indentation; **(right)** with scleral indentation

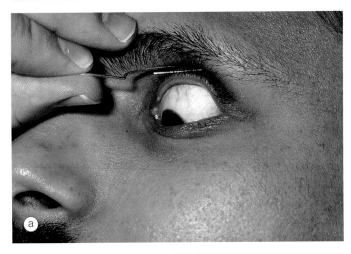

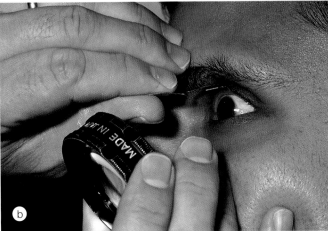

**Figure 1.15** Technique of scleral indentation

the same applies to the area of lattice degeneration between 1 o'clock and 2 o'clock (Fig. 1.17).

2. **Colour code** (Fig. 1.18)

- Have coloured pencils (red, blue, yellow, black and green) available.
- Record the boundaries of the retinal detachment (RD) by starting at the optic nerve and then extending to the periphery.
- Shade detached retina in blue and flat retina in red.
- Indicate the course of retinal veins with blue. Retinal arterioles are not usually drawn unless they serve as a special guide to an important lesion.
- Draw retinal breaks in red with blue outlines; the flat part of a retinal tear is also drawn in blue.
- Thin retina is indicated by red hatchings outlined in blue; lattice degeneration is shown as blue hatchings outlined in blue; retinal pigment is black; retinal exudates yellow; and vitreous opacities green.

# Psychophysiological Tests

## VISUAL ACUITY

This is the easiest to perform and most important test of visual function. Spatial visual acuity is the ability to distinguish separate elements of a target and identify it as a whole. It is quantified by the minimum angle of separation (subtended at the nodal point of the eye) between two objects that allows them to be perceived as separate.

1. **The Snellen** notation is described as the testing distance over the distance at which the letter would subtend 5 minutes of arc vertically. Thus, at 6 metres, a 6/6 letter

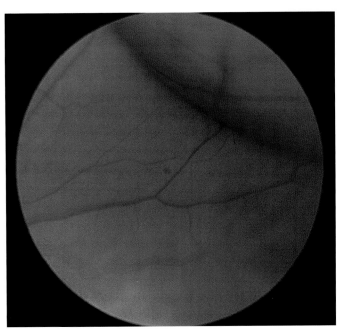

**Figure 1.16** Mound created by scleral indentation (Courtesy of N.E. Byer, from *The Peripheral Retina in Profile, a Stereoscopic Atlas*. Criterion Press, Torrance, California, 1982)

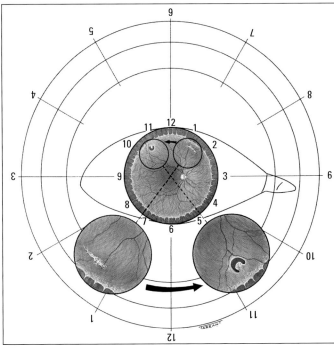

**Figure 1.17** Technique of drawing retinal lesions (see text)

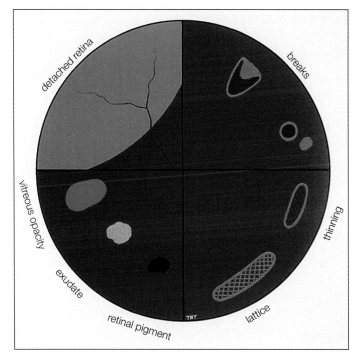

**Figure 1.18** Colour code for documenting retinal lesions

subtends 5 minutes of arc, a 6/12 letter subtends 10 minutes and a 6/60 letter 50 minutes. The Snellen fraction may also be expressed as a decimal (i.e. 6/6 = 1 and 6/12 = 0.5). Unfortunately, the Snellen chart (Fig. 1.19) has many shortcomings. For example, the letters on the lower lines are more crowded than are those towards the top, the spacing between each letter and each row bears no systematic relationship to the width or height of the letters, and the small number of larger letters limits the chart's usefulness.

2. **The Bailey–Lovie** chart (Fig. 1.20) is more accurate than the Snellen and is preferred in vision research. This records the minimum angle of resolution (MAR). The MAR relates to the resolution required to resolve the elements of a letter. Thus, 6/6 equates to a MAR of 1 minute of arc and 6/12 equates to 2 minutes. LogMAR is simply the log of the MAR. Each line of the chart comprises five letters, and the spacing between each letter and each row is related to the width and height of the letters, respectively. The results are usually recorded in terms of a logMAR score, with the notation 6/6 being equivalent to a logMAR of zero. As letter size changes by 0.1 logMAR units per row and there are five letters in each row, each letter can be assigned a score of 0.02. The final score takes account of every letter that has been read correctly, thus avoiding the shortcomings of the Snellen chart.

3. **The potential visual acuity meter** is used to test macular function in eyes with cataract. The instrument projects a standard Snellen chart onto the macula through a small chink of an immature cataract and the patient is asked to read the letters (Fig. 1.21).

## CONTRAST SENSITIVITY

1. **Principle.** Contrast sensitivity is a measure of the minimal amount of contrast required to distinguish a test object.

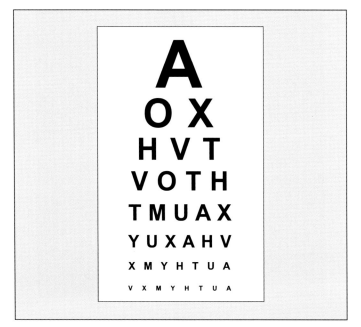

**Figure 1.19** Snellen chart

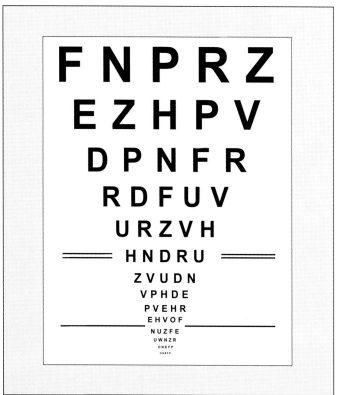

**Figure 1.20** Bailey–Lovie chart

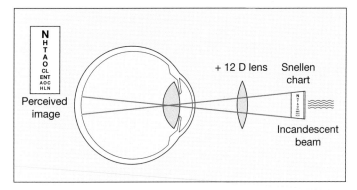

**Figure 1.21** Potential visual acuity meter (see text)

Although the test is capable of detecting very early visual dysfunction, even when Snellen visual acuity is normal, it is seldom performed in everyday clinical practice.

2. **The Pelli-Robson** contrast sensitivity letter chart (Fig. 1.22) is viewed at 1 metre and consists of rows of letters of equal size but with decreasing contrast of 0.15 log units for every group of three letters.

## AMSLER GRID

The Amsler grid charts evaluate the 20° of the visual field centred on fixation (Fig. 1.23) and are useful in screening and monitoring macular disease.

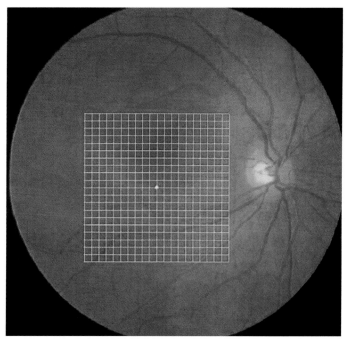

**Figure 1.23** Amsler grid superimposed onto the retina (Courtesy of A. Franklin)

1. **Charts.** There are seven charts, each consisting of a 10-cm square (Figs. 1.24 and 1.25).

   a. *Chart 1* is divided into 400 smaller 5-mm squares. When viewed at about one-third of a metre, each small square subtends an angle of 1°.
   b. *Chart 2* is similar to chart 1 but has diagonal lines that aid fixation in patients unable to see the central spot.

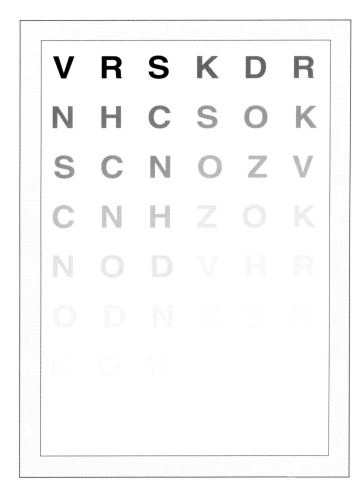

**Figure 1.22** Pelli–Robson contrast sensitivity letter chart

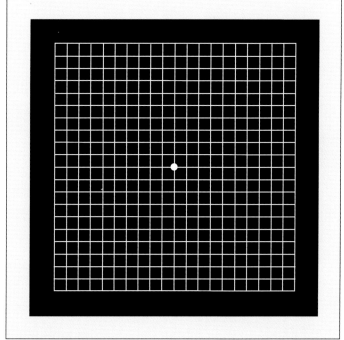

**Figure 1.24** Amsler grid chart 1 (Courtesy of A. Franklin)

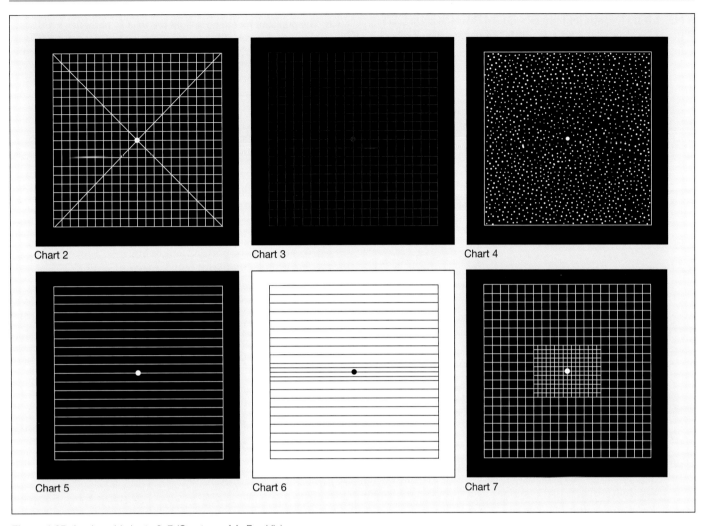

Chart 2

Chart 3

Chart 4

Chart 5

Chart 6

Chart 7

**Figure 1.25** Amsler grid charts 2–7 (Courtesy of A. Franklin)

c. *Chart 3* is identical to chart 1 but has red squares, which may be helpful in detecting colour desaturation in patients with optic nerve lesions.

d. *Chart 4* consisting only of random dots, reveals only scotomas, as there is no form to be distorted.

e. *Chart 5* consists of horizontal lines and is designed to detect metamorphopsia along specific meridians.

f. *Chart 6* is similar to chart 5 but has a white background, and the central lines are closer together.

g. *Chart 7* exhibits a fine central grid, each square subtending an angle of ½°, and is therefore more sensitive.

## 2. Technique

- Reading spectacles are worn, if appropriate, and one eye is covered.
- The patient is asked to look directly at the central dot with the uncovered eye and report any distortion, blurred areas or blank spots anywhere on the grid.
- Patients with macular disease often report that the lines are wavy whereas those with optic neuropathy often remark that some of the lines are missing or faint but not distorted (Fig. 1.26).

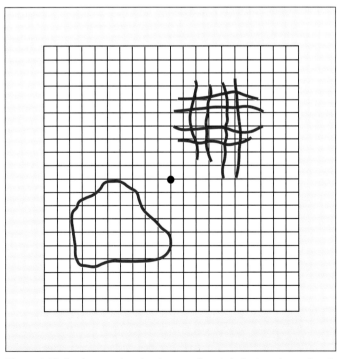

**Figure 1.26** Amsler recording showing wavy lines to indicate metamorphopsia and an outline of a relative scotoma (Courtesy of A. Franklin)

## THE LIGHT BRIGHTNESS COMPARISON TEST

This is essentially a test of optic nerve function, which is usually normal in retinal disease, unless very advanced. It is performed as follows:

- A light from an indirect ophthalmoscope is shone first into the normal eye and then the eye with suspected disease.
- The patient is asked whether the light is symmetrically bright in both eyes.
- In optic neuropathy, the patient will report that the light is less bright in the affected eye.
- The patient is asked to assign a relative value from 1 to 5 to the brightness of light in the diseased eye, as compared with the normal eye.

## PHOTOSTRESS TEST

1. **Principles.** Photostress testing is a gross test of dark adaptation in which the visual pigments are bleached by light. This causes a temporary state of retinal insensitivity perceived by the patient as a scotoma. The recovery of vision is dependent on the ability of the photoreceptors to re-synthesise visual pigments. The test may be useful in detecting maculopathy when ophthalmoscopy is equivocal, as in mild cystoid macular oedema or central serous retinopathy; it may also differentiate visual loss caused by macular disease from that caused by an optic nerve lesion.

2. **Technique**

- The best corrected distance visual acuity is determined.
- The patient fixates the light of a pen-torch or an indirect ophthalmoscope held about 3 cm away for about 10 seconds (Fig. 1.27a).
- The photostress recovery time (PSRT) is the time taken to read any three letters of the pre-test acuity line and is normally between 15 and 30 seconds (Fig. 1.27b).
- The test is performed on the other, presumably normal, eye and the results are compared.
- The PSRT is prolonged, relative to the normal eye, in macular disease (sometimes 50 seconds or more) but not in an optic neuropathy.

> **NB:** The pupillary reactions to light are usually normal in eyes with macular disease, although extensive retinal disease such as a retinal detachment or ischaemic central retinal vein occlusion may cause an afferent pupillary defect (APD). This is in contrast to optic neuropathy, in which an APD occurs even in mild cases.

## DARK ADAPTOMETRY

1. **Principle.** Dark adaptation (DA) is the phenomenon by which the visual system (pupil, retina and occipital cortex) adapts to decreased illumination. This test is particularly useful in the investigation of patients complaining of night-blindness (nyctalopia). The retina is exposed to an intense light for a time sufficient to bleach 25% or more of the rhodopsin in the retina. Following this, normal rods are insensitive to light and cones respond only to very bright stimuli. Subsequent recovery of light sensitivity can be monitored by placing the subject in the dark and periodically presenting spots of light of varying intensity in the visual field and asking the subject if they are perceived.

2. **Technique of Goldmann–Weekes adaptometry**

- The subject is exposed to an intense light that bleaches the photoreceptors and then is suddenly placed in the dark.
- The threshold at which the subject just perceives the light is plotted.
- The flashes are repeated at regular intervals; the sensitivity of the eye to light gradually increases.

3. **The sensitivity curve** is a plot of the light intensity of a minimally perceived spot versus time and is bipartite (Fig. 1.28).

   a. *The cone branch* of the curve represents the initial 5–10 minutes of darkness during which cone sensitivity rapidly improves. The rod photoreceptors are also recovering during this time, but more slowly.

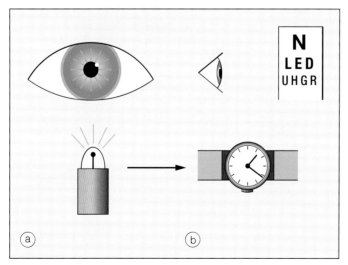

**Figure 1.27** Photostress test (see text)

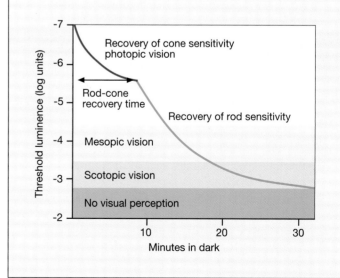

**Figure 1.28** Dark adaptation curve

b. The 'rod–cone' break in normal subjects occurs after 7–10 minutes, when cones achieve their maximum sensitivity, and the rods become perceptibly more sensitive than cones.

c. The rod branch of the curve is slower and represents the continuation of improvement of rod sensitivity. After 15–30 minutes, the fully dark-adapted rods allow the subject to perceive a spot of light over 100 times dimmer than would be possible with cones alone. If the flashes are focused onto the foveola (where rods are absent), only a rapid segment, corresponding to cone adaptation, is recorded.

## COLOUR VISION TESTS

These tests are sometimes useful in the clinical evaluation of hereditary fundus dystrophies, where impairment may be present prior to the development of visual acuity and visual field changes.

1. **Principles.** Colour vision is a function of three populations of retinal cones, each with its specific sensitivity; blue (tritan) at 414–424 nm, green (deuteran) at 522–539 nm and red (protan) at 549–570 nm. A normal person requires all these primary colours to match those within the spectrum. Any given cone pigment may be deficient (e.g. protanomaly – red weakness) or entirely absent (e.g. protanopia – red blindness). Trichromats possess all three types of cones (although not necessarily functioning perfectly), while absence of one or two types of cones renders an individual a dichromat or a monochromat, respectively. Most individuals with congenital colour defects are anomalous trichromats and use abnormal proportions of the three primary colours to match those in the light spectrum. Those with red–green deficiency caused by abnormality of red-sensitive cones are protanomalous, those with abnormality of green-sensitive cones are deuteranomalous, and those with blue–green deficiency caused by abnormality of blue-sensitive cones are tritanomalous.

> **NB: Acquired macular disease tends to produce blue–yellow defects, and optic nerve lesions red–green defects.**

2. **Ishihara** test is used mainly to screen for congenital protan and deuteran defects. It consists of a test plate followed by 16 plates each with a matrix of dots arranged to show a central shape or number, which the subject is asked to identify (Fig. 1.29). A colour-deficient person will only be able to identify some of the figs. Inability to identify the test plate (provided visual acuity is sufficient) indicates malingering.

3. **City University** test consists of 10 plates each containing a central colour and four peripheral colours (Fig. 1.30). The subject selects the peripheral colour that most closely matches the central colour.

4. **Hardy–Rand–Rittler** is similar to Ishihara but more sensitive, since it can detect all three congenital defects.

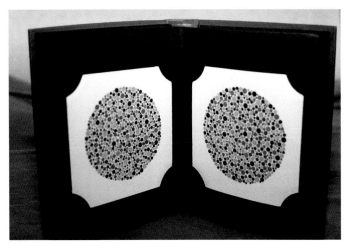

**Figure 1.29** Ishihara pseudo-isochromatic plates

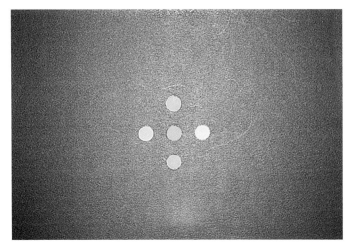

**Figure 1.30** City University colour vision test

5. **Farnsworth–Munsell 100-hue** is the most sensitive for both congenital and acquired colour defects but is seldom used in practice. Despite the name, it consists of 85 hue caps contained in four separate racks in each of which the two end caps are fixed while the others are loose so they can be randomised by the examiner (Fig. 1.31).

- The subject is asked to rearrange the loose randomised caps 'in their natural' order in one box.
- The box is then closed, turned upside down and then opened so that the markers on the inside of the caps become visible.
- The findings are then recorded in a simple cumulative manner on a circular chart.

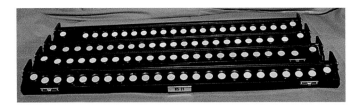

**Figure 1.31** Farnsworth–Munsell 100-hue test

- Each of the three forms of dichromatism is characterised by failure in a specific meridian of the chart (Fig. 1.32).

6. **Farnsworth D15 hue discrimination** test is similar to the Farnsworth–Munsell 100-hue test but utilises only 15 caps.

# Electrophysiological Tests

## ELECTRORETINOGRAPHY

***Principles.*** The electroretinogram (ERG) is the record of an action potential produced by the retina when it is stimulated by light of adequate intensity. The recording is made between an active electrode embedded in a contact lens placed on the patient's cornea, or a gold foil electrode placed on the eyelid, and a reference electrode on the patient's forehead. The potential between the two electrodes is then amplified and displayed (Fig. 1.33). The ERG is elicited both in the light-adapted (photopic) and dark-adapted (scotopic) states. The normal ERG is biphasic (Fig. 1.34):

1. **The a-wave** is the initial fast negative deflection directly generated by photoreceptors.
2. **The b-wave** is the next slower positive deflection with larger amplitude. Although it is generated from fluxes of potassium ions within and surrounding Muller cells, it is directly dependent on functional photoreceptors and its magnitude makes it a convenient measure of photoreceptor integrity. The amplitude of the b-wave is measured from the trough of the a-wave to the peak of the b-wave, and increases with both dark adaptation and increased light stimulus. The b-wave consists of b1 and b2 subcomponents. The former probably represents both rod and cone activity, and the latter mainly cone activity. It is possible to single out rod and cone responses with special techniques.

***Normal ERG*** consists of five recordings. The first three are elicited after 30 minutes of dark adaptation (scotopic), and the last two after 10 minutes of adaptation to moderately bright diffuse illumination (photopic) (Fig. 1.35).

1. **Scotopic ERG**

    a. *Rod* responses are elicited with a very dim flash of white light or a blue light, resulting in a large b-wave and a small or non-recordable a-wave.

    b. *Combined rod and cone* responses are elicited with a very bright white flash, resulting in a prominent a-wave and a b-wave.

    c. *Oscillatory potentials* are elicited by using a bright flash and changing the recording parameters. The oscillatory wavelets occur on the ascending limb of the b-wave and are generated by cells in the inner retina.

2. **Photopic ERG**

    a. *Cone* responses are elicited with a single bright flash, resulting in an a-wave and a b-wave with small oscillations.

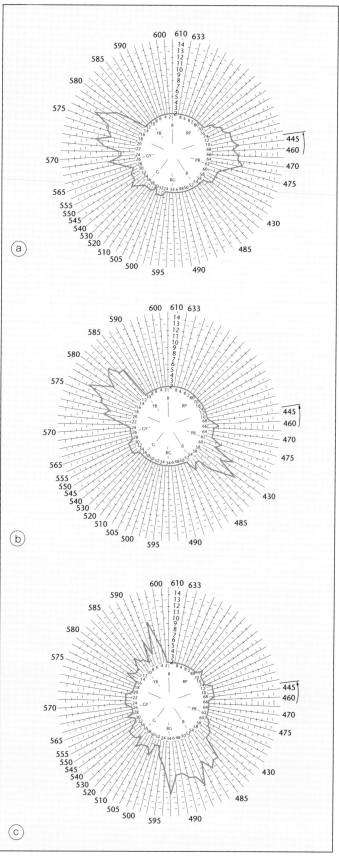

**Figure 1.32** Examples of Farnsworth–Munsell results of colour deficiencies. **(a)** Protan; **(b)** deuteran; **(c)** tritan

b. *Cone flicker* is used to isolate cones by using a flickering light stimulus at a frequency of 30 Hz to which

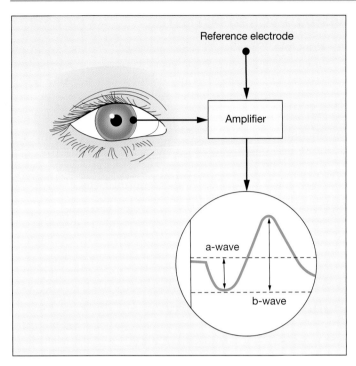

**Figure 1.33** Principles of electroretinography

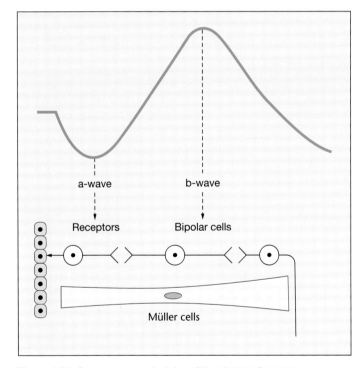

**Figure 1.34** Components and origins of the electroretinogram

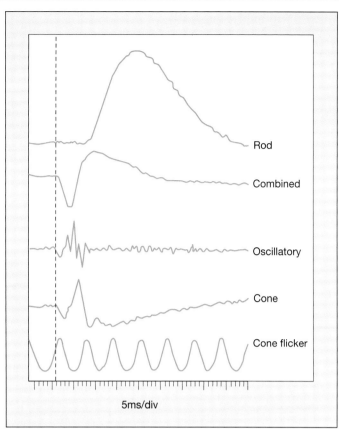

**Figure 1.35** Normal electroretinographic recordings

for variation in photoreceptor density across the retina; at the fovea, where the density of receptors is high, a smaller stimulus element is used than in the periphery, where receptor density is lower. As with conventional ERG, many types of measurements can be made at individual locations; both the amplitude and timing of the troughs and peaks can be measured and reported. The information can be summarised in the form of a three-dimensional plot which resembles the hill of vision. The technique can be used for almost any disorder that affects retinal function.

rods cannot respond. It provides a measure of the amplitude and implicit time of the cone b-wave. Cone responses can be elicited in normal eyes up to 50 Hz, after which point individual responses are no longer recordable (critical flicker fusion).

**Multifocal ERG** is a method of producing topographical maps of retinal function (Fig. 1.36). The stimulus is scaled

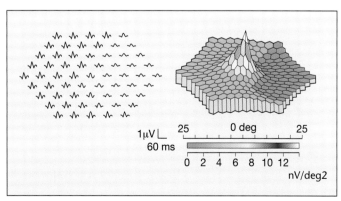

**Figure 1.36** Multifocal electroretinogram

## ELECTRO-OCULOGRAPHY

1. **Principle.** The electro-oculogram (EOG) measures the standing potential between the electrically positive cornea and the electrically negative back of the eye (Fig. 1.37). It reflects the activity of the RPE and the photoreceptors. This means that an eye blinded by lesions proximal to the photoreceptors will have a normal EOG. In general, diffuse or widespread disease of the RPE is needed to affect the EOG response significantly.

2. **Technique.** The test is performed in both light- and dark-adapted states.

   ● The electrodes are attached to the skin near the medial and lateral canthi.
   ● The patient is asked to look rhythmically from side to side, making excursions of constant amplitude. Each time the eye moves, the cornea makes the nearest electrode positive with respect to the other.
   ● The potential difference between the two electrodes is amplified and recorded.

3. **Interpretation.** As there is much variation in EOG amplitude in normal subjects, the result is calculated by dividing the maximal height of the potential in the light (light peak) by the minimal height of the potential in the dark (dark trough). This is expressed as a ratio (Arden ratio) or as a percentage. The normal value is over 1.85 or 185%.

## VISUAL EVOKED POTENTIAL

1. **Principle.** The visual evoked potential (VEP) is a recording of electrical activity of the visual cortex created by stimulation of the retina. The main indications are monitoring of visual function in babies and the investigation of optic neuropathy, particularly when associated with demyelination.

2. **Technique.** The stimulus is either a flash of light (flash VEP) or a black-and-white checker-board pattern, which periodically reverses polarity on a screen (pattern VEP) (Fig. 1.38). Several tests are performed and the average potential is calculated by a computer.

3. **Interpretation.** Both latency (delay) and amplitude of the VEP are assessed. In optic neuropathy, both parameters are affected, with prolongation of latency and decrease in amplitude.

# Fundus Angiography

## FLUORESCEIN ANGIOGRAPHY

### *Principles*

1. **Fluorescein** is an orange water-soluble dye that, when injected intravenously, remains largely intravascular and circulates in the bloodstream.

2. **Fluorescein angiography** (FA) involves photographic surveillance of the passage of fluorescein through the retinal and choroidal circulations following intravenous injection (Fig. 1.39).

3. **Fluorescein binding.** On intravenous injection, 70–85% of fluorescein molecules bind to serum proteins (bound fluorescein); the remainder remain unbound (free fluorescein) (Fig. 1.40a).

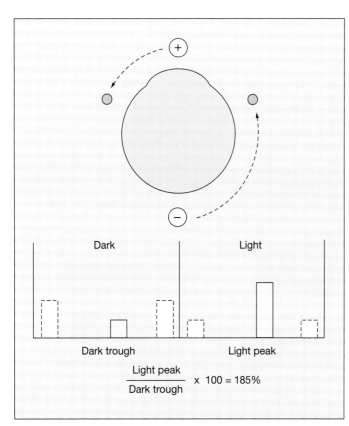

**Figure 1.37** Principles of electro-oculography

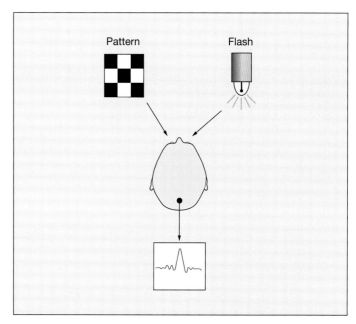

**Figure 1.38** Principles of visually evoked potential

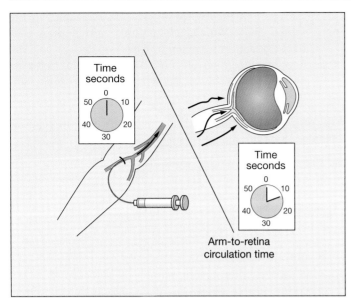

**Figure 1.39** Injection of fluorescein into the antecubital vein and its passage

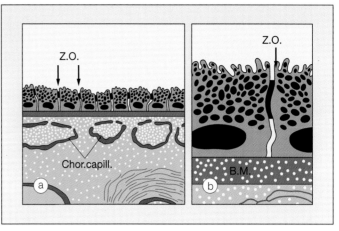

**Figure 1.41** The outer blood–retinal barrier (ZO = zonula occludens; BM = Bruch's membrane)

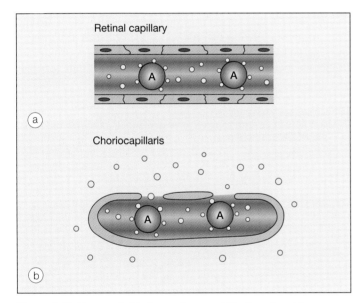

**Figure 1.40** Fluorescein binding and permeability (A = albumin)

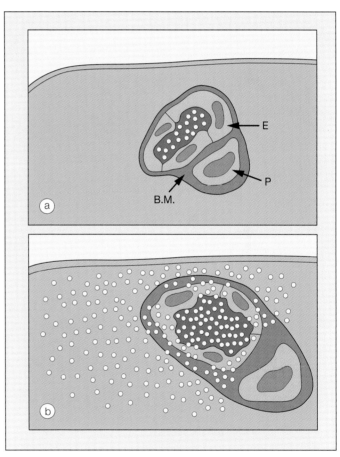

**Figure 1.42** The inner blood–retinal barrier (BM = basement membrane; P = pericyte; E = capillary endothelial cell). **(a)** Intact; **(b)** disrupted

4. **The outer blood–retinal barrier.** The major choroidal vessels are impermeable to both bound and free fluorescein. However, the walls of the choriocapillaris are extremely thin and contain multiple fenestrations through which free fluorescein molecules escape into the extravascular space (Fig. 1.40b). They then pass across Bruch's membrane but on reaching the RPE encounter tight junctional intercellular complexes termed zonula occludentes, which prevent the passage of free fluorescein molecules across the RPE (Fig. 1.41).

5. **The inner blood–retinal barrier** is composed of the tight junctions between retinal capillary endothelial cells across which neither bound nor free fluorescein can pass (Fig. 1.42a); fluorescein is therefore confined within the lumen of the retinal capillaries. The basement membrane and pericytes play only a minor role in this regard. Disruption of the inner blood–retinal barrier will permit leakage of both bound and free fluorescein into the extravascular space (Fig. 1.42b).

6. **Fluorescence** is the property of certain molecules to emit light of a longer wavelength when stimulated by light of a shorter wavelength. The excitation peak for fluorescein is

15

about 490 nm (blue part of the spectrum) and represents the maximal absorption of light energy by fluorescein. Molecules stimulated by this wavelength will be excited to a higher energy level and will emit light of a longer wavelength at about 530 nm (green part of the spectrum) (Fig. 1.43).

7. **Filters** of two types are used to ensure that blue light enters the eye and only yellow-green light enters the camera (Fig. 1.44).

   a. A *blue excitation filter* through which passes white light from the camera. The emerging blue light enters the eye and excites the fluorescein molecules in the retinal and choroidal circulations, which then emit light of a longer wavelength (yellow-green).

   b. A *yellow-green barrier filter* then blocks any reflected blue light from the eye, allowing only yellow-green light to pass through unimpaired to be recorded.

***Imaging technique.*** A good quality angiogram requires adequate pupillary dilatation and clear media.

- The patient is seated in front of the fundus camera.
- Fluorescein, usually 5 ml of a 10% solution, is drawn up into a syringe. In eyes with opaque media, 3 ml of a 25% solution may afford better results.
- A 'red-free' image is captured (Fig. 1.45).
- Fluorescein is injected intravenously over a few seconds.
- Images are taken at approximately 1-second intervals, 5–25 seconds after injection.
- After the transit phase has been photographed in one eye, control pictures are taken of the opposite eye. If appropriate, late photographs may also be taken after 10 minutes and, occasionally, 20 minutes if leakage is anticipated.

***Adverse effects.*** Discoloration of skin and urine is invariable. Mild side effects include nausea, vomiting, flushing of the skin, itching, hives and excessive sneezing. Serious but rare problems include syncope, laryngeal oedema, bronchospasm and anaphylactic shock.

> **NB: It is very important to have arrangements in place for managing these eventualities.**

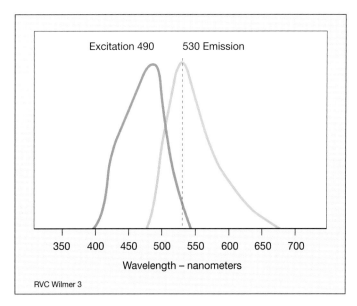

**Figure 1.43** Excitation and emission of fluorescence

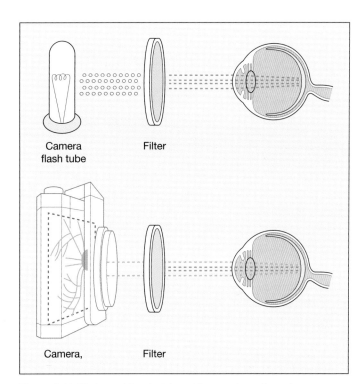

**Figure 1.44** Photographic principles of fluorescein angiography

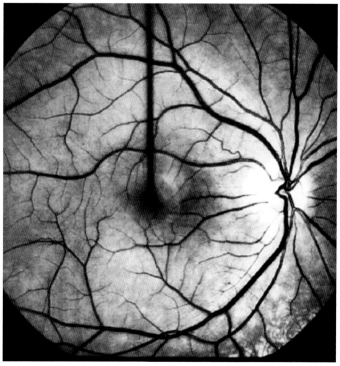

**Figure 1.45** Red-free photograph

***Phases of the angiogram.*** Fluorescein enters the eye through the ophthalmic artery, passing into the choroidal circulation through the short posterior ciliary arteries and into the retinal circulation through the central retinal artery. Because the route to the retinal circulation is slightly longer than that to the choroidal, the latter is filled about 1 second before the former (Fig. 1.46). In the choroidal circulation, precise details are often not discernible, mainly because of rapid leakage of free fluorescein from the choriocapillaris and also because the melanin in the RPE cells blocks choroidal fluorescence. The angiogram consists of the following overlapping phases (Fig. 1.47): (a) choroidal (pre-arterial), (b) arterial, (c) arteriovenous (capillary) (d) venous and (e) late (elimination).

### Normal angiogram

1.  **The choroidal (pre-arterial) phase** occurs 8–12 seconds after dye injection and is characterised by patchy filling of the choroid due to leakage of free fluorescein through the

fenestrated choriocapillaris. A cilioretinal artery, if present, will fill at this time (Fig. 1.48) because it is derived from the posterior ciliary circulation.

2.  **The arterial phase** shows arterial filling and the continuation of choroidal filling (Fig. 1.49).

3.  **The arteriovenous (capillary) phase** shows complete filling of the arteries and capillaries with early laminar flow in the veins, in which the dye appears to line the venous wall, leaving an axial hypofluorescent strip (Fig. 1.50). Choroidal filling continues and background choroidal fluorescence increases as free fluorescein continues to leak from the choriocapillaris into the extravascular space. In hypopigmented eyes, this may be so marked that details of the retinal capillaries may be obscured. In highly pigmented eyes, background choroidal fluorescence will be less obvious.

4.  **The venous phase**

    a.  *The early* phase exhibits complete arterial and capillary filling, and more marked laminar venous flow (Fig. 1.51).
    b.  *The mid* phase displays almost complete venous filling (Fig. 1.52).
    c.  *The late* phase shows complete venous filling with reducing concentration of dye in the arteries.

5.  **The late (elimination) phase** demonstrates the effects of continuous recirculation, dilution and elimination of the dye. With each succeeding wave, the intensity of fluorescence becomes weaker. Late staining of the disc is a normal finding (Fig. 1.53). Fluorescein is absent from the angiogram after 5–10 minutes and is usually totally eliminated from the body within several hours.

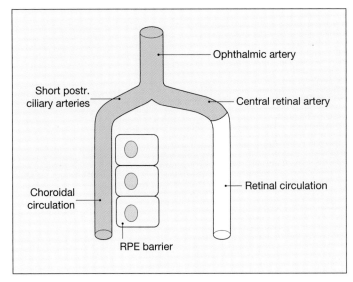

**Figure 1.46** Entry of fluorescein into the choroidal and retinal circulations

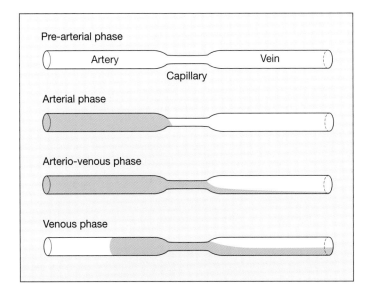

**Figure 1.47** Phases of the fluorescein angiogram

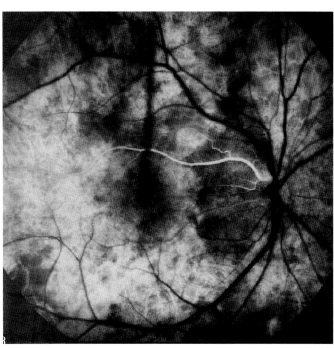

**Figure 1.48** Choroidal phase showing patchy choroidal filling as well as filling of a cilioretinal artery

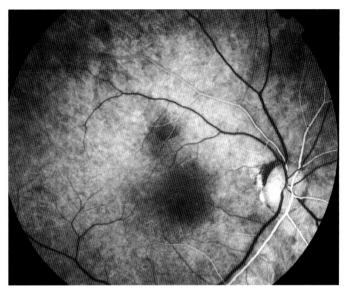

**Figure 1.49** Arterial phase showing filling of the choroid and retinal arteries

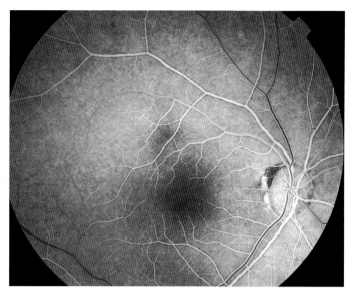

**Figure 1.51** Early venous phase showing marked lamellar venous flow

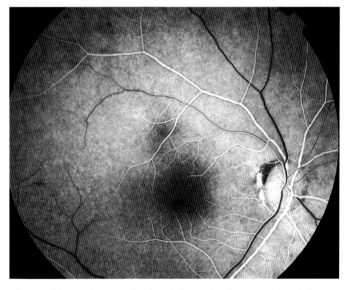

**Figure 1.50** Arteriovenous (capillary) phase showing complete arterial filling and early lamellar venous flow

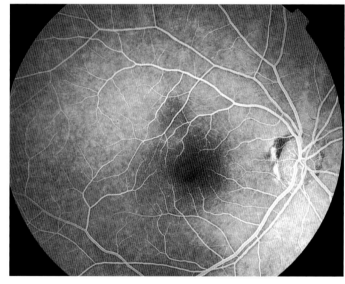

**Figure 1.52** Mid-venous phase showing complete venous filling

6. **The dark appearance of the fovea** (Fig. 1.54a) is caused by three phenomena (Fig. 1.54b).

   - Absence of blood vessels in the foveal avascular zone.
   - Blockage of background choroidal fluorescence due to increased density of xanthophyll at the fovea.
   - Blockage of background choroidal fluorescence by the RPE cells at the fovea, which are larger and contain more melanin than elsewhere.

**Causes of hyperfluorescence.** Increased fluorescence may be due to enhanced visualisation of a normal density of fluorescein in the fundus, or an absolute increase in the fluorescein content of the tissues.

1. **A transmission (window) defect** is caused by atrophy (Fig. 1.55a) or absence of the RPE, as in atrophic age-related macular degeneration. This results in unmasking of normal background choroidal fluorescence, characterised by early hyperfluorescence which increases in intensity and then fades without changing size or shape (Fig. 1.55b and c).

2. **Pooling** of dye in an anatomical space occurs due to breakdown of the outer blood–retinal barrier (RPE tight junctions).

   a. *In the subretinal space*, as in central serous retinopathy (Fig. 1.56a). This is characterised by early hyperfluorescence which increases in both area and intensity (Fig. 1.56b and c).

   b. *In the sub-RPE space*, as in a pigment epithelial detachment (PED) (Fig. 1.57a). This is characterised by early hyperfluorescence which increases in intensity but not in size (Fig. 1.57b and c).

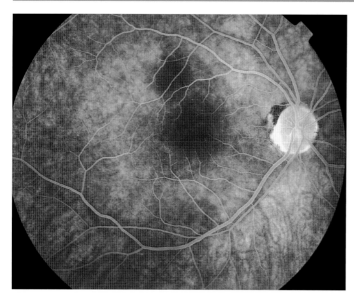

**Figure 1.53** Late (elimination) phase showing weak fluorescence and staining of the optic disc

3. **Leakage** of dye may occur from the following:

   a. *Abnormal choroidal vasculature* such as choroidal neo-vascularisation (CNV). This is characterised by an early lacy filling pattern of hyperfluorescence which increases in size and intensity due to leakage (see Fig. 3.19).

   b. *Breakdown of the inner blood-retinal barrier*, as in cystoid macular oedema. This is characterised by hyperfluorescence beginning in the arteriovenous phase, which increases in size and intensity, giving rise to the characteristic 'flower-petal' pattern seen in the late phase (see Fig. 3.73).

   c. *New vessels*, as in proliferative diabetic retinopathy. This is characterised by early hyperfluorescence due to rapid filling of the new vessels; the hyperfluorescence increases in intensity and area due to leakage (see Fig. 2.33).

4. **Staining** of tissues as a result of prolonged retention of dye (e.g. drusen, fibrous tissue, exposed sclera) may be seen in the late (elimination) phase of the angiogram after the dye has left the choroidal and retinal circulations.

***Causes of hypofluorescence.*** Reduction or absence of fluorescence may be due to: (a) optical obstruction (masking) of normal density of fluorescein in a tissue (Fig. 1.58); or (b) inadequate perfusion of tissue with resultant low fluorescein content.

1. **Blockage of retinal fluorescence** may be caused by lesions anterior to the retina. This may involve the large superficial vessels, the capillaries, or both, depending on the location of the lesion as follows:

   a. *Preretinal* lesions such as blood (Fig. 1.59a and b) will block all fluorescence (Fig. 1.59c).

   b. *Deep retinal* lesions such as intraretinal haemorrhages and hard exudates will block only capillary fluorescence, sparing that from the larger retinal vessels.

2. **Blockage of background choroidal fluorescence** is caused by all conditions that block retinal fluorescence as well as by the following, which block only choroidal fluorescence:

   a. *Subretinal or sub-RPE* lesions such as blood.

   b. *Increased density of the RPE* such as in congenital hypertrophy (Fig. 1.60).

   c. *Choroidal lesions* such as naevi.

3. **Filling defects** may result from:

   a. *Vascular occlusion*, which prevents access of dye to the tissues. The occlusion may involve the choroidal circulation or the retinal arteries, veins or capillaries (capillary drop-out) (see Fig. 2.75b).

   b. *Loss of the vascular bed*, which may occur in severe myopic degeneration or choroideremia (see Fig. 5.97b).

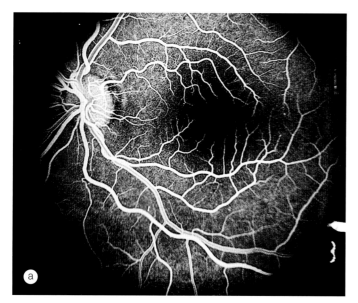

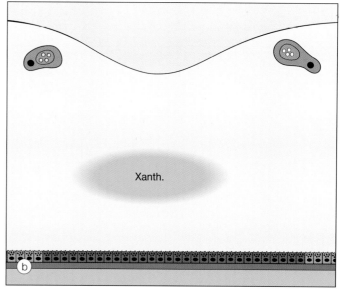

**Figure 1.54** Reason for the dark appearance of the fovea on fluorescein angiography (Xanth. = xanthophyll)

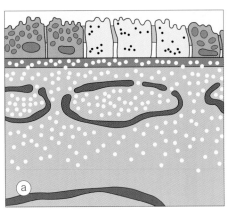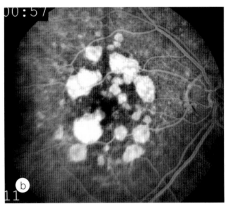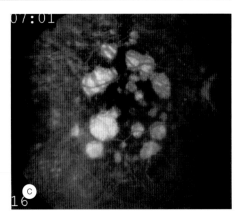

**Figure 1.55** Hyperfluorescence caused by a transmission (window) defect

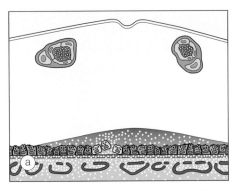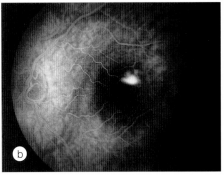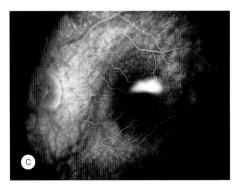

**Figure 1.56** Hyperfluorescence due to pooling of dye in the subretinal space

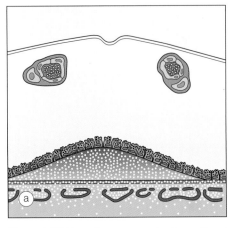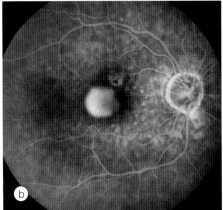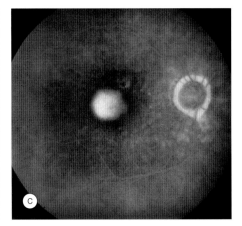

**Figure 1.57** Hyperfluorescence due to pooling of dye in the sub-RPE space

***Stepwise approach to reporting angiograms.*** A fluorescein angiogram should be interpreted systematically to optimise diagnostic accuracy, as follows:

- Indicate whether images of right, left or both eyes have been taken.
- Comment on the red-free images.
- Indicate any delay in filling as well as hyper- or hypofluorescence.

- Indicate any characteristic features such as a smoke-stack or lacy filling pattern.
- Indicate any evolution through the course of the angiogram in the area or intensity of fluorescence.

> **NB: It is important to take into consideration the patient's history and ophthalmoscopic findings before drawing conclusions from the angiogram.**

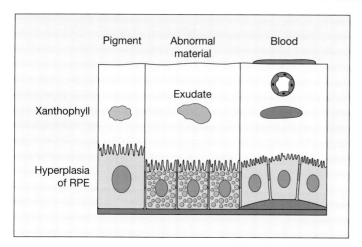

**Figure 1.58** Causes of blocked fluorescence

## INDOCYANINE GREEN ANGIOGRAPHY

***Principles.*** Whilst FA is an excellent method of demonstrating the retinal circulation against the uniform dark background of the RPE, it is not helpful in delineating the choroidal circulation. In contrast, indocyanine green (ICG) angiography is of particular value in studying the choroidal circulation and can be a useful adjunct to FA in the investigation of macular disease in some circumstances.

1. **ICG binding.** About 98% of ICG molecules bind to serum proteins (mainly albumin) on entering the circulation. This phenomenon reduces the passage of ICG through the fenestrations of the choriocapillaris, which are impermeable to the larger protein molecules.

2. **Fluorescence of ICG** is only 1/25 that of fluorescein. The excitation peak is at 805 nm and emission at 835 nm, in

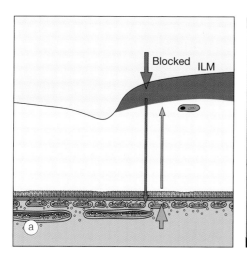
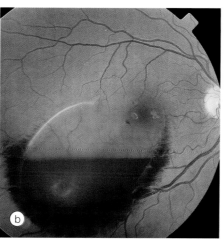
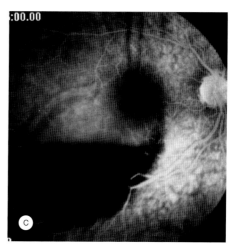

**Figure 1.59** Hypofluorescence due to blockage of all fluorescence by a preretinal haemorrhage

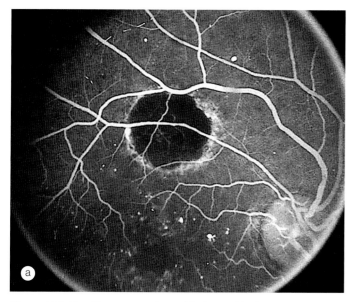
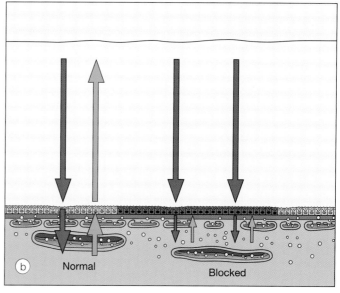

**Figure 1.60** Hypofluorescence due to blockage of background choroidal fluorescence by congenital hypertrophy of the RPE

the near-infrared spectrum. The filters used are infrared barrier and excitation. Infrared light absorbed and emitted by the dye readily penetrates ocular pigments such as melanin and xanthophyll, as well as exudates or thin layers of subretinal blood. Additionally, the near-infrared light is scattered to a less extent than visible light, making ICG superior to FA in eyes with media opacities.

### Imaging technique

- ICG powder is mixed with aqueous solvent to provide 40 mg in 2 ml.
- The patient is seated in front of the imaging system with one arm outstretched.
- A 'red-free' image is captured.
- Between 25 mg and 40 mg of dye is injected intravenously.
- Rapid serial photographs are taken initially and subsequently at about 3 minutes, 10 minutes and 30 minutes.
- Late phases yield the most useful information in ICG angiography because the dye remains in neovascular tissue after leaving the retinal and choroidal circulations.

If necessary, ICG angiography may be performed at exactly the same time as or sequentially to FA. ICG videoangiography (ICG-VA) is commonly used as a supplementary test to FA in the diagnosis and treatment of occult CNV. The two angiographic systems used in performing ICG-VA are the high-resolution digital fundus camera and the scanning laser ophthalmoscope. ICG-guided laser treatment of occult CNV is based on the detection of focal spots or plaques by the digital ICG-VA. The scanning laser ophthalmoscope is better at detecting the vascular net in the very early transit phase of the ICG-VA.

**Adverse effects** are less common than with FA. Because ICG contains 5% iodine it should not be given to patients allergic to iodine. Its use is also contraindicated in pregnancy. The most common side effects are staining of stools, nausea, vomiting, sneezing and pruritus. Less common manifestations include syncope, skin eruptions, pyrexia, backache and local injection site skin necrosis.

### Normal angiogram

1. **Early phase** (within 2–60 seconds of injection) (Fig. 1.61a)
   - Hypofluorescence of the optic disc associated with poor perfusion of the watershed zone.
   - Prominent filling of choroidal arteries and early filling of choroidal veins.
   - Retinal arteries are visible but not veins.

2. **Early mid phase** (1–3 minutes) (Fig. 1.61b)
   - Filling of the watershed zone.
   - Fading of choroidal arteries with increased prominence of choroidal veins.
   - Both retinal veins and arteries are visible.

3. **Late mid phase** (3–15 minutes) (Fig. 1.61c)
   - Fading of filling of choroidal vessels.

- Diffuse hyperfluorescence as the result of diffusion of dye from the choriocapillaris.
- Retinal vessels are still visible.

4. **Late phase** (15–30 minutes) (Fig. 1.61d)
   - Hypofluorescence of choroidal vasculature against a background of hyperfluorescence resulting from staining of extrachoroidal tissue.
   - Decreased visibility of retinal vasculature.
   - The dye may remain in neovascular tissue after it has left the choroidal and retinal circulations.

### Causes of abnormal fluorescence

1. **Hyperfluorescence**
   - RPE 'window' defect.
   - Leakage from the retinal or choroidal circulations, or the optic nerve head.
   - Abnormal blood vessels.

2. **Hypofluorescence**
   - Blockage of fluorescence by pigment, blood or exudate.
   - Obstruction of the circulation.
   - Loss of vascular tissue.
   - PED (hyperfluorescent on FA).

### Clinical indications

1. **Exudative age-related macular degeneration.** Whilst FA remains the method of choice for the identification of classic CNV, it may not be useful in the following situations:
   - Occult CNV in which FA in the early frames may show a suspicion of CNV and the later frames merely show multiple foci of punctate or diffuse hyperfluorescence. This presumed occult CNV can be identified more clearly with ICG as a focal hyperfluorescent 'hot spot', a plaque or a combination of both. Whilst plaques have a poor visual prognosis, 'hot spots' are potentially treatable by ICG-guided laser photocoagulation.
   - CNV associated with PED.
   - CNV associated with subretinal or sub-RPE blood.
   - Recurrent CNV adjacent to laser scars.
   - Identification of feeder vessels.

2. **Other indications** in which ICG may help establish a diagnosis include the following:
   - Polypoidal choroidal vasculopathy, in which ICG is generally superior to FA in lesion identification.
   - Chronic central serous retinopathy, in which it is often difficult to interpret the area or areas of leakage on FA. However, ICG shows choroidal leakage and the presence of dilated choroidal vessels. Previously unidentified lesions are also frequently visible using ICG.
   - Breaks in Bruch's membrane such as lacquer cracks in myopic eyes are more numerous and longer on ICG than the crack dimensions seen on FA. Angioid streaks are more obvious and appear longer on ICG than on FA.

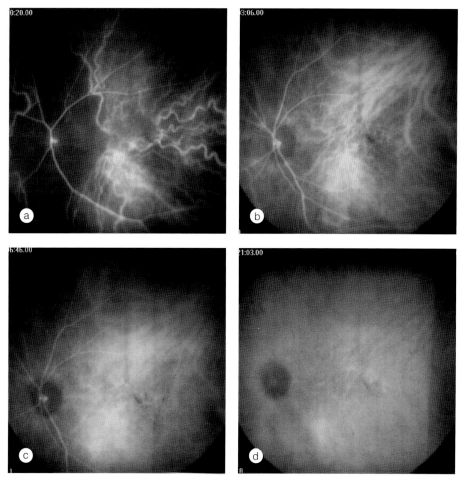

**Figure 1.61** Phase of an ICG angiogram

# Imaging Techniques

## ULTRASONOGRAPHY

### *Principles*

1. **Definitions.** Ultrasound is defined as sound that is beyond the range of human hearing. Ultrasonography uses high-frequency sound waves to produce echoes as they strike interfaces between acoustically distinct structures.

2. **Principles.** The pulsar sends an electric pulse to the transducer in the probe which changes electric energy into an ultrasonic signal. Signals reflected by tissues return through the probe and are sent again as electrical signals to the receiver. The signal is then processed and displayed as an echo on the screen. Amplification displays differences in the strengths of reflected echoes.

3. **A-scan** ultrasonography is performed with a stationary transducer (Fig. 1.62a). It produces a one-dimensional time–amplitude evaluation in the form of vertical spikes along a baseline. The height of the spikes is proportional to the strength of the echo. The greater the distance to the right, the greater the distance between the source of the sound and the reflecting surface. The distance between individual spikes can be precisely measured.

4. **B-scan** ultrasonography is performed with an oscillatory transducer (Fig. 1.62b). It produces a two-dimensional image which is easier to interpret by the non-expert. The amount of reflected sound is portrayed as a dot of light. The more sound reflected, the brighter the dot. Gain adjusts the amplification of the echo signal, similar to volume control of a radio. The higher the gain, the greater the sensitivity of the instrument in displaying weak echoes such as vitreous opacities. Lowering the gain only allows display of strong echoes such as the retina and sclera as well as improving resolution because it narrows the beam. B-scan ultrasonography provides topographic information concerning the size, shape and quality of a lesion as well as its relationship to other structures.

5. **Other types** of ultrasonography

   a. *High-frequency* is used for imaging the anterior segment.
   b. *Doppler*, which demonstrates blood flow. It is useful in assessing tumour response to radiotherapy.
   c. *Three-dimensional*, which can measure tumour volume and enhance plaque localisation over a tumour.

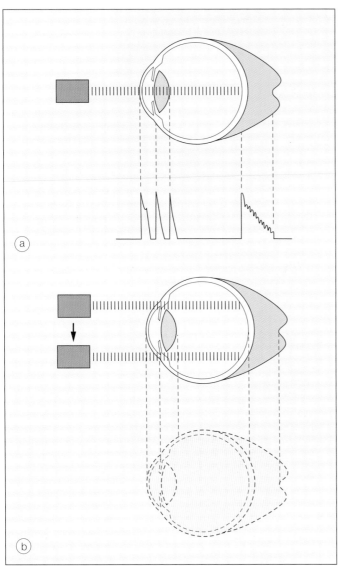

**Figure 1.62** Principles of ultrasonography. **(a)** A-scan; **(b)** B-scan

### Clinical indications in fundus disease

1. **Retinal detachment** evaluation in eyes with opaque media, particularly in those with recent dense vitreous haemorrhage which obscures visualisation of the fundus, as in proliferative diabetic retinopathy. In these cases, ultrasonography will help to differentiate a PVD (Fig. 1.63) from retinal detachment (Fig. 1.64). It may also be possible to detect the presence of a retinal tear in flat retina (Fig. 1.65). Dynamic ultrasonography, in which examination of intraocular structures is performed during eye movements, is helpful in assessing the mobility of the vitreous and retina, for instance in eyes with proliferative vitreoretinopathy.

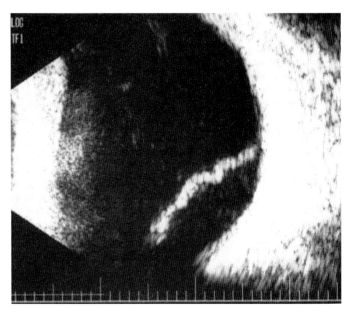

**Figure 1.64** Sagittal B-scan showing an inferior retinal detachment (Courtesy of K. Nischal)

**Figure 1.63** Axial B-scan showing a posterior vitreous detachment and an intragel vitreous haemorrhage (Courtesy of K. Nischal)

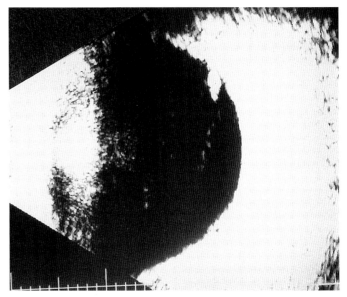

**Figure 1.65** Sagittal B-scan showing a flat superior retinal tear associated with posterior vitreous detachment (Courtesy of K. Nischal)

## 2. Intraocular tumour evaluation

- To detect tumours in eyes with opaque media.
- To define the shape of a tumour and detect possible extraocular extension.
- To measure tumour dimensions, particularly over time, to detect growth or regression.
- To demonstrate features characteristic that would suggest a specific diagnosis.

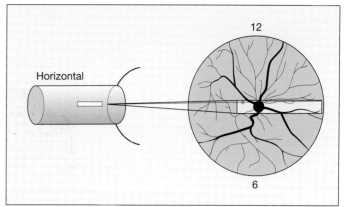

**Figure 1.67** Transverse scanning with the marker pointing rotated 90° away from the limbus

### *Technique*

- The patient should lie supine and be given a paper tissue for wiping away excess gel that may run down the cheeks.
- Sit behind the patient's head and hold the probe with your dominant hand and have the ultrasound machine within easy reach of your non-dominant hand.
- Dim the room lighting just enough to have a clear view of the image.

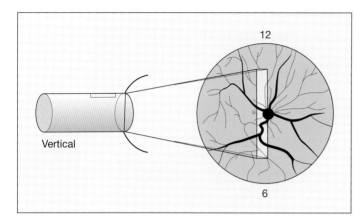

**Figure 1.66** Longitudinal scanning with the marker pointing towards the limbus

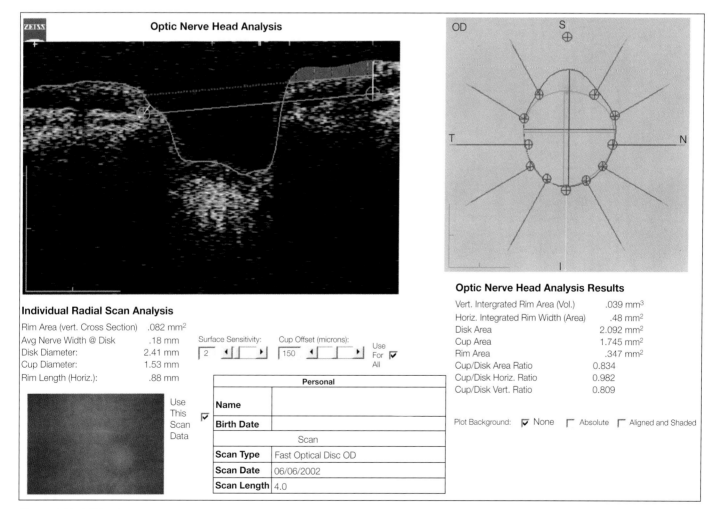

### Individual Radial Scan Analysis

| | |
|---|---|
| Rim Area (vert. Cross Section) | .082 mm² |
| Avg Nerve Width @ Disk | .18 mm |
| Disk Diameter: | 2.41 mm |
| Cup Diameter: | 1.53 mm |
| Rim Length (Horiz.): | .88 mm |

Surface Sensitivity: 2

Cup Offset (microns): 150

Use For All ☑

Use This Scan Data ☑

| Personal | |
|---|---|
| Name | |
| Birth Date | |
| Scan | |
| Scan Type | Fast Optical Disc OD |
| Scan Date | 06/06/2002 |
| Scan Length | 4.0 |

### Optic Nerve Head Analysis Results

| | |
|---|---|
| Vert. Intergrated Rim Area (Vol.) | .039 mm³ |
| Horiz. Integrated Rim Width (Area) | .48 mm² |
| Disk Area | 2.092 mm² |
| Cup Area | 1.745 mm² |
| Rim Area | .347 mm² |
| Cup/Disk Area Ratio | 0.834 |
| Cup/Disk Horiz. Ratio | 0.982 |
| Cup/Disk Vert. Ratio | 0.809 |

Plot Background: ☑ None ☐ Absolute ☐ Aligned and Shaded

**Figure 1.68** OCT optic nerve head display demonstrating gross damage

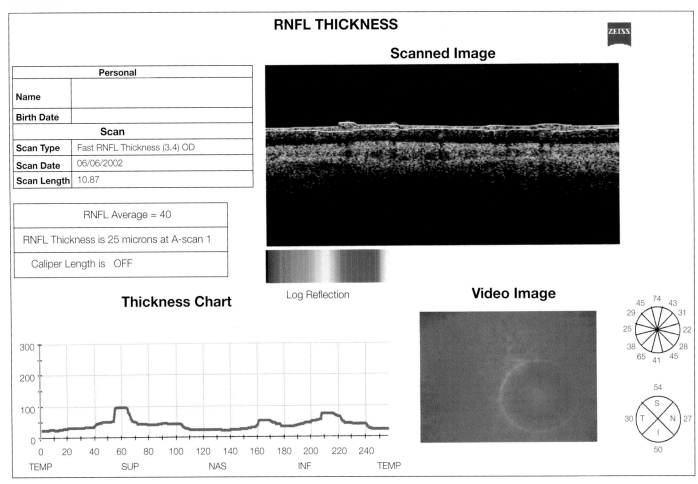

**Figure 1.69** OCT retinal nerve fibre display showing gross reduction in thickness

- Place a globule of methylcellulose or gel onto the tip of the probe.
- Hold the probe against the lower eyelid or the closed upper eyelid, steadying it by resting your outstretched finger on the patient's cheek.
- Perform longitudinal (anteroposterior) scanning with the marker pointing towards the limbus (Fig. 1.66).
- Perform transverse (circumferential) scanning with the marker rotated 90° from the limbus (Fig. 1.67).
- Perform axial (vertical, horizontal or oblique) scanning with the patient looking straight ahead. With vertical scans, the marker is conventionally placed superiorly, so that the superior part of the globe is orientated superiorly in the upper part of the image. With vertical scans, the marker may point towards the nose.
- Probe movements involve tilting in one direction, 'flapping' by tilting backwards and forwards, sliding the tip along the lids and twisting around its axis.

## OPTICAL COHERENCE TOMOGRAPHY

1. **Definition.** Optical coherence tomography (OCT) is a non-invasive, non-contact imaging system which provides high-resolution cross-sectional images analogous to B-scan ultrasonography but using light instead of sound waves.

2. **Principles.** Interferometry is used to assess the echo time delay of light scattered from different layers of the retina and produce an optical cross-section of the retina. Each B-scan OCT image is composed of 100 longitudinal A-scans taken in each pass of the scanning beam. The wavelength used (830 nm) is in the near infrared and is well tolerated by the patient. The practical limit of depth resolution is approximately 20 $\mu$m although this may be further improved with recently developed ultrahigh-resolution OCT allowing imaging of intraretinal morphological features. The commercially available OCT3 incorporates numerous software tools allowing detailed analysis of the optic nerve head (Fig. 1.68) and retinal nerve fibre layer thickness (Fig. 1.69).

3. **Clinical indications**

- Diagnosis and staging of macular holes.
- Objective assessment of macular thickness in cystoid macular oedema and response to treatment.
- Demonstration of occult vitreo-macular traction, particularly in diabetic eyes, which may benefit from surgical intervention.

## FURTHER READING

Drexler W, Sattmann H, Hermann B, et al. Enhanced visualization of macular pathology with the use of ultrahigh-resolution optical coherence tomography. *Arch Ophthalmol* 2003;121:695–706.

# Chapter 2

# RETINAL VASCULAR DISEASE

## Diabetic Retinopathy

### Introduction

#### DIABETES MELLITUS

***Classification.*** Diabetes mellitus is a common metabolic disorder characterised by sustained hyperglycaemia of varying severity secondary to lack or diminished efficacy of endogenous insulin. The disease affects about 2% of the population in the UK and can be classified into two types, with some degree of overlap.

1. **Type 1 diabetes** (insulin-dependent diabetes mellitus [IDDM], juvenile-onset diabetes) develops most frequently between the ages of 10 and 20 years, with acute polydipsia, polyuria, nocturia and weight loss. There is an association with HLA-DR3 and HLA-DR4. Autoimmune destruction of pancreatic islet cells is postulated as instrumental in pathogenesis. Type 1 diabetics are often lean and manifest a total lack of insulin.

2. **Type 2 diabetes** (non-insulin-dependent diabetes mellitus [NIDDM], maturity-onset diabetes), on the other hand, develops most frequently between the ages of 50 and 70 years. Type 2 diabetics are often overweight and manifest relative deficiency of insulin and/or peripheral insulin resistance. Type 2 diabetes is often asymptomatic and discovered by chance. Alternatively, it may present with recurrent infections of the skin, vulva or glans penis or with complications such as vitreous haemorrhage.

***Diagnostic tests***

- Fasting glucose >6.7 mmol/l.
- Random glucose >10.0 mmol/l.
- Glucose tolerance test is performed only if the diagnosis is uncertain.
- Glycosylated haemoglobin (HBA1c) reflects the average level of blood glucose over the preceding 6 weeks. Normally 4–8% of haemoglobin is glycosylated; values in excess of this reflect inadequacy of glycaemic control. It is a better indicator of the efficacy of treatment than is a single random glucose level.
- Urine testing for glycosuria is a crude and unsatisfactory means of monitoring diabetic control.

> **NB: Glycosuria per se does not necessarily imply diabetes as it may merely reflect a lowered renal threshold for glucose excretion.**

***Treatment.*** Type 1 diabetics require insulin; type 2 diabetics require a regimen involving weight reduction, physical exercise and diet control, often in combination with oral hypoglycaemic agents or insulin. Oral hypoglycaemic agents include sulphonylureas (e.g. gliclazide, glipizide) and biguanides (e.g. metformin). It is also important to aggressively treat any associated problems, particularly hypertension and hyperlipidaemia. Blood pressure should be maintained at or below 140/80 mmHg.

***Systemic complications***

1. **Renal.** Nephropathy is initially characterised by microscopic proteinuria. Severe renal disease may eventually result in renal failure requiring dialysis or transplantation.

2. **Vascular.** Accelerated atherosclerosis of coronary and lower limb arteries. Severe involvement of the legs may result in ischaemic ulceration and gangrene of the feet and toes (Fig. 2.1).

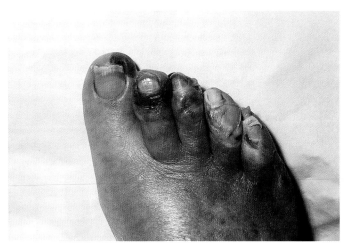

**Figure 2.1** Diabetic gangrene

### 3. Neurological

- Sensory polyneuropathy principally affects the feet in a 'glove and stocking' distribution and may give rise to painless neuropathic perforating ulcers at pressure points in the soles (Fig. 2.2) and degenerative arthropathy (Charcot joints) (Fig. 2.3).
- Cranial nerve palsies – classically a sixth-nerve palsy or a pupil-sparing third-nerve palsy – may occur due to small-vessel involvement.

### 4. Cutaneous

- Increased susceptibility to bacterial and fungal infections (Fig. 2.4).
- Blistering of the feet and toes.
- Necrobiosis lipoidica (Fig. 2.5).
- Lipodystrophy at sites of insulin injection (Fig. 2.6).
- Granuloma annulare (Fig. 2.7).

> **NB:** Neuropathy in combination with vascular insufficiency and increased susceptibility to infection commonly results in gangrene of the extremities (diabetic foot).

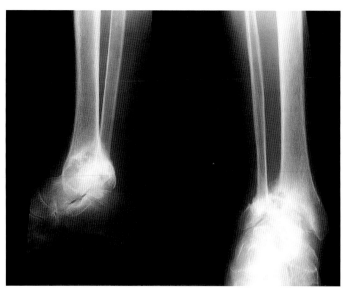

**Figure 2.3** Degenerative arthropathy (Charcot joints) of the ankles in diabetes

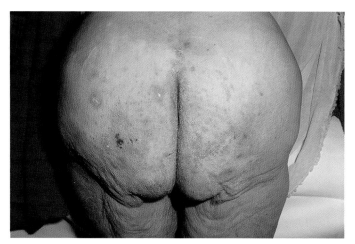

**Figure 2.4** Moniliasis in diabetes

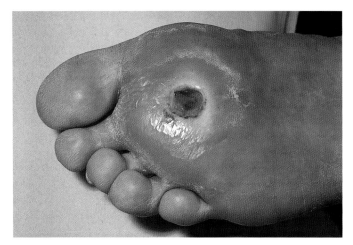

**Figure 2.2** Neuropathic ulceration in diabetes

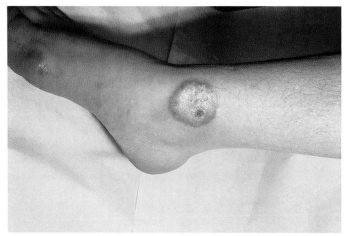

**Figure 2.5** Necrobiosis lipoidica

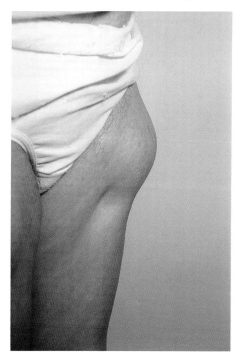

**Figure 2.6** Lipodystrophy at site of insulin injection

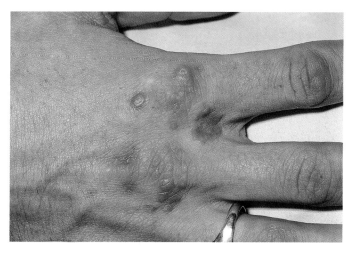

**Figure 2.7** Granuloma annulare

## *Ophthalmic complications*

### 1. Common

- Retinopathy.
- Iridopathy (increased iris transillumination).
- Unstable refraction.

### 2. Uncommon

- Recurrent styes.
- Xanthelasmata.
- Accelerated senile cataract.
- Rubeosis iridis which may lead to neovascular glaucoma.
- Ocular motor nerve palsies.
- Reduced corneal sensitivity.

### 3. Rare

- Papillopathy.
- Pupillary light-near dissociation.
- Wolfram syndrome: progressive optic atrophy and multiple neurological and systemic abnormalities.
- Acute-onset cataract.
- Rhino-orbital mucormycosis.

## RETINOPATHY RISK FACTORS

Diabetic retinopathy (DR) is commoner in type 1 (40%) than in type 2 (20%), and is the most common cause of legal blindness between the ages of 20 and 65 years.

1. **Duration of diabetes** is the most important risk factor. In patients diagnosed with diabetes before the age of 30 years, the incidence of DR after 10 years is 50% and after 30 years 90%. DR rarely develops within 5 years of the onset of diabetes or before puberty, but about 5% of type 2 diabetics have DR at presentation.

2. **Poor metabolic control** is less important than duration, but is nevertheless relevant to the development and progression of DR. It has been shown that tight blood glucose control, particularly when instituted early, can prevent or delay the development or progression of DR. It is, however, associated with an increased risk of hypoglycaemic events. Type 1 diabetic patients appear to obtain greater benefit from tight control than do those with type 2 diabetes. Unfortunately, perfect glycaemic control remains elusive in many patients.

3. **Pregnancy** is occasionally associated with rapid progression of DR. Predicating factors include poor pre-pregnancy control of diabetes, too rapid control during the early stages of pregnancy, and the development of pre-eclampsia and fluid imbalance.

4. **Hypertension** should be rigorously controlled in all patients with diabetes. Tight control appears to be particularly beneficial in type 2 diabetics with maculopathy.

5. **Nephropathy,** if severe, is associated with worsening of DR. Conversely, treatment of renal disease (e.g. renal transplantation) may be associated with improvement of retinopathy and a better response to photocoagulation.

6. **Other risk factors** include obesity, hyperlipidaemia and anaemia.

## CLASSIFICATION OF DIABETIC RETINOPATHY

DR is a microangiopathy primarily affecting pre-capillary arterioles, capillaries and post-capillary venules, although larger vessels may also be involved. Retinopathy exhibits features of both microvascular occlusion and leakage. Clinically, DR may be

1. **Background** (BDR) or **non-proliferative.**

2. **Preproliferative** (PPDR).

3. **Proliferative** (PDR).

## *Pathogenesis of diabetic retinopathy*

Hyperglycaemia appears to be the critical factor in the pathogenesis of DR and initiates the following downstream events.

### MICROVASCULAR OCCLUSION

#### *Pathogenesis*

1. **Capillary changes**

   - Loss of pericytes.
   - Thickening of basement membrane.
   - Proliferation of endothelial cells.

Fig. 2.8 shows a normal capillary bed with equal distribution between pericytes, with round dark nuclei, and endothelial cells, with elongated pale-staining nuclei. Fig. 2.9 shows a diabetic capillary bed in which many capillaries are acellular due to occlusion. The remaining capillaries are dilated and show loss of pericytes and an increase in number of endothelial cells.

2. **Haematological changes**

   - Deformation of erythrocytes and increased rouleaux formation.
   - Increased platelet stickiness and aggregation.

***Consequences.*** Retinal capillary non-perfusion results in retinal ischaemia, which initially develops in the retinal mid-periphery. Retinal hypoxia has two main effects:

1. **Arteriovenous** shunts, running from arterioles and venules, are associated with significant capillary occlusion ('dropout') and are referred to as 'intraretinal microvascular abnormalities' (IRMA).

2. **Neovascularisation** is thought to be caused by angiogenic growth factors elaborated by hypoxic retinal tissue in an attempt to re-vascularise hypoxic retina. These substances promote neovascularisation on the retina and optic nerve head (PDR) and occasionally on the iris (rubeosis iridis). Many angiogenic stimulators have been identified:

vascular endothelial growth factor (VEGF) appears to be of particular importance; others include placental growth factor and pigment epithelium-derived factor. Similarly, several endogenous inhibitors of angiogenesis have also been reported, such as endostatin, platelet factor 4 and angiostatin. It has been hypothesised that the net balance between VEGF and endostatin is associated with the activity of DR.

### MICROVASCULAR LEAKAGE

***Pathogenesis.*** Breakdown of the inner blood–retinal barrier leads to leakage of plasma constituents into the retina. Physical weakening of the capillary walls results in localised saccular outpouchings of the vessel wall, termed microaneurysms, which may leak or become thrombosed (Fig. 2.10).

***Consequences.*** Increased vascular permeability causes the development of intraretinal haemorrhages and oedema, which may be diffuse or localised.

1. **Diffuse** retinal oedema is caused by extensive capillary leakage.

2. **Localised** retinal oedema is caused by focal leakage from microaneurysms and dilated capillary segments. Chronic localised retinal oedema leads to the deposition of 'hard exudates' at the junction of normal and oedematous retina. These exudates, composed of lipoprotein and lipid-filled macrophages, typically surround leaking microvascular lesions in a circinate pattern. When leakage ceases, they absorb spontaneously over a period of months or years, either into the healthy surrounding capillaries or by phagocytosis of their lipid content. Chronic leakage leads to enlargement of the exudates and the deposition of cholesterol.

## *Background diabetic retinopathy*

Fig. 2.11 shows the location of the lesions within the retina.

### CLINICAL FEATURES

***Microaneurysms*** are located in the inner nuclear layer of the retina in association with capillaries linking the super-

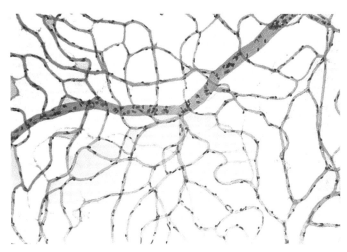

**Figure 2.8** Normal retinal capillary bed (see text)

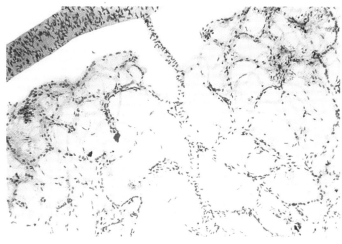

**Figure 2.9** Diabetic retinal capillary bed (see text)

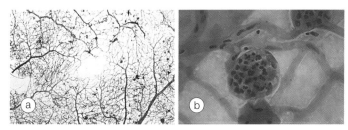

**Figure 2.10 (a)** Trypsin digest of diabetic retinopathy showing perifoveal microaneurysms with a predilection for the temporal zone of the fovea; **(b)** high-power view shows a microaneurysm containing many cells. (Courtesy of Wilmer Institute)

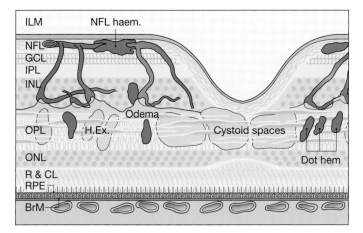

**Figure 2.11** Location of lesions in BDR (Courtesy of Wilmer Institute)

ficial and deep capillary networks. They are the earliest clinically detectable lesions of DR and appear as tiny, red dots, initially temporal to the fovea (Fig. 2.12). When coated with blood, they may be indistinguishable from dot haemorrhages.

**Hard exudates** lie within the outer plexiform layer.

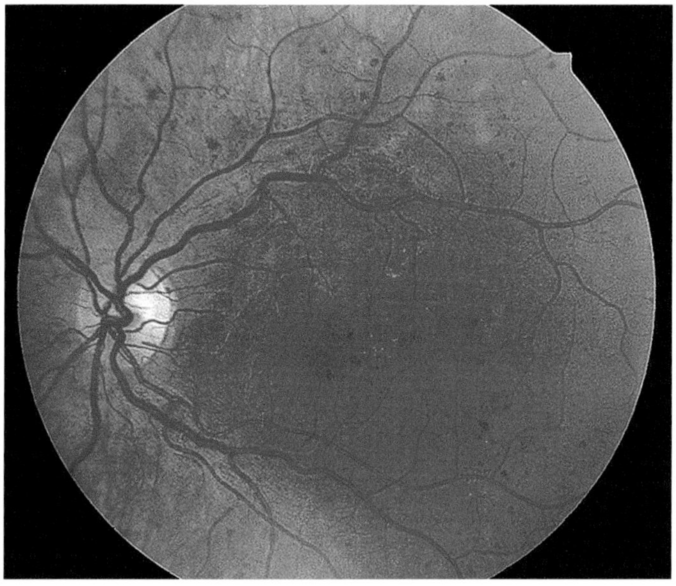

## 1. Signs

- Waxy, yellow lesions with relatively distinct margins, often arranged in clumps and/or rings at the posterior pole (Fig. 2.13 and 2.14).
- A ring of hard exudates often exhibits microaneurysms at its centre.
- With time, number and size tend to increase, and the fovea may be threatened or involved (Fig. 2.15).

## 2. FA shows hypofluorescence due to blockage of background choroidal fluorescence.

**Retinal oedema** is initially located between the outer plexiform and inner nuclear layers (Fig. 2.16a). Later it may also involve the inner plexiform and nerve fibre layers, until

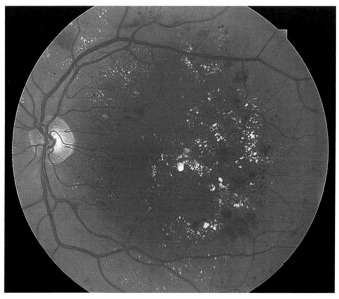

**Figure 2.13** Background DR with clumps of hard exudates and haemorrhages

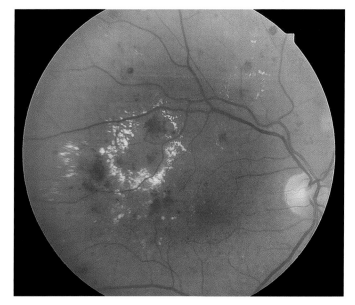

**Figure 2.12** Microaneurysms and dot haemorrhages in early background DR

**Figure 2.14** Background DR with a ring of hard exudates and haemorrhages

eventually the entire thickness of the retina becomes oedematous. With further accumulation of fluid, the fovea assumes a cystoid appearance (cystoid macular oedema).

1. **Signs.** Retinal thickening is best detected by slit-lamp biomicroscopy with a Goldmann lens.

2. **FA** shows diffuse late hyperfluorescence due to retinal capillary leakage (Fig. 2.16b).

### Haemorrhages

1. **Intraretinal** haemorrhages arise from the venous end of capillaries and are located in the compact middle layers of the retina with a resultant red, 'dot–blot' configuration.

2. **Retinal nerve fibre layer** haemorrhages arise from the larger superficial pre-capillary arterioles and, because of the architecture of the retinal nerve fibres, are flame-shaped.

## MANAGEMENT

Patients with mild BDR require no treatment but should be reviewed annually. In addition to optimal control of diabetes, associated factors such as hypertension, anaemia or renal failure should also be addressed. Patients with more severe BDR should be carefully assessed to determine whether they have clinically significant macular oedema (see below).

# Diabetic maculopathy

## DIAGNOSIS

Involvement of the fovea by oedema and hard exudates or ischaemia (diabetic maculopathy) is the most common cause of visual impairment in diabetic patients, particularly those with type 2 diabetes.

### Focal maculopathy

1. **Signs.** Well-circumscribed retinal thickening associated with complete or incomplete rings of perifoveal hard exudates (Fig. 2.17b).

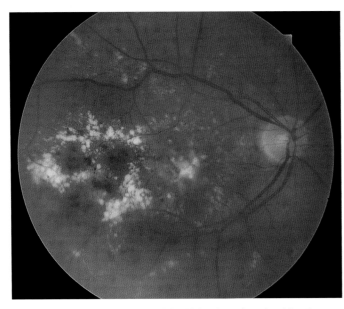

**Figure 2.15** Severe background DR with hard exudates involving the fovea

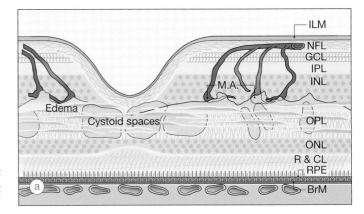

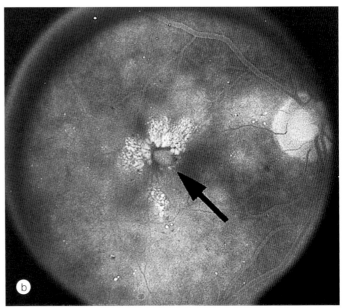

**Figure 2.16** Retinal oedema **(a)** location; **(b)** FA shows diffuse hyperfluorescence and a petalloid pattern at the fovea.

2. **FA** shows late, focal hyperfluorescence due to leakage and good macular perfusion (Fig. 2.17c).

### Diffuse maculopathy

1. **Signs**

   - Diffuse retinal thickening, which may be associated with cystoid changes.
   - Obliteration of landmarks by severe oedema may render localisation of the fovea impossible (Fig. 2.18a).

2. **FA** shows widespread spotty hyperfluorescence of microaneurysms (Fig. 2.18b) and late diffuse hyperfluorescence due to leakage, which is frequently more dramatic than on clinical examination, with a flower-petal pattern if cystoid macular oedema is present (Fig. 2.18c).

### Ischaemic maculopathy

1. **Signs**

   - Reduced visual acuity (VA) but a normal appearing fovea.
   - Associated PPDR is frequent and dark blot haemorrhages and cotton-wool spots may be seen (Fig. 2.19a).

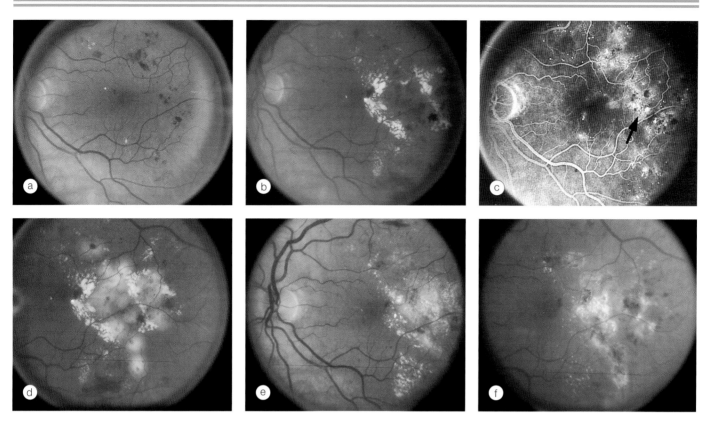

**Figure 2.17** Focal diabetic maculopathy. **(a)** Mild background DR; **(b)** severe retinopathy 2 years later with a ring of hard exudates; **(c)** FA shows focal leakage corresponding to the centre of the exudate ring; **(d)** immediately following focal laser photocoagulation to areas of leakage; **(e)** partial resolution of hard exudates 3 months later; **(f)** complete resolution of hard exudates 9 months later with residual laser scarring (Courtesy of Wilmer Institute)

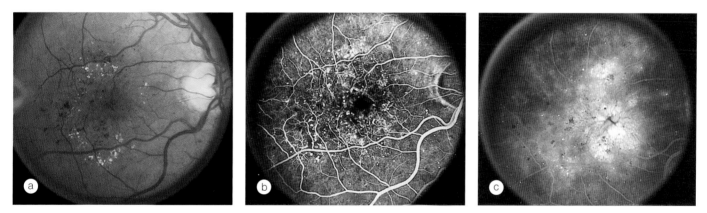

**Figure 2.18** Diffuse diabetic maculopathy. **(a)** A few hard exudates and dot haemorrhages; **(b)** FA early phase shows spotty hyperfluorescence of microaneurysms; **(c)** later phase shows extensive leakage with cystoid macular oedema (Courtesy of Wilmer Institute)

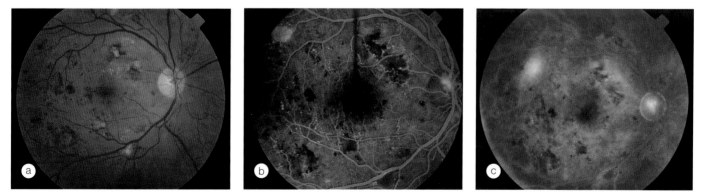

**Figure 2.19** Ischaemic diabetic maculopathy. **(a)** Dot and blot haemorrhages and cotton-wool spots; **(b)** & **(c)** FA shows enlargement of the foveal avascular zone and other areas of capillary non-perfusion at the posterior pole

2. **FA** shows capillary non-perfusion at the fovea, the severity of which does not always relate to the level of VA. Other areas of capillary non-perfusion are also frequently present at the posterior pole and periphery (Fig. 2.19b and c).

***Mixed maculopathy*** is characterised by features of ischaemia and exudation.

***Clinically significant macular oedema (CSMO)*** is defined as:

- Retinal oedema within 500 μm of the centre of the macula (Fig. 2.20a).
- Hard exudates within 500 μm of the centre of the macula, if associated with retinal thickening (which may be outside the 500-μm limit) (Fig. 2.20b).
- Retinal oedema one disc area (1500 μm) or larger, any part of which is within one disc diameter of the centre of the macula (Fig. 2.20c).

## LASER THERAPY

***Indications.*** All eyes with CSMO should be considered for laser photocoagulation irrespective of the level of VA, because treatment reduces the risk of visual loss by 50%. Pre-treatment FA is useful to delineate the area and extent of leakage and also to detect ischaemic maculopathy, which carries a poor prognosis and, if severe, is a contraindication to treatment.

### Technique

1. **Focal treatment** involves the application of laser burns to microaneurysms and microvascular lesions in the centre of rings of hard exudates located 500–3000 μm from the centre of the macula (see Fig. 2.17d). The spot size is 50–100 μm, with a duration of 0.1 seconds and sufficient power to obtain gentle whitening or darkening of the microaneurysm. Treatment of lesions up to 300 μm from the centre of the fovea may be considered if CSMO persists despite previous treatment and VA is less than 6/12. In these cases, a shorter exposure time of 0.05 seconds is recommended.

2. **Grid treatment** is used for areas of diffuse retinal thickening located more than 500 μm from the centre of the macula and 500 μm from the temporal margin of the optic disc. The spot size is 100 μm and exposure time

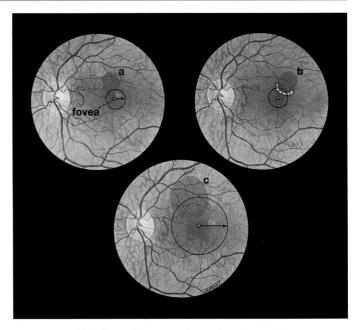

**Figure 2.20** Clinically significant macular oedema (see text)

0.1 seconds. The burns should be of very light intensity and one burn-width apart (Figs. 2.21 and 2.22).

***Results.*** Approximately 70% of eyes achieve stable VA, 15% show improvement and 15% subsequently deteriorate. Since it may take up to 4 months for the oedema to resolve (see Fig. 2.17f), re-treatment should not be considered prematurely.

### Poor prognostic factors

1. **Ocular**

   - Hard exudates involving the centre of the macula.
   - Diffuse macular oedema.
   - Cystoid macular oedema.
   - Mixed exudative–ischaemic maculopathy.
   - Severe retinopathy at presentation.

2. **Systemic**
   - Uncontrolled hypertension.
   - Renal disease.
   - Elevated glycosylated haemoglobin levels.

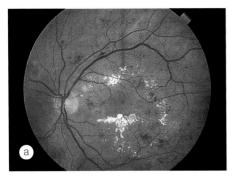
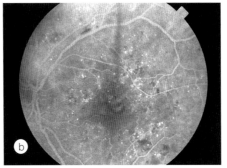
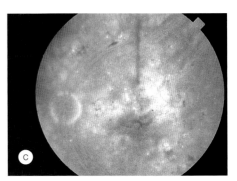

**Figure 2.21** Diffuse diabetic macular oedema prior to treatment

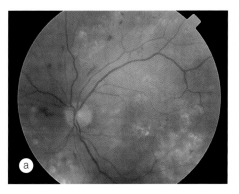
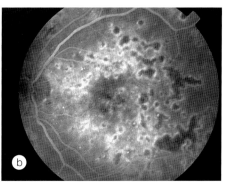
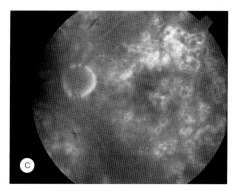

**Figure 2.22** Resolution of diffuse diabetic macular oedema following grid laser photocoagulation

## OTHER FORMS OF THERAPY

1. **Pars plana vitrectomy** may be indicated when macular oedema is associated with tangential traction from a thickened and taut posterior hyaloid. In these cases, laser therapy is of limited benefit but surgical release of traction may be beneficial. Clinically, a taut thickened posterior hyaloid is characterised by an increased glistening of the pre-macular vitreous face. Typically, FA shows diffuse leakage and prominent cystoid macular oedema. It has also been suggested that some eyes without a taut posterior hyaloid may too benefit from vitrectomy. Optical coherence tomography (OCT) may aid patient selection.

2. **Intravitreal triamcinolone acetonide** is a promising new therapy for the treatment of diffuse macular oedema that fails to respond to conventional laser photocoagulation.

## Preproliferative diabetic retinopathy

BDR that exhibits signs of imminent proliferative disease is termed preproliferative diabetic retinopathy (PPDR). The clinical signs of PPDR indicate progressive retinal ischaemia, seen on FA as extensive hypofluorescent areas representing retinal non-perfusion (capillary dropout) (Fig. 2.23). The risk of progression to proliferative disease appears proportional to the number of lesions (Fig. 2.24).

## DIAGNOSIS

*Cotton-wool spots* represent focal infarcts of the retinal nerve fibre layer due to occlusion of pre-capillary arterioles (Fig. 2.25a). Interruption of axoplasmic transport with subsequent build-up of transported material within the axons (axoplasmic stasis) is responsible for the white appearance of the lesions.

1. **Signs.** Small, whitish, fluffy superficial lesions which obscure underlying blood vessels and are clinically evident only in the post-equatorial retina, where the nerve fibre layer is of sufficient thickness to render them visible (Fig. 2.25b).

2. **FA** shows focal hypofluorescence due to blockage of background choroidal fluorescence frequently associated with adjacent capillary non-perfusion (Fig. 2.25c).

*Intraretinal microvascular abnormalities (IRMA)* run from retinal arterioles to venules, thus bypassing the capillary bed, and are therefore often seen adjacent to areas of capillary closure (Fig. 2.26).

1. **Signs.** Fine, irregular, red lines that run from arterioles to venules.

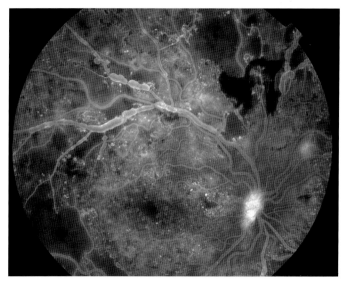

**Figure 2.23** FA shows extensive capillary dropout

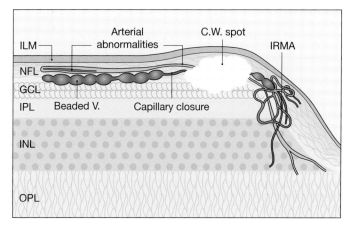

**Figure 2.24** Location of lesions in PPDR

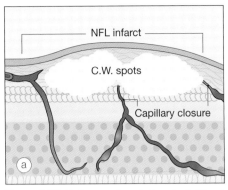

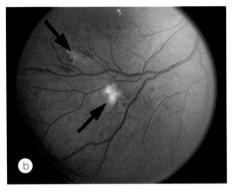

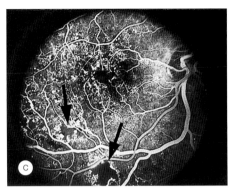

**Figure 2.25** Cotton-wool spots (see text). (Courtesy of Wilmer Institute)

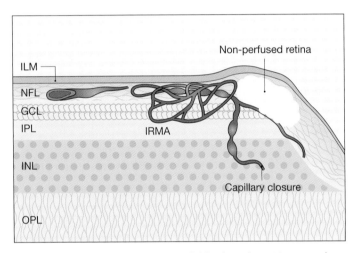

**Figure 2.26** IRMA located in the superficial retina adjacent to areas of capillary closure in PPDR

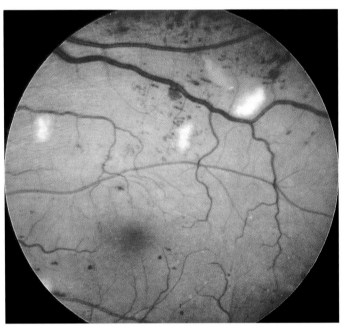

**Figure 2.27** Venous dilatation and tortuosity, cotton-wool spots and haemorrhages in PPDR

2. **FA** shows focal hyperfluorescence associated with adjacent areas of capillary closure.

> **NB:** The main distinguishing features of IRMA are their intraretinal location, their failure to cross major retinal blood vessels and absence of leakage on FA.

### Other features

1. **Venous changes** consist of dilatation and tortuosity (Fig. 2.27), looping (Fig. 2.28), beading and 'sausage-like' segmentation (Fig. 2.29).
2. **Arterial changes** include narrowing, silver-wiring and obliteration (Fig. 2.30) resembling a branch retinal artery occlusion.
3. **Dark blot haemorrhages** represent haemorrhagic retinal infarcts and are located within the middle retinal layers (Fig. 2.31).

### MANAGEMENT

PPDR should be watched closely because of the risk of PDR. Treatment is usually not appropriate unless regular follow-up is not possible, or vision in the fellow eye has been already lost due to proliferative disease.

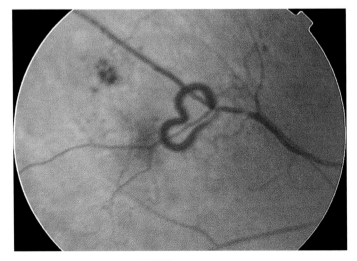

**Figure 2.28** Venous loop in PPDR

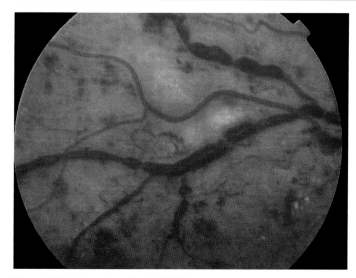

**Figure 2.29** Venous beading in PPDR

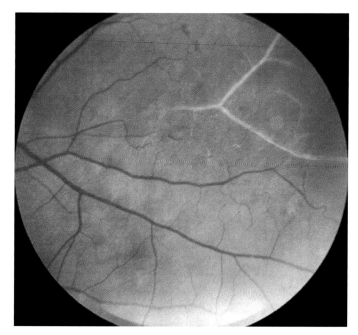

**Figure 2.30** Peripheral arteriolar occlusion in PPDR

## *Proliferative diabetic retinopathy*

PDR affects 5–10% of the diabetic population. Type 1 diabetics are at particular risk, with an incidence of about 60% after 30 years. Protective factors include ipsilateral carotid occlusion, posterior vitreous separation, high myopia and optic atrophy.

### DIAGNOSIS

1. **Signs.** Neovascularisation is the hallmark of PDR. New vessels may proliferate on or within one disc diameter of the optic nerve head (NVD = new vessels at disc), or along the course of the major vessels (NVE = new vessels elsewhere), or both. It has been estimated that over one-quarter of the retina has to be non-perfused before PDR develops. The absence of the internal limiting membrane

(ILM) at the optic nerve head may partially explain the predilection for neovascularisation at this site. New vessels start as endothelial proliferations, arising most frequently from veins; they then pass through defects in the ILM to lie in the potential plane between the retina and posterior vitreous cortex, using the latter as a 'scaffold' for their growth (Fig. 2.32).

2. **FA,** although not required to make the diagnosis, highlights the neovascularisation during the early phases of the angiogram and shows hyperfluorescence during the later stages, due to intense leakage of dye from neovascular tissue (Fig. 2.33).

### *Natural history*

1. The fibrovascular network proliferates between the ILM and the cortical vitreous gel to which it becomes adherent.

2. As a result of the strong attachments of the gel to areas of fibrovascular proliferation, traction at these sites by contracting vitreous gel causes elevation of the vessels above the plane of the retina (Fig. 2.34).

3. The fibrovascular tissue continues to proliferate along the posterior surface of the partially detached vitreous, and is

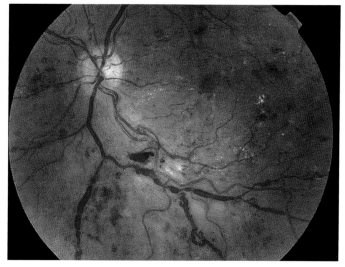

**Figure 2.31** Severe venous changes and blot haemorrhages in PPDR

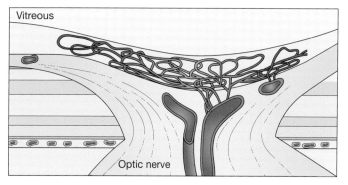

**Figure 2.32** Location of NVD

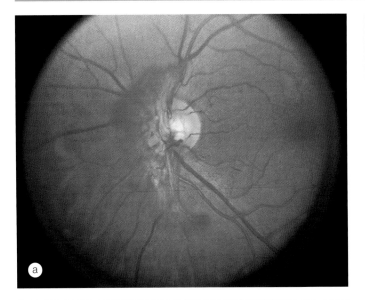

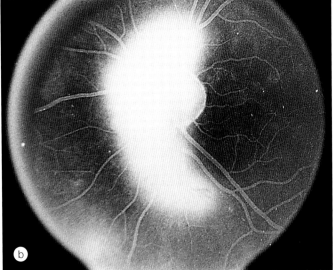

**Figure 2.33 (a)** Disc new vessels; **(b)** FA late phase shows intense hyperfluorescence due to leakage

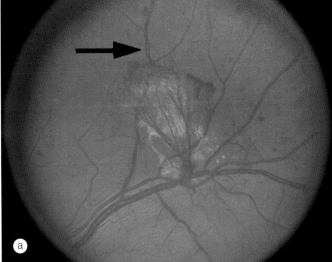

**Figure 2.34 (a)** Elevated NVE with fibrosis; **(b)** elevated NVE with partial vitreous separation

progressively pulled further into the vitreous cavity (Figs. 2.35 and 2.36) until bleeding occurs into either the vitreous gel or retrohyaloid space (Fig. 2.37). Until the occurrence of vitreous haemorrhage, PDR is asymptomatic and can be detected only by screening.

4. The burnt-out stage is characterised by a gradual increase in the fibrous component and a decrease in the vascular component of the neovascular proliferation, the blood vessels becoming non-perfused and no further proliferation occurring (Fig. 2.38).

### Clinical assessment

1. **Severity** of PDR is determined by the area covered with new vessels in comparison with the area of the disc. The severity of PDR is described as follows:

   - NVD are mild when less than one-third disc area in extent and severe when more than one-third disc area in extent (Fig. 2.39 and 2.40).

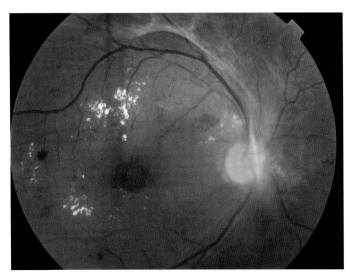

**Figure 2.35** Early fibrovascular proliferation along the superotemporal arcade in PDR

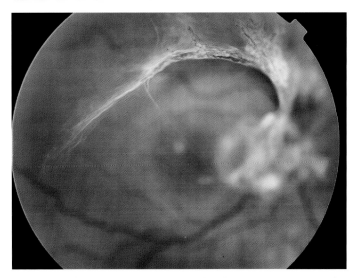

**Figure 2.36** Severe fibrovascular proliferation along the superotemporal arcade in PDR

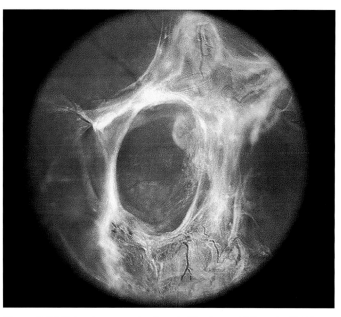

**Figure 2.38** Extensive avascular fibrosis (Courtesy of Wilmer Institute)

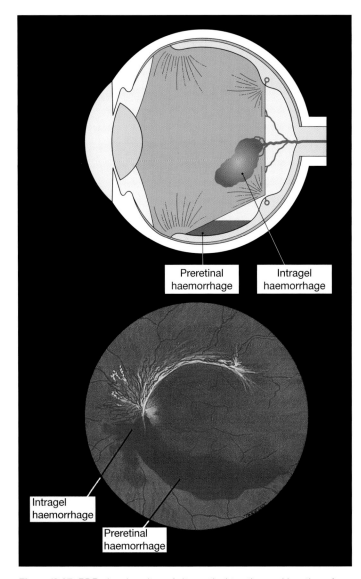

Preretinal haemorrhage

Intragel haemorrhage

Intragel haemorrhage

Preretinal haemorrhage

**Figure 2.37** PDR showing sites of vitreoretinal traction and location of preretinal and intragel haemorrhage

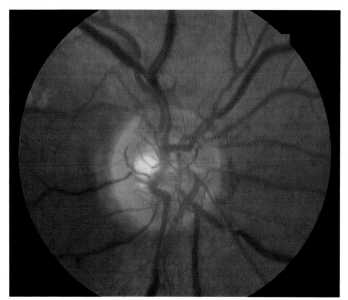

**Figure 2.39** Severe flat NVD

- NVE are mild if less than half disc area in extent and severe if half disc area or more in extent (Fig. 2.41).

2. **Elevated new vessels** (Fig. 2.42) are less responsive to laser therapy than flat new vessels.

3. **Fibrosis** associated with neovascularisation (Figs. 2.43 and 2.44) is important, since significant fibrous proliferation, although less likely to bleed, carries an increased risk of tractional retinal detachment (see Chapter 5).

4. **Haemorrhage** which may be preretinal (sub-hyaloid) (Fig. 2.45) or within the vitreous gel (Fig. 2.46) is an important risk factor for visual loss.

5. **High-risk characteristics.** The following signify a high risk of severe visual loss within 2 years, if left untreated:

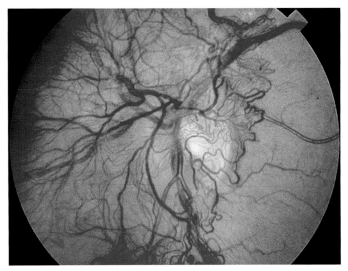

**Figure 2.40** Very severe flat NVD

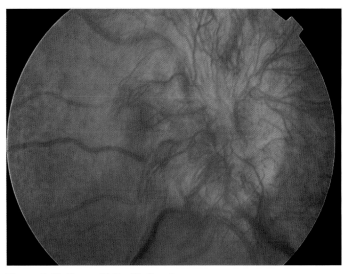

**Figure 2.43** Severe NVD with fibrosis

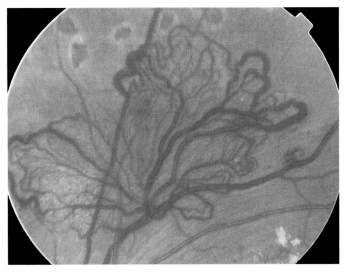

**Figure 2.41** Severe NVE

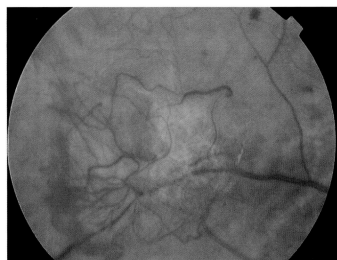

**Figure 2.44** Severe NVE with some fibrosis

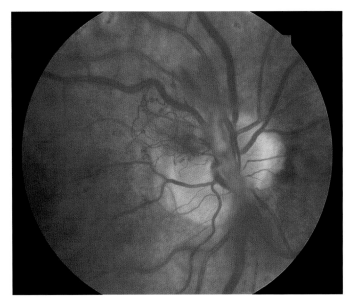

**Figure 2.42** Elevated NVD

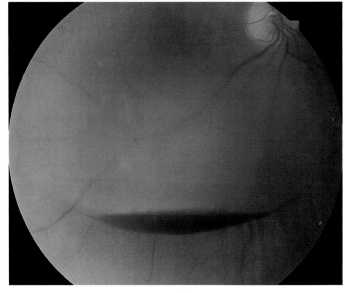

**Figure 2.45** Preretinal haemorrhage

- Mild NVD with haemorrhage carries a 26% risk of visual loss, which is reduced to 4% with treatment.
- Severe NVD without haemorrhage carries a 26% risk of visual loss, which is reduced to 9% with treatment.
- Severe NVD with haemorrhage carries a 37% risk of visual loss, which is reduced to 20% with treatment.
- Severe NVE with haemorrhage carries a 30% risk of visual loss, which is reduced to 7% with treatment.

NB: Unless the above criteria apply, it is reasonable to delay photo-coagulation and review the patient at 3-monthly intervals as suggested by the original trials. In practice, however, most ophthalmologists perform laser photocoagulation at the first sign of neovascularisation.

## TREATMENT

Laser therapy is aimed at inducing involution of new vessels and preventing visual loss from vitreous haemorrhage and tractional retinal detachment.

### Laser settings

1. **Spot size** depends on the contact lens used. With the Goldmann lens, spot size is set at 500 $\mu$m, but with a panfundoscopic lens it is set at 300 $\mu$m because of induced magnification. In the beginner's hands, a panfundoscopic lens is perhaps safer than the Goldmann three-mirror lens, since it is relatively easy to inadvertently photocoagulate the posterior pole through the latter, with disastrous consequences.

2. **Duration** of the burn is 0.02–0.10 seconds.

3. **Power** should be sufficient to produce only a light intensity burn (Fig. 2.47), with the intention of stimulating the retinal pigment epithelium (RPE) rather than ablating the retina.

NB: The main effect is related to the surface area of retina treated rather than the number of burns; a small variation in the size of the laser burn has a pronounced effect on the area treated.

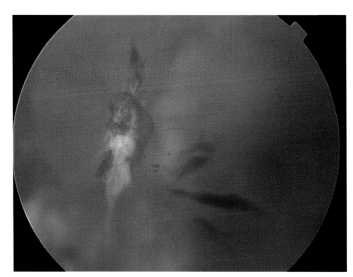

**Figure 2.46** Intragel haemorrhage

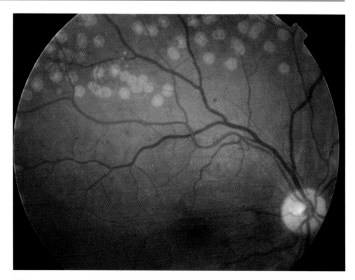

**Figure 2.47** Appropriate laser burns

***Initial treatment*** involves 1000–2000 burns in a scatter pattern extending from the posterior fundus to cover the peripheral retina in one or more sessions. Panretinal photo-coagulation (PRP) completed in a single session carries a slightly higher risk of complications. The amount of treatment during any one session is governed by the patient's pain threshold and ability to maintain concentration. Topical anaesthesia is adequate in most patients, although peribulbar or sub-Tenon anaesthesia may be necessary. The sequence is as follows:

- Step 1. Close to the disc (Fig. 2.48a); below the inferior temporal arcades (Fig. 2.48b and c).
- Step 2. Protective barrier around the macula (Fig. 2.49a and b) to prevent inadvertent treatment of the fovea; above the superotemporal arcade (Fig. 2.49c).

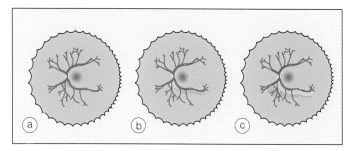

**Figure 2.48** PRP technique – step 1

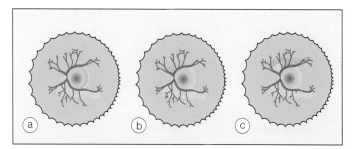

**Figure 2.49** PRP technique – step 2

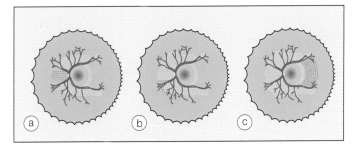

**Figure 2.50** PRP technique – step 3

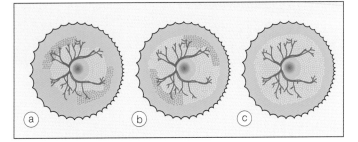

**Figure 2.51** PRP technique – step 4

- Step 3. Nasal to the disc (Fig. 2.50a and b); completion of posterior pole treatment (Fig. 2.50c).
- Step 4. Peripheral treatment (Fig. 2.51a and b) until completion (Fig. 2.51c).

> **NB: In very severe PDR, it is advisable to treat the inferior fundus first, since any vitreous haemorrhage will gravitate inferiorly and obscure this area, precluding further treatment.**

***Follow-up*** is after 4–6 weeks. In eyes with severe NVD, several treatment sessions involving 5000 or even more burns may be required. Occasionally, complete elimination of NVD may be difficult, but once the tips of the vessels start to fibrose and become inactive they pose much less of a threat to vision. Such fibrosed vessels can be observed without the need for further destructive laser surgery with associated field loss. However, it should be remembered that the commonest cause of visual loss is inadequate treatment to persistently active neovascular proliferation.

***Signs of involution*** are regression of neovascularisation leaving 'ghost' vessels or fibrous tissue (Fig. 2.52 and 2.53), decrease in venous changes, absorption of retinal haemorrhages, and disc pallor. In most eyes, once the retinopathy is quiescent, stable vision is maintained. In a few eyes, recurrences of PDR occur despite an initial satisfactory response; it is therefore necessary to re-examine the patient at intervals of approximately 6–12 months.

> **NB: PRP influences only the vascular component of the fibrovascular process. Eyes in which new vessels have regressed leaving only fibrous tissue should not be re-treated.**

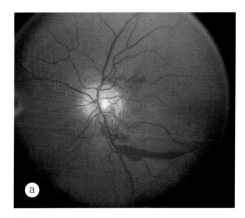

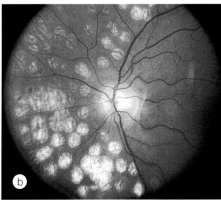

**Figure 2.52** Treatment of NVD. **(a)** Before treatment; **(b)** regression after treatment (Courtesy of Wilmer Institute)

***Treatment of recurrence*** may involve:

1. **Further laser photocoagulation,** filling in any gaps between previous laser scars or utilising indirect laser to treat very peripheral retina.

2. **Cryotherapy** to the anterior retina is occasionally useful when further photocoagulation is impossible as a result of inadequate visualisation of the fundus caused by opaque media. It also offers a means of treating areas of the retina spared by PRP. However, it is now very rarely required due to improved visualisation with indirect laser photocoagulation combined with peripheral retinal indentation.

3. **Vitrectomy and endolaser** is another option.

> **NB: It should be explained to patients that PRP may result in visual field defects of sufficient severity to legally preclude driving a motor vehicle.**

## Advanced diabetic eye disease

Serious vision-threatening complications of DR (advanced diabetic eye disease) occur in patients who have not had laser therapy or in whom laser photocoagulation has been unsuccessful or inadequate. One or more of the following complications may occur.

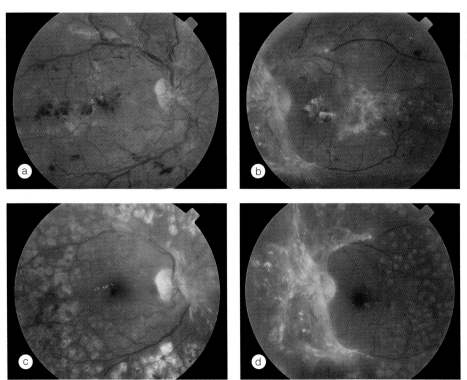

**Figure 2.53** Treatment of severe PDR. **(a)** & **(b)** Before treatment; **(c)** & **(d)** several months after treatment, showing residual fibrosis but absence of new vessels

## CLINICAL FEATURES

1. **Haemorrhage** may occur into the vitreous gel, the retro-hyaloid space (preretinal haemorrhage), or both (Fig. 2.54). A preretinal haemorrhage often has a crescentic shape which demarcates the level of posterior vitreous detachment. Occasionally, a preretinal haemorrhage may penetrate the vitreous gel. Intragel haemorrhages usually take longer to clear than preretinal haemorrhages because the former are usually the result of a more extensive bleed. In some eyes, altered blood becomes compacted on the posterior vitreous face to form an 'ochre membrane'. Patients should be warned that bleeding may be precipitated by severe physical exertion or straining, hypoglycaemia and direct ocular trauma. However, not infrequently, bleeding occurs while the patient is asleep.

2. **Tractional retinal detachment** (Fig. 2.55) is caused by progressive contraction of fibrovascular membranes over areas of vitreoretinal attachment (there may actually be small foci of abnormal attachment at sites of new vessels). Posterior vitreous detachment in eyes with PDR is often incomplete due to the strong adhesions between cortical vitreous and areas of fibrovascular proliferation (see Chapter 6).

3. **Tractional retinoschisis** with or without retinal detachment may also occur. Differentiation between retinoschisis and tractional retinal detachment is clinically difficult but very important, because the indications for surgery and visual prognosis may differ. Recovery of central vision after macular reattachment following surgery is better in eyes with tractional detachment than in retinoschisis. In this respect, OCT may be useful in the differentiation between these two conditions preoperatively. The differential diag-

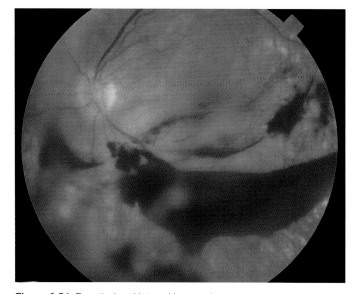

**Figure 2.54** Preretinal and intragel haemorrhage

nosis is often difficult to make due to the coexistence of macular oedema.

4. **Opaque fibrous membranes** may develop on the posterior surface of the detached hyaloid and stretch from the superior to the inferior temporal arcades (Fig. 2.56). Such membranes may obscure the macula and further impair VA.

5. **Rubeosis iridis** (iris neovascularisation) may occur in eyes with PDR, and, if severe (Fig. 2.57), may lead to neovascular glaucoma. Rubeosis is particularly common in eyes with severe retinal ischaemia or persistent retinal detachment following unsuccessful pars plana vitrectomy.

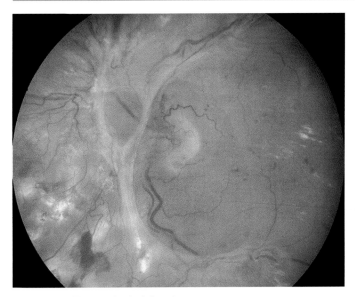

**Figure 2.55** Tractional retinal detachment

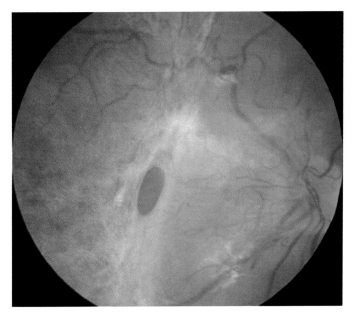

**Figure 2.56** Opaque fibrous membrane stretching between the vascular arcades

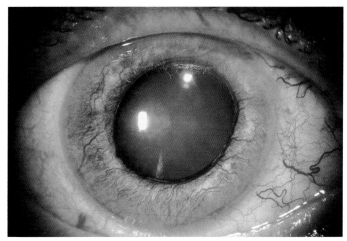

**Figure 2.57** Severe rubeosis iridis

2. **Progressive tractional retinal detachment** threatening or involving the macula must be treated without delay. However, extramacular tractional detachments may be observed, since they often remain stationary for prolonged periods of time.

3. **Combined tractional and rhegmatogenous retinal detachment** should be treated urgently, even if the macula is not involved, because subretinal fluid is likely to spread quickly to involve the macula.

4. **Premacular subhyaloid haemorrhage,** if dense (Fig. 2.58) and persistent, should be considered for vitrectomy, because, if untreated, the ILM or posterior hyaloid face may serve as a scaffold for subsequent fibrovascular proliferation and consequent tractional macular detachment or macular epiretinal membrane formation.

5. **Macular oedema** may occasionally benefit from pars plana vitrectomy, as previously mentioned.

## TREATMENT

Pars plana vitrectomy is the main method of treating severe complications of PDR.

### *Indications*

1. **Severe persistent vitreous haemorrhage** is the most common indication. In these cases, the density of the haemorrhage precludes adequate PRP. In the absence of rubeosis iridis, vitrectomy should be considered within 3 months of the initial vitreous haemorrhage in type 1 diabetics and at about 6 months in type 2 diabetics, although earlier intervention may be considered in selected cases such as dense bilateral haemorrhage.

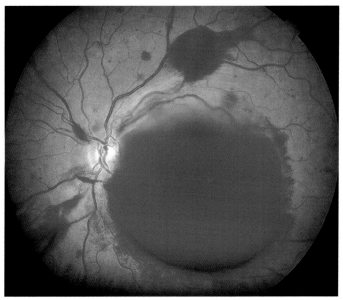

**Figure 2.58** Large subhyaloid haemorrhage obscuring the posterior pole

## Aims

1. **Removal of vitreous gel,** thus eliminating the scaffold along which further fibrovascular tissue can proliferate. If this goal is achieved, involution of existing neovascular tissue also frequently occurs.

2. **Removal of vitreous haemorrhage.**

3. **Repair of retinal detachment** by excising tractional membranes and removing fibrovascular tissue from the retinal surface. Any retinal breaks should also be sealed.

4. **Prevention of further neovascularisation** by laser endophotocoagulation.

## Complications

1. **Progressive rubeosis iridis** is the most common anterior segment complication resulting in failure. It has an increased incidence in aphakic eyes and in those with residual areas of detached retina. In eyes with total retinal detachments, the incidence of rubeosis is virtually 100%.

2. **Cataract** formation is virtually inevitable at some point following vitrectomy, and may be the result of progression of pre-existing lens opacities or surgical trauma.

3. **Glaucoma** may be secondary to rubeosis or may be due to 'ghost' cell or red cell trabecular meshwork obstruction.

4. **Recurrent vitreous haemorrhage** may be caused by fresh fibrovascular proliferation.

5. **Retinal detachment** may be caused by operative complications, such as traction on the vitreous base or the inadvertent creation of fresh breaks with the cutter or other instruments. It may also occur later as a result of fresh fibrovascular proliferation.

**Visual results** depend on the specific indications for surgery and the complexity of pre-existing vitreoretinal abnormalities. In general, about 70% of cases achieve visual improvement, about 10% are made worse and the rest are unchanged. It appears that the first few postoperative months are vital. If an eye is doing well after 6 months, then the long-term outlook is good because the incidence of subsequent vision-threatening complications is low. Favourable prognostic factors are:

- Good preoperative visual function.
- Age of 40 years or less.
- Absence of preoperative rubeosis iridis and glaucoma.
- Previous PRP of at least one-quarter of the fundus.

# Screening for diabetic retinopathy

All diabetic patients aged over 12 years and/or entering puberty should be screened, and those with risk factors for visual loss referred to an ophthalmologist. Screening involves measurement of VA for distance and near, and fundus examination following pupillary dilatation.

1. **Annual review**

   - Normal fundus.
   - Mild BDR with small haemorrhages and/or small hard exudates more than one disc diameter from the fovea.

2. **Routine referral**

   - BDR with large exudates within the major temporal arcades but not threatening the fovea.
   - BDR without maculopathy but with reduced VA, in order to determine the cause of visual impairment.

3. **Early referral**

   - BDR with hard exudates and/or haemorrhages within one disc diameter from the fovea.
   - PPDR.

4. **Urgent referral**

   - PDR.
   - Preretinal or vitreous haemorrhage.
   - Rubeosis iridis.
   - Retinal detachment.

## FURTHER READING

Aiello LP, Cahill MT, Wong JS. Systemic considerations in the management of diabetic retinopathy. *Am J Ophthalmol* 2001;132:760–776.

Aiello LM. Perspectives on diabetic retinopathy. *Am J Ophthalmol* 2003;136:122–135.

Cai J, Boulton M. The pathogenesis of diabetic retinopathy: old concepts and new questions. *Eye* 2002;16:242–260.

Donaldson M, Dodson PM. Medical treatment of diabetic retinopathy. *Eye* 2003;17:550–562.

Jonas JB, Kreissig I, Sofker A, et al. Intravenous injection of triamcinolone for diffuse diabetic macular edema. *Arch Ophthalmol* 2003;121:57–61.

Kaiser PK, Reimann CD, Sears JE, et al. Macular traction detachment and diabetic macular edema associated with posterior hyaloid traction. *Am J Ophthalmol* 2001;131:44–49.

Klein R, Klein BEK. Blood pressure control and diabetic retinopathy. *Br J Ophthalmol* 2002;86:365–367.

Lewis H, Abrams GW, Blumenkranz MS, et al. Vitrectomy for diabetic macular traction and edema associated with posterior hyaloidal traction. *Ophthalmology* 1992;99:753–759.

Massin P, Duguid G, Erginay A, et al. Optical coherence tomography for evaluating diabetic macular edema before and after vitrectomy. *Am J Ophthalmol* 2003;135:169–177.

Martidis A, Duker JS, Greenberg PB, et al. Intravitreal triamcinolone for refractory diabetic macular edema. *Ophthalmology* 2002;109:920–927.

Noma H, Funatsu H, Yamashita H, et al. Regulation of angiogenesis in diabetic retinopathy. *Arch Ophthalmol* 2002;120:1075–1080.

Otani T, Kishi S. A controlled study of vitrectomy for diabetic macular edema. *Am J Ophthalmol* 2002;134:214–219.

Prendergast SD, Hassan TS, Williams GA, et al. Vitrectomy for diffuse diabetic macular edema associated with a taut premacular posterior hyaloid. *Am J Ophthalmol* 2000;130:178–186.

Tachi N, Ogino N. Vitrectomy for diffuse macular edema in cases of diabetic retinopathy. *Am J Ophthalmol* 1996;122:258–260.

Yamamoto T, Akabane N, Takeuchi S. Vitrectomy for diabetic macular edema: the role of posterior vitreous detachment and epimacular membrane. *Am J Ophthalmol* 2001;132:369–377.

# Retinal Venous Occlusive Disease

## PATHOGENESIS

Arteriolosclerosis is an important causative factor for branch retinal vein occlusion (BRVO). Because a retinal arteriole and its corresponding vein share a common adventitial sheath, thickening of the arteriole appears to compress the vein. This causes secondary changes, including venous endothelial cell loss, thrombus formation and potential occlusion. Similarly, the central retinal vein and artery share a common adventitial sheath posterior to the lamina cribrosa, so that atherosclerotic changes of the artery may compress the vein and precipitate central retinal vein occlusion (CRVO). It therefore appears that both arterial and venous disease contribute to retinal vein occlusion. Venous occlusion causes elevation of venous and capillary pressure with stagnation of blood flow. Stagnation results in hypoxia of the retina drained by the obstructed vein, which, in turn, results in damage to the capillary endothelial cells and extravasation of blood constituents. The tissue pressure is increased, causing further stagnation of the circulation and hypoxia, so that a vicious cycle is established.

## PREDISPOSING FACTORS

### Common

1. **Advancing age** is the most important factor; over 50% of cases occur in patients over the age of 65 years.

2. **Hypertension** is present in up to 64% patients over the age of 50 years and in 25% of younger patients with retinal vein occlusion. It is most prevalent in patients with BRVO, particularly when the site of obstruction is at an arteriovenous crossing. Inadequate control of hypertension may also predispose to recurrence of retinal vein occlusion in the same eye or to fellow eye involvement.

3. **Hyperlipidaemia** (cholesterol >6.5 mmol/l) is present in 35% of patients, irrespective of age.

4. **Diabetes mellitus** is present in about 10% of cases over the age of 50 years but is uncommon in younger patients. This may be due to an increase of other cardiovascular risk factors such as hypertension, which is present in 70% of type 2 diabetics.

5. **Raised intraocular pressure** increases the risk of CRVO, particularly when the site of obstruction is at the edge of the optic cup.

**Uncommon** predispositions (listed below) may assume more importance in patients under the age of 50 years.

1. **Myeloproliferative disorders**

   - Polycythaemia.
   - Abnormal plasma proteins (e.g. myeloma, Waldenström macroglobulinaemia).

2. **Acquired hypercoagulable states**

   - Hyperhomocysteinaemia.

- Lupus anticoagulant and antiphospholipid antibodies.
- Dysfibrinogenaemia.

3. **Inherited hypercoagulable states**

   - Activated protein C resistance (factor V Leiden mutation).
   - Protein C deficiency.
   - Protein S deficiency.
   - Antithrombin deficiency.
   - Prothrombin gene mutation.

4. **Inflammatory disease** associated with occlusive periphlebitis

   - Behçet disease.
   - Sarcoidosis.
   - Wegener's granulomatosis.
   - Goodpasture syndrome.

5. **Miscellaneous**

   - Sickling haemoglobinopathies.
   - Oral contraceptives.
   - Chronic renal failure.
   - Causes of secondary hypertension (e.g. Cushing syndrome) or hyperlipidaemia (e.g. hypothyroidism).

> **NB:** Factors that appear to decrease the risk of venous occlusion include increased physical activity and moderate alcohol consumption.

## MEDICAL INVESTIGATIONS

### All patients

1. **Blood pressure.**

2. **ECG.**

3. **Blood**

   - Full blood count and erythrocyte sedimentation rate (ESR).
   - Fasting blood glucose and lipids.
   - Plasma protein electrophoresis.

### Selected patients

1. **Chest x-ray.**

2. **Blood**

   - Thrombophilia screen.
   - Autoantibodies – anticardiolipin, lupus anticoagulant, antinuclear (ANA) and anti-DNA.
   - Angiotensin-converting enzyme (ACE).
   - Homocysteine.

## BRANCH RETINAL VEIN OCCLUSION

### Classification

1. **Major BRVO** may be subdivided as follows:

   - First-order temporal branch at the optic disc (Fig. 2.59).
   - First-order temporal branch away from the disc but involving the branches to the macula (Fig. 2.60).

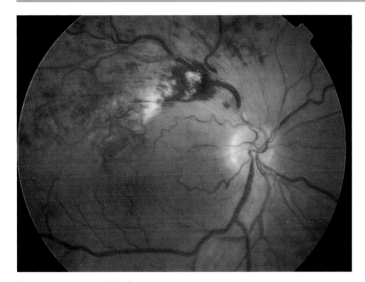

**Figure 2.59** Major BRVO at the disc

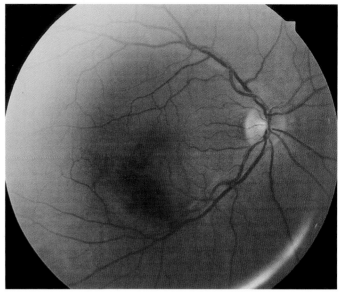

**Figure 2.61** Minor macular BRVO

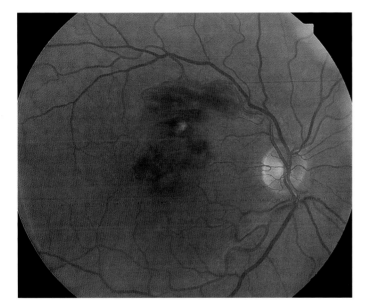

**Figure 2.60** Major BRVO away from the disc

2. **Minor macular BRVO** involving only a macular branch (Fig. 2.61).

3. **Peripheral BRVO** not involving the macular circulation.

### Diagnosis

1. **Presentation** depends on the amount of macular drainage compromised by the occlusion. Patients with macular involvement often present with sudden onset of blurred vision and metamorphopsia or a relative visual field defect. Patients with peripheral occlusions may be asymptomatic.

2. **Signs**

   a. *VA* is variable and dependent on the extent of macular involvement.

   b. *Fundus* (Fig. 2.62a)

   - Dilatation and tortuosity of the venous segment distal to the site of occlusion and attenuation proximal to the occlusion.
   - Flame-shaped and dot–blot haemorrhages, retinal oedema, and cotton-wool spots affecting the sector of the retina drained by the obstructed vein.

3. **FA** shows variable blockage by haemorrhages, leakage, capillary drop-out, staining of the vein wall and 'pruning' of vessels in ischaemic areas (Fig. 2.62b and c).

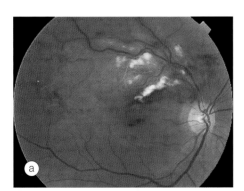 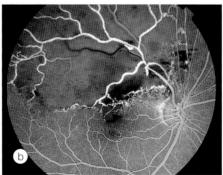 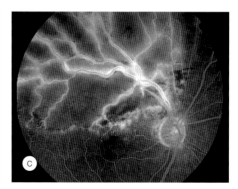

**Figure 2.62 (a)** BRVO; **(b)** FA venous phase shows extensive hypofluorescence, due to capillary non-perfusion, and 'pruning' of vessels; **(c)** late phase shows staining of the vein wall

**4. Course.** The acute features take 6–12 months to resolve and may be replaced by the following:

- Venous sheathing and sclerosis peripheral to the site of obstruction, with variable residual haemorrhage (Fig. 2.63).
- Collateral venous channels, characterised by slightly tortuous vessels, develop locally (Fig. 2.64) or across the horizontal raphe between the inferior and superior vascular arcades (Fig. 2.65).
- Microaneurysms and hard exudates (Fig. 2.66) may be associated with cholesterol crystal deposition.
- The macula may show RPE changes or epiretinal gliosis.

*Prognosis* is reasonably good. Within 6 months, about 50% of eyes develop efficient collaterals, with return of VA to 6/12 or better. Eventual visual recovery depends on the amount of venous drainage involved by the occlusion (which is related to the site and size of the occluded vein) and the severity of macular ischaemia. The two main vision-threatening complications are:

1. **Chronic macular oedema** which is the most common, cause of persistent poor VA after BRVO. Some patients with VA of 6/12 or worse may benefit from laser photocoagulation, provided the macula is oedematous rather than significantly ischaemic.

2. **Neovascularisation.** NVD develops in about 10% and NVE in 20–30% of eyes that show at least one quadrant of capillary non-perfusion. NVE usually develops at the border of the triangular sector of ischaemic retina drained by the occluded vein. Neovascularisation usually appears within 6–12 months but may develop at any time within the first 3 years. It is a serious complication because it can lead to recurrent vitreous and preretinal haemorrhage, and, occasionally, tractional retinal detachment.

*Follow-up* should at 6–12 weeks with FA, provided the retinal haemorrhages have cleared sufficiently. Further management depends on VA and angiographic findings.

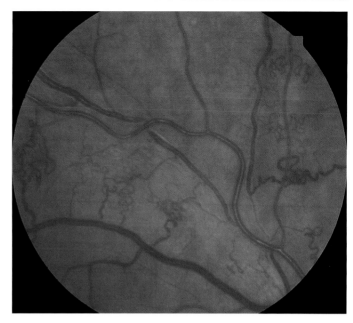

**Figure 2.64** Local collaterals following BRVO

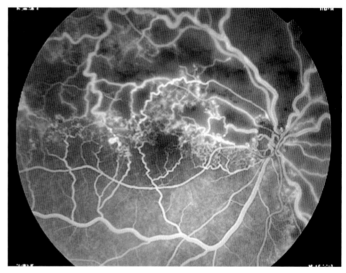

**Figure 2.65** FA shows severe ischaemia and collaterals extending across the horizontal raphe between the superior and inferior vascular arcades

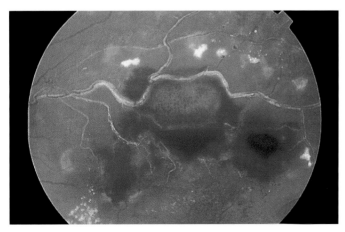

**Figure 2.63** Old superotemporal BRVO showing venous sclerosis, residual haemorrhages and a few hard exudates

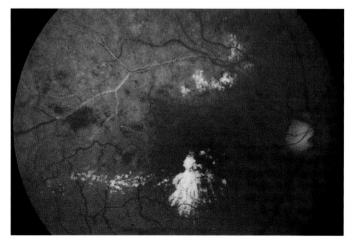

**Figure 2.66** Hard exudates following an old superotemporal BRVO

- If there is good macular perfusion and VA is improving, no treatment is required.
- If there is macular oedema associated with good macular perfusion (Fig. 2.67) and VA continues to be 6/12 or worse after 3–6 months, laser photocoagulation should be considered. Prior to treatment, the FA should be studied carefully to identify the leaking areas. It is also very important to identify shunts, which do not leak fluorescein, because they must not be treated.
- If there is macular non-perfusion (Fig. 2.68) and VA is poor, laser treatment will not improve vision. However, if the FA shows five or more disc areas of non-perfusion, the patient should be reviewed at 4-monthly intervals for 12–24 months because of the risk of neovascularisation.

---

NB: Patients with VA of less than 6/60 or those with symptoms for over a year are unlikely to benefit from laser therapy.

---

### Treatment

1. **Macular oedema** is treated by grid laser photocoagulation (100–200 μm burns, 0.1 second duration and spaced one burn width apart) to produce a gentle reaction to the area of leakage as identified on FA. The burns should extend no closer to the fovea than the edge of the foveal avascular zone (FAZ) and be no more peripheral than the major vascular arcades. Care should be taken to avoid treating over intraretinal haemorrhage. Follow-up should be after 3 months. If macular oedema persists, re-treatment may be considered, although the results are frequently disappointing.

2. **Neovascularisation** is not normally treated unless vitreous haemorrhage occurs, because early treatment does not appear to affect the visual prognosis. If appropriate, scatter laser photocoagulation (200–500 μm spots, 0.05–0.10 second

duration and spaced one burn width apart) is performed with sufficient energy to achieve a medium reaction covering the entire involved sector (Fig. 2.69) as defined by the colour photograph and FA. A quadrant usually requires 400–500 burns. Follow-up should be after 4–6 weeks. If neovascularisation persists, re-treatment is frequently effective in inducing regression.

### IMPENDING CENTRAL RETINAL VEIN OCCLUSION

Impending (partial) CRVO is an uncommon, poorly described condition which may resolve or progress to complete obstruction.

1. **Presentation** is with mild blurring of vision which is characteristically worse on waking and then improves during the day.

2. **Signs.** Mild venous dilatation and tortuosity with a few widely scattered flame-shaped haemorrhages (Fig. 2.70).

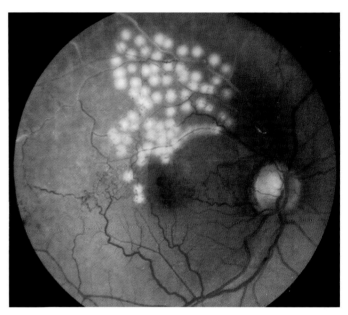

**Figure 2.69** Laser photocoagulation for neovascularisation following BRVO

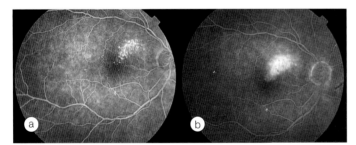

**Figure 2.67** FA of an old superotemporal BRVO showing progressive hyperfluorescence due to macular oedema but good retinal perfusion

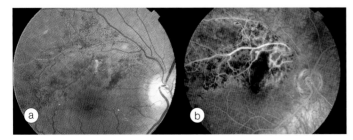

**Figure 2.68 (a)** Old superotemporal BRVO; **(b)** FA shows macular hypofluorescence due to non-perfusion

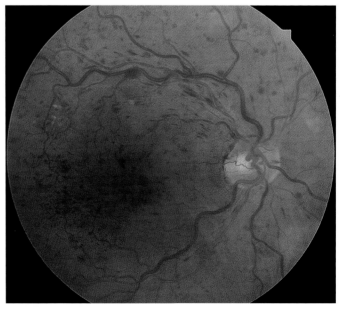

**Figure 2.70** Impending CRVO

49

3. **FA** shows increased retinal circulation time.

4. **Treatment** is aimed at preventing complete occlusion by correcting any predisposing systemic conditions and lowering intraocular pressure to improve perfusion. A short course of systemic carbonic anhydrase inhibitors may be tried, but their efficacy has not been tested in clinical trials.

## NON-ISCHAEMIC CENTRAL RETINAL VEIN OCCLUSION

Non-ischaemic CRVO is the most common type, accounting for about 75% of all cases.

### Diagnosis

1. **Presentation** is with sudden, unilateral blurred vision.

2. **Signs**

   a. *VA* is impaired to a moderate–severe degree.
   b. *APD* (afferent pupillary defect) is absent or mild (in contrast with ischaemic CRVO).
   c. *Fundus* (Fig. 2.71a)

   - Tortuosity and dilatation of all branches of the central retinal vein (CRV), dot–blot and flame-shaped haemorrhages throughout all four quadrants and most numerous in the periphery, and cotton-wool spots.
   - Optic disc and macular oedema are common.

3. **FA** shows delayed venous return good retinal capillary perfusion and late leakage (Fig. 2.71b and c).

**Course.** Most acute signs resolve over 6–12 months. Residual findings include disc collaterals (Fig. 2.72), epiretinal gliosis and pigmentary changes at the macula. Conversion to ischaemic CRVO occurs in 15% of cases within 4 months and in 34% within 3 years.

**Prognosis** in cases that do not subsequently become ischaemic is reasonably good, with return of vision to normal or near normal in about 50%. The main cause for poor vision is chronic cystoid macular oedema (Fig. 2.73), which may lead to secondary RPE changes. To a certain extent, the prognosis is related to initial VA as follows:

- If initial VA is 6/18 or better, it is likely to remain so.

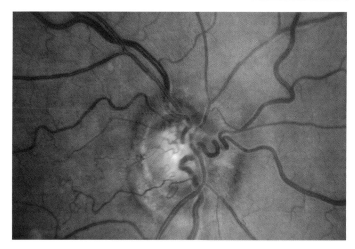

**Figure 2.72** Disc collateral following non-ischaemic CRVO

- If VA is 6/24–6/60, the clinical course is variable, and vision may subsequently improve, remain the same, or worsen.
- If VA at the onset is worse than 6/60, improvement is unlikely.

**Treatment** is currently very inadequate. Laser photocoagulation for macular oedema is not beneficial. The following experimental therapies require further evaluation.

1. **Laser-induced chorioretinal venous anastomosis** which bypasses the site of obstruction to venous outflow may be beneficial in some cases but is not without potential risks such as fibrous proliferation at the laser site (Fig. 2.74), and haemorrhage from the ruptured vein or from vessels in the choroid. This technique has not been widely adopted despite initial encouraging reports.

2. **Cannulation** and infusion of tissue plasminogen activator (t-PA) into the vein is a new modality.

3. **Intravitreal triamcinolone acetonide** for chronic macular oedema may be a viable treatment option that requires further investigation. This technique has shown good initial results and is increasingly popular, although randomised controlled trials are needed.

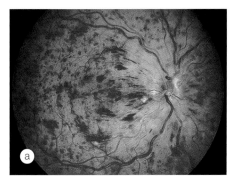 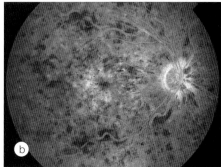 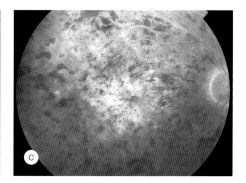

**Figure 2.71** **(a)** Recent non-ischaemic CRVO; **(b)** FA late venous phase shows hyperfluorescence at the macula due to leakage; **(c)** late phase shows increasing hyperfluorescence due to progressive leakage.

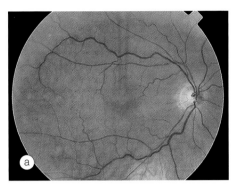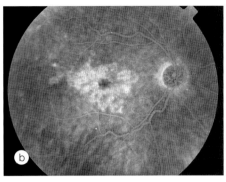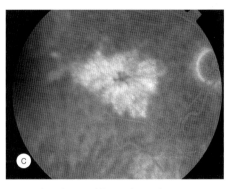

**Figure 2.73** **(a)** Old non-ischaemic CRVO; **(b)** and **(c)** FA shows progressive hyperfluorescence due to severe chronic cystoid macular oedema

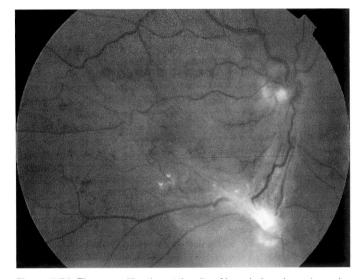

**Figure 2.74** Fibrous proliferation at the site of laser-induced anastomosis for non-ischaemic CRVO

## ISCHAEMIC CENTRAL RETINAL VEIN OCCLUSION

Ischaemic CRVO is characterised by rapid-onset venous obstruction resulting in decreased retinal perfusion, capillary closure and retinal hypoxia. This may lead to profound vascular leakage, rubeosis iridis and raised intraocular pressure. Neovascular glaucoma is one of the most common indications for enucleation in the western world.

### Diagnosis

1. **Presentation** is with sudden and severe visual impairment.

2. **Signs**

   *a.* *VA* is usually counting fingers (CF) or worse.
   *b.* *APD* is marked.
   *c.* *Fundus* (Fig. 2.75a)

   - Severe tortuosity and engorgement of all branches of the CRV, extensive dot–blot and flame-shaped haemorrhages involving the peripheral retina and posterior pole, cotton-wool spots, macular oedema and haemorrhage.
   - Severe optic disc oedema and hyperaemia.

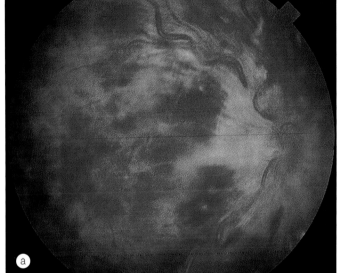

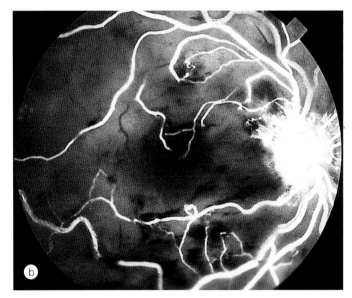

**Figure 2.75** **(a)** Ischaemic CRVO; **(b)** FA shows extensive hypofluorescence due to capillary non-perfusion

3. **FA** shows central masking by retinal haemorrhages, extensive areas of capillary non-perfusion and vessel wall staining (Fig. 2.75b).

4. **ERG** is reduced.

**Course.** Most acute signs resolve over 9–12 months. Residual findings include disc collaterals and macular epiretinal gliosis and pigmentary changes. Rarely, subretinal fibrosis resembling that associated with exudative age-related macular degeneration may develop.

**Prognosis** is extremely poor due to macular ischaemia. Rubeosis iridis (see Fig. 2.57) develops in about 50% of eyes, usually between 2 and 4 months (100-day glaucoma), and unless vigorous PRP is performed, there is a high risk of neovascular glaucoma. The development of opticociliary shunts (retinochoroidal collateral veins) may protect the eye from anterior segment neovascularisation. Retinal neovascularisation occurs in about 5% of eyes and is therefore much less common than with BRVO.

**Follow-up** should be monthly for 6 months to detect anterior segment neovascularisation. Angle neovascularisation, while not synonymous with eventual neovascular glaucoma, is the best clinical predictor of the eventual risk of neovascular glaucoma because it may occur in the absence of neovascularisation at the pupillary margin. Routine gonioscopy of eyes at risk should therefore be performed and the pupillary margin should be examined prior to mydriasis.

**Treatment** with laser PRP (Fig. 2.76) should be performed without delay in eyes with angle or iris neovascularisation. This involves the application of 1500–3000 burns (0.05–0.10 seconds, spaced one burn width apart), with sufficient energy to produce a moderate reaction in the periphery but avoiding areas of haemorrhage. Some cases require further treatment if rubeosis fails to regress or progresses. Prophylactic laser therapy is appropriate only if regular follow-up is not possible.

> **NB:** Control of systemic cardiovascular risk factors is extremely important in order to reduce systemic morbidity and to reduce the risk of another ocular venous event.

## PAPILLOPHLEBITIS

Papillophlebitis (optic disc vasculitis) is an uncommon condition which typically affects otherwise healthy individuals under the age of 50 years. It is thought that the underlying lesion is optic disc swelling with resultant secondary venous congestion rather than venous thrombosis occurring at the level of the lamina cribrosa as occurs in older patients.

### Diagnosis

1. **Presentation** is with relatively mild blurring of vision, typically worst on waking.

2. **Signs**

   a. *VA* reduction is mild to moderate.
   b. *APD* is absent.
   c. *Fundus* (Fig. 2.77)

   - Disc oedema, which may be associated with cotton-wool spots, is the dominant finding.
   - Venous dilatation and tortuosity with variable amount of retinal haemorrhages, usually confined to the peripapillary area and posterior fundus.

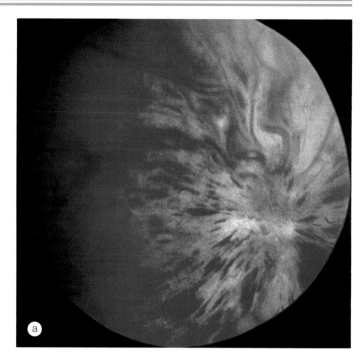

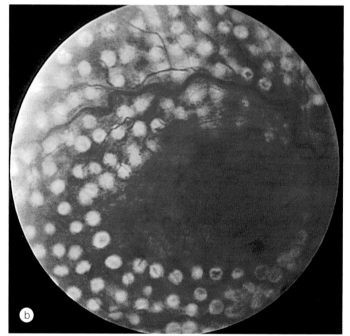

**Figure 2.76 (a)** Ischaemic CRVO; **(b)** following PRP

   - Enlargement of the physiological blind spot.

3. **FA** shows delay in venous filling, hyperfluorescence due to leakage and good capillary perfusion.

**Prognosis** is excellent despite the lack of treatment. Eighty per cent of cases achieve a final VA of 6/12 or better. The remainder suffer significant and permanent visual impairment as a result of macular oedema.

## HEMIRETINAL VEIN OCCLUSION

Hemiretinal vein occlusion is less common than both BRVO and CRVO. It involves occlusion of the superior or inferior branch of the CRV. A hemispheric occlusion blocks a major

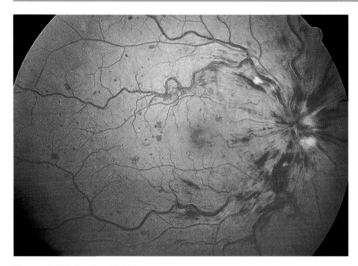

**Figure 2.77** Papillophlebitis

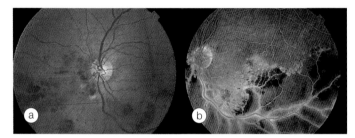

**Figure 2.78 (a)** Inferior hemiretinal vein occlusion; **(b)** FA shows extensive hypofluorescence due to ischaemia

branch of the CRV at or near the optic disc. A hemicentral occlusion, which is less common, involves one trunk of a dual-trunked CRV, which persists in the anterior part of the optic nerve head as a congenital variant.

1. **Presentation** is with sudden-onset altitudinal visual field defect.

2. **Signs**

   a. *VA* reduction is variable.
   b. *Fundus* shows the features of BRVO, involving the superior or inferior hemisphere (Fig. 2.78a).

3. **FA** shows masking by haemorrhages, hyperfluorescence due to leakage and variable capillary non-perfusion (Fig. 2.78b).

4. **Management** depends on the severity of retinal ischaemia. Extensive retinal ischaemia carries the risk of neovascular glaucoma and should be managed in the same way as ischaemic CRVO.

## FURTHER READING

Beaumont PE, Kang HK. Clinical characteristics of retinal venous occlusion occurring at different sites. *Br J Ophthalmol* 2002; 86:572–580.

Brown BA, Marx JL, Ward TP, et al. Homocysteine: a risk factor for retinal venous occlusive disease. *Ophthalmology* 2002;109: 287–290.

Central Vein Occlusion Study Group. Baseline and early natural history report: the central vein occlusion study. *Arch Ophthalmol* 1993;111:1087–1095.

Central Retinal Vein Occlusion Study Group. Evaluation of grid pattern photocoagulation for macular edema in central vein occlusion. The Central Vein Occlusion Study Group M report. *Ophthalmology* 1995;102:1425–1433.

Central Vein Occlusion Study Group. A randomized clinical trial of early panretinal photocoagulation for ischemic central vein occlusion. The Central Vein Occlusion Study Group N report. *Ophthalmology* 1995;102:1434-1444.

Central Vein Occlusion Study Group. Natural history and clinical management of central retinal vein occlusion. *Arch Ophthalmol* 1997;115:486–491.

Christoffersen NLB, Larsen M. Pathophysiology and hemodynamics of branch retinal vein occlusion. *Ophthalmology* 1999;106:2054–2062.

Fegan CD. Central retinal vein occlusion and thrombophilia. *Eye* 2002;11;98–106.

Fong ACO, Schatz H. Central retinal vein occlusion in young adults. *Surv Ophthalmol* 1993;37:393–417.

Fuller JJ, Mason JO III, White MF Jr, et al. Retinochoroidal collateral veins protect against anterior segment neovascularization after central retinal vein occlusion. *Am J Ophthalmol* 2003;121:332–336.

Hayreh SS, Heyreh MS. Hemi-central retinal vein occlusion. Pathogenesis, clinical features, and natural history. *Arch Ophthalmol* 1980;98:14–22.

Kumar B, Yu D-Y, Morgan WH, et al. The distribution of architectural changes within the vicinity of arteriovenous crossing in branch retinal vein occlusion. *Ophthalmology* 1998;105:424–427.

Lahey JM, Tunc M, Kearney J, et al. Laboratory evaluation of hypercoagulability states in patients with central retinal vein occlusion who are less than 56 years of age. *Ophthalmology* 2002; 109:126–131

Leonard BC, Coupland SG, Kertes PJ, et al. Long-term follow-up of a modified technique for laser-induced chorioretinal venous anastomosis in nonischemic central retinal vein occlusion. *Ophthalmology* 2003;110:948–954.

Lunz MH, Schenker HI. Retinal vascular accidents in glaucoma and ocular hypertension. *Surv Ophthalmol* 1980;25:163–167.

Martin SC, Butcher A, Martin N, et al. Cardiovascular risk assessment in patients with retinal vein occlusion. *Br J Ophthalmol* 2002;86:774–776.

McAllister IL, Douglas JP, Constable IJ, et al. Laser-induced chorioretinal venous anastomosis for nonischemic central retinal vein occlusion: evaluation of the complications and their risk factors. *Am J Ophthalmol* 1998;126:219–229.

Sperduto RD, Hiller R, Chew E, et al. Risk factors for hemiretinal vein occlusion. Comparison with risk factors for central and branch retinal vein occlusion. The Eye Disease Case-Control Study. *Ophthalmology* 1998;105:765–771.

The Eye Disease Case-Control Study Group. Risk factors for central retinal vein occlusion. *Arch Ophthalmol* 1996;114:545–554.

Weiss JN, Bynoe LA. Injection of tissue plasminogen activator into a branch retinal vein in eyes with central retinal vein occlusion. *Ophthalmology* 2002;108:2249–2257.

Williamson TH. Central retinal vein occlusion; what's the story? Perspectives. *Br J Ophthalmol* 1997;81:698–704.

# Retinal Arterial Occlusive Disease

## CAUSES

### Common

1. **Atherosclerosis-related** thrombosis at the level of the lamina cribrosa is by far the most common underlying cause of central retinal artery occlusion (CRAO), accounting for about 80% of cases.

**2. Carotid embolism** originating from the bifurcation of the common carotid artery. This is a vulnerable site for atheromatous ulceration and stenosis (Fig. 2.79). Retinal emboli from the carotid arteries may be of the following types:

a. *Cholesterol* emboli (Hollenhorst plaques) appear as intermittent showers of minute, bright, refractile, golden to yellow-orange crystals, often located at arteriolar bifurcations (Fig. 2.80). They rarely cause significant obstruction to the retinal arterioles and are frequently asymptomatic.

b. *Fibrin–platelet* emboli are dull grey, elongated particles which are usually multiple and occasionally fill the entire lumen (Fig. 2.81). They may cause a retinal transient ischaemic attack (TIA), with resultant amau-

rosis fugax, and, occasionally, complete obstruction. Amaurosis fugax is characterised by painless transient unilateral loss of vision, often described as a curtain coming down over the eye, usually from top to bottom, but occasionally vice versa. Visual loss, which may be complete, usually lasts a few minutes. Recovery is in the same pattern as the initial loss, although usually more gradual. Frequency of attacks may vary from several times a day to once every few months. The attacks may be associated with ipsilateral cerebral TIA with contralateral signs.

c. *Calcific* emboli may originate from atheromatous plaques in the ascending aorta or carotid arteries, as well as from calcified heart valves. They are usually single, white, non-scintillating and often on or close to the disc (Fig. 2.82). When located on the disc itself,

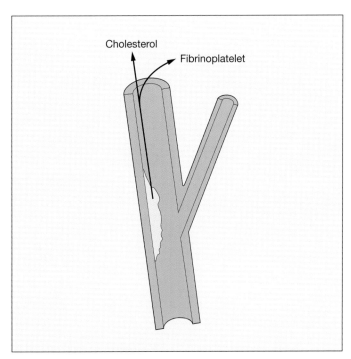

**Figure 2.79** Embolism from carotid artery disease

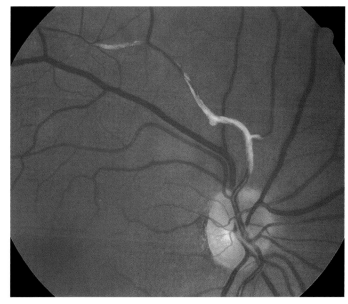

**Figure 2.81** Fibrinoplatelet emboli

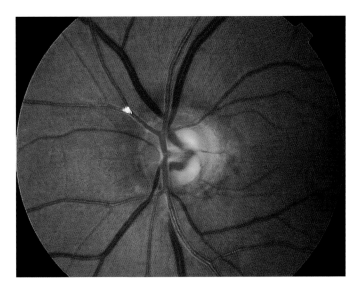

**Figure 2.80** Cholesterol embolus (Hollenhorst plaques)

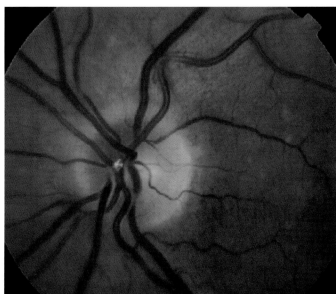

**Figure 2.82** Calcific embolus

they may be easily overlooked because they tend to merge with the disc. Calcific emboli are much more dangerous than the other two kinds because they may cause permanent occlusion of the central retinal artery or one of its main branches.

3. **Giant-cell arteritis.**

## *Uncommon*

1. **Cardiac embolism.** Since the ophthalmic artery is the first branch of the internal carotid artery, embolic material from the heart and carotid arteries has a fairly direct route to the eye. Emboli originating from the heart and its valves may be of the following four types (Fig. 2.83):

   *a. Calcific emboli* from the aortic or mitral valves.
   *b. Vegetations* from cardiac valves in bacterial endocarditis.
   *c. Thrombus* from the left side of the heart, consequent to myocardial infarction (mural thrombi), and mitral stenosis associated with atrial fibrillation or mitral valve prolapse.
   *d. Myxomatous material* from the very rare atrial myxoma.

2. **Periarteritis** associated with dermatomyositis, systemic lupus erythematosus, polyarteritis nodosa, Wegener's granulomatosis and Behçet disease may occasionally be responsible for branch retinal artery occlusion (BRAO), which may be multiple (Fig. 2.84).

3. **Thrombophilic disorders** that may be associated with retinal artery occlusion in young individuals include hyper-homocysteinaemia, antiphospholipid antibody syndrome and inherited defects of natural anticoagulants.

4. **Sickling haemoglobinopathies.**

5. **Retinal migraine** may very rarely be responsible for retinal artery occlusion in young individuals. However, the diagnosis should be made only after other more common causes have been excluded.

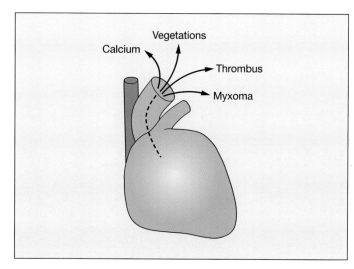

**Figure 2.83** Cardiac embolism

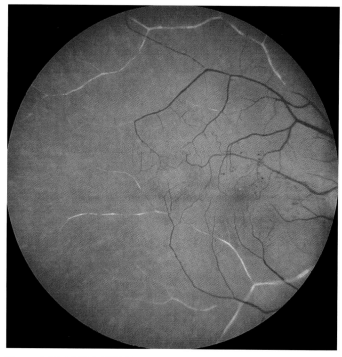

**Figure 2.84** Multiple BRAO in polyarteritis nodosa

6. **Susac syndrome,** which is characterised by the triad of retinal artery occlusion, sensorineural deafness and encephalopathy.

## MEDICAL INVESTIGATIONS

### *All patients*

1. **Pulse** to detect atrial fibrillation.

2. **Blood pressure.**

3. **Carotid evaluation** for stenosis by auscultation to detect a bruit, and Duplex scanning.

4. **ECG.**

5. **Blood**
   - Full blood count, ESR and CRP.
   - Fasting glucose and lipids.

### *Selected patients*

1. **Echocardiogram.**

2. **MRI angiography.**

3. **Blood**
   - Thrombophilia screen.
   - Autoantibodies – anticardiolipin, lupus anticoagulant, ANA, anti-DNA and antinuclear cytoplasmic (ANCA).
   - Homocysteine.

## BRANCH RETINAL ARTERY OCCLUSION

### *Diagnosis*

1. **Presentation** is with sudden and profound altitudinal or sectoral visual field loss.

**2. Signs**

 *a.* *VA* is variable.

 *b.* *Fundus* (Fig. 2.85a)

- Retinal cloudiness corresponding to the area of ischaemia resulting from oedema.
- Narrowing of arteries and veins with sludging and segmentation of the blood column.
- One or more emboli may be present.

**3. FA** shows delay in arterial filling and masking of background fluorescence by retinal swelling which is confined to the involved sector (Fig. 2.85b).

***Prognosis*** is poor unless the obstruction can be relieved within a few hours (see below). The visual field defect is permanent and the affected artery remains attenuated. Occasionally, however, recanalisation of the obstructed artery may leave subtle or absent ophthalmoscopic signs.

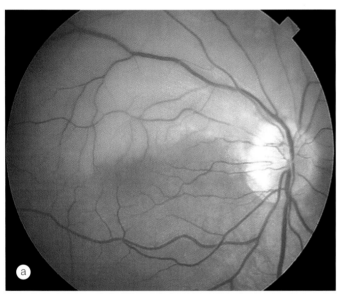

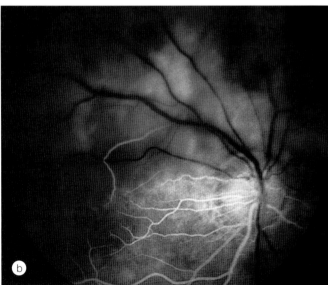

**Figure 2.85 (a)** Superotemporal BRAO; **(b)** FA shows hypofluorescence of the involved sector due to absence of arterial filling and blockage of background fluorescence by oedema

# CENTRAL RETINAL ARTERY OCCLUSION

## *Diagnosis*

**1. Presentation** is with sudden and profound loss of vision.

**2. Signs**

 *a.* *VA* is severely reduced except when a portion of the papillomacular bundle is supplied by a cilioretinal artery, when central vision may be preserved.

 *b.* *APD* is profound or total (amaurotic pupil).

 *c.* *Fundus*

- Attenuation of arteries and veins with sludging and segmentation of the blood column ('cattle-trucking') (Fig. 2.86).
- Extensive retinal cloudiness at the posterior pole; the orange reflex from the intact choroid stands out at the

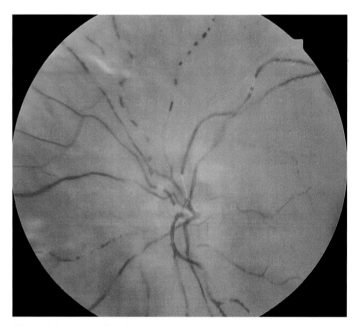

**Figure 2.86** Acute CRAO showing vascular attenuation and segmentation of the blood column ('cattle-trucking')

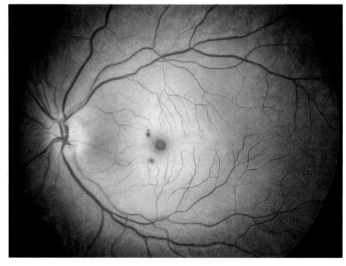

**Figure 2.87** Acute CRAO with a cherry-red spot at the foveola (Courtesy of C. Barry)

thin foveola, in contrast to the surrounding pale retina, giving rise to the 'cherry-red spot' appearance (Fig. 2.87); in eyes with a cilioretinal artery, the macula will remain of normal colour (Fig. 2.88a).

3. **FA** shows delay in arterial filling and masking of background choroidal fluorescence by retinal swelling. However, a patent cilioretinal artery will fill during the early phase (Fig. 2.88b).

***Prognosis*** is poor due to retinal infarction. After a few weeks, the retinal cloudiness and the 'cherry-red spot' gradually disappear, although the arteries remain attenuated (Fig. 2.89).

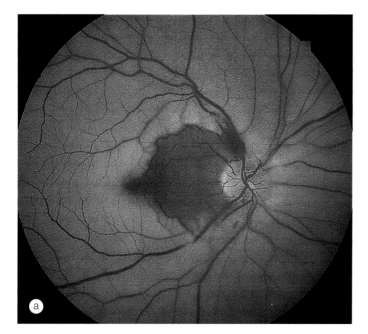

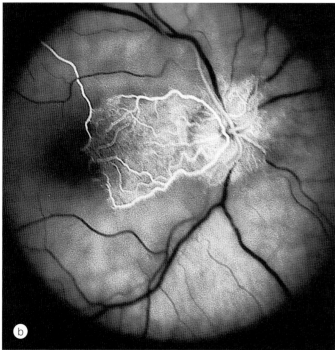

**Figure 2.88 (a)** Acute CRAO with sparing of a cilioretinal artery; **(b)** FA shows perfusion only of the macula

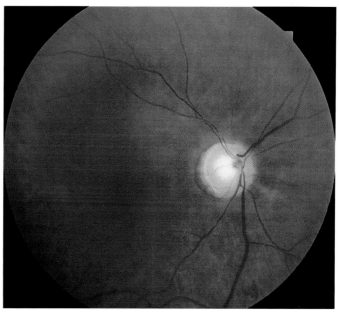

**Figure 2.89** Vascular attenuation and consecutive optic atrophy following CRAO

The inner retinal layers become atrophic and consecutive optic atrophy results in permanent loss of all useful vision. Some eyes develop rubeosis iridis, which may require PRP, and about 2% develop NVD.

## CILIORETINAL ARTERY OCCLUSION

A cilioretinal artery, present in 20% of the population, arises from the posterior ciliary circulation but supplies the retina, commonly in the area of the macula and papillomacular bundle.

1. **Classification**

    *a. Isolated* (Fig. 2.90) typically affects young patients with an associated systemic vasculitis.

    *b. Combined with CRVO* (Fig. 2.91) has a similar prognosis to non-ischaemic CRVO.

    *c. Combined with anterior ischaemic optic neuropathy* (Fig. 2.92) typically affects patients with giant-cell arteritis and carries a very poor prognosis.

2. **Presentation** is with acute, severe loss of central vision.

3. **Signs.** Cloudiness localised to that part of the retina normally perfused by the vessel.

4. **FA** shows a corresponding filling defect (see Fig. 2.90b).

## TREATMENT OF ACUTE RETINAL ARTERY OCCLUSION

Retinal artery occlusion is an emergency because it causes irreversible visual loss unless the retinal circulation is re-established prior to the development of retinal infarction. It appears that the prognosis for occlusions caused by calcific emboli is worse than for those resulting from either cholesterol or platelet emboli. Theoretically, timely dislodgement of emboli of the latter two types may prevent subsequent visual loss. The following treatment may be tried in patients with occlusions of less than 48 hours duration at presentation.

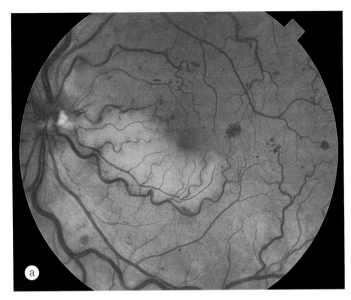

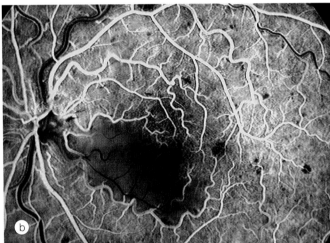

**Figure 2.90 (a)** Isolated cilioretinal artery occlusion; **(b)** FA shows hypofluorescence at the macula due to ischaemia

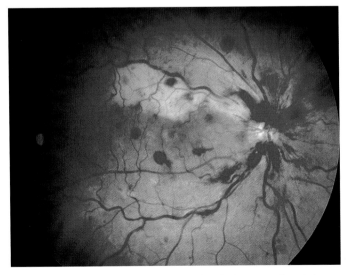

**Figure 2.91** Combined occlusion of the cilioretinal artery and central retinal vein

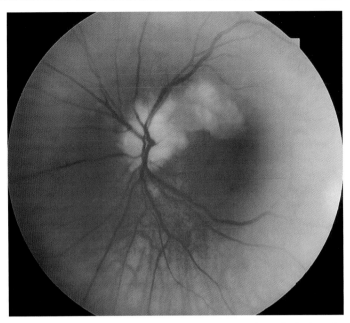

**Figure 2.92** Combined cilioretinal artery occlusion and anterior ischaemic optic neuropathy

1. **Ocular massage** using a three-mirror contact lens for approximately 10 seconds, to obtain central retinal artery pulsation or cessation of flow (for BRAO), followed by 5 seconds of release. The aim is to mechanically collapse the arterial lumen and cause prompt changes in arterial flow.

2. **Anterior chamber paracentesis** should be carried out.

3. **Intravenous acetazolamide** to obtain a more prolonged lowering of intraocular pressure with repeated paracentesis, if this was initially successful but flow has ceased.

## FURTHER READING

Augsburger JJ, Magargal LE. Visual prognosis following treatment of acute central retinal artery occlusion. *Br J Ophthalmol* 1980;64:913–917.

Egan RA, Nguyen TH, Gass JDM, et al. Retinal arterial wall plaques in Susac syndrome. *Am J Ophthalmol* 2003;135:483–486.

Greven CM, Slusher MM, Waever RG. Retinal artery occlusion in young adults. *Am J Ophthalmol* 1995;120:776–783.

Haase CG, Buchner T. Microemboli are not a prerequisite in retinal artery occlusive diseases. *Eye* 1998;12:659–662.

Johnson MW, Thomley ML, Huang SS, et al. Idiopathic recurrent branch retinal artery occlusion. Natural history and laboratory evaluation. *Ophthalmology* 1994;101:480–489.

Salomon O, Huna-Baron R, Moisseiev J, et al. Thrombophilia as a cause for central and branch retinal artery occlusion in patients without an apparent embolic source. *Eye* 2001;15:511–514.

## Ocular Ischaemic Syndrome

Ocular ischaemic syndrome is an uncommon condition which is the result of chronic ocular hypoperfusion secondary to severe ipsilateral atherosclerotic carotid stenosis. It typically affects patients during the seventh decade and may be associated with diabetes, hypertension, ischaemic heart disease and cerebrovascular disease. The 5-year mortality is in the order of 40%, most frequently from cardiac disease.

Patients with ocular ischaemic syndrome may also give a history of amaurosis fugax due to retinal embolism.

## DIAGNOSIS

The ocular ischaemic syndrome is unilateral in 80% of cases and affects both anterior and posterior segments. The signs are variable and may be subtle such that the condition is missed or misdiagnosed.

1. **Presentation** is usually with gradual loss of vision over several weeks or months, although, occasionally, visual loss may be sudden.

2. **Signs**

   *a. Anterior segment*

   - Diffuse episcleral injection and corneal oedema.
   - Aqueous flare with few if any cells (ischaemic pseudoiritis).
   - Iris atrophy and a mid-dilated and poorly reacting pupil.
   - Rubeosis iridis is common and often progresses to neovascular glaucoma.
   - Cataract in very advanced cases.

   *b. Fundus* (Fig. 2.93)

   - Venous dilatation, with or without mild tortuosity, and arteriolar narrowing; dot–blot haemorrhages and occasionally cotton-wool spots.
   - Proliferative retinopathy with NVD and occasionally NVE.
   - Spontaneous arterial pulsation, most pronounced near the optic disc, is present in most cases or may be easily induced by exerting gentle pressure on the globe (digital ophthalmodynamometry).
   - In diabetic patients, proliferative retinopathy may be more advanced ipsilateral to the carotid stenosis.

3. **FA** shows delayed and patchy choroidal filling, prolonged arteriovenous transit time, retinal capillary non-perfusion, late leakage and prominent arterial staining.

4. **Carotid imaging** may involve colour Doppler ultrasonography (Fig. 2.94), digital subtraction angiography (Fig. 2.95) and MRI angiography (Fig. 2.96).

## MANAGEMENT

1. **Anterior segment manifestations** are treated with topical steroids and mydriatics.

2. **Neovascular glaucoma** may be treated medically or surgically.

3. **Proliferative retinopathy** requires PRP, although the results are less favourable than in diabetic retinopathy.

4. **Carotid endarterectomy** may be beneficial for proliferative retinopathy.

## DIFFERENTIAL DIAGNOSIS

1. **Non-ischaemic CRVO** is also characterised by unilateral retinal haemorrhages, venous dilatation and cotton-wool spots. However, haemorrhages are more numerous and mainly flame-shaped, and disc oedema is often present.

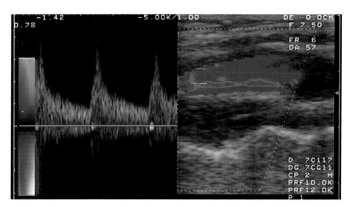

**Figure 2.94** Colour Doppler sonogram showing carotid stenosis

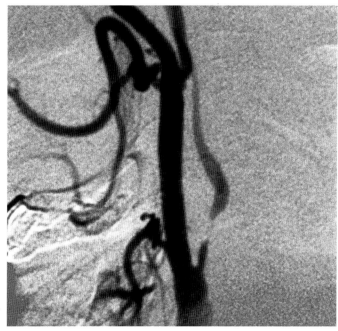

**Figure 2.95** Digital subtraction angiogram showing carotid occlusion

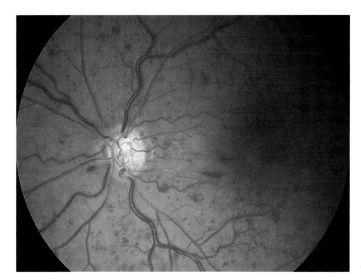

**Figure 2.93** Arteriolar attenuation, venous dilatation, haemorrhages and NVD in ocular ischaemic syndrome

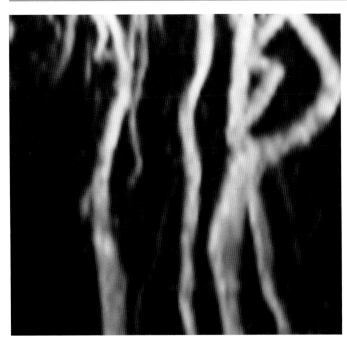

**Figure 2.96** MRI angiogram showing severe right carotid stenosis

2. **Diabetic retinopathy** is also characterised by dot–blot retinal haemorrhages, venous tortuosity and proliferative retinopathy. However, it is usually bilateral and hard exudates are present.

3. **Hypertensive retinopathy** is also characterised by arteriolar attenuation and focal constriction, haemorrhages and cotton-wool spots. However, it is invariably bilateral and venous changes are absent.

## FURTHER READING

Brown G, Magargal L. The ocular ischemic syndrome. Clinical, fluorescein angiographic and carotid angiographic features. *Int Ophthalmol* 1988;11:239–251.

Malhotra R, Gregory-Evans K. Management of ocular ischaemic syndrome. *Br J Ophthalmol* 2000;84:1428–1431.

Mizener JB, Podhajsky P, Hayreh SS. Ocular ischemic syndrome. *Ophthalmology* 1997;104:859–864.

Riordan-Eva R, Restori M, Hamilton AMP, et al. Orbital ultrasound in the ocular ischaemic syndrome. *Eye* 1994;8:93–96.

# Hypertensive Disease

## SYSTEMIC HYPERTENSION

### Clinical features

Hypertension is most commonly idiopathic (essential) and occasionally secondary to a renal or metabolic disorder.

1. **Presentation** is usually in the fifth to sixth decades.

2. **Signs.** Blood pressure >140/90 mmHg.

3. **Complications**

   - Ventricular hypertrophy and subsequent failure.

   - Increased risk of atherosclerosis resulting in coronary heart disease and stroke, particularly in those with hypertensive retinopathy.
   - Renal disease.

4. **Treatment** options include lifestyle modification (exercise, weight reduction, diminished salt intake and alcohol consumption) and drug therapy (diuretics, beta-blockers, calcium channel blockers, ACE inhibitors, angiotensin II receptor antagonists and alpha-blockers).

### Ophthalmic features

1. **Common.** Retinal arteriolosclerosis and BRVO.

2. **Uncommon.** Retinopathy, retinal artery occlusion, retinal artery macroaneurysm, anterior ischaemic optic neuropathy, choroidal infarcts and ocular motor nerve palsies.

3. **Rare.** Exudative retinal detachment (e.g. in eclampsia).

## FUNDUS CHANGES

***Hypertensive retinopathy*** consists of a spectrum of retinal vascular changes that are pathologically related to both transient and persistent microvascular damage from elevated blood pressure. The primary response of the retinal arterioles to systemic hypertension is narrowing (vasoconstriction). However, the degree of narrowing is dependent on the amount of pre-existing replacement fibrosis (involutional sclerosis). For this reason, hypertensive narrowing is seen in its pure form only in young individuals. In older patients, rigidity of retinal arterioles due to involutional sclerosis prevents the same degree of narrowing seen in young individuals. In sustained hypertension, the inner blood–retinal barrier is disrupted in small areas, with increased vascular permeability. The fundus picture of hypertensive retinopathy is therefore characterised by the following:

1. **Arteriolar narrowing** may be focal (Fig. 2.97) or generalised (Fig. 2.98). Ophthalmoscopic diagnosis of generalised narrowing is difficult, although the presence of focal narrowing makes it highly probable that blood pressure is raised. Severe hypertension may lead to obstruction of the

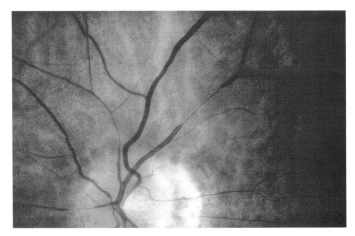

**Figure 2.97** Focal arteriolar attenuation in hypertension

precapillary arterioles and the development of cotton-wool spots (Fig. 2.99). It appears that the presence of retinal arteriolar narrowing is related to the risk of coronary heart disease in women.

2. **Vascular leakage** leads to flame-shaped retinal haemorrhages and retinal oedema (Fig. 2.100). Chronic retinal oedema may result in the deposition of hard exudates around the fovea in the Henle layer with a macular star configuration (Fig. 2.101). Swelling of the optic nerve head is the hallmark of malignant hypertension (Figs. 2.102 and 2.103).

3. **Arteriolosclerosis** involves thickening of the vessel wall characterised histologically by intimal hyalinisation, medial hypertrophy and endothelial hyperplasia. The most important clinical sign is the presence of changes at arteriovenous crossings (AV nipping) (Fig. 2.104); although not necessarily indicative of the severity of hypertension, their presence makes it probable that hypertension has been

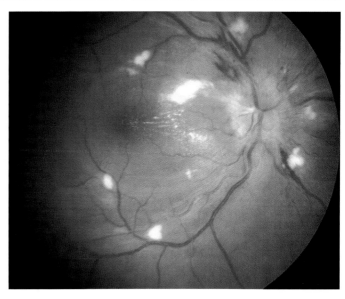

**Figure 2.100** Severe hypertensive retinopathy with cotton-wool spots, flame-shaped haemorrhages, early macular star formation and mild disc swelling (Courtesy of J. Salmon)

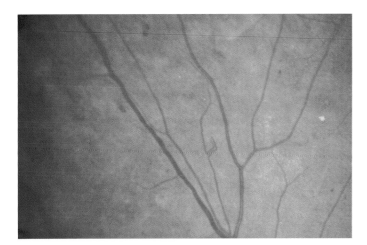

**Figure 2.98** Generalised arteriolar attenuation in hypertension

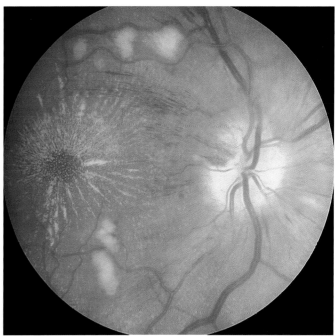

**Figure 2.101** Severe hypertensive retinopathy with a fully developed macular star, cotton-wool spots, a few flame-shaped haemorrhages and moderate disc swelling

present for many years. Mild changes at arteriovenous crossings are seen in patients with involutional sclerosis in the absence of hypertension. The grading of arteriolosclerosis is as follows (Fig. 2.105):

*Grade 1.* Subtle broadening of the arteriolar light reflex, mild generalised arteriolar attenuation, particularly of small branches, and vein concealment.

*Grade 2.* Obvious broadening of the arteriolar light reflex and deflection of veins at arteriovenous crossings (Salus sign).

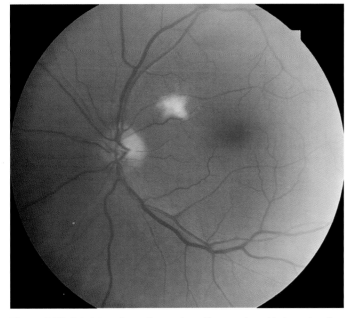

**Figure 2.99** Arteriolar attenuation and a cotton-wool spot in hypertension

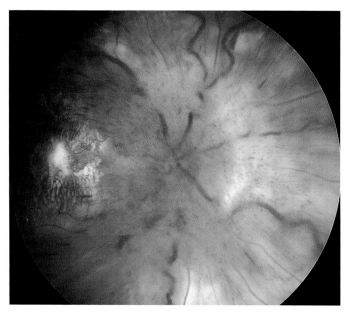

**Figure 2.102** Very severe hypertensive retinopathy with severe disc oedema and a macular star

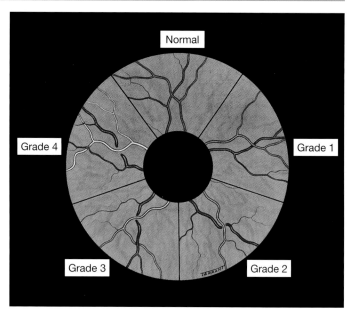

**Figure 2.105** Grading of retinal arteriolosclerosis (see text)

*Grade 3.*

- Copper-wiring of arterioles.
- Banking of veins distal to arteriovenous crossings (Bonnet sign).
- Tapering of veins on both sides of the crossings (Gunn sign) and right-angled deflection of veins.

*Grade 4.* Silver-wiring of arterioles associated with grade 3 changes.

> **NB: The presence of generalised retinal arteriolar narrowing and possibly arteriovenous nicking are related to previously elevated blood pressure, independent of concurrent blood pressure level.**

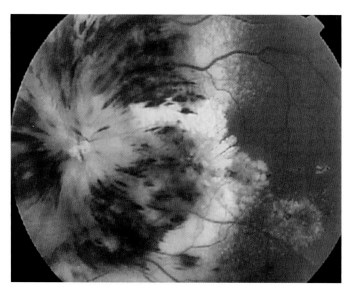

**Figure 2.103** Very severe retinopathy in a patient with severe hypertension, diabetes and hyperlipidaemia

***Choroidopathy*** is rare but may occur as the result of an acute hypertensive crisis (accelerated hypertension) in young adults.

1. **Elschnig spots** are small, black spots surrounded by yellow halos (Fig. 2.106) which represent focal choroidal infarcts.

2. **Siegrist streaks** are flecks arranged linearly along choroidal vessels (Fig. 2.107) which are indicative of fibrinoid necrosis associated with malignant hypertension.

3. **Exudative retinal detachment,** sometimes bilateral, may occur in severe acute hypertension such as that associated with toxaemia of pregnancy.

## FURTHER READING

Duncan BB, Wong TY, Tyroler HA, et al. Hypertensive retinopathy and incident coronary heart disease in high risk men. *Br J Ophthalmol* 2002;86:1002–1006.

Hubbard LD, Brothers RJ, King WN, et al. Methods for evaluation of retinal micro-vascular abnormalities associated with hypertension/sclerosis in the Atherosclerosis Risk in Communities (ARIC) Study. *Ophthalmology* 1999;106:2269–2280.

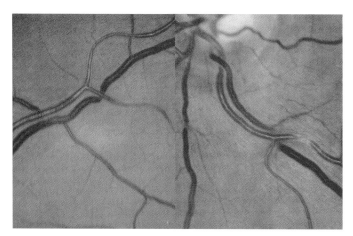

**Figure 2.104** Hypertensive changes at arteriovenous crossings

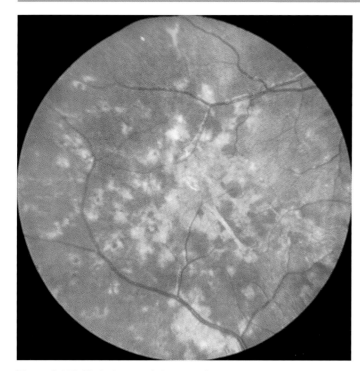

**Figure 2.106** Elschnig spots in hypertension

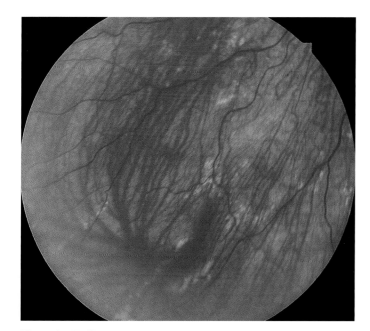

**Figure 2.107** Siegrist lines in hypertension

Ramsay LE, Williams B, Johnston GD, et al. British Hypertension Society guidelines for hypertensive management 1999; summary. *BMJ* 1999;319:630–635.

Wong TY, Klein R, Couper DJ, et al. Retinal microvascular abnormalities and incident stroke. The Atherosclerosis Risk in the Communities Study. *Lancet* 2001;358:1134–1140.

Wong TY, Klein R, Klein BEK, et al. Retinal microvascular abnormalities and their relations with hypertension, cardiovascular disease and mortality. *Surv Ophthalmol* 2001;46:59–80.

Wong TY, Klein R, Sharrett AR, et al. Retinal arteriolar narrowing and risk of coronary heart disease in men and women: the Atherosclerosis Risk in Communities Study. *JAMA* 2002;287:1153–1159.

Wong TY, Hubbard LD, Klein R, et al. Retinal microvascular abnormalities and blood pressure in older people: the Cardiovascular Health Study. *Br J Ophthalmol* 2002;86:1007–1013.

Yu T, Mitchell P, Berry G, et al. Retinopathy in older persons without diabetes and its relationship to hypertension. *Arch Ophthalmol* 1998;116:83–89.

## Sickle-Cell Retinopathy

Sickling haemoglobinopathies are caused by one, or a combination of, abnormal haemoglobins which cause the red blood cell to adopt an anomalous shape (Fig. 2.108) under conditions of hypoxia and acidosis. Because these deformed red blood cells are more rigid than healthy cells, they may become impacted in and obstruct small blood vessels. The sickling disorders in which the mutant haemoglobins S and C are inherited as alleles of normal haemoglobin A have important ocular manifestations. These abnormal haemoglobins may occur in combination with normal haemoglobin A or in association with each other, as indicated below.

1. **SS** (sickle-cell disease, sickle-cell anaemia) affects 0.4% of black Americans and is caused by a point mutation on the beta-globulin gene. The disease is characterised by severe chronic haemolytic anaemia and periodic, potentially fatal crises due to vaso-occlusive disease involving most organs, resulting in liver necrosis, painful crises (largely bone marrow infarcts), abdominal pain, acute chest syndrome and CNS symptoms. Despite the severity of systemic manifestations, ocular complications are usually mild and asymptomatic.

2. **AS** (sickle-cell trait) is present in about 10% of black Americans. It is the mildest form and usually requires severe hypoxia or other abnormal conditions to produce sickling.

3. **SC** (sickle-cell C disease) is present in 0.2% of black Americans. It is characterised by haemolytic anaemia and infarctive crises that are less severe than in SS disease but may be associated with severe retinopathy.

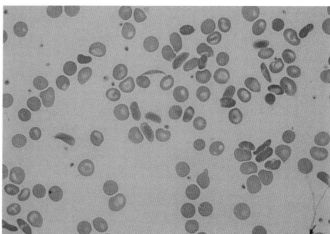

**Figure 2.108** Blood film in sickle-cell anaemia

**4. SThal** (sickle-cell thalassaemia) is characterised by mild anaemia but may be associated with severe retinopathy.

NB: Retinopathy is most severe in SC and SThal disease.

## PROLIFERATIVE RETINOPATHY

### *Grading* (Fig. 2.109)

**Stage 1** is characterised by occlusion of peripheral arteries.

### Stage 2

- Peripheral arteriovenous anastomoses which appear to be dilated pre-existent capillary channels (Fig. 2.110).

- The peripheral retina beyond the point of vascular occlusion is largely avascular and non-perfused.

### Stage 3

- Sprouting of new vessels from the anastomoses which have a 'sea-fan' configuration and are usually fed by a single arteriole and drained by a single vein (Fig. 2.111 and see Fig. 2.115a).
- Between 40% and 50% of 'sea-fans' spontaneously involute as a result of auto-infarction and appear as greyish fibrovascular lesions (Fig. 2.112).
- In other cases, the neovascular tufts continue to proliferate, become adherent to the cortical vitreous gel and may bleed as a result of vitreoretinal traction (Fig. 2.113).

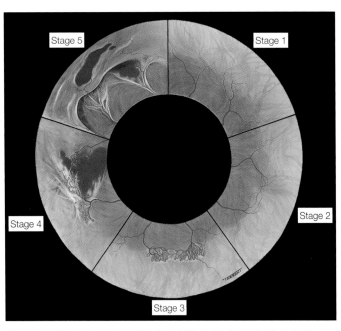

**Figure 2.109** Grading of proliferative sickle-cell retinopathy (see text)

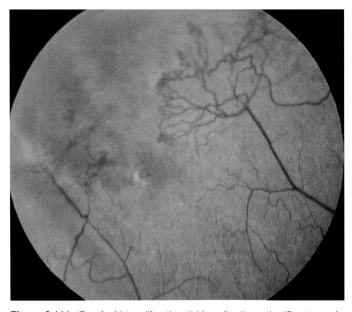

**Figure 2.111** 'Sea-fan' in proliferative sickle-cell retinopathy (Courtesy of R. Marsh)

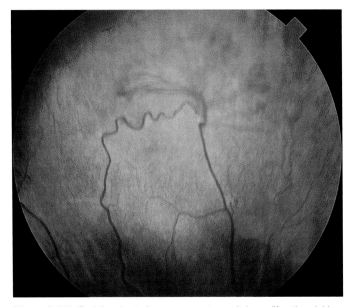

**Figure 2.110** Peripheral arteriovenous anastomosis in proliferative sickle-cell retinopathy (Courtesy of R. Marsh)

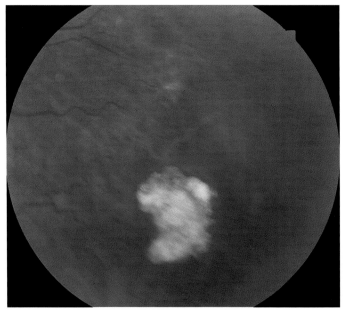

**Figure 2.112** Spontaneous involution of a neovascular tuft in proliferative sickle-cell retinopathy

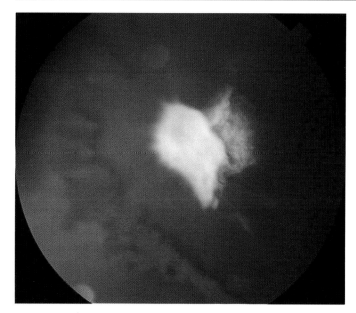

**Figure 2.113** Haemorrhage due to traction on a neovascular tuft

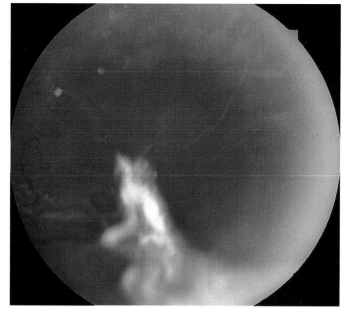

**Figure 2.114** Peripheral retinal detachment in proliferative sickle-cell retinopathy

**Stage 4** is characterised by vitreous haemorrhage.

**Stage 5** is characterised by fibrovascular proliferation and retinal detachment (Fig. 2.114).

*FA* shows extensive capillary non-perfusion of the peripheral retina (Fig. 2.115b) and late leakage from neovascularisation (Fig. 2.115c).

*Treatment* is not required in most cases because new vessels tend to auto-infarct and involute spontaneously without treatment. Occasionally, vitreoretinal surgery may be required for tractional retinal detachment and/or persistent vitreous haemorrhage.

## NON-PROLIFERATIVE RETINOPATHY

### Asymptomatic lesions

1. **Venous tortuosity** is one of the first ophthalmic signs of sickling and is due to peripheral arteriovenous shunts.

2. **Silver-wiring of arterioles** in the peripheral retina which represent previously occluded vessels.

3. **Salmon patches** are pink, preretinal (Fig. 2.116) or superficial intraretinal haemorrhages at the equator, which lie adjacent to arterioles and usually resolve without sequelae.

4. **Black sunbursts** are patches of peripheral RPE hyperplasia (Fig. 2.117).

5. **Macular depression sign** is an oval depression of the bright central macular reflex due to atrophy and thinning of the sensory retina.

6. **Peripheral retinal holes** and areas of whitening similar to 'white-without-pressure' are occasionally seen (Fig. 2.118).

### Symptomatic lesions

1. **Macular arteriolar occlusion** occurs in about 30% of patients.

2. **Acute CRAO** is rare.

3. **Retinal vein occlusion** is uncommon.

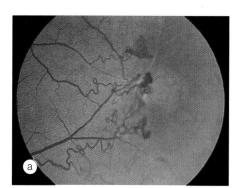
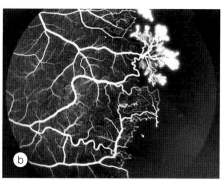
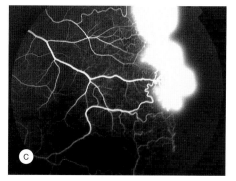

**Figure 2.115 (a)** Proliferative sickle-cell retinopathy stage 3; **(b)** FA early phase shows filling of new vessels ('sea-fans') and extensive peripheral retinal capillary non-perfusion; **(c)** late phase shows leakage from new vessels

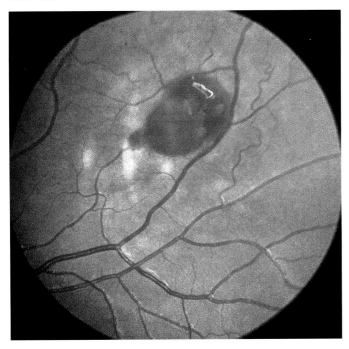

Figure 2.116 Preretinal haemorrhage (salmon patch) in sickle-cell retinopathy

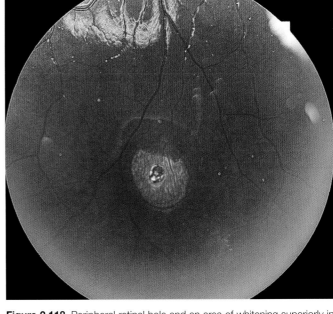

Figure 2.118 Peripheral retinal hole and an area of whitening superiorly in sickle-cell retinopathy

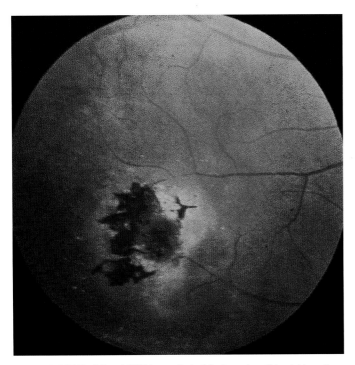

Figure 2.117 Peripheral RPE hyperplasia (black sunburst) in sickle-cell retinopathy

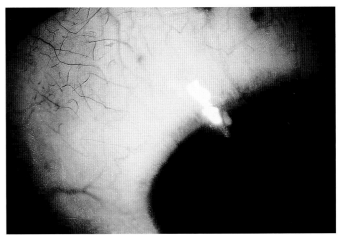

Figure 2.119 Conjunctival vascular lesions in sickle-cell disease (Courtesy of R. Marsh)

2. **Iris** lesions consist of circumscribed areas of ischaemic atrophy, usually at the pupillary edge and extending to the collarette. Rubeosis may be seen occasionally.

## FURTHER READING

Jampol LM, Ebroon DA, Goldbaum MH. Peripheral proliferative retinopathies: an update on angiogenesis, etiologies and management. *Surv Ophthalmol* 1994;38:519–540.

Mathews MK, McLeod DS, Merges C, et al. Neutrophils and leucocyte adhesion molecules in sickle cell retinopathy. *Br J Ophthalmol* 2002;86:684–690.

McLeod D, Goldberg M, Lutty G. Dual perspective analysis of vascular formations in sickle cell retinopathy. *Arch Ophthalmol* 1993;111:1234–1245.

McLeod DS, Merges C, Fukushima A, et al. Histopathological features of neovascularization in sickle cell retinopathy. *Am J Ophthalmol* 1997;124:473–487.

4. **Choroidal vascular occlusion** may be seen occasionally, particularly in children.

5. **Angioid streaks** occur in a minority of patients.

## ANTERIOR SEGMENT FEATURES

1. **Conjunctival** lesions are characterised by isolated dark-red vascular anomalies shaped like commas or corkscrews involving small-calibre vessels (Fig. 2.119).

# Retinopathy of Prematurity

Retinopathy of prematurity (ROP) is a proliferative retinopathy affecting premature infants of very low birth weight, who have often been exposed to high ambient oxygen concentrations. The retina is unique among tissues in that it has no blood vessels until the fourth month of gestation, at which time vascular complexes emanating from the hyaloid vessels at the optic disc grow towards the periphery. These vessels reach the nasal periphery after 8 months of gestation, but do not reach the temporal periphery until about 1 month after delivery (Fig. 2.120). The incompletely vascularised retina is particularly susceptible to oxygen damage in the premature infant. A model of ROP suggests that the avascular retina produces vascular endothelial growth factor (VEGF) which in utero is the stimulus for vessel migration in the developing retina. With premature birth, the production of VEGF is downregulated by the relative hyperoxia and vessel migration is halted. Subsequently, the increased metabolic demand of the growing eye allows excessive VEGF production, which leads to the neovascular complications of ROP.

## ACUTE RETINOPATHY OF PREMATURITY

***Location*** is determined according to three zones centred on the optic disc (Fig. 2.121).

> **Zone 1** is bounded by an imaginary circle, the radius of which is twice the distance from the disc to the macula.
> **Zone 2** extends concentrically from the edge of zone 1; its radius extends from the centre of the disc to the nasal ora serrata.
> **Zone 3** consists of a residual temporal crescent anterior to zone 2.

***Extent*** of involvement is determined by the number of clock hours of retina involved.

***Grading*** (Fig. 2.122)

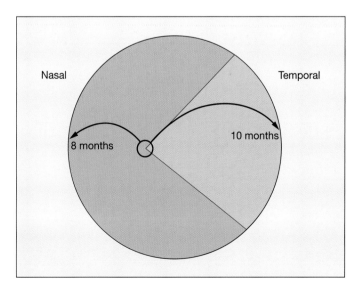

**Figure 2.120** Vascularisation of the peripheral retina (see text)

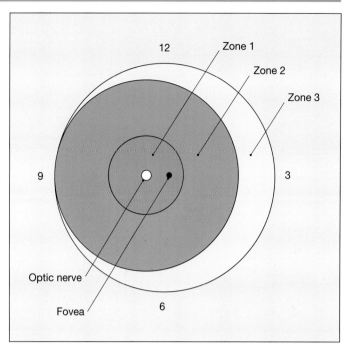

**Figure 2.121** Grading of ROP according to location (see text)

**Stage 1** (demarcation line).

- A thin, tortuous, grey-white line running roughly parallel with the ora serrata which separates avascular immature peripheral retina from vascularised posterior retina.
- The line is more prominent in the temporal periphery and may have abnormal branching blood vessels leading up to it.

**Stage 2** (ridge).

- The demarcation line develops into an elevated ridge, which represents a mesenchymal shunt joining arterioles with veins.
- Blood vessels enter the ridge and small isolated neovascular tufts may be seen posterior to it (Fig. 2.123).

**Stage 3** (ridge with extraretinal fibrovascular proliferation).

- The ridge develops a pink colour due to fibrovascular proliferation which grows along the surface of the retina and into the vitreous (Fig. 2.124). This stage is often associated with 'plus' disease (see below).
- Retinal haemorrhage is common, and vitreous haemorrhage may develop. The highest incidence of this stage is around the post-conceptual age of 35 weeks.

**Stage 4** (partial retinal detachment) typically develops at about 10 weeks.

- In stage 4a, the macula is not involved (Fig. 2.125).
- In stage 4b, the macula is involved.

**Stage 5** is characterised by a total retinal detachment.

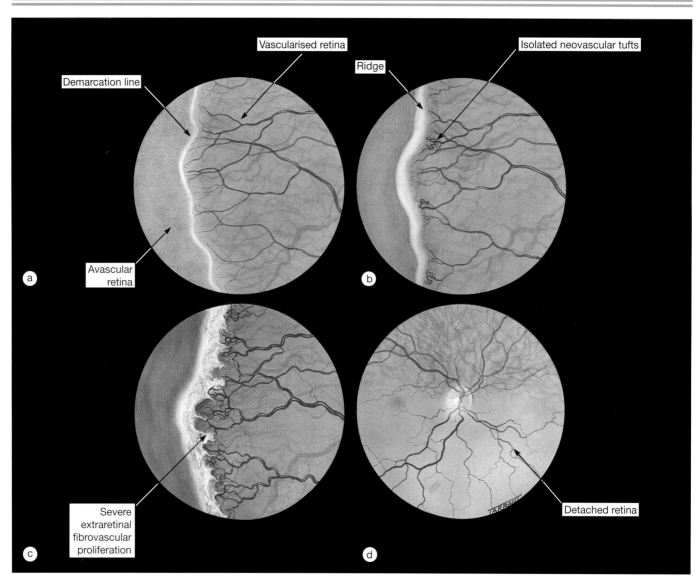

**Figure 2.122** Progression of ROP (see text)

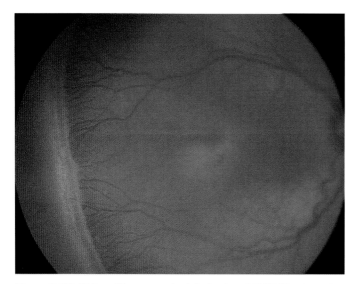

**Figure 2.123** Ridge with neovascular tufts in stage 2 ROP (Courtesy of P. Watts)

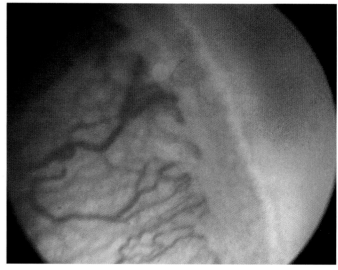

**Figure 2.124** Ridge with severe fibrovascular proliferation in stage 3 ROP (Courtesy of J. Arnold)

NB: Although the clinical features of ROP usually take several weeks to develop, rarely the disease can progress from stage 1 to stage 4 within a few days ('rush disease'). In about 80% of infants, ROP regresses spontaneously, leaving few if any residua. Spontaneous regression may even occur in patients with partial retinal detachments.

**'Plus' disease** signifies a tendency to progression and is characterised by the following:

- Failure of the pupil to dilate associated with gross vascular engorgement of the iris.
- Vitreous haze.
- Dilatation of veins and tortuosity of the arteries in the posterior fundus (Fig. 2.126).

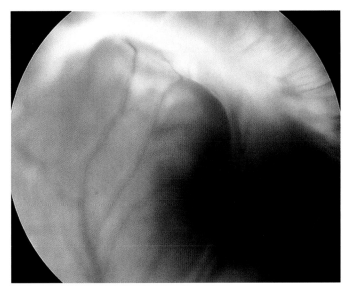

**Figure 2.125** Severe fibrovascular proliferation and early peripheral retinal detachment in stage 4a ROP

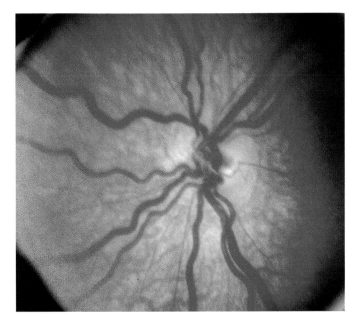

**Figure 2.126** Vascular dilatation in 'plus' disease

- Increasing preretinal and vitreous haemorrhage.

When these changes are present, a plus sign is added to the stage number.

**Threshold disease** is defined as five contiguous clock hours or eight cumulative clock hours of extraretinal neovascularisation (stage 3 disease) in zone 1 or zone 2, associated with plus disease, and is an indication for treatment.

### Screening

Babies born at or before 31 weeks gestational age, or weighing 1500 g or less, should be screened for ROP by an ophthalmologist with expertise in ROP. This may involve indirect ophthalmoscopy and a 28 dioptre or a 2.2 panfunduscopic Volk lens or a wide-field retinal camera (RetCam 120°). Screening should begin at 4–7 weeks' post-natal age to detect the onset of threshold disease. Subsequent review should be at 1- to 2-weekly intervals, depending on the severity of the disease, until retinal vascularisation reaches zone 3. The pupils in a premature infant are dilated using 0.5% cyclopentolate with 2.5% phenylephrine.

NB: Only about 8% of babies screened actually require treatment.

### Treatment

1. **Ablation** of avascular immature retina by cryotherapy or laser (indirect or transcleral) photocoagulation (Fig. 2.127) is recommended in infants with threshold disease. This is successful in 85% of cases, but the remainder progress to retinal detachment in spite of treatment. Overall, laser-treated eyes appear to have a better structural and functional outcome compared with those treated by cryotherapy. Laser-treated eyes are also less myopic.

2. **Vitreoretinal surgery** for tractional retinal detachment usually has a poor visual outcome.

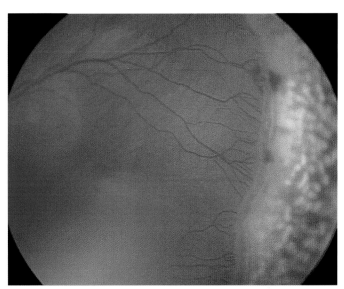

**Figure 2.127** Laser photocoagulation burns in ROP (Courtesy of P. Watts)

## CICATRICIAL RETINOPATHY OF PREMATURITY

About 20% of infants with active ROP develop cicatricial complications, which range from innocuous to extremely severe. In general, the more advanced or the more posterior the proliferative disease at the time of involution, the worse the cicatricial sequelae.

**Stage 1.** Myopia associated with mild peripheral retinal pigmentary disturbance and haze at the vitreous base.

**Stage 2.** Temporal vitreoretinal fibrosis (Fig. 2.128) with 'dragging' of the macula and disc (Fig. 2.129), which may lead to a pseudo-exotropia, due to resultant exaggeration of angle kappa.

**Stage 3.** More severe peripheral fibrosis with contracture and a falciform retinal fold (Fig. 2.130).

**Stage 4.** Partial ring of retrolental fibrovascular tissue with partial retinal detachment.

**Stage 5.**

- Complete ring of retrolental fibrovascular tissue with total retinal detachment (Fig. 2.131), a picture formerly known as 'retrolental fibroplasia'.
- Secondary angle-closure glaucoma may develop due to progressive shallowing of the anterior chamber caused by a forward movement of the iris–lens diaphragm and the development of anterior synechiae.
- Treatment involving lensectomy and anterior vitrectomy may be tried but the results are often poor.

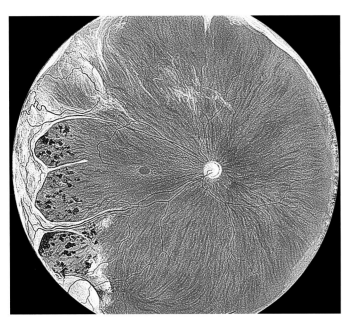

**Figure 2.128** Peripheral fibrous proliferation and pigmentary changes with straightening of temporal blood vessels in ROP

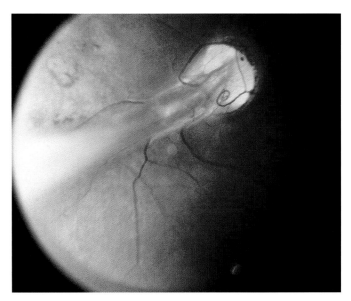

**Figure 2.130** Falciform vitreoretinal fold with inferotemporal dragging of the disc in ROP

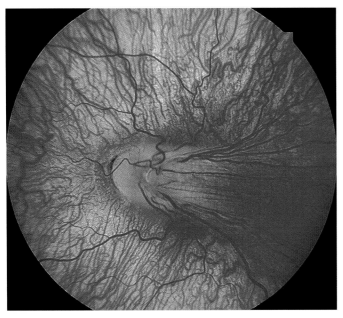

**Figure 2.129** Temporal dragging of the disc and macula in ROP

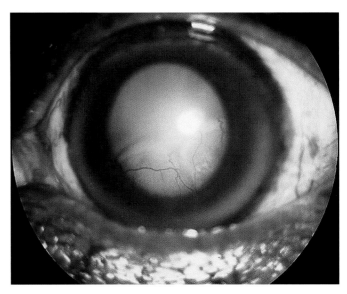

**Figure 2.131** Total retinal detachment in ROP

NB: Very low birth weight infants, especially those treated for ROP, are at a higher risk of developing strabismus and myopia than term infants and require follow-up until the age of visual maturity.

## FURTHER READING

Andruscavage L, Weissgold DJ. Screening for retinopathy of prematurity. *Br J Ophthalmol* 2002;86:1127–1130.

Connolly BP, McNamara JA, Sharma S, et al. A comparison of laser photocoagulation with trans-scleral cryotherapy in the treatment of threshold retinopathy of prematurity. *Ophthalmology* 1998;105:1628–1631.

Connolly BP, Ng EYJ, McNamara JA, et al. A comparison of laser photocoagulation with cryotherapy for threshold retinopathy of prematurity at 10 years. Part 2. Refractive outcome. *Ophthalmology* 2002;109:936–941.

Cryotherapy for Retinopathy of Prematurity Cooperative Group. Multicenter Trial of Cryotherapy for Retinopathy of Prematurity: ophthalmological outcomes at 10 years. *Arch Ophthalmol* 2001;119:1110–1118.

Darlow BA, Clemett RS, Horwood LJ, Mogridge N. Prospective study of New Zealand infants with birth weight less than 1500g and screened for retinopathy of prematurity: visual outcome at 7-8 years. *Br J Ophthalmol* 1997;81:935–940.

Editorial Committee; for the Cryotherapy for Retinopathy of Prematurity Cooperative Group. Multicenter trial of cryotherapy for retinopathy of prematurity. *Am J Ophthalmol* 2002;120: 595–599.

Fielder AR, Haines L, Scrivener R, et al. Retinopathy of prematurity in the UK II: Audit of national guidelines for screening and treatment. *Br J Ophthalmol* 2002;16:285–291.

Fielder AR. Time for a fresh look at ROP screening. *Eye* 2003;17:117–118.

Goble RR, Jones HS, Fielder AR. Are we screening too many babies for retinopathy of prematurity? *Eye* 1997;11:509–514.

Kent D, Pennie F, Laws D, et al. The influence of retinopathy of prematurity on ocular growth. *Eye* 2000;14:23–29.

Larsson E, Holdstrom G. Screening for retinopathy of prematurity: evaluation and modification of guidelines. *Br J Ophthalmol* 2002; 86:1399–1402.

Ng EYJ, Connolly BP, McNamara JA, et al. A comparison of laser photocoagulation with cryotherapy for threshold retinopathy of prematurity. Part 1. Visual function and structural outcome. *Ophthalmology* 2002;109:928–935.

O'Keefe M, O'Reilly J, Janigan B. Longer term visual outcome of eyes with retinopathy of prematurity with cryotherapy or diode laser. *Br J Ophthalmol* 1998;82:1246–1248.

Pearce IA, Pennie FC, Gannon LM, et al. Three-year visual outcome for treated stage 3 retinopathy of prematurity. *Br J Ophthalmol* 1998;82:1254–1259.

Quinn GE, Dobson V, Kilvin J, et al. Prevalence of myopia between 3 months and 5 1/2 years in preterm infants with and without retinopathy of prematurity. *Ophthalmology* 1998;105: 1292–1300.

Repka MX, Palmer EA, Tung B, for the Cryotherapy for Retinopathy of Prematurity Cooperative Group. Involution of retinopathy of prematurity. *Arch Ophthalmol* 2000;118:645–649.

Reynolds JD, Dobson V, Quinn GE, et al. Evidence-based screening criteria for retinopathy of prematurity. *Am J Ophthalmol* 2002; 120:1470–1476.

Shalev B, Farr AK, Repka MX. Randomized comparison of diode laser photocoagulation versus cryotherapy for threshold retinopathy of prematurity. *Am J Ophthalmol* 2001;132:76–80.

# Eales Disease

The eponym 'Eales disease' is used to describe patients with bilateral, idiopathic, occlusive, peripheral periphlebitis and

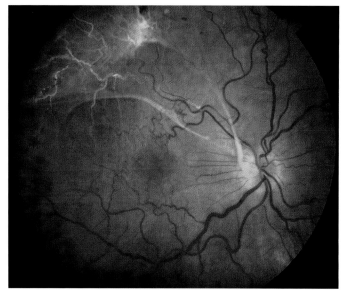

**Figure 2.132** Peripheral vascular occlusion in Eales disease (Courtesy of Western Eye Hospital)

neovascularisation. The disease is rare in Caucasians but is an important cause of visual morbidity in young Asian males and is strongly associated with tuberculoprotein hypersensitivity.

### *Diagnosis*

1. **Presentation** is usually in the third to fifth decades with vitreous haemorrhage.

2. **Signs,** in chronological order:

   ● Peripheral sheathing of retinal venules and arterioles associated with peripheral capillary non-perfusion, particularly superotemporally (Fig. 2.132).

   ● Peripheral neovascularisation, similar in shape to the 'sea-fans' in sickle-cell retinopathy, between perfused and non-perfused retina.

   ● Recurrent vitreous haemorrhage, tractional retinal detachment, rubeosis iridis, glaucoma and cataract.

3. **FA** shows peripheral retinal capillary non-perfusion and leakage from new vessels, if present.

***Treatment*** involving either scatter or feeder vessel photocoagulation is useful in active disease. Persistent vitreous haemorrhage or tractional detachment may require vitreo-retinal surgery. The visual prognosis is good in the majority of cases.

## FURTHER READING

Bissau J, Therese L, Maharani H. Use of polymerase chain reaction in detection of Mycobacterium tuberculosis complex DNA from vitreous samples in Eales' disease. *Br J Ophthalmol* 1999; 83:994.

El-Asar AMA, Al-Karachi SA. Full panretinal photocoagulation and early vitrectomy improve prognosis of retinal vasculitis associated with tuberculoprotein hypersensitivity (Eales' disease). *Br J Ophthalmol* 2002;86:1248–1251.

# Retinal Artery Macroaneurysm

A retinal artery macroaneurysm is a localised dilatation of a retinal arteriole which usually occurs in the first three orders of the arterial tree. It has a predilection for elderly hypertensive women and involves one eye in 90% of cases.

### Diagnosis

1. **Presentation** may be in one of the following ways:

   - Detection by chance of an asymptomatic lesion.
   - Insidious impairment of central vision due to macular oedema and hard exudate formation.
   - Sudden visual loss resulting from vitreous haemorrhage is uncommon.

2. **Signs**

   - A saccular or fusiform arteriolar dilatation, most frequently occurring at a bifurcation or an arteriovenous crossing along the temporal vascular arcades. The aneurysm may enlarge to several times the diameter of the artery.

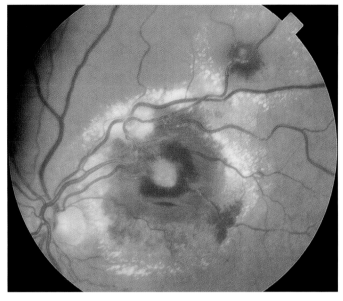

**Figure 2.134** Two retinal artery macroaneurysms

   - Associated retinal haemorrhage is present in 50% of cases (Fig. 2.133).
   - Multiple macroaneurysms along the same or different arterioles may occasionally be present (Fig. 2.134).

3. **FA** findings are dependent on the patency of the lesion and any associated haemorrhage. The typical appearance is that of immediate uniform filling of the macroaneurysm (Fig. 2.135b) with late leakage (Fig. 2.135c). Incomplete filling is due to partial or complete obliteration of the lumen by thrombosis.

### Course

- Rupture with haemorrhage, which may be subretinal, intraretinal, preretinal or vitreous. In these cases, the underlying lesion may be overlooked and the diagnosis missed (Fig. 2.136).
- Spontaneous involution following thrombosis and fibrosis is very common. This may follow the development of leakage or haemorrhage (Fig 2.137).

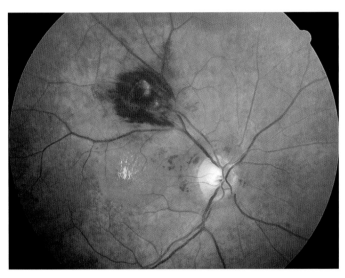

**Figure 2.133** Retinal artery macroaneurysm with localised haemorrhage

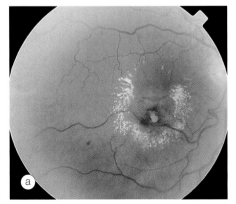
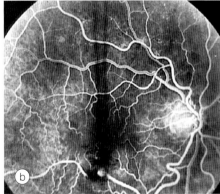
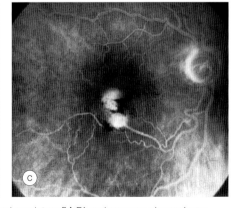

**Figure 2.135** **(a)** Leaking retinal artery macroaneurysm with a small haemorrhage and surrounding hard exudates; **(b)** FA early venous phase shows filling; **(c)** late phase shows leakage

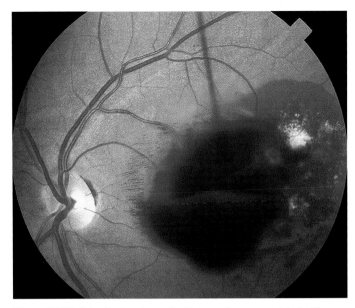

**Figure 2.136** Subretinal and preretinal haemorrhage associated with a retinal artery macroaneurysm

- Chronic leakage resulting in retinal oedema with accumulation of hard exudates at the fovea is common and may result in permanent loss of central vision.

### Management

1. **Observation** in anticipation of spontaneous involution is indicated in eyes with good VA in which the macula is not threatened and those with mild retinal haemorrhage without significant oedema or exudation.

2. **Laser photocoagulation** may be considered if oedema or hard exudates threaten or involve the fovea (Fig. 2.138a), particularly if there is documented visual deterioration. The burns may be applied to the lesion itself, the surrounding area, or both (Fig. 2.138b). It may take several months for the oedema and hard exudates to absorb.

3. **YAG laser hyaloidotomy** may be considered in eyes with large non-absorbing preretinal haemorrhage overlying the macula in order to disperse the blood into the vitreous cavity from where it may be absorbed more quickly.

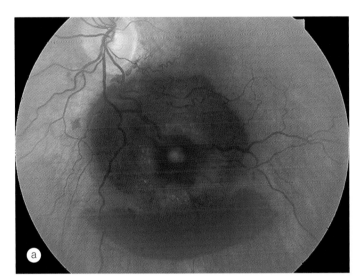
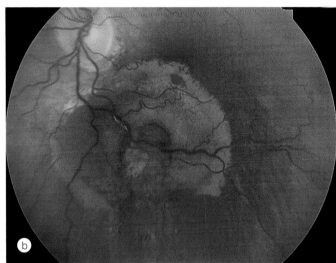

**Figure 2.137 (a)** Subretinal haemorrhage associated with retinal artery macroaneurysm; **(b)** several months later there is spontaneous absorption of blood and the macroaneurysm has fibrosed

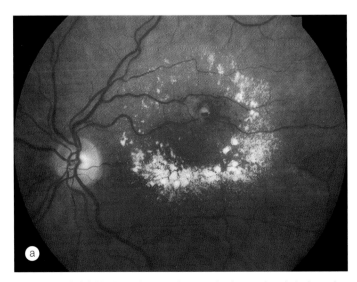
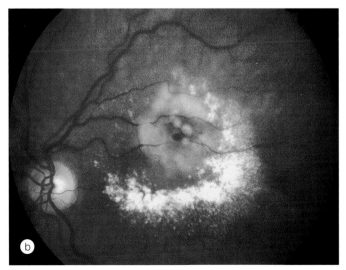

**Figure 2.138 (a)** Hard exudates at the macula due to chronic leakage from a retinal artery macroaneurysm; **(b)** immediately following laser photocoagulation

**4. Intravitreal injection** of expandable gas with face-down positioning to shift the haemorrhage away from the macula, with or without t-PA.

## FURTHER READING

Lavin MJ, Marsh RJ, Peart S, et al. Retinal artery macroaneurysms: a retrospective study of 40 patients. *Br J Ophthalmol* 1987; 71:817–825.

Rabb MF, Gagliano DA, Teske MP. Retinal artery macroaneurysms. *Surv Ophthalmol* 1988;33:73–96.

# Primary Retinal Telangiectasis

Primary retinal telangiectasis comprises a group of rare, idiopathic, congenital or acquired retinal vascular anomalies characterised by dilatation and tortuosity of retinal blood vessels, multiple aneurysms, vascular leakage and the deposition of hard exudates. Retinal telangiectasis involves the capillary bed, although the arterioles and venules may also be involved. The vascular malformations often progress and become symptomatic later in life as a result of haemorrhage, oedema or lipid exudation.

## IDIOPATHIC JUXTAFOVEOLAR RETINAL TELANGIECTASIS

Idiopathic juxtafoveolar telangiectasis is a rare, congenital or acquired condition which can be divided into the following types.

### Group 1A. Unilateral congenital juxtafoveolar telangiectasis

1. **Presentation** is typically in a middle-aged man with mild-to-moderate blurring of vision.

2. **Signs.** Telangiectasis involving an area about 1.5 disc diameter, temporal to the fovea, frequently associated with hard exudates (Fig. 2.139a). Fig. 2.139b shows leakage and hard exudate deposition within the middle retinal layers.

3. **FA** shows capillary dilatation and late leakage (Fig. 2.139c).

4. **Treatment** by laser photocoagulation to areas of leakage may be beneficial in preventing visual loss from chronic cystoid macular oedema and exudation, but results are often disappointing.

### Group 1B. Unilateral idiopathic focal juxtafoveolar telangiectasis

1. **Presentation** is similar to type 1A.

2. **Signs.** Telangiectasis confined to one clock hour at the edge of the FAZ (Fig. 2.140a). Fig. 2.140b shows telangiectasis within the middle retinal layers.

3. **FA** shows absence of leakage (Fig. 2.140c).

4. **Treatment** is not appropriate and the prognosis good.

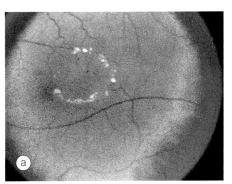 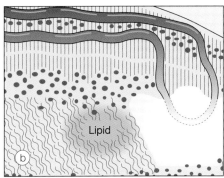 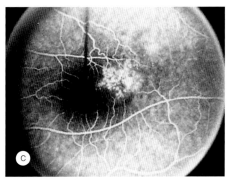

**Figure 2.139** Idiopathic juxtafoveolar retinal telangiectasis – group 1A (see text: Courtesy of Wilmer Institute)

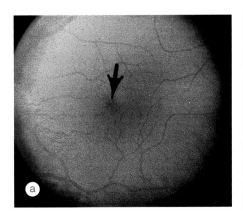 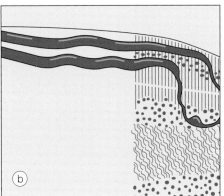 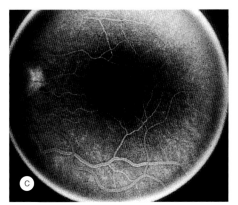

**Figure 2.140** Idiopathic juxtafoveolar retinal telangiectasis – group 1B (see text: Courtesy of Wilmer Institute)

### Group 2A. Bilateral idiopathic acquired juxtafoveolar telangiectasis

1. **Presentation** is in the sixth decade with mild, slowly progressive disturbance of central vision in one or both eyes. Both sexes are affected equally.

2. **Signs**

   - Symmetrical telangiectasis, one disc area or less, involving all or a part of the parafoveal area without hard exudates (Fig. 2.141a).
   - Stellate pigmented plaques of RPE hyperplasia.
   - Multiple refractile white juxtafoveolar dots and solitary small yellow central deposits may be present.
   - Subretinal choroidal neovascularisation may develop in advanced cases.

3. **FA** shows capillary dilatation outside the FAZ (Fig. 2.141b) and late leakage (Fig. 2.141c).

4. **Prognosis** is guarded. Conventional laser photocoagulation for choroidal neovascularisation is usually unsuccessful, although photodynamic therapy may be beneficial.

### Group 2B. Bilateral familial occult juxtafoveolar telangiectasis is similar to type 2A but presents earlier and is associated with neither superficial retinal refractile deposits nor stellate pigmented plaques.

### Group 3A. Idiopathic occlusive juxtafoveolar telangiectasis is the most severe form, which is frequently associated with systemic diseases such as polycythaemia, multiple myeloma and chronic lymphatic leukaemia.

1. **Presentation** is in the sixth decade with slowly progressive loss of central vision.

2. **Signs**

   - Marked aneurysmal dilatation of terminal capillaries and progressive occlusion of parafoveal capillaries.
   - Optic atrophy may be present.

3. **FA** shows widening of the FAZ but absence of leakage.

4. **Prognosis** is usually poor as there is no effective treatment.

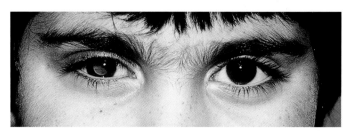

**Figure 2.142** Leukocoria in advanced Coats disease

### Group 3B. Idiopathic occlusive juxtafoveolar telangiectasis associated with CNS vasculopathy is similar to type 3A but is associated with neurological disease.

## COATS DISEASE

Coats disease is an idiopathic, non-hereditary, retinal telangiectasis with intraretinal and subretinal exudation, and frequently exudative retinal detachment. About 75% of patients are males and the vast majority have involvement of only one eye. It is now considered that Coats disease and Leber miliary aneurysms represent a spectrum of the same disease, the latter being more localised and carrying a better visual prognosis.

### Diagnosis

1. **Presentation** is most frequently in the first decade of life (average 5 years), but may be later, with unilateral visual loss, strabismus or a leukocoria (Fig. 2.142).

2. **Signs,** in chronological order:

   - Retinal telangiectasis (Fig. 2.143), most often in the inferior and temporal quadrants between the equator and ora serrata, and sometimes posterior to the equator towards the vascular arcades.
   - Intraretinal and subretinal yellowish exudation often affecting areas remote from the vascular abnormalities, particularly the macula (Fig. 2.144).
   - Progression of subretinal exudate deposition (Fig. 2.145).

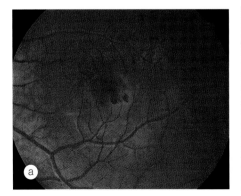
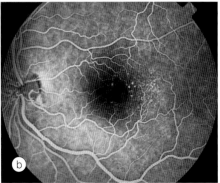
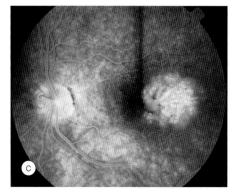

**Figure 2.141** Idiopathic juxtafoveolar retinal telangiectasis - group 2 (see text)

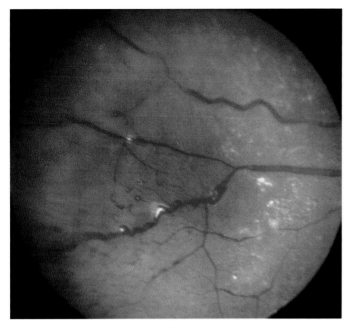

**Figure 2.143** Retinal telangiectasis in early Coats disease

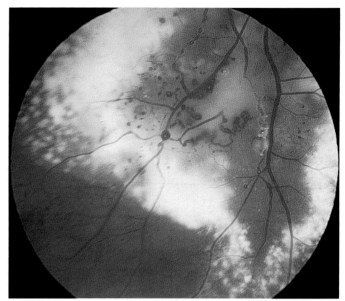

**Figure 2.145** Subretinal exudate deposition in Coats disease

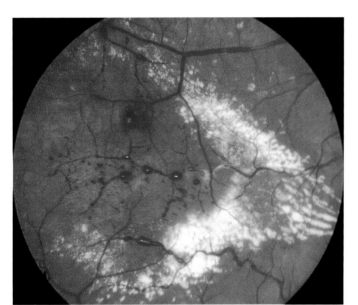

**Figure 2.144** Retinal exudates in Coats disease

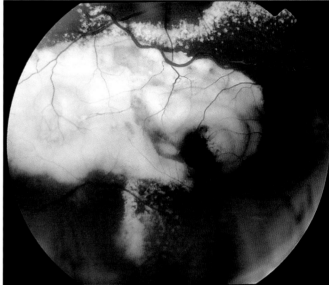

**Figure 2.146** Massive subretinal exudate deposition in Coats disease

- Massive subretinal exudation (Fig. 2.146).
- Complications include exudative retinal detachment (Fig. 2.147), rubeosis iridis, glaucoma, uveitis, cataract and phthisis bulbi. Anterior chamber cholesterolosis may occur in eyes with total retinal detachments (Fig. 2.148).

3. **FA** shows early hyperfluorescence of the telangiectasia, hypofluorescence of exudation and variable capillary non-perfusion in the region of telangiectasia (Fig. 2.149).

4. **Ultrasonography** in eyes with advanced disease shows a linear echo typical of retinal detachment with acoustically clear subretinal fluid. These findings are useful in differentiating Coats disease from exophytic retinoblastoma.

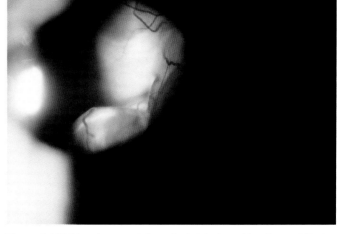

**Figure 2.147** Very deep exudative retinal detachment in advanced Coats disease

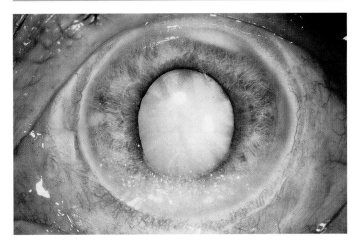

**Figure 2.148** Cataract and cholesterolosis in the anterior chamber in end-stage Coats disease

## Treatment

1. **Observation** in patients with mild, non-vision-threatening disease and in those with a comfortable eye with total retinal detachment in which there is no hope of restoring useful vision.

2. **Laser photocoagulation** to areas of telangiectasia should be considered if progressive exudation is documented. Frequently, more than one treatment session is required to obliterate the peripheral telangiectasia and induce resolution of remote exudation at the macula (Fig. 2.150). Photocoagulation is most effective in eyes without retinal detachment.

3. **Cryotherapy,** with a double freeze-thaw method, in eyes with extensive exudation or subtotal retinal detachment may result in marked reaction with increased leakage; therefore, laser photocoagulation is still the preferred option if at all possible.

4. **Vitreoretinal surgery** may be considered in eyes with total retinal detachments and a poor visual prognosis because successful retinal re-attachment often prevents the subsequent development of neovascular glaucoma.

5. **Enucleation** may be required in painful eyes with neovascular glaucoma.

*Prognosis* is variable and dependent on the severity of involvement at presentation. Young children, particularly those under 3 years of age, frequently have a more aggressive

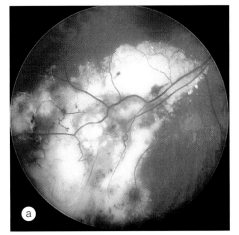
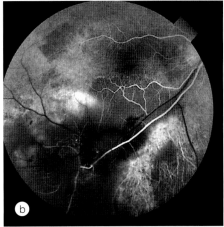
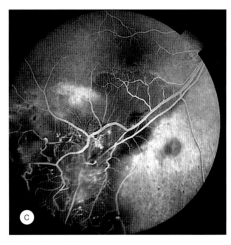

**Figure 2.149 (a)** Coats disease; **(b)** and **(c)** FA shows hyperfluorescence of telangiectasis and blockage by hard exudates

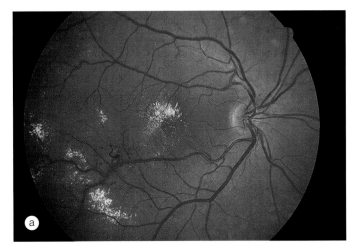
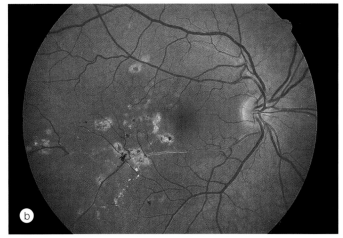

**Figure 2.150 (a)** Hard exudates in early Coats disease; **(b)** absorption several months after laser photocoagulation

clinical course and often already have extensive retinal detachment at presentation. However, older children and young adults have a more benign disease with less likelihood of progressive exudation and retinal detachment and in some cases spontaneous regression may occur.

***Differential diagnosis*** includes other causes of unilateral leukocoria and retinal detachment in children, such as late-onset retinoblastoma, toxocariasis, incontinentia pigmenti and retinal capillary haemangioma.

## HEREDITARY HAEMORRHAGIC TELANGIECTASIS

Hereditary haemorrhagic telangiectasis, also known as Rendu–Osler–Weber disease, is an autosomal dominant condition characterised by telangiectasis of skin, mucous membranes (Fig. 2.151) and various internal vascular beds. These vascular lesions are composed of multiple dilatations of capillaries and venules that frequently have thinned vessel walls, making them friable and prone to bleeding.

1. **Systemic manifestations** include epistaxis, gastrointestinal bleeding and haemoptysis. Death may result from severe internal bleeding.

2. **Ocular manifestations**

   ● Conjunctival telangiectasis.
   ● Fundus lesions are rare and include retinal vascular tortuosity (Fig. 2.152), retinal telangiectasia, localised arteriovenous malformation, neovascularisation and vitreous haemorrhage.

3. **Indocyanine green angiography** may also show choroidal involvement.

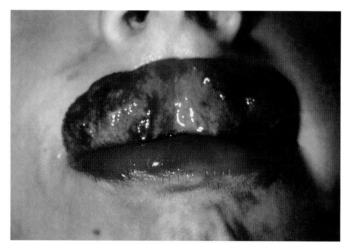

**Figure 2.151** Telangiectasis of the tongue in hereditary haemorrhagic telangiectasis

## FURTHER READING

Brant AM, Schachat AP, White RI. Ocular manifestations in hereditary hemorrhagic telangiectasia (Rendu-Osler-Weber disease). *Am J Ophthalmol* 1989;107:642–646.

Davis DG, Smith JL. Retinal involvement in hereditary hemorrhagic telangiectasia. *Arch Ophthalmol* 1971;85:618–623.

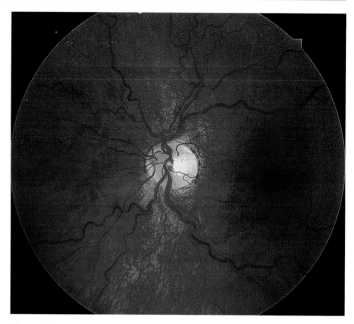

**Figure 2.152** Vascular tortuosity in hereditary haemorrhagic telangiectasis

Gass JDM, Blodi BA. Idiopathic juxtafoveolar retinal telangiectasis. Update of classification and follow-up study. *Ophthalmology* 1993;100:1536–1546.

Lee AL. Bilateral subretinal neovascular membrane in idiopathic juxtafoveolar retinal telangiectasis. *Retina* 1996;16:344–346.

Shields JA, Shields CL, Honavar SG, et al. Clinical variations and complications of Coats disease in 150 cases: The 2000 Sandford Gifford Memorial Lecture. *Am J Ophthalmol* 2001;131:561–571.

Shields JA, Shields CL, Honavar SG, et al. Classification and management of Coats disease: The 2000 Proctor Lecture. *Am J Ophthalmol* 2001;131:572–583.

Tsai DC, Wang AG, Lee AF, et al. Choroidal telangiectasia in a patient with hereditary haemorrhagic telangiectasia. *Eye* 2002;16:92–94.

# Radiation Retinopathy

Radiation retinopathy may develop following treatment of intraocular tumours by plaque therapy (brachytherapy) or external beam irradiation of sinus, orbital or nasopharyngeal malignancies. It is characterised by delayed retinal microvascular changes with endothelial cell loss, capillary occlusion and microaneurysm formation. As with diabetic retinopathy, its progress may be accelerated by pregnancy.

## Diagnosis

1. **Presentation.** The time interval between exposure and disease is variable and unpredictable, although commonly between 6 months and 3 years.

2. **Signs,** in chronological order:

   ● Discrete capillary occlusion with the development of collateral channels and microaneurysms, best seen on FA (Fig. 2.153).
   ● Macular oedema, hard exudates and retinal haemorrhages (Fig. 2.154).

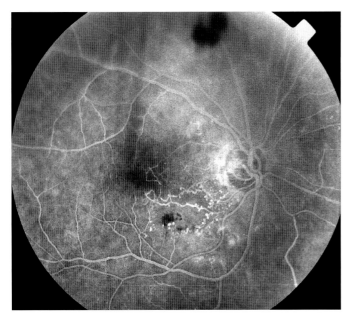

**Figure 2.153** FA of early radiation retinopathy showing focal retinal capillary non-perfusion associated with microvascular changes

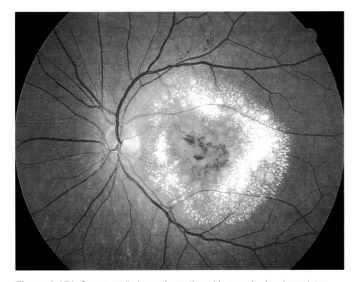

**Figure 2.154** Severe radiation retinopathy with macular hard exudates and haemorrhages

- Papillopathy, widespread arteriolar occlusion and cotton-wool spots.
- Proliferative retinopathy and tractional retinal detachment.

**Treatment** involving laser photocoagulation may be beneficial for macular oedema but proliferative retinopathy responds very poorly. Papillopathy is treated with systemic steroids.

**Prognosis** depends on the severity of involvement. Poor prognostic features include papillopathy and proliferative retinopathy, which may result in vitreous haemorrhage and tractional retinal detachment.

## FURTHER READING
Gunduz K, Shields CL, Shields JA, et al. Radiation retinopathy following plaque radiotherapy for posterior uveal melanoma. *Arch Ophthalmol* 1999;117:609–614.

# Purtscher Retinopathy

Purtscher retinopathy is caused by microvascular damage with occlusion and ischaemia associated with severe trauma, especially to the head and chest compressive injury. Other causes include embolism (fat, air or amniotic fluid) and systemic diseases (acute pancreatitis, pancreatic carcinoma, connective tissue diseases, lymphomas, thrombotic thrombocytopenic purpura and following bone marrow transplantation). Cases not associated with trauma are sometimes referred to as 'Purtscher-like retinopathy'.

## DIAGNOSIS

1. **Presentation** is with sudden visual loss.
2. **Signs.** Multiple, unilateral or bilateral, superficial, white retinal patches, resembling large cotton-wool spots, often associated with superficial peripapillary haemorrhages (Fig. 2.155).
3. **FA** shows variable capillary non-perfusion and blockage of background choroidal fluorescence by haemorrhages and oedema (Fig. 2.156).

**Treatment** of the underlying cause is desirable but not always possible.

**Prognosis** is guarded, because although the acute fundus changes usually resolve within a few weeks, permanent variable visual impairment occurs in approximately 50% of cases as a result of macular or optic nerve damage.

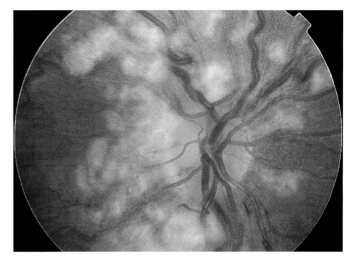

**Figure 2.155** Purtscher retinopathy

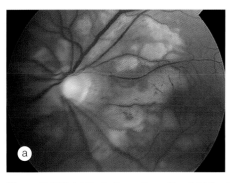 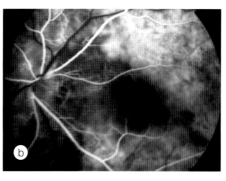 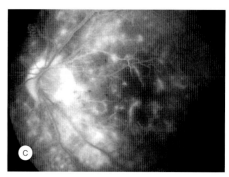

**Figure 2.156** **(a)** Purtscher retinopathy; **(b)** FA arterial phase shows slow choroidal filling and hypofluorescence at the macula; **(c)** late venous phase shows capillary non-perfusion at the fovea and staining of retinal vessels

# Benign Idiopathic Haemorrhagic Retinopathy

This distinct rare form of retinopathy is important because it has a good prognosis without treatment.

## DIAGNOSIS

1. **Presentation** is in adult life at any age with acute unilateral visual impairment.

2. **Signs**

   - Unilateral, multiple, large intraretinal haemorrhages at the posterior pole and around the optic disc (Fig. 2.157).
   - Absence of significant vascular signs or abnormal optic discs.

3. **FA** shows normal arteriovenous flow, with neither capillary non-perfusion nor vascular leakage.

4. **Course.** Vision recovers within 4 months.

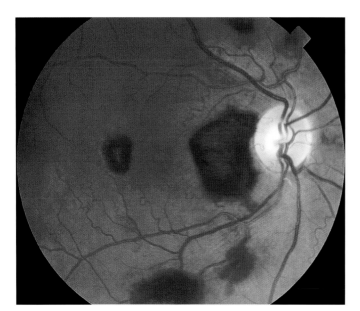

**Figure 2.157** Benign idiopathic haemorrhagic retinopathy

## *Differential diagnosis*

- Terson syndrome, which is associated with subarachnoid haemorrhage.
- Benign retinal vasculitis.
- Valsalva retinopathy.
- High-altitude retinopathy.

## FURTHER READING
Baker GRC, Grey RHB. Benign idiopathic haemorrhagic retinopathy. *Eye* 2001;15:267–273.

# Idiopathic Retinal Vasculitis, Aneurysms, and Neuroretinitis (IRVAN) Syndrome

IRVAN is a rare entity characterised predominantly by the presence of multiple leaking aneurysmal dilatations along the retinal arteriolar tree and over the optic nerve. The aneurysms may increase in number and leak and then some may spontaneous regress. Treatment by laser photocoagulation may be beneficial.

## FURTHER READING
Chang TS, Aylward GW, Davis JUL, et al. Idiopathic retinal vasculitis, aneurysms, and neuroretinitis. *Ophthalmology* 1995;102:1089–1097.
Owens SL, Gregor ZJ. Vanishing retinal arterial aneurysms: a case report. *Br J Ophthalmol* 1992;76:637–638.
Sashihara H, Hayashi H, Oshima K. Regression of retina arterial aneurysms in a case of idiopathic vasculitis, aneurysms, and neuroretinitis (IRVAN). *Retina* 1999;19:250–251.

# Takayasu Disease

Takayasu disease is a chronic autoimmune, inflammatory obstructive vascular disease affecting the major branches of the aorta and is considered to occur most often in young Asian women.

1. **Systemic features** include common carotid artery insufficiency, vertebrobasilar ischaemia, cardiac ischaemia and renal artery involvement with associated systemic hypertension.

2. **Ocular features** include microaneurysms, retinal arteriovenous anastomoses, proliferative retinopathy, epiretinal membranes, neovascular glaucoma and ischaemic optic neuropathy.

## FURTHER READING

Chun YK, Park SJ, Park IK, et al. The clinical and ocular manifestations of Takayasu arteritis. *Retina* 2001;21:132–140.

Kuwahara C, Imamura Y, Okamura N, et al. Severe proliferative retinopathy progressing to blindness in a Japanese woman with Takayasu disease. *Am J Ophthalmol* 2003;135:722–723.

# Retinopathy in Blood Disorders

## ANAEMIA

The anaemias are a group of disorders characterised by a decrease in the number of circulating red blood cells, or a decrease in the amount of haemoglobin in each cell, or both. Retinal changes in anaemia are usually innocuous and rarely of diagnostic importance.

1. **Retinopathy** is characterised by dot–blot and flame-shaped haemorrhages, which may have white centres (Roth spots), cotton-wool spots and venous tortuosity (Fig. 2.158). The duration and type of anaemia do not influence the occurrence of these changes, which are more common with coexistent thrombocytopenia.

2. **Optic neuropathy** with centrocaecal scotomas may occur in patients with pernicious anaemia. Unless treated with vitamin B12 supplements, permanent optic atrophy may ensue. Pernicious anaemia may also cause dementia, peripheral neuropathy and subacute combined degeneration of the spinal cord characterised by posterior and lateral column disease.

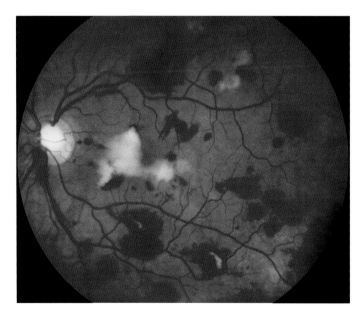

**Figure 2.158** Retinopathy in severe anaemia with Roth spots

## LEUKAEMIA

The leukaemias are a group of neoplastic disorders characterised by abnormal proliferation of white blood cells (Figs. 2.159 and 2.160). Ocular involvement is more commonly seen in the acute than in the chronic forms and virtually any ocular structure may be involved. It is, however, important to distinguish the fairly rare primary leukaemic infiltration from the more common secondary changes such as those associated with anaemia, thrombocytopenia, hyperviscosity and opportunistic infections.

1. **Fundus changes**

   - Choroidal deposits may cause a 'leopard skin' RPE appearance (Fig. 2.161), serous retinal detachment and ciliochoroidal effusion.
   - Retinal deposits may manifest as: vascular sheathing; discrete white nodules obscuring the retinal blood vessels; cotton-wool spots, which are probably due to vascular occlusion by leukaemic cells; and Roth spots in which the white centre is composed either of leukaemic cells or platelet–fibrin emboli.

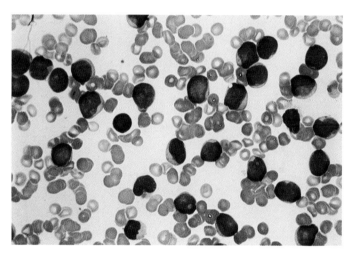

**Figure 2.159** Bone marrow aspirate in acute myeloid leukaemia showing immature blast cells

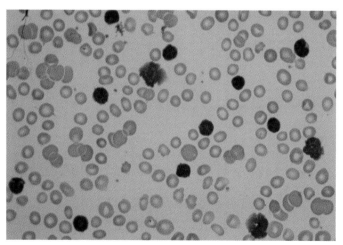

**Figure 2.160** Peripheral blood smear in chronic lymphatic leukaemia showing many mature lymphocytes

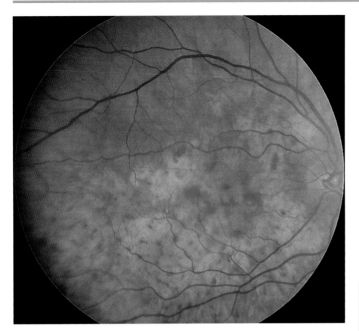

**Figure 2.161** 'Leopard spot fundus' in chronic leukaemia

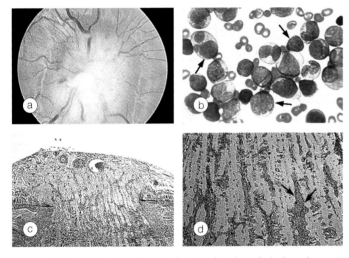

**Figure 2.162** Optic nerve infiltration in acute lymphocytic leukaemia.
**(a)** Infiltration of the optic nerve head resulting in greyish-white elevation; **(b)** blood smear shows lymphoblasts; **(c)** disc elevation due to infiltration by leukaemic cells; **(d)** high-power section of retrolaminar optic nerve showing leukaemic infiltration (Courtesy of Wilmer Institute)

- Peripheral retinal neovascularisation is an occasional feature of chronic myeloid leukaemia.
- Optic nerve infiltration may cause swelling and visual loss (Fig. 2.162).

### 2. Other ocular features

- Orbital involvement, particularly in children.
- Iris thickening, iritis and pseudo-hypopyon (Fig. 2.163).
- Spontaneous subconjunctival haemorrhage and hyphaema.

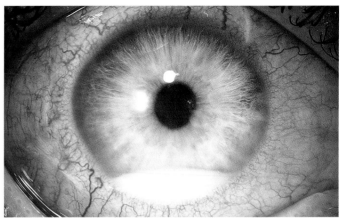

**Figure 2.163** Pseudo-hypopyon in acute leukaemia

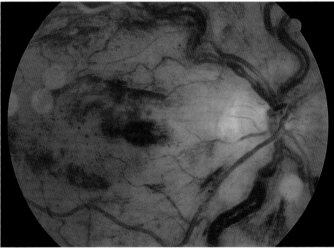

**Figure 2.164** Retinal haemorrhages and gross venous dilatation and haemorrhages in hyperviscosity

## HYPERVISCOSITY

The hyperviscosity states are a diverse group of rare disorders characterised by increased blood viscosity due to polycythaemia or abnormal plasma proteins as in Waldenström macroglobulinaemia and myeloma. Retinopathy is characterised by venous dilatation, segmentation and tortuosity, retinal haemorrhages and, occasionally, venous occlusion (Fig. 2.164).

## FURTHER READING

Fletcher ME, Farber MD, Cohen SB, et al. Retinal abnormalities associated with anemia. *Arch Ophthalmol* 1984;102:358.

Gordon KB, Rugo HS, Duncan JL, et al. Ocular manifestations of leukemia. Leukemic infiltration versus infectious process. *Ophthalmology* 2002;108:2293–2300.

Guyer DR, Schachat AP, Vitale S, et al. Leukemic retinopathy. Relationship between fundus lesions and hematologic parameters at diagnosis. *Ophthalmology* 1989;96:860–864.

Incorvaia C, Parmeggiani F, Costagliola C, et al. Quantitative evaluation of the retinal venous tortuosity in chronic anaemic patients affected by beta-thalassaemia major. *Eye* 2003;17:324–329.

Schachat AP, Markowitz JA, Guyer DR, et al. Ophthalmic manifestations of leukemia. *Arch Ophthalmol* 1989;107:697–700.

# Chapter 3

# ACQUIRED MACULAR DISORDERS AND RELATED CONDITIONS

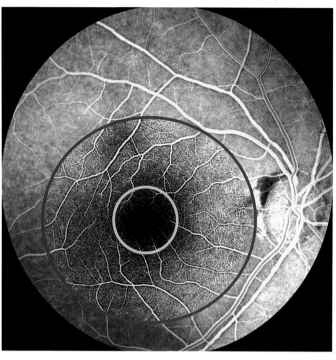

**Figure 3.1** Anatomical landmarks. Macula (blue circle); fovea (yellow circle)

## Introduction

### APPLIED ANATOMY

***Anatomical landmarks*** (Figs. 3.1 and 3.2)

1. **The macula** is a round area at the posterior pole measuring approximately 5.5 mm in diameter. Histologically, it contains xanthophyll pigment and more than one layer of ganglion cells.

2. **The fovea** is a depression in the inner retinal surface at the centre of the macula with a diameter of 1.5 mm (about one optic disc) (Fig. 3.3). Ophthalmoscopically, it gives rise to an oval light reflex (Fig. 3.4) because of the increased thickness of the retina and internal limiting membrane (ILM) at its border.

3. **The foveola** forms the central floor of the fovea and has a diameter of 0.35 mm. It is the thinnest part of the retina, is devoid of ganglion cells, and consists only of cones and their nuclei.

4. **The foveal avascular zone** (FAZ) is located within the fovea but extends beyond the foveola. The exact diameter is variable and its limits can be determined with accuracy only by fluorescein angiography (FA) (Fig. 3.5).

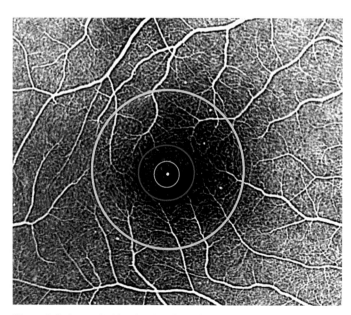

**Figure 3.2** Anatomical landmarks. Fovea (yellow circle); foveal avascular zone (red circle); foveola (lilac circle); umbo (central white spot)

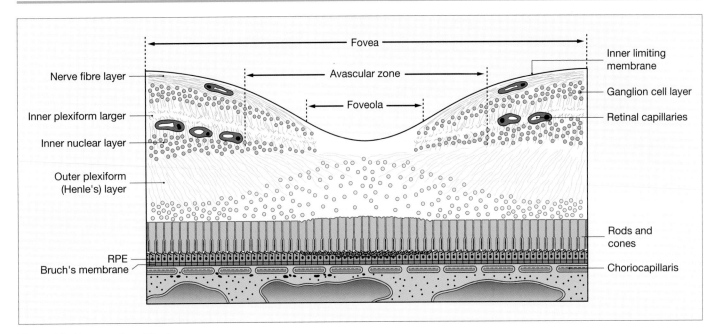

**Figure 3.3** Cross-section of the fovea

5. **The umbo** is a tiny depression in the very centre of the foveola which corresponds to the foveolar reflex, loss of which may be an early sign of damage.

***The retinal pigment epithelium*** (RPE) is a single layer of hexagonal cells, the apices of which manifest villous processes that envelop the outer segments of the photoreceptors. The RPE cells at the fovea are taller, thinner and contain more and larger melanosomes than elsewhere in the retina. The adhesion between the RPE and sensory retina is weaker than that between the RPE and Bruch's membrane, which underlies the RPE. The potential space between the RPE and sensory retina is the subretinal space. The RPE prevents the accumulation of subretinal fluid in two ways:

- The RPE cells and the intervening tight junctional complexes (zonula occludentes) constitute the outer blood–retinal barrier (see Fig. 1.41), preventing extracellular fluid, which normally leaks from the choriocapillaris, from entering the subretinal space.
- It also actively pumps ions and water out of the subretinal space.

***Bruch's membrane*** separates the RPE from the choriocapillaris. On electron microscopy, it consists of five elements:

- Basal lamina of the RPE.
- Inner collagenous layer.
- Thicker band of elastic fibres.
- Outer collagenous layer.
- Basal lamina of the inner layer of the choriocapillaris.

Changes in Bruch's membrane are relevant to the pathogenesis of many macular disorders.

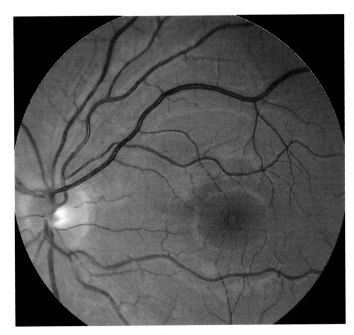

**Figure 3.4** Normal foveal light reflex

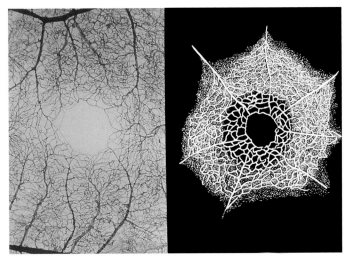

**Figure 3.5** Foveal avascular zone (Courtesy of Wilmer Institute)

## SYMPTOMS

1. **Impairment of central vision** is the main symptom. Patients with macular disease complain of 'something obstructing central vision' (positive scotoma) in contrast to those with optic neuropathy, who may notice 'something missing' or a hole in their central vision (negative scotoma).

2. **Metamorphopsia,** distortion of perceived images, is a common symptom of macular disease not present in optic neuropathy.

3. **Micropsia,** a decrease in image size caused by spreading apart of foveal cones, is less common.

4. **Macropsia,** an increase in image size due to crowding together of foveal cones, is uncommon.

> **NB: Colour desaturation is not present in early macular disease, but is common in mild optic neuropathy.**

# Age-Related Macular Degeneration

## Introduction

### Definition

1. **Age-related maculopathy** (ARM) is a 'normal' ageing process characterised by:

   - Discrete yellow spots at the macula (drusen).
   - Hyperpigmentation or depigmentation of the RPE associated with drusen.

2. **Age-related macular degeneration** (AMD) is a more advanced, sight-threatening stage of ARM characterised by one or more of the following:

   - Geographic atrophy of the RPE with visible underlying choroidal vessels.
   - Pigment epithelial detachment (PED) with or without neurosensory detachment.
   - Subretinal or sub-RPE choroidal neovascularisation (CNV).
   - Fibroglial scar tissue, haemorrhage and exudates.

**Prevalence.** AMD is the most common cause of irreversible visual loss in the developed world in individuals over 50 years of age. The prevalence of severe visual loss increases with age. In the USA, at least 10% of individuals between the ages of 65 and 75 years have lost some central vision as a result of AMD. Among those over 75, 30% are affected to some degree. End-stage (blinding) AMD occurs in about 1.7% of all individuals aged over 50 years and in about 18% of those over 85 years.

### Risk factors for age-related macular degeneration

1. **Age** is the main risk factor.

2. **ARM,** particularly when associated with soft drusen (see below).

3. **Race** – the condition is most prevalent in Caucasians.

4. **Positive family history.**

5. **Cigarette smoking.**

6. **Hypertension.**

7. **Cataract,** particularly nuclear opacity, is a risk factor for AMD. Cataract surgery may be associated with progression of macular disease in some patients with pre-existing high-risk characteristics such as confluent soft drusen. It is difficult to prove a link between surgery and progression of AMD, however, since advanced disease often coexists in patients with cataracts sufficiently advanced to require surgery.

## *Drusen*

### HISTOPATHOLOGY

Loss of central vision in AMD is the result of changes that occur in response to deposition of abnormal material in Bruch's membrane. This material is derived from the RPE, and its accumulation is thought to result from failure to clear the debris discharged into this region. Drusen consist of discrete deposits of the abnormal material located between the basal lamina of the RPE and the inner collagenous layer of Bruch's membrane (Fig. 3.6). Thickening of Bruch's membrane is compounded by excessive production of basement membrane-like material by the RPE. It has been postulated that the lipid content of drusen may be a determinant for subsequent behaviour.

### DIAGNOSIS

Drusen appear as yellow excrescences beneath the RPE, distributed symmetrically at both posterior poles. They may vary in number, size, shape, degree of elevation and extent of associated RPE changes. In some patients, drusen may be confined to the region of the fovea, whereas in others the deposits encircle but spare the fovea itself. Drusen are rarely clinically visible before the age of 45 years; they are not uncommon between the ages of 45 and 60 years and are almost universal thereafter. With advancing age, they increase in size and number.

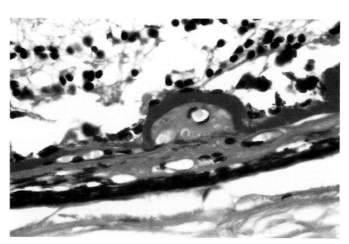

**Figure 3.6** Histopathology of drusen (Courtesy of Wilmer Institute)

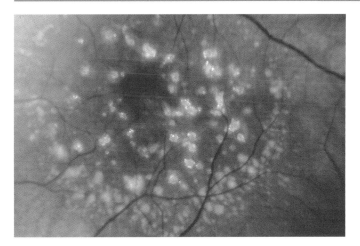

**Figure 3.7** Hard drusen

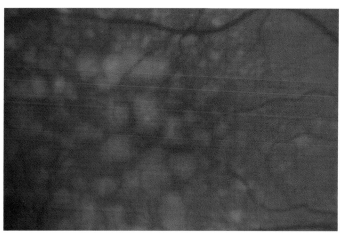

**Figure 3.8** Soft drusen

## Signs

1. **Hard drusen** are small, round, discrete, yellow-white spots (Fig. 3.7) associated with focal dysfunction of the RPE and are usually innocuous but may occasionally precede the development of atrophic AMD.

2. **Soft drusen** are larger greyish-white or pale-yellow nodules with indistinct margins (Fig. 3.8). Coalescence of soft macular drusen is a common precursor of atrophic and exudative AMD.

**FA** findings depend on the state of the overlying RPE and the degree of staining of drusen.

1. **Hyperfluorescence** is caused both by a window defect due to atrophy of the overlying RPE (Fig. 3.9a and b) and by late staining (Fig. 3.9c and d). The centre of the macula

also shows a 'drusenoid' detachment of the RPE due to coalescence of soft drusen, which is a common precursor of atrophic and exudative AMD. It has been postulated that hyperfluorescent drusen are hydrophilic (low lipid content) and predispose to CNV.

2. **Hypofluorescent** drusen are hydrophobic (high lipid content) and, if large and confluent, predispose to subsequent detachment of the RPE. A prolonged filling phase of the choroid may indicate diffuse thickening of Bruch's membrane.

## DRUSEN AND AGE-RELATED MACULAR DEGENERATION

Although many patients with drusen maintain normal vision throughout life, a significant number of elderly patients

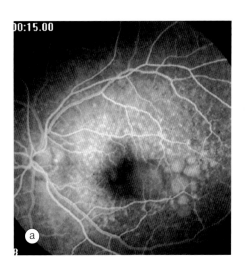

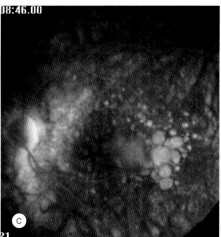

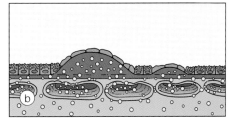

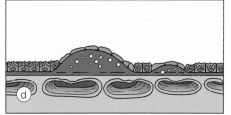

**Figure 3.9** FA of drusen. **(a and b)** Early hyperfluorescence; **(c and d)** late staining

develop AMD. The exact role of drusen in the pathogenesis of AMD is still unclear, although their chemical composition may be relevant. Features associated with an increased risk of subsequent visual loss include large soft and/or confluent drusen, and focal hyperpigmentation of the RPE, particularly if the other eye has already developed AMD.

## PROPHYLACTIC TREATMENT

1. **Laser photocoagulation** to drusen has been targeted at two types of patients: (a) those with bilateral drusen and good visual acuity (VA); and (b) those with drusen and good VA in one eye but exudative AMD in the other. Low-dose photocoagulation of drusen appears to be effective in causing drusen regression. This can be seen as early as 3 months after treatment, but is generally apparent at 6 months and continues throughout the first year. Drusen located near the burn tend to disappear before those located more remotely. It has been proposed that the laser burns cause defects in the RPE, the adjacent cells hypertrophy to cover up the defects, and, in so doing, their metabolic activity is increased such that they remove the debris. Whilst the majority of treated eyes tend to have stable vision, there is a suggestion that in some cases such treatment may predispose to CNV. Prophylactic treatment is therefore currently not recommended.

2. **Supplemental antioxidants** (vitamin C, vitamin E and beta carotene) and zinc may protect eyes at high risk of developing AMD. Those patients with high-risk characteristics (visual loss in one eye or large drusen) seem to benefit, achieving a 25% reduction in their risk of severe visual loss. Current advice is for such patients to take the formulation on a long-term basis.

## Atrophic age-related macular degeneration

Atrophic AMD is caused by slowly progressive atrophy of the photoreceptors, RPE and choriocapillaris, although occasionally it may follow subsidence of an RPE detachment (see later).

### Diagnosis

1. **Presentation** is with a gradual impairment of vision over months or years. Both eyes are usually affected but often asymmetrically.

2. **Signs,** in chronological order:
   - Focal hyperpigmentation or atrophy of the RPE in association with macular drusen (Fig. 3.10).
   - Sharply circumscribed, circular areas of RPE atrophy associated with variable loss of the choriocapillaris (Fig. 3.11).
   - Enlargement of the atrophic areas within which the larger choroidal vessels may become visible and pre-existing drusen disappear (geographic atrophy) (Fig. 3.12). VA is severely impaired if the fovea is involved.

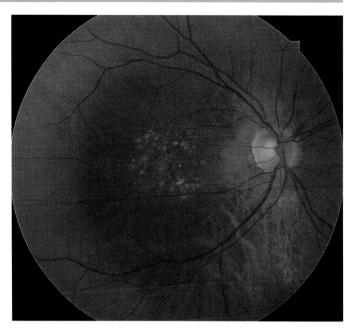

**Figure 3.10** Drusen and mild RPE changes in early atrophic AMD

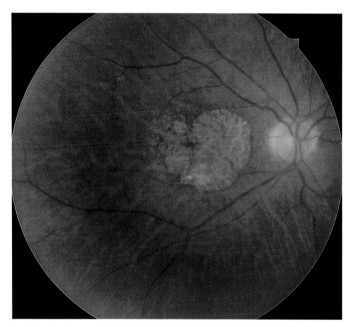

**Figure 3.11** Focal RPE atrophy in moderate atrophic AMD

3. **FA** shows a window defect characterised by hyperfluorescence due to unmasking of background choroidal fluorescence (Fig. 3.13) which may be more extensive than that apparent clinically, if the underlying choriocapillaris is still intact.

**Treatment** is not possible although low vision aids (Fig. 3.14) may be useful.

## Retinal pigment epithelial detachment

PED is thought to be caused by reduction of hydraulic conductivity of the thickened Bruch's membrane, thus impeding movement of fluid from the RPE towards the choroid.

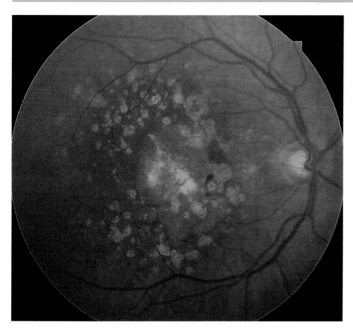

**Figure 3.12** Geographic atrophy in advanced disease

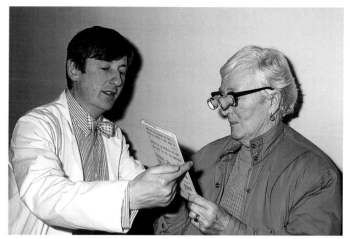

**Figure 3.14** Patient trying out a low vision aid

## Diagnosis

1. **Presentation** is with unilateral metamorphopsia and impairment of central vision.

2. **Signs**
   - Sharply circumscribed, dome-shaped elevation of varying size at the posterior pole (Fig. 3.15a).
   - The sub-RPE fluid is usually clear but may be turbid.

3. **FA** (Fig. 3.15b–3.15d) shows a well-demarcated oval area of hyperfluorescence which increases in density but not in area due to pooling of dye under the detachment.

4. **Indocyanine green (ICG)** angiography (Fig. 3.15e and 3.15f) demonstrates an oval area of hypofluorescence with a faint ring of surrounding hyperfluorescence. Occult CNV is detected in 96% of cases.

> NB: Laser photocoagulation should not be performed for PED as it may result in visual loss secondary to an RPE rip or sudden collapse of the PED with associated RPE atrophy.

***Course*** is variable and may follow one of the following patterns:

1. **Spontaneous resolution** without residua, particularly in younger patients.

2. **Geographic atrophy** may develop following spontaneous resolution in a minority of patients.

3. **Detachment of the sensory retina** may occur due to breakdown of the outer blood–retinal barrier, allowing passage of fluid into the subretinal space. Because of the relatively loose adhesion between the RPE and sensory retina, the subretinal fluid spreads more widely and is less well defined than in a pure PED.

4. **RPE tear formation** (see next).

## Retinal pigment epithelial tear

A tear of the RPE may occur at the junction of attached and detached RPE if tangential stress becomes sufficient to rupture the detached tissue. Tears may occur spontaneously or following laser photocoagulation of CNV in eyes with PED (Fig. 3.16).

## Diagnosis

1. **Presentation** is with sudden worsening of central vision.

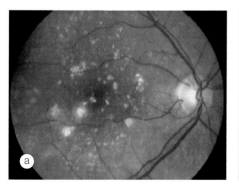
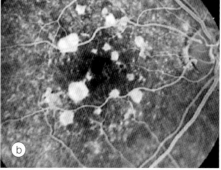
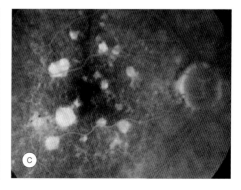

**Figure 3.13** **(a)** Dry AMD; **(b)** and **(c)** FA shows multiple RPE window defects

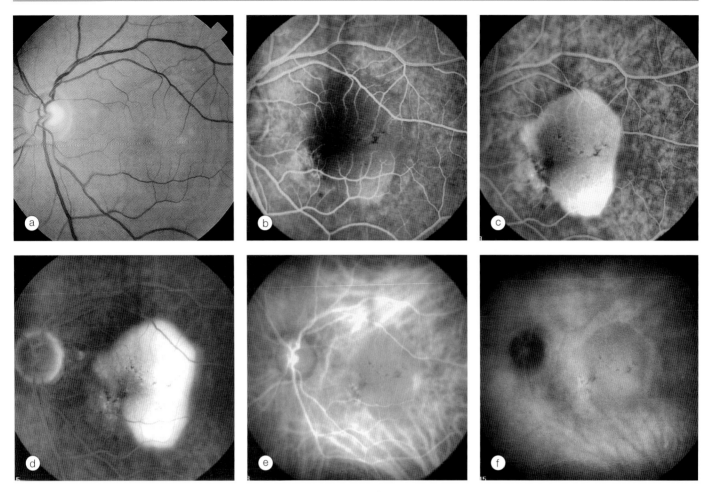

**Figure 3.15** **(a)** Pigment epithelial detachment; **(b)–(d)** FA; **(e)** & **(f)** ICG (see text)

2. **Signs.** Crescent-shaped RPE dehiscence at the edge of a prior serous detachment with a retracted and folded flap (see Fig. 3.16c).

3. **FA** shows hypofluorescence over the flap due to the folded-over and thickened RPE, with adjacent hyperfluorescence due to the exposed choriocapillaris.

4. **ICG** shows a linear area of hypofluorescence with a hyperfluorescent outline (see Fig. 3.16d).

***Prognosis*** of subfoveal tears is poor. Detachments of the RPE progressing to tears have an especially poor prognosis and are at particular risk of developing visual loss in the fellow eye. A minority of eyes maintain good VA despite RPE tears, particularly if the fovea is spared.

## Exudative age-related macular degeneration

Exudative AMD is caused by CNV originating from the choriocapillaris which grows through defects in Bruch's membrane. CNV may remain confined to the sub-RPE space (type 1) or extend into the subretinal space (type 2).

### CLINICAL FEATURES

1. **Presentation** is with metamorphopsia, a positive scotoma and blurring of central vision due to leakage of fluid from the CNV. At this stage, argon laser treatment or photodynamic therapy may be beneficial.

2. **Signs.** Many membranes cannot be identified ophthalmoscopically.

   ● Sub-RPE (type 1) CNV may occasionally be detected clinically as a grey-green or pinkish-yellow, slightly elevated lesion (Fig. 3.17).
   ● Subretinal (type 2) CNV may form a subretinal halo or pigmented plaque.
   ● The most frequent signs are caused by leakage from CNV resulting in serous retinal elevation, foveal thickening, cystoid macular oedema, subretinal haemorrhage and hard exudates (Fig. 3.18).

### FLUORESCEIN ANGIOGRAPHY

FA is important for the detection and precise localisation of CNV in relation to the centre of the FAZ and should be performed urgently in patients with recent onset of symptoms.

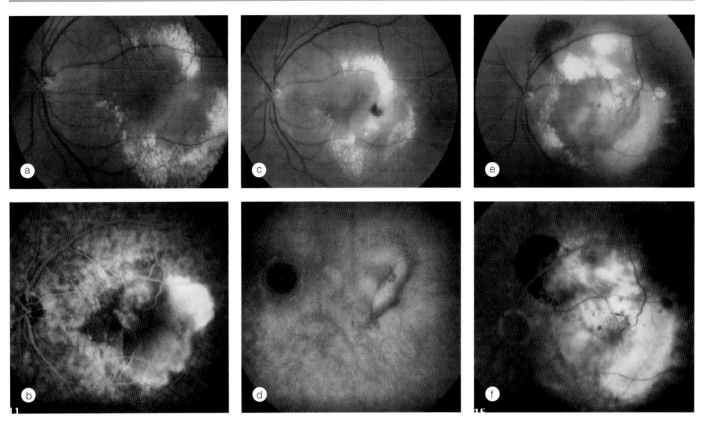

**Figure 3.16** RPE tear following laser photocoagulation:
1. At presentation. **(a)** Retinal oedema and hard exudates; **(b)** FA shows juxtafoveal CNV with adjacent PED
2. Two months following laser photocoagulation to CNV. **(c)** There is less exudation but a crescent elevation just lateral to the fovea and a blot haemorrhage are present; **(d)** ICG shows a hyperfluorescent area with a hypofluorescent outline, representing an RPE tear
3. Four months later. **(e)** & **(f)** show worsening of exudation and subretinal bleeding

***Classic*** CNV is a well-defined membrane which fills with dye in a 'lacy' pattern during the very early phase of dye transit (Fig. 3.19b), fluoresces brightly during peak dye transit (Fig. 3.19c), and then leaks into the subretinal space and around the CNV within 1–2 minutes. The fibrous tissue within the CNV then stains with dye with late hyperfluorescence (Fig. 3.19d). Classic CNV is classified according to its rela-tion to the centre of FAZ as follows:

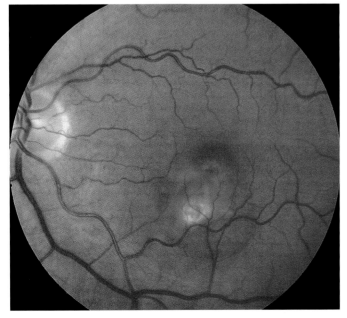

**Figure 3.17** Type 1 CNV below the fovea

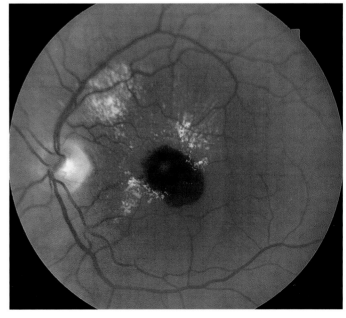

**Figure 3.18** Hard exudates and haemorrhage associated with CNV

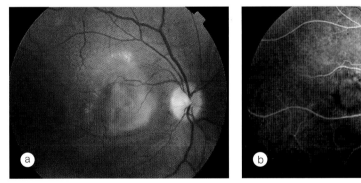

**Figure 3.19** FA of classic CNV (see text)

1. **Extrafoveal,** in which the CNV is more than 200 $\mu$m from the centre of the FAZ.

2. **Subfoveal,** in which the centre of the FAZ is involved either by extension from an extrafoveal area or by originating directly under the centre (Fig. 3.20). About 70% of

CNV extend under the fovea within 1 year and have a very poor prognosis.

3. **Juxtafoveal,** in which the CNV is closer than 200 $\mu$m from the centre of the FAZ but does not involve it (Fig. 3.21).

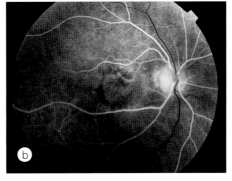

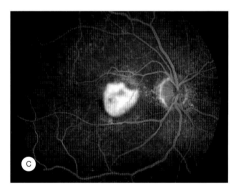

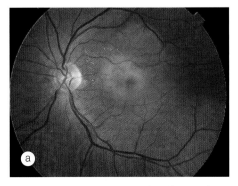

**Figure 3.20** FA of subfoveal CNV (see text)

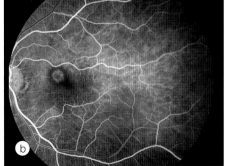

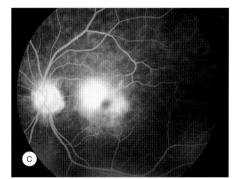

**Figure 3.21** FA of juxtafoveal CNV (see text)

**Occult** CNV is a poorly defined membrane with less precise features on the early frames but gives rise to late, diffuse or multifocal leakage (Fig. 3.22).

**Fibrovascular PED** is a combination of CNV and PED. The CNV fluoresces brighter ('hot spot') than the detachment. In other cases, the CNV may be obscured by blood or turbid fluid.

## INDOCYANINE GREEN ANGIOGRAPHY

ICG angiography may be superior to FA under certain circumstances. The longer, near-infrared wavelengths can penetrate the RPE and choroid, and are less absorbed by haemoglobin. These properties allow greater transmission of ICG fluorescence than that of fluorescein and are of particu-lar value in the following circumstances:

- Occult or poorly defined CNV.
- Distinguishing serous from vascularised portions of a fibrovascular PED (Fig. 3.23).
- CNV associated with overlying haemorrhage, pigment or exudate (Fig. 3.24).
- Recurrent CNV adjacent to an old photocoagulation scar.

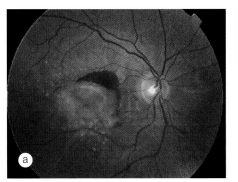 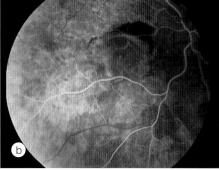 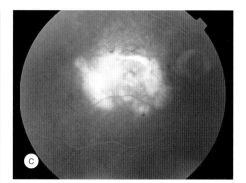

**Figure 3.22** FA of occult CNV (see text)

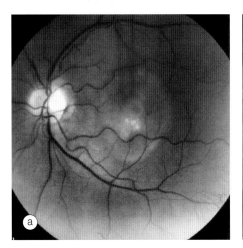 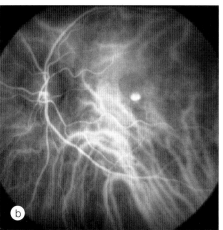 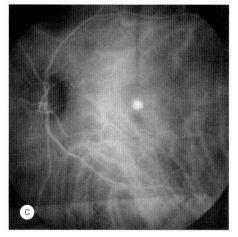

**Figure 3.23** ICG of a fibrovascular PED. **(a)** Red-free; **(b)** and **(c)** hypofluorescence of the detachment associated with a focal area of hyperfluorescence ('hot spot') corresponding to CNV

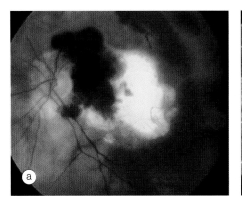 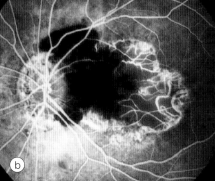 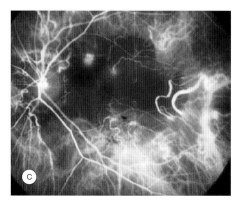

**Figure 3.24 (a)** Haemorrhage and scarring in AMD; **(b)** FA shows hypofluorescence corresponding to the haemorrhage; **(c)** ICG shows a 'hot spot' associated with CNV superotemporal to the disc

## COURSE

The course of untreated CNV is often relentless and the prognosis very poor due to the following complications:

1. **Haemorrhagic PED** caused by rupture of blood vessels within the CNV. Initially, the blood is confined to the sub-RPE space and appears as a dark elevated mound (Fig. 3.25). The haemorrhage may then break into the subretinal space and assume a more diffuse outline and a lighter red colour which may surround or be adjacent to the PED (Fig. 3.26).

2. **Vitreous haemorrhage** may rarely occur when blood under a sensory haemorrhagic detachment breaks through into the vitreous cavity.

3. **Subretinal (disciform) scarring** follows the haemorrhagic episode in which there is gradual organisation of the blood, and further ingrowth of new vessels from the choroid (Fig. 3.27). Eventually, a fibrous disciform scar at the fovea causes permanent loss of central vision (Fig. 3.28).

4. **Massive exudation,** both intra- and subretinal, may develop in some eyes with disciform scars as a result of chronic leakage from the CNV (Fig. 3.29). If severe, subretinal fluid may spread beyond the macula and destroy peripheral vision (Fig. 3.30).

## ARGON LASER PHOTOCOAGULATION

Treatment of CNV reduces the risk of severe visual loss in selected cases. The aim is to destroy the CNV whilst avoiding damage to the foveola. Because a lesion is more likely to be treatable if detected early, prompt identification with the daily use of the Amsler grid in patients at risk is essential.

***Indications*** are extrafoveal or juxtafoveal CNV with well-defined margins (i.e. classic membranes).

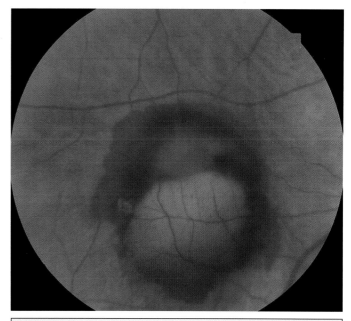

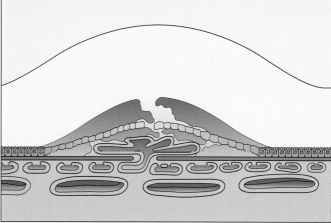

**Figure 3.26** Haemorrhagic PED with adjacent subretinal haemorrhage in exudative AMD

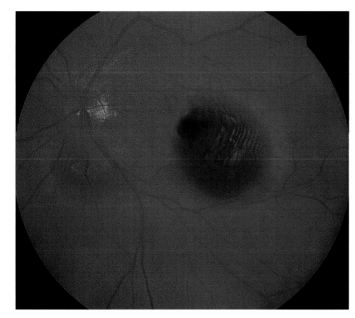

**Figure 3.25** Haemorrhagic PED in exudative AMD

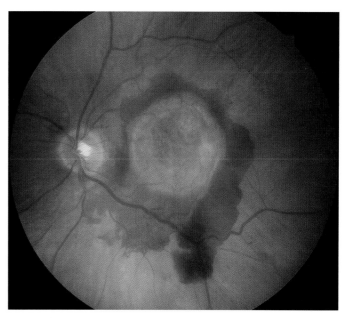

**Figure 3.27** Subretinal scarring surrounded by haemorrhage in exudative AMD

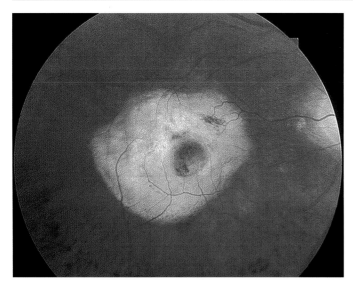

**Figure 3.28** Disciform scar in exudative AMD

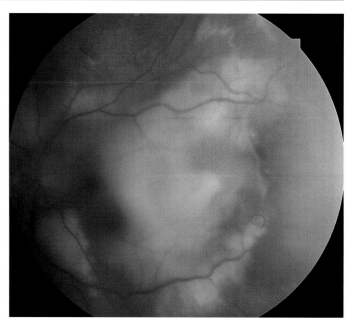

**Figure 3.30** Exudative retinal detachment in exudative AMD

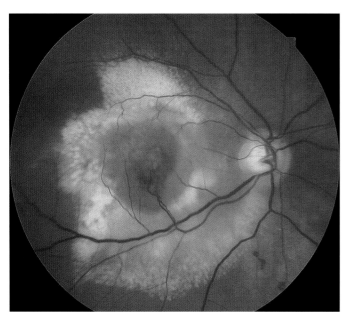

**Figure 3.29** Massive subretinal exudation in exudative AMD

3. A good quality FA, not more than 72 hours old, should be available. Selected frames of the FA are projected onto a screen so that the CNV can be precisely localised in relation to visible retinal landmarks.
4. The perimeter of the lesion is treated with overlapping 200 $\mu$m (0.2–0.5 second) burns and then the entire area is covered with high-energy burns (Fig. 3.31). Treatment must extend beyond the margins of the membrane and produce a confluent, intense white burn.
5. A post-treatment fundus photograph is taken to document the extent of treatment.

***Follow-up*** should be meticulous so that persistent or recurrent CNV is detected early. Initial follow-up is after 1–2 weeks with an FA to ensure adequacy of treatment.

Re-treatment is indicated if there is true persistence or recurrence of CNV more than 200 $\mu$m from the centre of the fovea (Fig. 3.32).

> **NB: Because recurrences can occur several years after initially successful treatment, it is important for the patient to continue to self-monitor progress with the regular use of the Amsler grid. On detection of any fresh distortion or scotoma, immediate examination should be arranged.**

***Results*** are frequently disappointing for the following reasons:

1. Using FA as a guide, only a very small proportion of eyes are eligible for treatment.
2. Even after treatment in eligible eyes, the recurrence rate is greater than 50% – most recurrent lesions are subfoveal.

## PHOTODYNAMIC THERAPY

***Principles.*** Verteporfin is a photosensitiser or light-activated compound that is preferentially taken up by dividing cells, in

### Contraindications

1. **Poorly defined CNV,** because the membrane is either occult or obscured by blood and/or serous RPE detachment. In these cases, treatment, if attempted, is often incomplete because the extent of the CNV cannot be accurately determined.
2. **Poor VA** (6/36 or less) is often a contraindication, because the CNV is likely to be subfoveal. In fact, less than 10% of eyes are suitable for treatment with argon photocoagulation at first presentation.

### Technique

1. VA is measured for near and distance.
2. The area of the scotoma or visual distortion is documented on the Amsler grid.

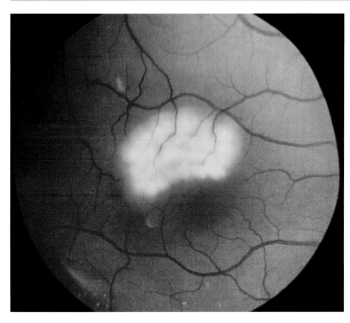

**Figure 3.31** Appearance immediately following laser photocoagulation of CNV

this instance neovascular tissue. It is injected intravenously and is then activated focally by illumination with light from a diode laser source at a wavelength (689 nm) that corresponds to an absorption peak of the compound. The main advantage of photodynamic therapy is the ability to selectively damage tissue, attributable to both preferential localisation of the photosensitiser to the CNV and irradiation confined to the target tissue. The CNV is irradiated with light levels far lower than those required for thermal destruction by argon laser therapy, enabling treatment of subfoveal CNV with relative sparing of healthy tissue.

### Indications

1. **Definite indications** are subfoveal (Fig. 3.33), predominantly classic CNV (area of classic CMV $\geq$ 50% of the area of the entire lesion), not larger than 5400 $\mu$m, in eyes with a VA of 6/60 or better. The results are encouraging in this group, with stability and, sometimes, improvement of VA in 60% of cases over 3 years.

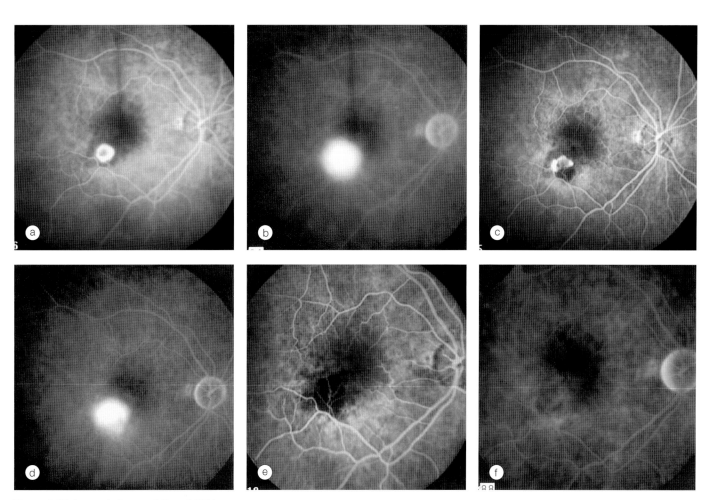

**Figure 3.32** Laser photocoagulation of CNV:
1. At presentation. **(a)** & **(b)** FA shows classic extrafoveal CNV
2. Three weeks following laser photocoagulation to CNV. **(c)** The venous phase shows hypofluorescence corresponding to the laser scar, with adjacent hyperfluorescence due to persistence and extension of CNV; **(d)** the late phase shows increased hyperfluorescence due to leakage from CNV
3. Six weeks following re-treatment. **(e)** Early and **(f)** late frames show absence of leakage

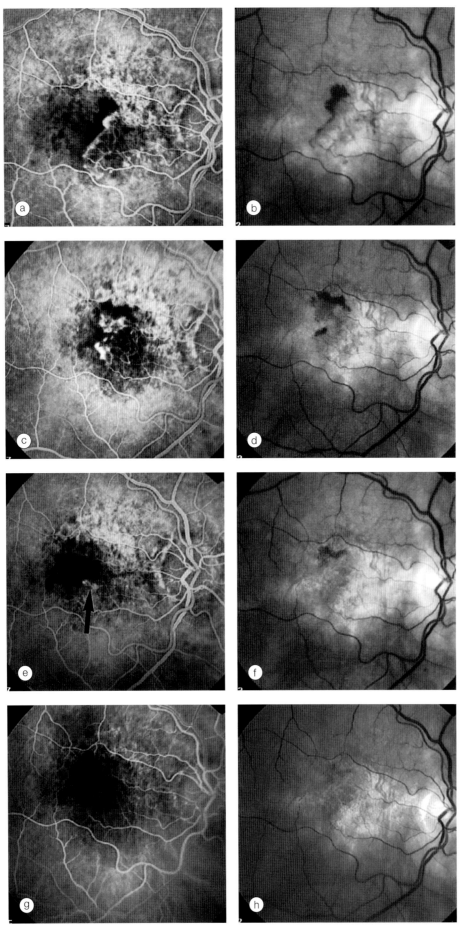

**Figure 3.33** Photodynamic and conventional laser treatment of CNV:

1. At presentation. **(a)** FA shows a well-defined subfoveal CNV which was treated by photodynamic therapy; **(b)** red-free image shows subretinal haemorrhage
2. Three months later. **(c)** FA shows persistent CNV which was re-treated by photodynamic therapy; **(d)** red-free image shows subretinal haemorrhage but in a different distribution
3. Two months later, following re-treatment. **(e)** FA shows shrinkage of CNV apart from a small extrafoveal inferonasal area (arrow), which was treated by conventional laser photocoagulation; **(f)** red-free image shows a small subretinal haemorrhage
4. One month later. **(g)** FA shows complete resolution of CNV; **(h)** red-free image shows absence of haemorrhage

### 2. Possible indications

*a.* Small, pure occult lesions (Fig. 3.34) associated with a documented decrease in VA may also stabilise with photodynamic therapy, although the results are not as encouraging as for predominately classic lesions.

*b.* Lesions greater than 5400 $\mu$m, juxtapapillary CNV with subfoveal extension.

### 3. Contraindications are PEDs and lesions with <50% classic CNV.

### Technique

1. Verteporfin (6 mg/kg body weight) is infused intravenously over 10 minutes.

2. Five minutes later, non-thermal laser is applied to the CNV for 83 seconds.

3. Re-treatment is applied to areas of persistent or new leakage at 3-monthly intervals until the entire CNV is obliterated.

**Side effects** include transient lower backache during infusion, transient decrease in vision, injection site reaction, and sensitivity to bright light for 24–48 hours.

## EXPERIMENTAL THERAPIES

### Surgery

1. **Submacular** surgery involves vitrectomy, posterior retinotomy and removal of the subfoveal CNV (Fig. 3.35).

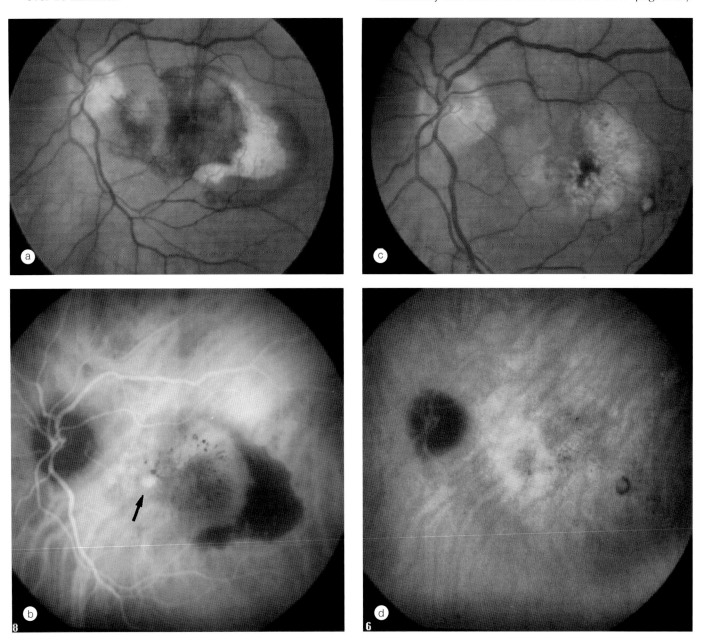

**Figure 3.34** Photodynamic therapy of occult CNV:
1. At presentation. **(a)** Serosanguinous detachment at the macula with subretinal plaque of hard exudates; **(b)** ICG shows hypofluorescence corresponding to blood and lipid and a small round area of hyperfluorescence ('hot spot') nasal to the fovea (arrow), which was treated by photodynamic therapy
2. Three months later. **(c)** Atrophic changes are present but there is absence of blood and lipid; **(d)** ICG shows absence of hyperfluorescence

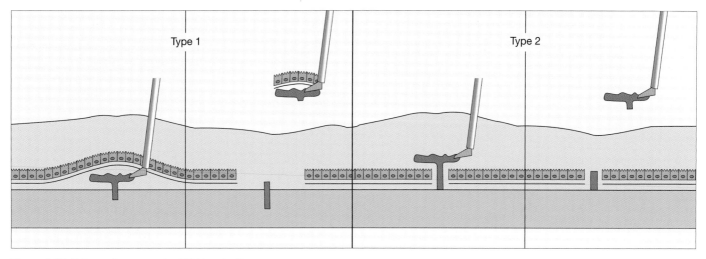

**Figure 3.35** Submacular surgery for CNV (see text)

Preliminary results suggest a high recurrence rate. The procedure also causes a large central scotoma because in type 1 CNV it is impossible to remove the membrane without also removing the overlying RPE. Therefore, CNV removal is not normally carried out for patients with AMD, although results are more encouraging in younger patients with type 2 CNV in which the CNV lies anterior and separate to the RPE.

2. **Macular translocation** is aimed at surgically moving the fovea away from the CNV. Indications and techniques for this type of surgery are still evolving and the procedures are not without risk, but early results have been encouraging in selected cases.

   a. *Limited macular translocation* can be carried out via vitrectomy followed by subretinal infusion of balanced salt solution to induce a temporal retinal detachment. The underlying sclera is then imbricated (i.e. overlapped like the tiles of a roof) to produce a shortening relative to the retina (Fig. 3.36). Fluid–air exchange is performed, followed by postoperative upright positioning to displace the fovea away from the CNV which can then be photocoagulated without the risk of foveal damage. Success is dependent on effective transposition of the fovea away from the leaking CNV complex and the degree of preoperative foveal function. Unfortunately, only relatively small displacements of the fovea are possible which may not be sufficient to allow laser of the CNV, and the risk of recurrence is high. In cases that have been successfully translocated, with recovery of central vision the patient will require extensive extraocular muscle surgery to correct the severe torsional diplopia.

   b. *Large retinotomy techniques.* A more promising technique of macular translocation involves vitrectomy, the creation of a total retinal detachment and 360° peripheral retinectomy. With easy access to the subretinal space beneath the reflected retina, the CNV can be removed surgically. The retina is then rotated with

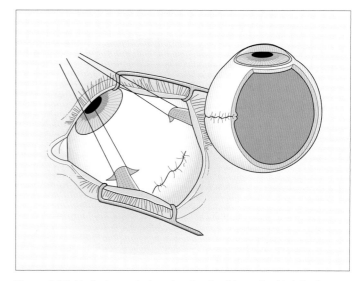

**Figure 3.36** Limited macular translocation involving scleral imbrication

the assistance of heavy liquids, and laser retinopexy combined with silicone oil tamponade is used to secure it in its new position. In addition to torsional diplopia, the main complications are retinal detachment and proliferative vitreoretinopathy.

3. **Pneumatic displacement** of submacular haemorrhage involves injection of gas into the vitreous cavity followed by face-down posturing in order to displace the blood from the fovea. The procedure may also be combined with insertion of a fibrinolytic agent called tissue plasminogen activator (t-PA) to aid displacement of the blood, although there is some doubt as to whether the t-PA molecule is small enough to cross the blood–retinal barrier.

***Transpupillary thermotherapy*** with a diode laser (810 nm) may be used for predominantly occult CNV. The diode laser has a theoretical advantage over other wavelengths of light as there is little absorption in the xanthophyll layer and thus damage to the sensory retina is minimal. Additionally, the diode laser is poorly absorbed by haemoglobin, allowing an improved ability to treat through preretinal and subretinal haemorrhage. The wavelength of the diode laser is mainly absorbed by melanin in the RPE and choroid, enabling treat-ment of CNV. The large spot size (3000–6000 $\mu$m) of the diode laser also ensures that the treatment will cover large, multifocal or diffuse occult CNV.

***Antiangiogenic*** therapy with intravitreal steroids (triamcinolone acetonide) and anti-vascular endothelial growth factor (anti-VEGF) are undergoing evaluation and show promising results. It is possible that triamcinolone may be of particular value for recurrent subfoveal neovascularisation, thus avoiding additional vision loss from laser re-treatment, as well as being an adjunct to other forms of treatment such as argon laser or photodynamic therapy.

# Retinal angiomatous proliferation

Retinal angiomatous proliferation (RAP) is an uncommon manifestation of exudative AMD in which the neovascular process originates from the retinal vasculature as opposed to the choriocapillaris.

## Diagnosis

1. **Presentation** is similar to that of AMD.

2. **Signs,** in chronological order:

   - Intraretinal neovascularisation, similar to intrarctinal microvascular abnormalities (IRMA) in diabetic retinopathy, which originates from the deep paramacular capillary plexus and which is often accompanied by intraretinal haemorrhage and oedema.
   - Subretinal neovascularisation beyond the photoreceptor layer into the subretinal space, associated with increasing oedema, intraretinal and preretinal haemorrhage and serous PED.
   - CNV associated with fibrovascular PED and retinochoroidal anastomoses.

3. **FA** is similar to purely occult or minimally classic CNV.

4. **ICG** shows a hot spot in mid or late frames.

***Treatment*** with conventional laser photocoagulation is usually ineffective although photodynamic therapy with adjunctive intravitreal injection of triamcinolone may be successful. Surgical section of the feeder artery and draining vcin is a rccently described experimental option.

## FURTHER READING

Abdel-Meguid A, Lappas A, Hartmann K, et al. One year follow up of macular translocation with 360 degree retinotomy in patients with age related macular degeneration. *Br J Ophthalmol* 2003; 87:615–621.

Abdelsalam A, Del Priore L, Zarbin MA. Drusen in age-related macular degeneration; pathogenesis, natural course and laser photocoagulation-induced regression. *Surv Ophthalmol* 1999; 44:1–25.

Age-Related Eye Disease Study Research Group. A randomized, placebo-controlled, clinical trial of high-dose supplementation with vitamins C and E, beta carotene, and zinc for age-related macular degeneration and vision loss: AREDS report no. 8. *Arch Oph almol* 2001; 119:1417–1436.

Age-Related Eye Disease Study Research Group. The Age-Related Eye Disease Study system for classifying age-related macular degeneration from stereoscopic color fundus photographs: the Age-Related Eye Disease Study Report Number 6. *Am J Ophthalmol* 2001; 132:668–681.

Aisenbrey S, Lafaut BA, Szurman P, et al. Macular translocation with 360 degree retinotomy for exudative age-related macular degeneration. *Arch Ophthalmol* 2002;120:451–459.

Bird AC. Towards an understanding of age-related macular disease. Bowman Lecture. *Eye* 2003;17:457–466.

Bird AC. The ageing macula. *Eye* 2001;15:369–370.

Bird AC, Bressler NM, Bressler SB, et al. An international classification and grading system for age-related maculopathy and age-related macular degeneration. *Surv Ophthalmol* 1995;39:367–374.

Choroidal Neovascularization Prevention Trial Research Group. Laser treatment in fellow eyes with large drusen: updated findings from a pilot randomized clinical trial. *Ophthalmology* 2003; 110:971–978.

Choroidal Neovascularization Prevention Trial Research Group. Choroidal neovascularization in the Choroidal Neovascularization Prevention Trial. *Ophthalmology* 1998;105:1364–1372.

Choroidal Neovascularization Prevention Trial Research Group. Laser treatment in eyes with large drusen. Short-term effects seen in a pilot randomized clinical trial. *Ophthalmology* 1998;105:11–23.

Ciulla TA, Danis RP, Harris A. Age-related macular degeneration: a review of experimental treatments. *Surv Ophthalmol* 1998;43: 134–146.

Eyetech Study Group. Anti-vascular endothelial growth factor therapy for subfoveal choroidal neovascularization secondary to age-related macular degeneration. Phase II study results. *Ophthalmology* 2003;110:976–986.

Fine SL. Photodynamic therapy with verteporfin is effective for selected patients with neovascular age-related macular degeneration [Editorial]. *Arch Ophthalmol* 1999;117:1400–1402.

Fujii GY, De Huan E Jr, Pieramici DJ, et al. Inferior limited macular translocation for subfoveal choroidal neovascularization secondary to age-related macular degeneration: 1-year visual outcome and recurrence report. *Am J Ophthalmol* 2002;134:69–74.

Gillies MC, Simpson JM, Luo W, et al. A randomized clinical trial of a single dose of intravitreal triamcinolone acetonide for neovascular age-related macular degeneration. *Arch Ophthalmol* 2003; 121:667–673.

Grossniklaus HE, Gass JD. Clinicopathologic correlations of surgically excised type 1 and type 2 submacular choroidal neovascular membranes. *Am J Ophthalmol* 1998;126:59–69.

Haddad WM, Coscas G, Soubrane G. Eligibility for treatment and angiographic features at the early stage of exudative age related macular degeneration. *Br J Ophthalmol* 2002;86:663–669.

Lafaut BA, Bartz-Schmidt KU, Vanden Broecke C, et al. Clinicopathological correlation in exudative age related macular degeneration: histological differentiation between classic and occult choroidal neovascularization. *Br J Ophthalmol* 2000; 84:239–243.

Jampol LM, Scott L. Treatment of juxtafoveal and extrafoveal choroidal neovascularization in the era of photodynamic therapy with verteporfin [Editorial]. *Am J Ophthalmol* 2002;134:99–101.

Jonas JB, Kreissig I, Hugger P, et al. Intravitreal triamcinolone acetonide for exudative age related macular degeneration. *Br J Ophthalmol* 2003;87:462–468.

Lai JC, Lapolice DJ, Stinnett SS, et al. Visual outcomes following macular translocation with 360 degree peripheral retinectomy. *Arch Ophthalmol* 2002;120:1317–1324.

Lois N, Owens SL, Coco R, et al. Fundus autofluorescence in patients with age-related macular degeneration and high risk of visual loss. *Am J Ophthalmol* 2002;133:341–349.

Merrill PT, LoRusso FJ, Lomeo MD, et al. Surgical removal of subfoveal choroidal neovascularization in age-related macular degeneration. *Ophthalmology* 1999;106:782–789.

Moshfeighi DM, Kaiser PK, Grossniklaus HE, et al. Clinicopathologic study after submacular removal of choroidal neovascular membranes treated with verteporfin ocular photodynamic therapy. *Am J Ophthalmol* 2003;135:343–350.

Pieramici DJ, De Juan Jr E, Fujii GY, et al. Limited inferior macular translocation for the treatment of subfoveal choroidal neovascularization secondary to age-related macular degeneration. *Am J Ophthalmol* 2000;130:419–428.

Ranson NT, Danis RP, Cuilla TA, et al. Intravitreal triamcinolone in subfoveal recurrence of choroidal neovascularization after laser treatment in macular degeneration. *Br J Ophthalmol* 2002;86: 527–529.

Regallo CD, Blade KA, Custis PH, et al. Evaluation of persistent and recurrent choroidal neovascularization. *Ophthalmology* 1998; 105:1821–1826.

Rodanant N, Friberg TR, Cheng L, et al. Predictors of drusen reduction after threshold infrared (810 nm) diode laser macular grid photocoagulation for non-exudative age-related macular degeneration. *Am J Ophthalmol* 2002;134:577–585.

Schmidt-Erfurth U, Hasan T. Mechanisms of action of photodynamic therapy with verteporfin for the treatment of age-related macular degeneration. *Surv Ophthalmol* 2000;45:195–214.

Soubrane G, Bressler NM. Treatment of subfoveal choroidal neovascularization in age related macular degeneration: focus on clinical application of verteporfin photodynamic therapy. *Br J Ophthalmol* 2001;85:483–495.

Spaide RF. Fundus autofluorescence and age-related macular degeneration. *Ophthalmology* 2003;110:392–399.

Submacular Surgical Trials Pilot Study Investigators. Submacular surgery trials randomized pilot trial of laser photocoagulation versus surgery for recurrent choroidal neovascularization secondary to age-related macular degeneration: ophthalmic outcomes. *Am J Ophthalmol* 2000;130:387–407.

Sunness JS, Gonzalez-Baron J, Applegate CA, et al. Enlargement of atrophy and visual loss in the geographic atrophy form of age-related macular degeneration. *Ophthalmology* 1999;106: 1768–1779.

TAP Study Group. Photodynamic therapy of subfoveal choroidal neovascularization in age-related macular degeneration with verteporfin. One-year results of two randomized clinical trials – TAP report 1. *Arch Ophthalmol* 1999;117:1329–1345.

TAP Study Group. Photodynamic therapy of subfoveal choroidal neovascularization in age-related macular degeneration with verteporfin. Two-year results of two randomized clinical trials – TAP report 2. *Arch Ophthalmol* 2001;119:198–207.

TAP Study Group. Verteporfin therapy of subfoveal choroidal neovascularization in patients with age-related macular degeneration. TAP report no. 3. *Arch Ophthalmol* 2002;120:1443–1454.

TAP Study Group. Verteporfin therapy for subfoveal choroidal neovascularization in age-related macular degeneration. TAP report no. 5. *Am J Ophthalmol* 2002;120:1307–1314.

van Leeuwen R, Klaver CCW, Vingerling JR, et al. The risk and natural course of age-related maculopathy. *Arch Ophthalmol* 2003;121:519–526.

Yannuzzi LA, Negrao S, Iida T, et al. Retinal angiomatous proliferation in age related macular degeneration. *Retina* 2001; 21:416–434.

# Polypoidal Choroidal Vasculopathy

Polypoidal choroidal vasculopathy (PCV), also described as posterior uveal bleeding syndrome or multiple serosanguinous RPE detachment syndrome, is a relatively uncommon, idiopathic condition. The inner choroidal vessels consist of a dilated network and multiple terminal aneurysmal protrubences in a polypoidal configuration.

## *Diagnosis*

1. **Presentation** is in old age with sudden onset of unilateral visual impairment.

2. **Signs** are often bilateral but asymmetrical in severity. Most frequently, the lesions occur at the macula; 20% are peripapillary and 15% extramacular. Classically there is lack of significant drusen. The two main patterns of PCV are:

   a. *The exudative* pattern, characterised by serous PED and serous retinal detachment associated with intraretinal lipid deposits in the macula (Fig. 3.37).

   b. *The haemorrhagic* pattern, characterised by haemorrhagic PED and subretinal haemorrhage in the macula.

3. **ICG** is required to make a definitive diagnosis of PCV. This shows a branching vascular network from the choroidal circulation and polypoidal and aneurysmal dilatations at the terminals of the branching vessels that fill slowly and then leak intensely (Fig. 3.38).

4. **Course.** The condition develops slowly and persists for a long time. The prognosis is good in 50% of cases, with eventual spontaneous resolution of exudation and haemorrhage. In the remainder, the disorder persists for a long time, with occasional repeated bleeding and leakage, resulting in macular damage and visual loss. Eyes with a cluster of grape-like vascular polypoidal dilatations have a high risk of visual loss.

***Treatment*** involving laser photocoagulation is occasionally used to try and decrease serosanguinous leakage threatening the fovea. Unfortunately, in some cases, extensive subretinal exudation and haemorrhage can leave an eye with bare perception of light and loss of peripheral vision, in contrast to AMD-related CNV, which is very rarely severe enough to affect peripheral vision.

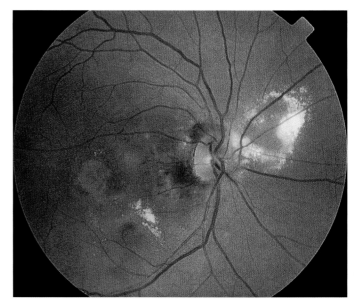

**Figure 3.37** Exudative type of polypoidal choroidal vasculopathy (Courtesy of R. Spaide)

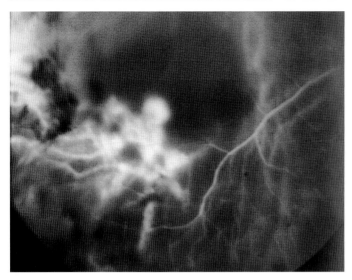

**Figure 3.38** ICG of idiopathic polypoidal choroidal vasculopathy, showing hyperfluorescence of polyp-like bulbs

### Differential diagnosis

- Exudative pattern PCV may mimic chronic central serous retinopathy in the elderly.
- Haemorrhagic pattern PCV may mimic exudative AMD.

### FURTHER READING

Ahuja RA, Stanga PE, Vingerling JR, et al. Polypoidal vasculopathy in exudative and haemorrhagic pigment epithelial detachments. *Br J Ophthalmol* 2000;84:479–484.

Moorthy RS, Lyon AT, Rabb MF, et al. Idiopathic polypoidal choroidal vasculopathy of the macula. *Ophthalmology* 1998;105:1380–1385.

Okuba A, Sameshima M, Uemura A, et al. Clinicopathological correlation of polypoidal choroidal vasculopathy revealed by ultrastructural study. *Br J Ophthalmol* 2002;86:1093–1098.

Rosa RH Jr, Davis JL, Eifrig CWG. Clinicopathologic correlation of idiopathic polypoidal choroidal vasculopathy. *Arch Ophthalmol* 2002;120:502–508.

Schneider U, Gelisken F, Kreissig I. Indocyanine green angiography and idiopathic polypoidal choroidal vasculopathy. *Br J Ophthalmol* 1998;82:98–99.

Uyama M, Wada M, Nagai Y, et al. Polypoidal choroidal vasculopathy: natural history. *Am J Ophthalmol* 2002;133:639–648.

Yannuzzi LA, Ciardella A, Spaide RF, et al. The expanding clinical spectrum of idiopathic polypoidal choroidal vasculopathy. *Arch Ophthalmol* 1997;115:478–485.

## Age-Related Macular Hole

Age-related (idiopathic) full-thickness macular holes (FTMH) are a relatively common cause of visual loss, affecting approximately three in 1000 individuals. Those affected are characteristically female, in the sixth or seventh decade, with normal refractive errors. Presentation is with severe impairment of central vision or as a relatively asymptomatic deterioration, first noticed when the fellow eye is closed. The risk of involvement of the fellow eye at 5 years is about 15%.

***Staging.*** A macular hole results from the centrifugal displacement of photoreceptors from a central dehiscence of the umbo. The primary event is probably an abnormal vitreo-foveolar attachment, with resultant anteroposterior traction initiating the following sequence (Fig. 3.39).

1. **Stage 1a** (impending) macular hole is rarely seen clinically and is usually detected in a patient with an FTMH in the other eye. It is characterised by a yellow spot with loss of the foveolar reflex (Fig. 3.40) representing a foveal cyst.

2. **Stage 1b** (occult) macular hole results from centrifugal displacement of the foveolar retina and xanthophyll. It is characterised by a yellow ring with a bridging interface of vitreous cortex. These findings may be associated with a mild decrease in VA or metamorphopsia. About 50% of stage 1 holes resolve following spontaneous vitreofoveolar separation.

3. **Stage 2** (early FTMH) is characterised by an eccentric, oval, crescentic or horseshoe-shaped retinal defect less than 400 $\mu$m in diameter with or without an overlying prefoveal opacity (pseudo-operculum) (Fig. 3.41). True opercula are rare and the pseudo-operculum is formed by

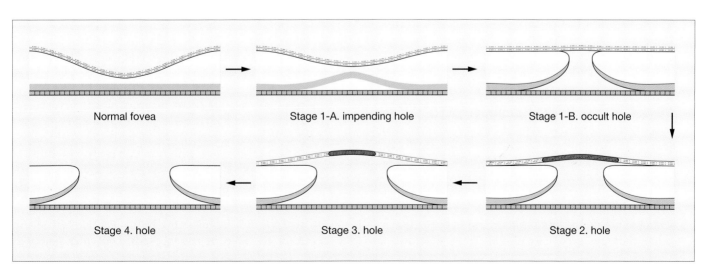

Normal fovea | Stage 1-A. impending hole | Stage 1-B. occult hole

Stage 4. hole | Stage 3. hole | Stage 2. hole

**Figure 3.39** Stages of age-related macular hole (see text)

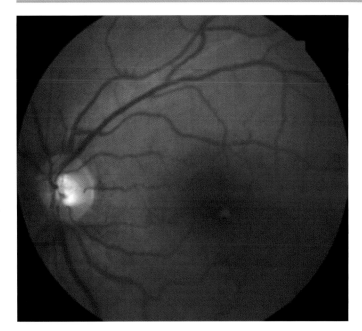

**Figure 3.40** Stage 1a macular hole

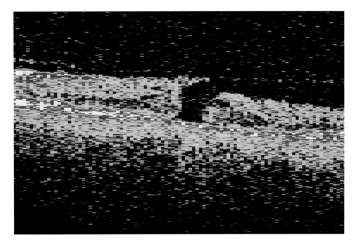

**Figure 3.41** OCT of stage 2 macular hole

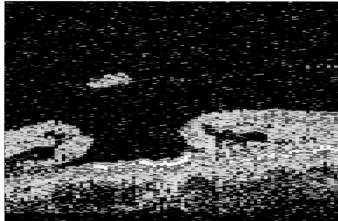

**Figure 3.42** OCT of stage 3 macular hole with an operculum

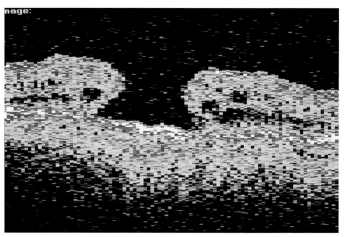

**Figure 3.43** OCT of stage 4 macular hole

the contracted prefoveal cortical vitreous. Progression from stage 1 to stage 2 takes between 1 week and several months.

4. **Stage 3** (established FTMH) is characterised by a round retinal defect greater than 400 $\mu$m in diameter with an attached posterior vitreous face with or without an overlying pseudo-operculum (Fig. 3.42).

5. **Stage 4** is characterised by enlargement of the round defect which is now surrounded by a cuff of subretinal fluid (Fig. 3.43) and exhibits tiny yellowish deposits at the base of the crater (Fig. 3.44). The posterior vitreous is completely detached, often evidenced by a Weiss ring. VA is decreased primarily due to the absence of photoreceptors within the central defect, with a resultant absolute central scotoma. In addition, the surrounding cuff of subretinal fluid and secondary retinal elevation cause a surrounding area of relative scotoma. Vision tends to deteriorate progressively, stabilising at 6/60 or worse as the hole reaches its maximal diameter. Some patients may achieve better acuity by employing eccentric fixation.

NB: An FTMH may rarely spontaneously resolve, with improvement of VA, due to spontaneous posterior vitreous detachment with release of vitreomacular traction.

## Diagnostic tests

1. **Watzke–Allen** test is performed by projecting a narrow slit beam over the centre of the hole both vertically and horizontally, ideally with a Goldman fundus contact lens. A patient with a macular hole will report that the beam is thinned or broken. The vast majority of patients report a thinned beam, as the photoreceptors displaced to the edge of the hole are still functioning, albeit poorly, and are displaced over a wider area, with resultant micropsia. Patients with a pseudo-hole or cyst usually see a beam of uniform thickness which is distorted or bent rather than thinned.

2. **Laser aiming beam** test is performed by projecting a 50-$\mu$m spot of a laser aiming beam (e.g. He-Ne) at the centre of the hole. A patient with a macular hole will report that the spot has disappeared, whereas those with a pseudo-hole or cyst will still be able to see the beam.

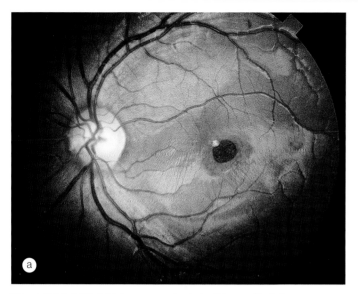
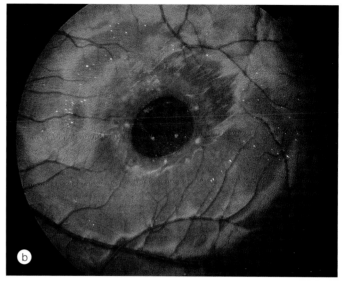

**Figure 3.44** **(a)** Full-thickness macular hole; **(b)** magnified view

3. **FA** shows a corresponding area of hyperfluorescence (Fig. 3.45a) resulting from unmasking of background choroidal fluorescence caused by a defect in xanthophyll due to centrifugal displacement (Fig. 3.45b). However, a similar appearance can also be seen with pseudo-holes and cysts, so FA is not usually helpful in differential diagnosis.

4. **Optical coherence tomography (OCT)** provides high-resolution optical sections of the retina and affords measurement of retinal thickness. It is useful in the diagnosis and staging of macular holes. It can even measure the volume of an FTMH.

### Surgical treatment

1. **Indications** are FTMH of stage 2 and above, associated with a VA worse than 6/9. Best results are achieved with holes of less than 1 year's duration. However, it is possible to close holes of several years' duration, with associated improvement in VA and decreased distortion, particularly if ILM peeling techniques are used.

2. **Technique** consists of removal of the cortical vitreous, relief of vitreomacular traction, with or without ILM peel, and gas tamponade, followed by strict postoperative face-down positioning. The potential for dramatic improvement in VA, together with the restoration of normal foveal architecture on OCT scanning, suggests that closure of the hole is the result of centripetal movement of previously displaced paracentral photoreceptors and not simply re-approximation of the retinal edges to the RPE.

3. **Results.** Following successful surgery, visual improvement is achieved in 80–90% of eyes, with a final VA of 6/12 or better in up to 65%. Fig. 3.46a shows an FTMH

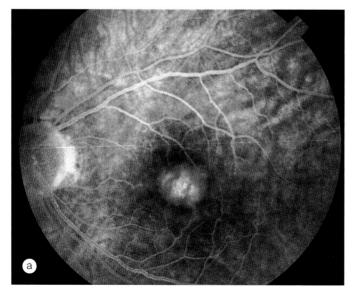
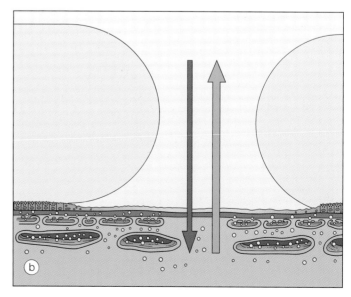

**Figure 3.45** FA of full-thickness macular hole

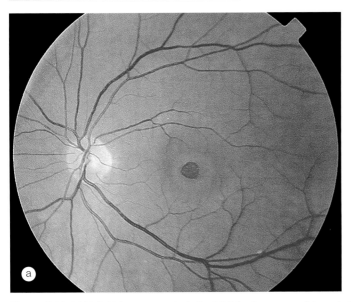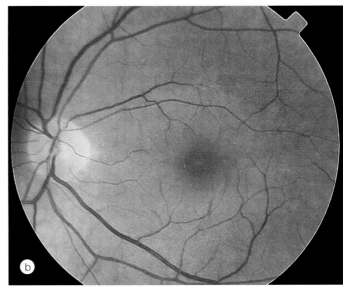

**Figure 3.46** **(a)** Full-thickness macular hole; **(b)** following successful surgical closure

and Fig. 3.46b the postoperative appearance following successful surgery.

4. **Complications** are those associated with vitrectomy, such as retinal detachment, pigment hyperplasia and acceleration of cataract. Increasingly, cataract surgery is combined with vitrectomy surgery to speed up the patient's visual rehabilitation. Occasionally, inferotemporal visual field defects may develop secondary to prolonged infusion of dry air into the ocular cavity.

### Differential diagnosis

1. **Other causes of true macular holes**

   a. *High myopia*, if associated with posterior staphyloma, may be associated with macular hole formation which can lead to retinal detachment. The subretinal fluid is confined to the posterior pole and seldom spreads to the equator.

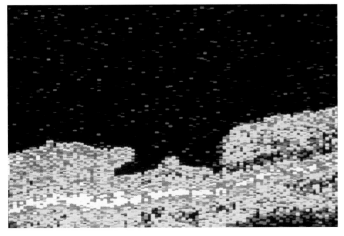

**Figure 3.47** OCT of a lamellar macular hole

   b. *Blunt ocular trauma* may cause a macular hole as a result of either vitreous traction or commotio retinae in which there is disruption of photoreceptors and subsequent hole formation.

2. **Macular pseudo-holes**

   a. *Hole within premacular fibrosis.*
   b. *Lamellar hole* resulting from longstanding severe cystoid macular oedema (Fig. 3.47).
   c. *White dot fovea* is an uncommon asymptomatic condition. White dots may be arranged diffusely or in the form of a ring along the margin of the foveola. The latter pattern simulates the appearance of a true macular hole with a cuff of fluid.

### FURTHER READING

Chew EY, Sperduto RD, Hiller R, et al. Clinical course of macular holes: the Eye Disease Case-Control Study. *Arch Ophthalmol* 1999;117:242–246.

Eye Disease Case-Control Study Group. Risk factors for idiopathic macular holes. *Am J Ophthalmol* 1994;118:754–761.

Ezra E. Idiopathic full-thickness macular hole; natural history and pathogenesis. *Br J Ophthalmol* 2001;85:102–108.

Fine SL. Macular hole. A continuing saga [Editorial]. *Arch Ophthalmol* 1999;117: 248–249.

Gass JDM. Muller cell cone, an overlooked part of the anatomy of the fovea centralis. Hypotheses concerning its role in the pathogenesis of macular hole and foveomacular retinoschisis. *Arch Ophthalmol* 1999;117:821–823.

Gass JDM. Reappraisal of biomicroscopic classification of stages of development of a macular hole. *Am J Ophthalmol* 1995;119: 752–759.

Ho AC, Guyer DR, Fine SL. Macular hole. *Surv Ophthalmol* 1998; 42:393–416.

Kelly NE, Wendel RT. Vitreous surgery for idiopathic macular holes. Results of a pilot study. *Arch Ophthalmol* 1991;109:654–659.

Lai JC, Stinnett SS, McCuen BW. Comparison of silicone oil versus gas tamponade in the treatment of idiopathic full-thickness macular hole. *Ophthalmology* 2003;110:1170–1174.

Mester V, Kuhn F. Internal limiting membrane removal of full-thickness macular holes. *Am J Ophthalmol* 2000;129:769–777.

Scott RAH, Ezra E, West JF, et al. Visual and anatomical results of surgery for long standing macular holes. *Br J Ophthalmol* 2000; 84:150–153.

Scott IU, Moraczewski AL, Smiddy WE, et al. Long-term anatomic and visual acuity outcomes after initial anatomic success with macular hole surgery. *Am J Ophthalmol* 2003;135:633–640.

Spaide RF, Wong D, Fisher Y, et al. Correlation of vitreous attachment and foveal deformation in early macular hole states. *Am J Ophthalmol* 2002;133:226–229.

Tanner V, Williamson TH. Watzke-Allen slit beam test in macular holes confirmed by optical coherence tomography. *Arch Ophthalmol* 2000;118:1059–1063.

Tanner V, Chauhan DS, Jackson TL, et al. Optical coherence tomography of the vitreoretinal interface in macular hole formation. *Br J Ophthalmol* 2001;85:1092–1097.

Wendel RT, Patel AC, Kelly NE, et al. Vitreous surgery for macular holes. *Ophthalmology* 1993;100:1671–1676.

# Central Serous Retinopathy

Central serous retinopathy (CSR), also known as central serous chorioretinopathy, is a sporadic, self-limited disease typically affecting young or middle-aged men with type A personality. It is characterised by a usually unilateral, localised detachment of the sensory retina at the macula secondary to focal RPE defects. Factors reported to induce or aggravate CSR include emotional stress, hypertension, systemic lupus erythematosus, organ transplantation, Cushing disease, and the administration of steroids, both by inhalation and orally. Women with CSR tend to be older than affected men and it is also associated with pregnancy.

## TYPICAL CENTRAL SEROUS RETINOPATHY

### Diagnosis

1. **Presentation** is with unilateral blurred vision associated with a positive relative scotoma and micropsia and/or metamorphopsia. Occasionally the condition is extrafoveal and asymptomatic.

2. **Signs**

    a. *VA* is usually reduced to 6/9–6/12 and often correctable to 6/6 with a weak 'plus' lens. The elevation of the sensory retina gives rise to an acquired hypermetropia with disparity between the subjective and objective refraction of the eye.

    b. *Fundus*

    ● A round or oval detachment of the sensory retina is present at the macula, which may be associated with a small PED (Figs. 3.48 and 3.49).

    ● The subretinal fluid may be clear or turbid and small precipitates may be present on the posterior surface of the sensory detachment. Occasionally, an abnormal focus in the RPE, through which fluid has leaked from the choriocapillaris into the subretinal space, can be detected.

    ● Rare findings include yellowish subretinal deposits forming a leopard-spot pattern, as well as intraretinal or subretinal lipid.

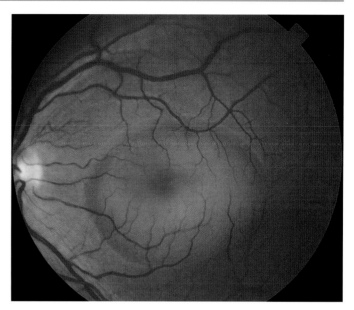

**Figure 3.48** Central serous retinopathy centred on the fovea

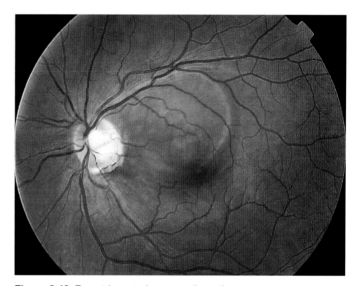

**Figure 3.49** Eccentric central serous retinopathy

3. **FA** shows one of the following patterns:

    a. *Ink-blot* appearance evolves as follows:

    ● The early phase shows a small hyperfluorescent spot (Fig. 3.50b).

    ● The spot gradually enlarges centrifugally (Fig. 3.50c and 3.50d) until the entire detachment is filled with dye.

    b. *Smoke-stack* appearance is more common and evolves as follows:

    ● The early phase shows a small hyperfluorescent spot due to leakage of dye through the RPE (Fig. 3.51a). More than one leak may be present.

    ● During the late venous phase, fluorescein passes into the subretinal space and ascends vertically (like a smoke-stack) (Fig. 3.51b) from the point of leakage until the upper border of the detachment (Fig. 3.51c).

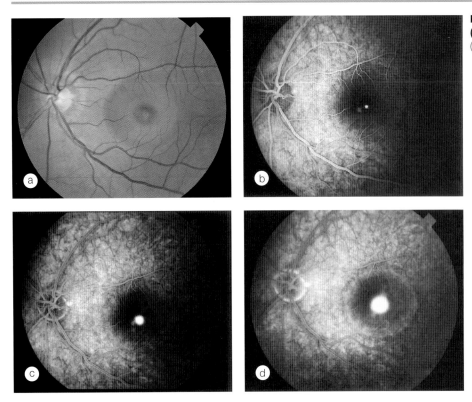

**Figure 3.50 (a)** Central serous retinopathy; **(b)**–**(d)** FA showing an 'ink-blot' appearance (see text)

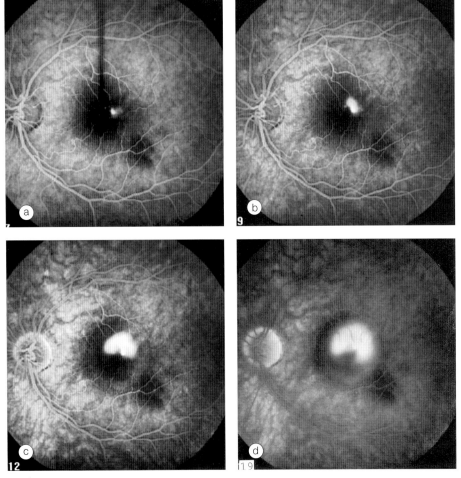

**Figure 3.51** FA of central serous retinopathy, showing a 'smoke-stack' appearance

**NB:** There is also an area of hypofluorescence inferotemporal to the macula due to blockage of background fluorescence by a choroidal naevus

- The dye then spreads laterally, taking on a 'mushroom' or 'umbrella' configuration (Fig. 3.51d), until the entire area of detachment is filled.

4. **ICG** in the early phase shows dilated choroidal vessels at the posterior pole (Fig. 3.52a) followed by diffuse hyperfluorescence due to choroidal hyperpermeability (Fig. 3.52b–3.52d).

5. **OCT** shows a serous detachment of the sensory retina (Fig. 3.53).

## Course

1. **Short** course. Most commonly, spontaneous absorption of subretinal fluid occurs within 1–6 months, with return to normal, or near normal, VA.

2. **Prolonged** course. In some patients, CSR lasts longer than 6 months but spontaneously resolves within 12 months. Even if VA returns to normal, some degree of subjective visual impairment such as micropsia may persist, but seldom causes any significant disability.

3. **Chronic** course. In a minority of cases, the condition lasts longer than 12 months and is characterised by progressive RPE changes, often without manifest retinal detachment, resulting in permanent impairment of VA. Secondary CNV is an uncommon occurrence. FA shows granular hyperfluorescence with one or more leaks (Fig. 3.54). This may be a consequence of either multiple recurrent attacks or prolonged detachment, although a minority of patients do not have a past history of typical CSR, and in some the changes are bilateral.

***Treatment*** is not required in most cases. Argon laser photocoagulation to the RPE leak or detachment achieves speedier resolution and lowers the recurrence rate but does not influence the final visual outcome. It is advisable to wait for 4 months before considering treatment of the first attack and 1 or 2 months for recurrences. Treatment is contra-indicated if the leak is near or within the FAZ. Two or three low- to moderate-intensity burns are applied to the leakage site (200 $\mu$m, 0.2 seconds) to produce mild greying of the RPE (Fig. 3.55).

> **NB: Careful follow-up is required, as 2–5% of treated eyes subsequently develop CNV.**

### Differential diagnosis of sensory macular detachment

1. **Congenital optic disc anomalies,** most frequently optic disc pit and occasionally tilted disc, may be associated with serous macular detachment. Unless the optic disc is examined carefully, the diagnosis may be missed.

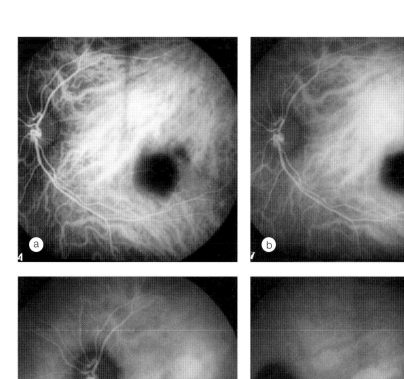

**Figure 3.52** ICG of the same eye, showing hyperfluorescence at the macula due to choroidal hyperpermeability and a round area of hypofluorescence corresponding to the choroidal naevus

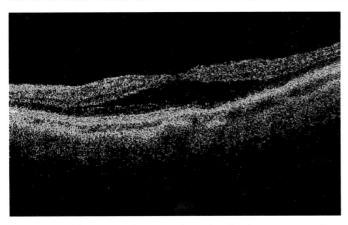

**Figure 3.53** OCT of central serous retinopathy, showing serous macular separation

2. **Choroidal tumours** with a predilection for the posterior pole, such as circumscribed choroidal haemangioma and metastatic carcinoma.

3. **Unilateral acute idiopathic maculopathy** is a rare self-limiting condition that typically causes sudden uni-lateral visual loss in a young person (see Chapter 4).

4. **CNV,** particularly if idiopathic.

5. **Harada disease** during the stage of multifocal detachments of the sensory retina may mimic multifocal CSR (see Chapter 4).

## BULLOUS CENTRAL SEROUS RETINOPATHY

Bullous CSR is characterised by large, single or multiple, serous retinal and RPE detachments (Fig. 3.56) that are

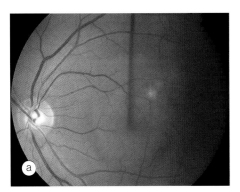
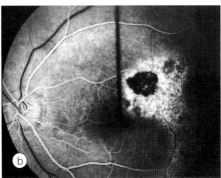
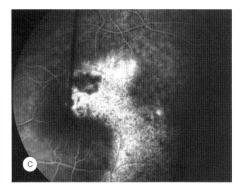

**Figure 3.54  (a)** Chronic central serous retinopathy; **(b)** and **(c)** FA shows granular hyperfluorescence due to diffuse RPE dysfunction

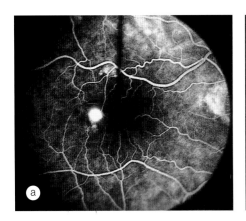
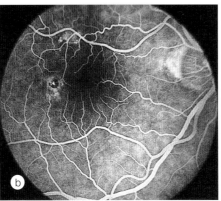

**Figure 3.55** Laser treatment of central serous retinopathy. **(a)** FA before treatment showing site of leakage which is outside the foveal avascular zone; **(b)** following closure of the leak

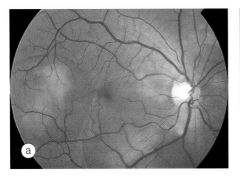
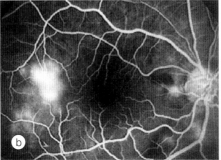
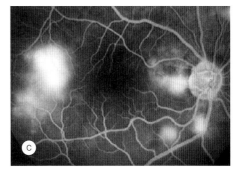

**Figure 3.56** Multiple serous retinal detachments (see text)

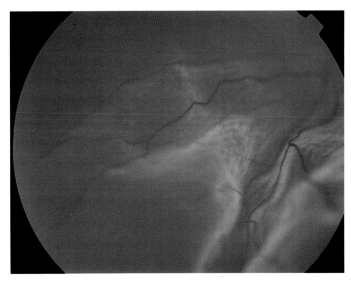

**Figure 3.57** Inferior bullous retinal detachment (see text)

# Degenerative Myopia

High myopia is defined as an eye with a refractive error >-6D and an axial length of the globe >26 mm (Fig. 3.58). It affects approximately 0.5% of the general population and 30% of myopic eyes. Pathological or degenerative myopia is characterised by progressive and excessive anteroposterior elongation of the globe which is associated with secondary changes involving the sclera, retina, choroid and optic nerve head. Maculopathy is the most common cause of visual loss in highly myopic patients.

## Chorioretinal changes

1. **A pale tessellate** (tigroid) appearance due to attenuation of the RPE (Fig. 3.59).

2. **Peripapillary chorioretinal atrophy,** which may surround a tilted optic disc (Fig. 3.60).

associated with an inferior bullous exudative retinal detachment (Fig. 3.57). This appearance may lead to the inappropriate diagnosis of rhegmatogenous retinal detachment, or exudative detachment from some other cause.

## FURTHER READING

Burumcek E, Mudum A, Karacorlu S, et al. Laser photocoagulation for persistent central serous retinopathy. Results of a long-term follow-up. *Ophthalmology* 1997;104:616–622.

Carvalho-Recchia CA, Yannuzzi LA, Negrao S, et al. Corticosteroids and central serous chorioretinopathy *Ophthalmology* 2002;109: 1834–1837.

Gass JDM, Little H. Bilateral bullous exudative retinal detachment complicating idiopathic central serous chorioretinopathy. *Ophthalmology* 1995;102:737–747.

Gilbert CM, Owens SL, Smith PD, et al. Long-term follow-up of central serous chorioretinopathy. *Br J Ophthalmol* 1984;68: 815–820.

Haimovici R, Rumelt S, Melby J. Endocrine abnormalities in patients with central serous chorioretinopathy. *Ophthalmology* 2003;110: 698–703.

Iida T, Spaide RF, Haas A, et al. Leopard-spot pattern yellowish subretinal deposits in central serous chorioretinopathy. *Arch Ophthalmol* 2002;120:37–42.

Jumper JM. Central serous chorioretinopathy [Editorial]. *Br J Ophthalmol* 2003;87:663.

Muzzaca D, Benson W. Central serous retinopathy: variants. *Surv Ophthalmol* 1986;31:170–174.

Perkins SL, Kim JE, Pollack JS, et al. Clinical characteristics of central serous chorioretinopathy in women. *Ophthalmology* 2002;109: 262–266.

Sahu DK, Namperumalsamy P, Hilton GF, et al. Bullous variant of idiopathic central serous chorioretinopathy. *Br J Ophthalmol* 2000;84:485–492.

Spahn C, Wiek J, Burger T, et al. Psychosomatic aspects in patients with central serous chorioretinopathy. *Br J Ophthalmol* 2003; 87:704–708.

Tittl MK, Spaide RF, Wong D, et al. Systemic findings associated with central serous chorioretinopathy. *Am J Ophthalmol* 1999; 128:63–68.

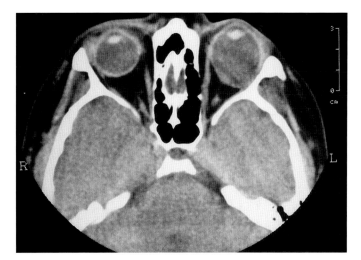

**Figure 3.58** Axial CT scan showing a very myopic left eye with a posterior staphyloma

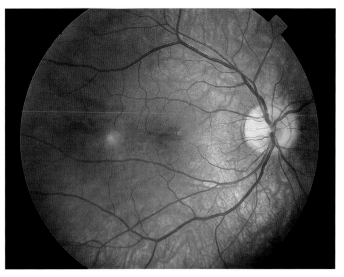

**Figure 3.59** Pale tessellate (tigroid) fundus in myopia

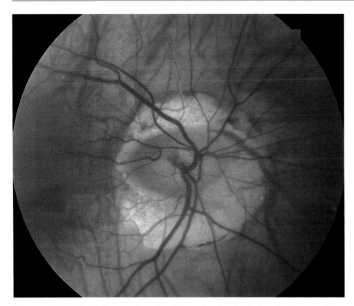

**Figure 3.60** Tilted disc and peripapillary chorioretinal atrophy in myopia

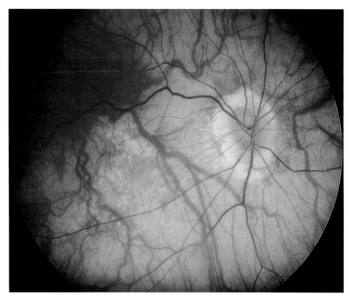

**Figure 3.62** Severe diffuse chorioretinal atrophy in myopia

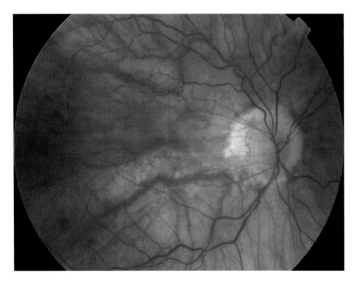

**Figure 3.61** Mild diffuse chorioretinal atrophy in myopia

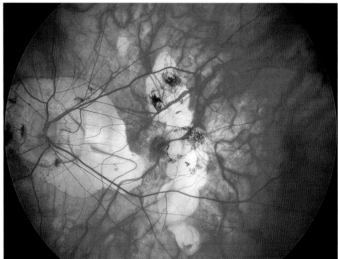

**Figure 3.63** Extreme chorioretinal atrophy with visibility of the sclera in high myopia (Courtesy of C. Barry)

3. **Chorioretinal atrophy involving the posterior pole,** characterised by visibility of the larger choroidal vessels (Figs. 3.61 and 3.62) and eventually the sclera (Fig. 3.63).

4. **Peripheral changes** include pavingstone degeneration, lattice degeneration (Fig. 3.64), retinal breaks, areas of white-without- pressure and pigmentary degeneration (see Chapter 6).

5. **'Lacquer cracks'** consist of ruptures in the RPE–Bruch's membrane–choriocapillaris complex, characterised clinically by fine, irregular, yellow lines, often branching and criss-crossing at the posterior pole (Fig. 3.65). They are potentially sight threatening as they precede development of CNV and geographic atrophy.

***Maculopathy*** may take one of the following forms:

1. **Geographic atrophy** of the RPE and choriocapillaris involving the macula (Fig. 3.66).

2. **CNV,** which may develop in association with 'lacquer cracks' and areas of patchy atrophy (Fig. 3.67). The prognosis for central vision is, however, often better than in exudative AMD, because CNV in highly myopic eyes tends to be relatively self-limited and not associated with the subsequent formation of subretinal fibrovascular scarring (Fig. 3.68). The visual prognosis is also influenced by age. Older patients with CNV tend to have a poorer visual outcome than do younger patients. The long-term results of thermal laser for juxtafoveal and extrafoveal CNV are extremely poor, mainly because of a high rate of recurrences as well as late-onset expansion of the laser scar to involve the fovea ('atrophic creep'). Due to the limitations

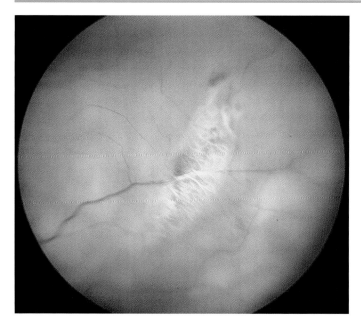

**Figure 3.64** Lattice degeneration (Courtesy of P. Morse)

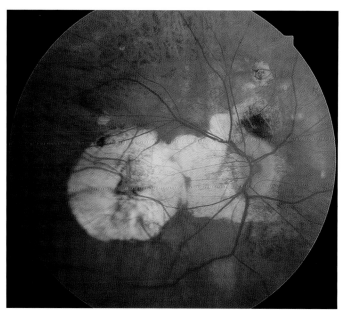

**Figure 3.66** Geographic macular atrophy in high myopia

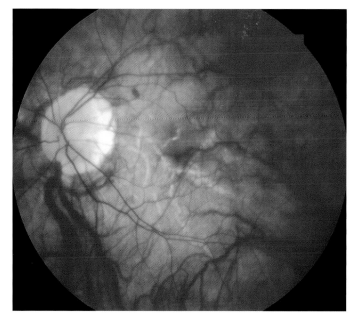

**Figure 3.65** Lacquer cracks in high myopia

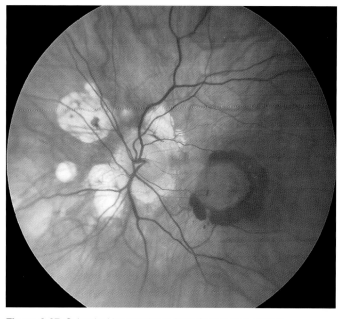

**Figure 3.67** Subretinal haemorrhage from CNV in high myopia

of thermal laser therapy, alternative modalities are being investigated, including photodynamic therapy, transpupillary thermotherapy and macular translocation.

3. **A Fuchs spot** is a raised, circular, pigmented lesion that may develop after a macular haemorrhage has absorbed (Fig. 3.69).

4. **Subretinal 'coin' haemorrhages,** which may be intermittent, may develop from lacquer cracks in the absence of CNV (Fig. 3.70).

5. **Macular hole formation,** which may result in retinal detachment.

### Other features

1. **Staphylomas** are due to expansion of the globe and scleral thinning (see Fig. 3.58). They may be peripapillary or involve the posterior pole and be associated with macular hole formation.

2. **Rhegmatogenous retinal detachment** may occur due to vitreous liquefaction, increased frequency of posterior vitreous detachment, lattice degeneration, asymptomatic atrophic holes, macular holes and, occasionally, giant retinal tears. The prevalence of retinal detachment appears to be related to the severity of myopia.

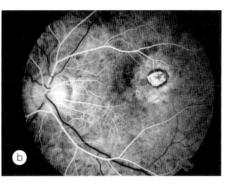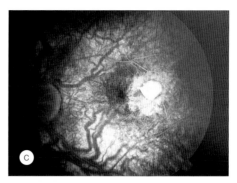

**Figure 3.68** Self-limiting CNV in myopia. **(a)** Raised chorioretinal scar just temporal to the fovea with a hyperpigmented outline which is itself surrounded by a larger halo of RPE loss; **(b)** FA arteriovenous phase shows a round area of hyperfluorescence encircled by a hypofluorescent ring which is itself surrounded by a larger area of hyperfluorescence due to a window defect; **(c)** late phase shows more intense hyperfluorescence of both the central area and the surrounding halo

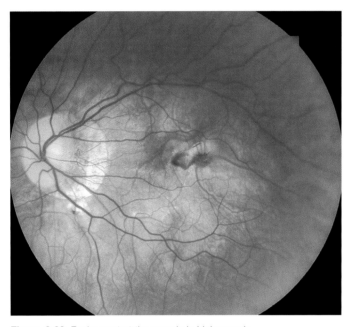

**Figure 3.69** Fuchs spot at the macula in high myopia

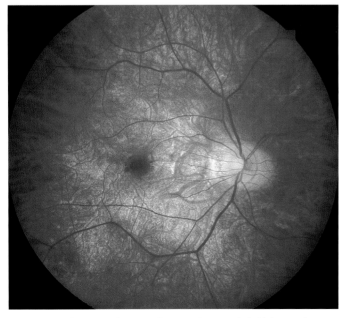

**Figure 3.70** Small 'coin' haemorrhage at the macula in high myopia

3. **Foveal retinoschisis** and retinal detachment without macular hole formation may occur in highly myopic eyes with posterior staphylomas as a result of vitreous traction. Retinoschisis is better characterised by OCT than by biomicroscopy.

4. **Peripapillary detachment** is an asymptomatic, innocuous, yellow-orange elevation of the RPE and sensory retina at the inferior border of the myopic conus. It should be distinguished from more serious fundus pathology such as a tumour or CNV.

### Associations

1. **Ocular**

   - Cataract, which may be either posterior subcapsular or early onset of nuclear sclerosis.
   - Increased prevalence of primary open-angle glaucoma, pigmentary glaucoma and steroid responsiveness.
   - Retinopathy of prematurity may be associated with the subsequent development of myopia.
   - Amblyopia is uncommon but may develop when there is a significant difference in myopia between the two eyes.

2. **Systemic**

   - Stickler syndrome.
   - Marfan syndrome.
   - Ehlers–Danlos syndrome.
   - Pierre Robin syndrome.

*Differential diagnosis* of other disorders characterised by extensive chorioretinal atrophy include the following:

1. **Choroideremia.** Differences include nyctalopia, absence of peripapillary changes and sparing of the macula until late in the disease.

2. **Gyrate atrophy.** Differences include early onset, lesions have typically scalloped edges and late macular sparing.

3. **Diffuse choroidal atrophy.** Differences include diffuse chorioretinal changes rather than punched-out lesions as in myopia.

4. **Progressive bifocal chorioretinal atrophy.** Differences include early onset, specific atrophic areas confined to the macular and nasal fundus.

## FURTHER READING

Akiba J, Konno S, Yoshida A. Retinal detachment associated with a macular hole in severely myopic eyes. *Am J Ophthalmol* 1999; 128:654–655

Baba T, Ohno-Matsui K, Futagami S, et al. Prevalence and characteristics of foveal retinal detachment without macular hole in high myopia. *Am J Ophthalmol* 2003;135:338–342.

Curtin BJ. Myopia; a review of its etiology, pathogenesis and treatment. *Surv Ophthalmol* 1970;15:1–17.

Freund KB, Ciardella AP, Yannuzzi LA, et al. Peripapillary detachment in pathologic myopia. *Arch Ophthalmol* 2003;121:197–204.

Hamelin N, Glacet-Bernard A, Brindeau C, et al. Surgical treatment of subfoveal neovascularisation in myopia: macular translocation vs surgical removal. *Am J Ophthalmol* 2002;133:530–536.

Ichibe M, Imai K, Ohta M, et al. Foveal translocation with scleral imbrication in patients with myopic neovascular maculopathy. *Am J Ophthalmol* 2001;132:164–171.

Montero JA, Ruiz-Moreno JM. Verteporfin photodynamic therapy in highly myopic subfoveal choroidal neovascularization. *Br J Ophthalmol* 2003;87:173–176.

Ohno-Mtsui K, Yoshida T, Futagami S, et al. Patchy atrophy and lacquer cracks predispose to the development of choroidal neovascularization in pathologic myopia. *Br J Ophthalmol* 2003;87:570–573.

Ruiz-Moreno JM, de la Vega C. Surgical removal of subfoveal choroidal neovascularization in highly myopic eyes. *Br J Ophthalmol* 2001; 85:1041–1043.

Tano Y. Pathologic myopia: where are we now? LIX Edward Jackson Memorial Lecture. *Am J Ophthalmol* 2002;134:645–660.

Uemura A, Thomas MA. Subretinal surgery for choroidal neovascularization in patients with high myopia. *Arch Ophthalmol* 2000; 118:344–350.

Verteporfin in Photodynamic Therapy (VIP) Study Group. Verteporfin therapy of subfoveal choroidal neovascularization in pathologic myopia. 2-year results of a randomized clinical trial – VIP report No. 3. *Ophthalmology* 2003;110:667–673.

Vongphanit J, Mitchell P, Wang JJ. Prevalence and progression of myopic retinopathy in an older population. *Ophthalmology* 2002; 109:704–711.

Yoshida T, Ohno-Matsui K, Ohtake Y, et al. Long-term visual prognosis of choroidal neovascularization in high myopia. *Ophthalmology* 2002;109:712–719.

# Cystoid Macular Oedema

Cystoid macular oedema (CMO) is the result of accumulation of fluid in the outer plexiform and inner nuclear layers of the retina with the formation of fluid-filled cyst-like changes. In the short term, CMO is usually innocuous; however, long-standing cases usually lead to coalescence of the microcystic spaces into large cavities and subsequent lamellar hole formation at the fovea with irreversible damage to central vision (Fig. 3.71). CMO is a common and non-specific condition that may occur with any type of macular oedema.

## *Diagnosis*

1. **Presentation** varies with the cause. VA may already be impaired by pre-existing disease such as branch vein occlusion. In other cases without pre-existing disease, such as after cataract surgery, the patient complains of impairment of central vision associated with a positive central scotoma.

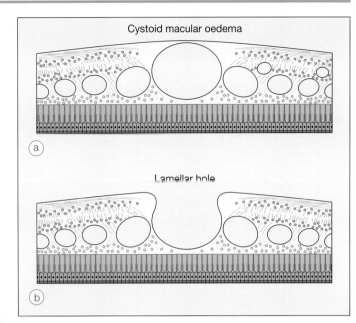

**Figure 3.71** Cystoid macular oedema resulting in lamellar hole formation

2. **Signs**

- Slit-lamp biomicroscopy shows loss of the foveal depression, thickening of the retina and multiple cystoid areas in the sensory retina (Fig. 3.72).
- In early cases, cystoid changes may be difficult to discern and the main finding is a yellow spot at the foveola.

3. **FA**

- The arteriovenous phase shows small hyperfluorescent spots due to early leakage (Fig. 3.73b).
- The late venous phase shows increasing hyperfluorescence and coalescence of the focal leaks (Fig. 3.73c).

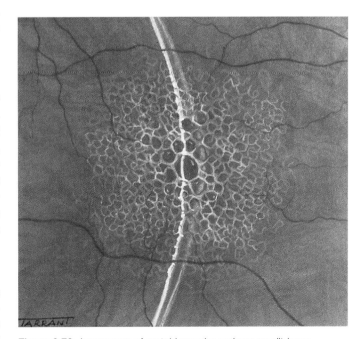

**Figure 3.72** Appearance of cystoid macular oedema on slit-lamp biomicroscopy

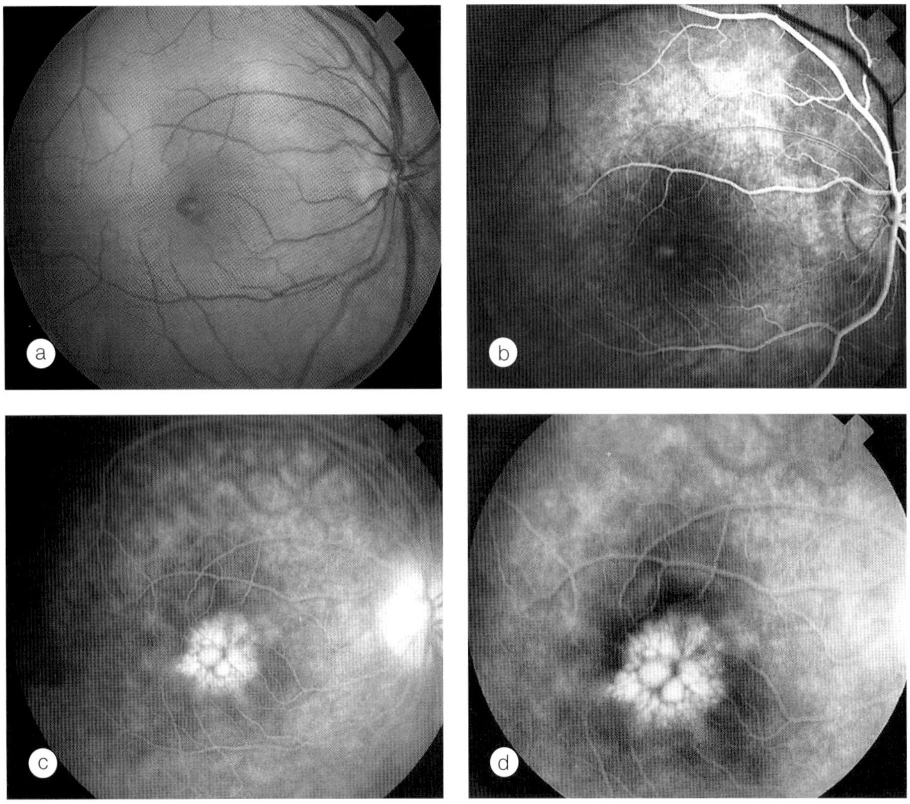

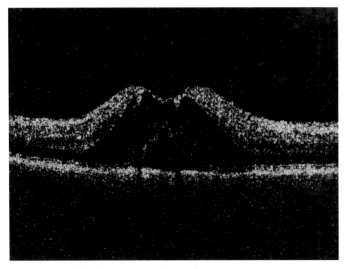

**Figure 3.73 (a)** Cystoid macular oedema; **(b)–(d)** FA (see text)

- The recirculation phase shows a 'flower-petal' pattern of hyperfluorescence (Fig. 3.73d) caused by accumulation of dye within microcystic spaces in the outer plexiform layer of the retina, with its radial arrangement of fibres about the centre of the foveola (Henle layer).

4. **OCT** (Fig. 3.74) may be used to monitor response to treatment.

### Causes and treatment

1. **Retinal vascular disease** (see Chapter 2)

**Figure 3.74** OCT of severe cystoid macular oedema

a. *Causes* include diabetic retinopathy, retinal vein occlusion, idiopathic retinal telangiectasis, retinal artery macroaneurysm and radiation retinopathy.

b. *Treatment* by laser photocoagulation may be appropriate in selected cases.

2. **Intraocular inflammation** (see Chapter 4)

a. *Causes* include intermediate uveitis, birdshot retinochoroidopathy, multifocal choroiditis with panuveitis, toxoplasmosis, cytomegaloviral retinitis, Behçet disease and scleritis.

b. *Treatment* is aimed at controlling the inflammatory process with steroids or immunosuppressive agents. Systemic carbonic anhydrase inhibitors may be beneficial in CMO associated with intermediate uveitis.

3. **Post-cataract surgery.** CMO is rare following uncomplicated surgery, and, when it does occur, spontaneous resolution is the rule.

a. *Risk factors* for visually significant CMO include operative complications such as posterior capsular rupture (Fig. 3.75), vitreous loss and vitreous incarceration into the incision site (Fig. 3.76), anterior chamber intraocu-lar lens (IOL) implantation, secondary IOL implantation, diabetes and a history of CMO in the other eye. Peak incidence is at 6–10 weeks after surgery, although the interval may be much longer.

b. *Treatment* involves correction of the underlying cause, if possible. For example, vitreous incarceration in the anterior segment may be amenable to anterior vitrec-

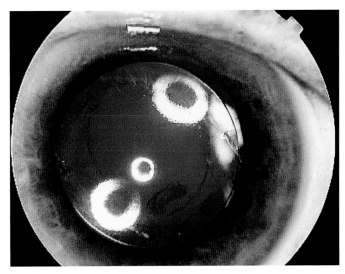

**Figure 3.75** Intraocular implant and a posterior capsular tear

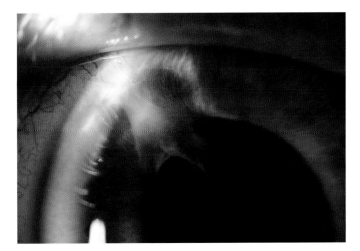

**Figure 3.76** Vitreous incarceration in the incision site following vitreous loss at the time of cataract surgery

tomy or YAG laser disruption of vitreous adhesions. As a last resort, it may be necessary to remove an anterior chamber IOL. If a correctable cause is not present, treatment is difficult, although many cases resolve spontaneously within 6 months. Treatment of persistent CMO involves the following measures:

- Systemic carbonic anhydrase inhibitors.
- Steroids, given topically or by posterior periocular injection, combined with topical non-steroidal anti-inflammatory drugs (NSAIDS) such as ketorolac 0.5% (Acular) administered q.i.d., which may be beneficial even in longstanding and clinically significant CMO. Unfortunately, in many cases CMO recurs when treatment is discontinued, so long-term medication may be required. Intravitreal triamcinolone has recently been reported to reduce CMO in those unresponsive to sub-Tenon injections.

- Pars plana vitrectomy may be useful for CMO refractory to medical therapy, even in eyes without apparent vitreous disturbance.

**4. Other surgical procedures**

a. *Causes* include YAG laser capsulotomy, peripheral retinal cryotherapy and laser photocoagulation. The risk of CMO may be reduced if capsulotomy is delayed for 6 months or more after cataract surgery. Rarely, CMO may develop following scleral buckling, penetrating keratoplasty and glaucoma filtration surgery.

b. *Treatment* is unsatisfactory although the CMO is often mild and self-limited.

**5. Drug-induced**

a. *Causes* include topical adrenaline 2%, especially in the aphakic eye, topical latanoprost and systemic nicotinic acid.

b. *Treatment* involves cessation of medication.

**6. Retinal dystrophies** (see Chapter 4)

a. *Causes* include retinitis pigmentosa, gyrate atrophy and dominantly inherited CMO.

b. *Treatment* with systemic carbonic anhydrase inhibitors may be beneficial in CMO associated with retinitis pigmentosa.

**7. Miscellaneous**

a. *Vitreomacular traction syndrome* is characterised by partial peripheral vitreous separation with persistent posterior attachment to the macula. This results in anteroposterior and tangential traction vectors. Chronic CMO due to anteroposterior traction is common and may respond to vitrectomy.

b. *Macular epiretinal membranes* may occasionally cause CMO by disrupting the perifoveal capillaries. Surgical excision of the membrane may be beneficial in selected cases.

c. *CNV* may be associated with foveal thickening and CMO, the presence of which constitutes an adverse prognostic factor.

## FURTHER READING

Antcliff RJ, Spalton DJ, Stanford MR, et al. Intravitreal triamcinolone for uveitis cystoid macular edema: an optical coherence tomography study. *Ophthalmology* 2001;108:765–772.

Cox SN, Bird AC. Treatment of chronic cystoid macular edema with acetazolamide. *Arch Ophthalmol* 1988;106:1190–1195.

Kent D, Vonores SA, Campocharino PA. Macular oedema: the role of soluble mediators. *Br J Ophthalmol* 2000;84:542–545.

Munera JM, Garcia-Layana A, Maldonaldo MJ, et al. Optical coherence tomography in successful surgery of vitreomacular traction syndrome. *Arch Ophthalmol* 1998;116:1388–1389.

Pendergast SD, Margherio RR, Williams GA, et al. Vitrectomy for chronic pseudophakic cystoid macular edema. *Am J Ophthalmol* 1999;128:317–323.

Rosetti L, Chaudhuri J, Dickersin K. Medical prophylaxis and treatment of cystoid macular edema after cataract surgery: the results of meta-analysis. *Ophthalmology* 1998;105:397–405.

Thach AB, Dugel PU, Findall RJ, et al. A comparison of retrobulbar versus sub-Tenon's corticosteroid injection for cystoid macular edema refractory to topical therapy. *Ophthalmology* 1997;104: 2003–2008.

Ting TD, Oh MO, Cox TA, et al. Decreased visual acuity associated with cystoid macular edema in neovascular age-related macular degeneration. *Arch Ophthalmol* 2002;120:731–737.

Wand M, Shields BM. Cystoid macular edema in the era of ocular hypotensive lipids. *Am J Ophthalmol* 2002;133:393–397.

Weisz JM, Bressler NM, Bressler SB, et al. Ketorolac treatment of pseudophakic cystoid macular edema identified more than 24 months after cataract extraction. *Ophthalmology* 1999;106: 1656–1659.

# Macular Epiretinal Membrane

***Pathogenesis.*** Macular epiretinal membranes that develop at the vitreoretinal interface consist of proliferation of retinal glial cells which have gained access to the retinal surface through breaks in the ILM. It has been postulated that these breaks may be created when the posterior vitreous detaches from the macula. The causes are as follows:

1. **Idiopathic** membranes predominantly affect otherwise healthy elderly individuals and are bilateral in about 10% of cases.

2. **Secondary** membranes may be associated with the following conditions:

   a. *Retinal procedures* such as detachment surgery, photo-coagulation and cryotherapy may either induce or worsen a pre-existing macular epiretinal membrane. Untreated, these membranes usually cause a variable but permanent reduction of vision. Very occasionally, however, the membrane may separate spontaneously from the retina.

   b. *Other* causes include retinal vascular disease, intraocular inflammation and ocular trauma.

> **NB:** The clinical appearance of epiretinal membranes depends on their density and any associated distortion of the retinal vasculature. It is convenient to divide the condition into (a) *cellophane maculopathy* and (b) *macular pucker*.

***Cellophane maculopathy*** consists of a thin layer of epiretinal cells. It is common and usually secondary to a posterior vitreous detachment. If no posterior vitreous detachment is seen, the peripheral retina should be examined carefully to exclude the presence of telangiectatic vessels.

1. **Presentation** may be with mild metamorphopsia, although frequently the condition is asymptomatic and is discovered by chance.

2. **Signs**

   a. *VA* may be normal or slightly reduced.

   b. *Fundus*

   - An irregular light reflex or sheen is present at the macula.
   - The membrane itself is translucent and is best detected using 'red-free' light, but, as it thickens and contracts, it becomes more obvious and may cause distortion of blood vessels (Fig. 3.77a), which is highlighted on FA (Fig. 3.77b).

3. **Treatment** is not appropriate.

***Macular pucker*** is caused by thickening and contraction of the membrane. It is much less common than cellophane maculopathy and may be idiopathic or secondary.

1. **Presentation** is with metamorphopsia and blurring of central vision.

2. **Signs**

   a. *VA* is reduced to 6/12 or worse, depending on severity.

   b. *Fundus*

   - The macula shows severe distortion of the blood vessels, retinal wrinkling and white striae which may obscure underlying blood vessels (Figs. 3.78 and 3.79).
   - Associated findings are macular pseudo-holes within the membrane (Fig. 3.80) and, occasionally, CMO.

3. **Treatment** by surgical removal of the membrane (Fig. 3.81) usually improves or eliminates distortion, and improves VA in about 50% of cases.

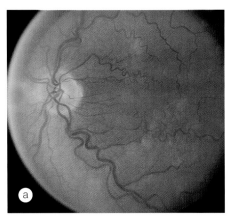
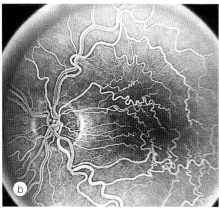

**Figure 3.77** Cellophane maculopathy (see text) (Courtesy of Wilmer Institute)

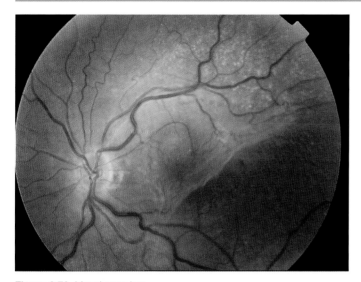

**Figure 3.78** Macular pucker

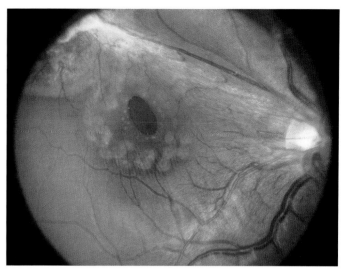

**Figure 3.80** Macular pseudo-hole in an epiretinal membrane

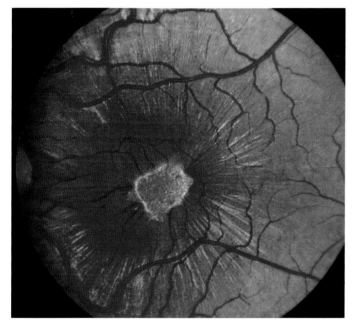

**Figure 3.79** Severe macular pucker

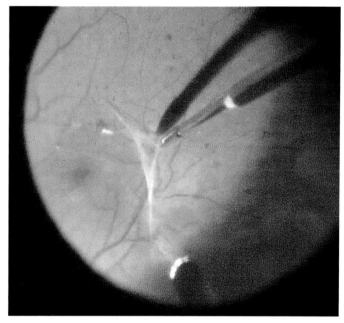

**Figure 3.81** Peeling of an epiretinal membrane

## FURTHER READING

Banaach MJ, Hasasan TS, Cox MS, et al. Clinical course and surgical treatment of macular epiretinal membranes in young subjects. *Ophthalmology* 2001;108:23–26.

Benhamou N, Massin P, Spolaore R, et al. Surgical management of epiretinal membranes in young patients. *Am J Ophthalmol* 2002; 133:358–364.

Fraser-Bell S, Guzowski M, Rochtchina E, et al. Five-year cumulative incidence and progression of epiretinal membranes. The Blue Mountains Eye Study. *Ophthalmology* 2003;110:34–40.

Massin P, Paques M, Masri H, et al. Visual outcomes of surgery for epiretinal membranes with macular pseudoholes. *Ophthalmology* 1999;106:580–585.

Mitchell P, Smith W, Chey T, et al. Prevalence and associations of epiretinal membranes. The Blue Mountains Eye Study, Australia. *Ophthalmology* 1997;104:1033–1040.

Park DW, Dugel PU, Garda J, et al. Macular pucker removal with and without internal limiting membrane peeling: pilot study. *Ophthalmology* 2003;110: 62–64.

Smiddy WE, Maguire AM, Green WR, et al. Idiopathic epiretinal membranes; ultrastructural characteristics and clinicopathologic correlation. *Ophthalmology* 1989;96:811–821.

# Choroidal Folds

***Causes.*** Choroidal folds are parallel grooves or striae involving the inner choroid, Bruch's membrane, the RPE and sometimes the outer sensory retina. Possible mechanisms include choroidal congestion, scleral folding and contraction of Bruch's membrane. The main causes are the following:

1. **Idiopathic** folds may occur for no apparent reason in both eyes of healthy hypermetropic patients with normal or near-normal VA.

2. **Orbital diseases** such as retrobulbar tumours and thyroid ophthalmopathy may cause choroidal folds that impair VA.

3. **Choroidal tumours** such as melanomas may mechanically displace the surrounding choroid and cause folding.

4. **Ocular hypotony** may occur following filtration surgery, particularly if associated with the use of antifibrotic agents. Prolonged very low intraocular pressure (i.e. 5 mmHg or less) may result in maculopathy and choroidal folds.

5. **Miscellaneous** uncommon causes include chronic papilloedema, posterior scleritis and scleral buckle for repair of retinal detachment.

### Diagnosis

1. **Presentation** is often with metamorphopsia although the patient may be asymptomatic. Initially, visual dysfunction is caused by distortion of overlying retinal receptors, but in longstanding cases, permanent changes may develop in the RPE and sensory retina.

2. **Signs**

   a. *VA* may be normal or variably impaired.
   b. *Fundus*

   ● Parallel lines, grooves or striae typically located at the posterior pole. The folds are usually horizontally orientated (Fig. 3.82a) but may be vertical, oblique or irregular.
   ● The crest (elevated portion) of a fold is yellow and less pigmented as a result of stretching and thinning of the RPE and the trough is darker due to compression of the RPE.

3. **FA** shows alternating hyperfluorescent and hypofluorescent streaks at the level of the RPE (Fig. 3.82b). The hyperfluorescence corresponds to the crests as a result of increased background choroidal fluorescence showing through the stretched and thinned RPE, and the hypofluorescence corresponds to the troughs owing to blockage of choroidal fluorescence by the compressed and thickened RPE (Fig. 3.82c).

### FURTHER READING

Cassidy LM, Sanders MD. Choroidal folds and papilloedema. *Br J Ophthalmol* 1999;83:1139–1143.

Fannin LA, Schiffman JC, Budenz DL. Risk factors for hypotony maculopathy. *Ophthalmology* 2003;110:1185–1191.

Griebel SP, Kosmorsky GS. Choroidal folds associated with increased intracranial pressure. *Am J Ophthalmol* 2000;129:513–516.

Leahey AB, Brucker AK, Wyszynski RE, et al. Chorioretinal folds. A comparison of unilateral and bilateral cases. *Arch Ophthalmol* 1993;111:357–359.

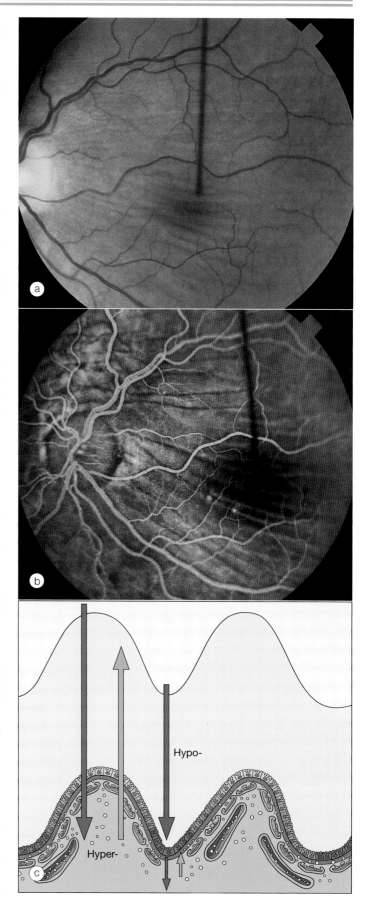

**Figure 3.82** Choroidal folds (see text)

Schubert HD. Postsurgical hypotony: relationship to fistulization, inflammation, chorioretinal lesions, and the vitreous. *Surv Ophthalmol* 1996;41:97–125.

# Vitreomacular Traction Syndrome

1. **Pathogenesis** – persistent attachment of the vitreous at the macula in eyes with incomplete posterior vitreous detachment. The most common morphological configuration is vitreous separation peripheral to a zone where the cortical vitreous remains attached to the retina at the macula and the optic nerve head.

2. **Presentation** is usually in adult life with decreased vision, metamorphopsia, photopsia and micropsia.

3. **Signs**

   - Partial posterior vitreous detachment with persistent attachment of vitreous to the macula.
   - The macula may show retinal surface wrinkling, distortion, an epiretinal membrane or CMO.

NB: Occult vitreomacular traction is best seen on OCT (Figure 3.83).

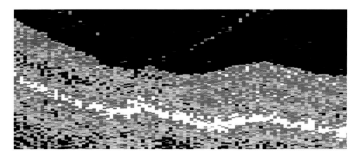

**Figure 3.83** OCT showing vitreomacular traction syndrome

4. **Treatment** involving pars plana vitrectomy to relieve macular traction is often successful.

## FURTHER READING

McDonald HR, Johnson RN, Schatz H. Surgical results in the vitreomacular traction syndrome. *Ophthalmology* 1994;101: 1397–1402.

Melberg NS, Williams DF, Balles MW, et al. Vitrectomy for vitreoretinal traction syndrome with macular detachment. *Retina* 1995; 15:192–197.

Smiddy WE, Michels RG, Glaser BM, et al. Vitrectomy for macular traction caused by incomplete vitreous separation. *Arch Ophthalmol* 1988;106:624–628.

# Angioid Streaks

Angioid streaks are the result of crack-like dehiscences in thickened, calcified and abnormally brittle collagenous and elastic portions of Bruch's membrane with secondary changes in the RPE and choriocapillaris.

## *Diagnosis*

1. **Signs**

   - 'Peau d'orange' (orange skin), consisting of mottled pigmentation of the posterior pole (Fig. 3.84), may occasionally antedate the appearance of angioid streaks.
   - Linear, grey or dark-red linear lesions with irregular serrated edges that lie beneath the normal retinal blood vessels. They may initially be very subtle and easily overlooked (Fig. 3.85) and later become more obvious (Fig. 3.86)

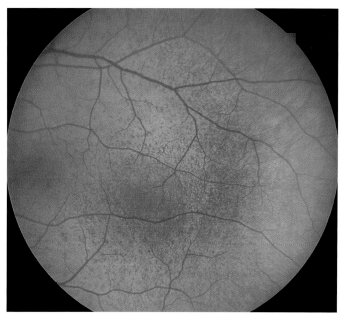

**Figure 3.84** Mottled pigmentation ('peau d'orange')

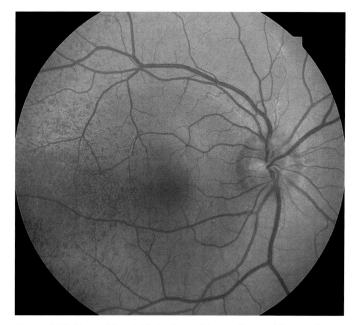

**Figure 3.85** Very mild angioid streaks and 'peau d'orange' temporal to the fovea

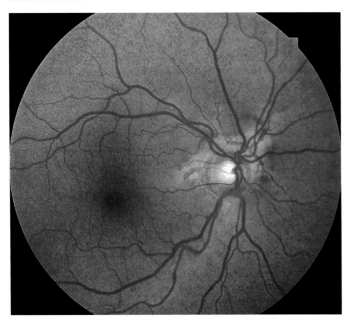

**Figure 3.86** More evident angioid streaks and more extensive 'peau d'orange'

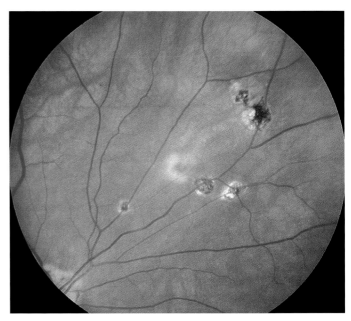

**Figure 3.88** Peripheral chorioretinal scars

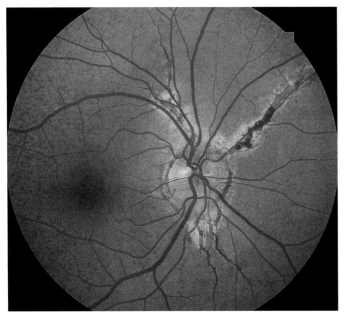

**Figure 3.87** Advanced angioid streaks

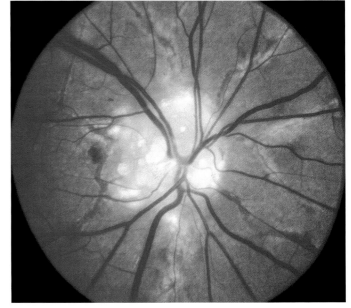

**Figure 3.89** Optic disc drusen in an eye with angioid streaks

- Longstanding streaks develop secondary RPE atrophy or hyperplasia. They intercommunicate in a ring-like fashion around the optic disc and then radiate outwards from the peripapillary area (Fig. 3.87).
- Peripheral, focal chorioretinal scars ('salmon spots') (Fig. 3.88).
- Optic nerve drusen (Fig. 3.89) occur more frequently in eyes with angioid streaks than in those without.

2. **FA** shows hyperfluorescence caused by RPE window defects over the streaks, associated with variable hypofluorescence corresponding to RPE hyperplasia (Fig. 3.90).

***Prognosis*** is guarded because visual impairment occurs in over 70% of patients as a result of one or more of the following:

1. **CNV** is by far the most common cause of visual loss (Fig. 3.91). Conventional thermal laser photocoagulation may be successful in certain juxtafoveal and extrafoveal lesions, although there is a high risk of aggressive recurrence. The results of photodynamic therapy for subfoveal CNV are often disappointing.

2. **Choroidal rupture,** which may occur following relatively trivial ocular trauma and result in a subfoveal haemorrhage (Fig. 3.92) and subsequent scarring (Fig. 3.93).

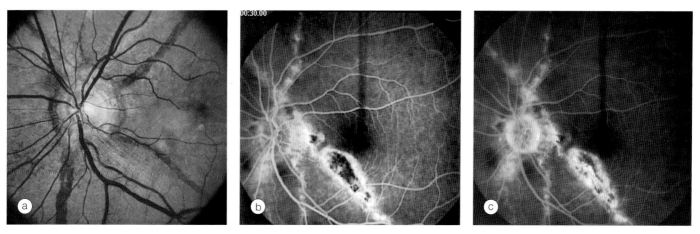

**Figure 3.90** **(a)** Angioid streaks; **(b)** and **(c)** FA (see text)

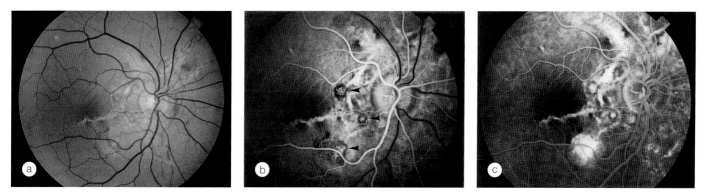

**Figure 3.91** **(a)** Angioid streaks; **(b)** FA arteriovenous phase shows hyperfluorescence of angioid streaks and three round areas of hyperfluorescence (arrows) associated with CNV; **(c)** venous phase shows increase in hyperfluorescence

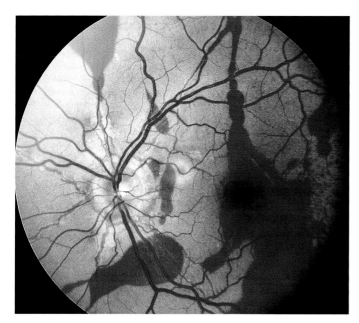

**Figure 3.92** Extensive haemorrhage caused by traumatic choroidal rupture in an eye with angioid streaks

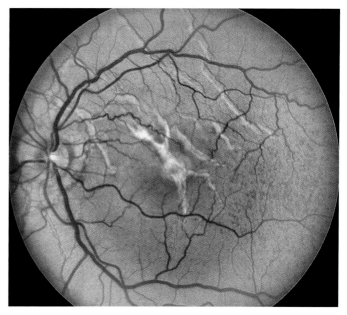

**Figure 3.93** Subretinal scarring following absorption of haemorrhage

Because eyes with angioid streaks are very fragile, patients should be warned against participating in contact sports and advised to use protective spectacles for ball games.

3. **Foveal involvement** by a streak.

***Systemic associations*** are present in approximately 50% of patients with angioid streaks.

1. **Pseudoxanthoma elasticum** (PXE) is by far the most common association of angioid streaks. Approximately 85% of patients develop ocular involvement, usually after the second decade of life. The combination of the two is referred to as 'Groenblad–Strandberg syndrome'. PXE is an uncommon, inherited, generalised disorder of connective tissue. It affects the elastin in the dermis, arterial walls and Bruch's membrane, resulting in abnormal mineralisation and deposition of phosphorus in the fibrils. There are four main types, of which two are dominant and two recessive, with varying severity of systemic and ocular manifestations. The following are the main clinical features of PXE:

   a. *Skin lesions* consist of yellow papules arranged in a linear or reticulate pattern, giving rise to a 'chicken-skin' appearance. The lesions are most frequently located on the neck (Fig. 3.94), antecubital fossae, axillae (Fig. 3.95), groins, and the paraumbilical area (Fig. 3.96). The affected areas of skin are loose (see Fig. 3.94), and may also be delicate and hyperelastic. Occasionally the condition is subclinical and can be diagnosed only by skin biopsy.
   b. *Cardiovascular disease*, which is characterised by accelerated atherosclerosis resulting in coronary artery disease and intermittent claudication, hypertension from renovascular disease, and mitral incompetence.

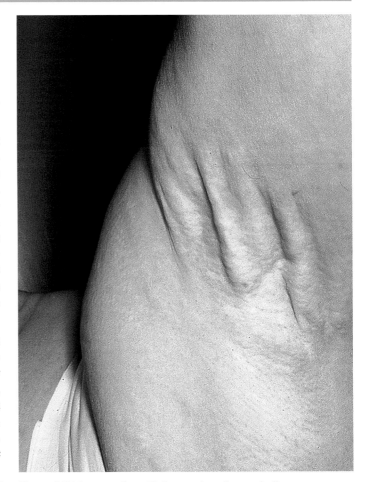

**Figure 3.95** Loose axillary skin in pseudoxanthoma elasticum

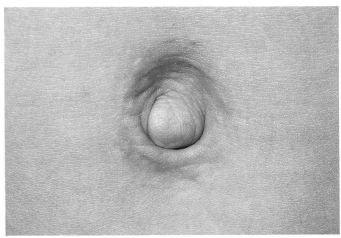

**Figure 3.96** Pseudoxanthoma elasticum involving the paraumbilical skin

   c. *Gastrointestinal haemorrhage*, which may be life threatening, and may occur as early as the first decade of life.

2. **Ehlers–Danlos syndrome type 6** (ocular sclerotic) is a rare, usually autosomal dominant, disorder of collagen caused by deficiency of procollagen lysyl hydroxylase. There are 11 subtypes but only type 6 is associated with ocular features. Systemic features include the following:

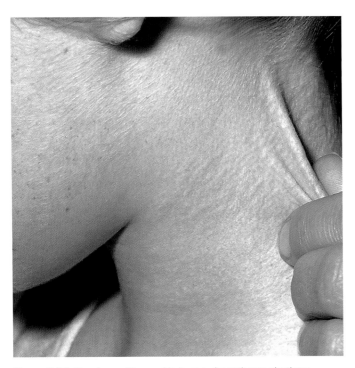

**Figure 3.94** Papules and loose skin in pseudoxanthoma elasticum

a. *The skin* is thin, hyperelastic (Fig. 3.97) and heals poorly.

b. *The joints* are hypermobile with lax ligaments (Fig. 3.98). This may lead to recurrent dislocation, repeated falls, hydroarthrosis and pseudotumour formation over the knees and elbows.

c. *Cardiovascular disease* consists of a bleeding diathesis, dissecting aneurysms, spontaneous rupture of large blood vessels and mitral prolapse.

d. *Other systemic problems* include scoliosis, diaphragmatic hernias and diverticula of the gastrointestinal and respiratory tracts.

e. *Other ocular features* include epicanthic folds, ocular fragility to trauma, keratoconus, high myopia, retinal detachment, blue sclera and lens subluxation.

3. **Paget disease** is a chronic, progressive metabolic bone disease characterised by excessive and disorganised resorption and formation of bone. Angioid streaks are uncommon, occurring in only about 2%. Systemic features include the following:

a. *Bone deformities,* such as enlargement of the skull (Fig. 3.99) and anterior bowing of the tibias (Fig. 3.100).

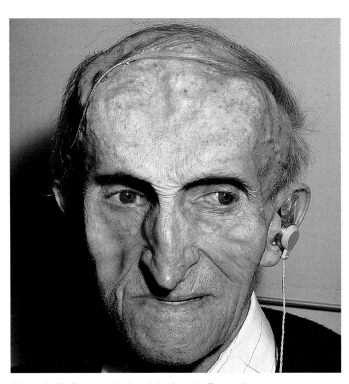

**Figure 3.99** Enlarged skull and deafness in Paget disease

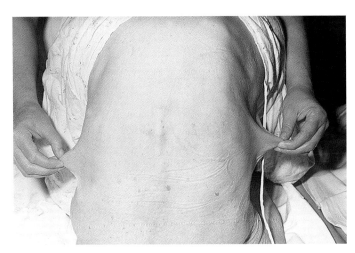

**Figure 3.97** Hyperelastic skin in Ehlers–Danlos syndrome

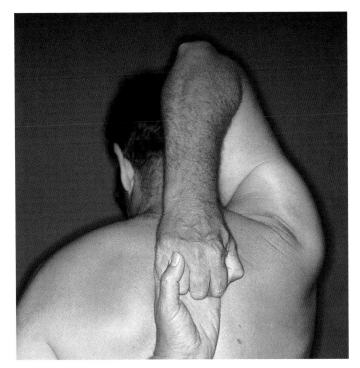

**Figure 3.98** Hypermobile joints in Ehlers–Danlos syndrome

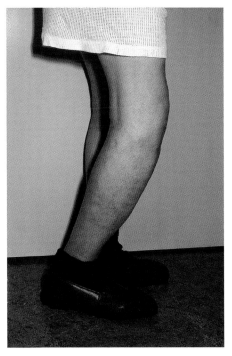

**Figure 3.100** Anterior bowing of the tibias in Paget disease

b. *Systemic complications* include deafness (see Fig. 3.99), arthropathy, kyphoscoliosis, fractures, compression of spinal and cranial nerves, heart failure and increased risk of osteosarcoma.

c. *Other ocular features* include optic atrophy, proptosis and ocular motor nerve palsies.

4. **Haemoglobulinopathies** occasionally associated with angioid streaks are: homozygous sickle-cell disease (HbSS), sickle-cell trait (HbAS), sickle-cell thalassaemia (HbS thalassaemia), sickle-cell haemoglobin C disease (HbSC), haemoglobin H disease (HbH), homozygous beta-thalassaemia major, beta-thalassaemia intermedia and beta-thalassaemia minor.

## FURTHER READING

Clarkson JG, Altman RD. Angioid streaks. *Surv Ophthalmol* 1982; 26:235–246.

Dabbs TR, Skjodt K. Prevalence of angioid streaks and other ocular complications of Paget's disease of bone. *Br J Ophthalmol* 1990; 74:579–582.

Karacorlu M, Karacorlu S, Ozdemir H, et al. Photodynamic therapy with verteporfin for choroidal neovascularization in patients with angioid streaks. *Am J Ophthalmol* 2002;134:360–366.

Lim JI, Bressler NM, Marsh MJ, et al. Laser treatment of choroidal neovascularization in patients with angioid streaks. *Am J Ophthalmol* 1993;116:414–423.

Mansour AM. Systemic associations of angioid streaks. *Ophthalmology* 1993;207:57–61.

Shaikh S, Ruby AL, Williams GA. Photodynamic therapy using verteporfin for choroidal neovascularization in angioid streaks. *Am J Ophthalmol* 2003;135:1–6.

# Idiopathic Choroidal Neovascularisation

Idiopathic CNV is an uncommon condition which affects patients under the age of 50 years. The diagnosis is one of exclusion of other possible associations of CNV such as AMD, angioid streaks, high myopia and presumed ocular histoplasmosis. Idiopathic CNV carries a better visual prognosis than that associated with AMD, and, in some cases, spontaneous resolution may occur. The CNV is of type 2 and lies predominantly above the RPE, often encircled by reactive RPE growth.

## FURTHER READING

Cohen SY, Laroche A, Leguen Y, et al. Etiology of choroidal neovascularization in young patients. *Ophthalmology* 1996;103:1241–1244.

Ho AC, Yannuzzi LA, Pisicano K, et al. The natural history of idiopathic subfoveal neovascularization. *Ophthalmology* 1995; 102:782–789.

Lindblom B, Andersson T. The prognosis of idiopathic choroidal neovascularization in persons younger than 50 years of age. *Ophthalmology* 1998;105:1816–1820.

Macular Photocoagulation Study Group. Krypton laser photocoagulation for idiopathic neovascular lesions. Results of a randomized clinical trial. *Arch Ophthalmol* 1990;108:832–837.

Spaide RF, Martin ML, Slakter J, et al. Treatment of idiopathic subretinal choroidal neovascular lesions using photodynamic therapy with verteporfin. *Am J Ophthalmol* 2002;134:62–68.

# Traumatic Retinopathies

## COMMOTIO RETINAE

1. **Pathogenesis** – concussion of the sensory retina resulting in cloudy swelling.

2. **Signs** – the involved retina has an opaque grey appearance (Fig. 3.101).

3. **Prognosis** in mild cases is good, with spontaneous resolution within a few weeks without sequelae. More severe involvement of the macula (Fig. 3.102) may be asso-ciated with subsequent macular hole formation.

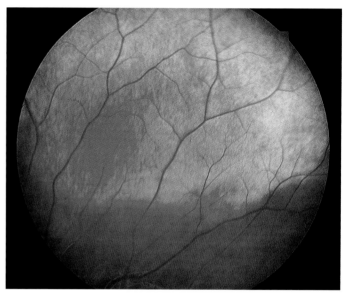

**Figure 3.101** Peripheral commotio retinae

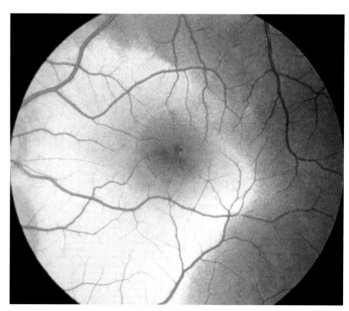

**Figure 3.102** Commotio retinae involving the macula

# CHOROIDAL RUPTURE

**Pathogenesis** – tearing involving the choroid, Bruch's membrane and RPE caused by either blunt or penetrating ocular trauma. Large ruptures may be associated with subretinal haemorrhage and in some cases the blood may break through the ILM and result in subhyaloid or vitreous haemorrhage.

## Diagnosis

1. **Types**

   a. *Direct* ruptures are located anteriorly to the site of impact and oriented parallel to the ora serrata.

   b. *Indirect* ruptures occur opposite the site of impact.

2. **Signs of indirect rupture**

   a. A *fresh* rupture appears as a crescent-shaped, vertical lesion concentric with the optic disc, which frequently involves the macula. Its exact location and extent may be difficult to determine because of masking by subretinal haemorrhage (Fig. 3.103).

   b. *An old* rupture is characterised by a white crescentic streak of exposed sclera (Fig. 3.104).

3. **FA** during the acute stage may not be helpful in showing the severity of the rupture if it is obscured by haemorrhage (Fig. 3.105b and 3.105c).

4. **ICG** may show the extent of the lesion.

**Prognosis** depends on the absence or presence (Fig. 3.106) of foveal involvement. An uncommon late complication is secondary CNV, which may result in bleeding and further visual deterioration.

# VALSALVA RETINOPATHY

1. **Pathogenesis** – transmission of a sudden and severe increase in intrathoracic or intra-abdominal pressure to the eye, resulting in intraocular bleeding.

2. **Signs** – small, unilateral or bilateral, macular haemorrhages which are most frequently preretinal (Fig. 3.107).

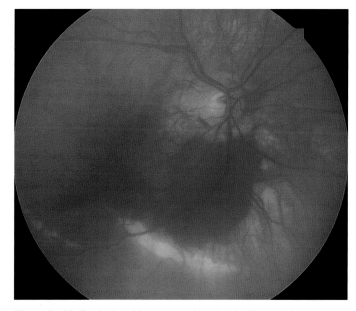

**Figure 3.103** Fresh choroidal rupture with subretinal haemorrhage

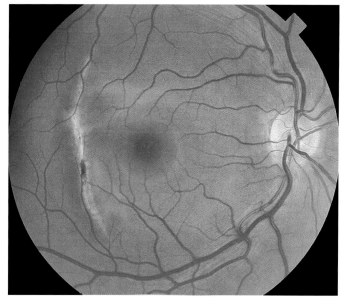

**Figure 3.104** Old choroidal rupture not involving the fovea

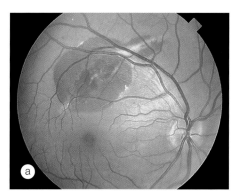
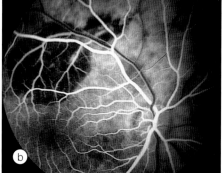
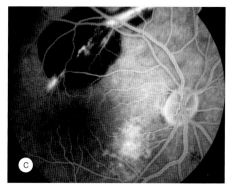

**Figure 3.105** **(a)** Acute choroidal rupture and haemorrhage; **(b)** and **(c)** FA shows hypofluorescence of the rupture due to an RPE window defect and hypofluorescence due to blockage by blood

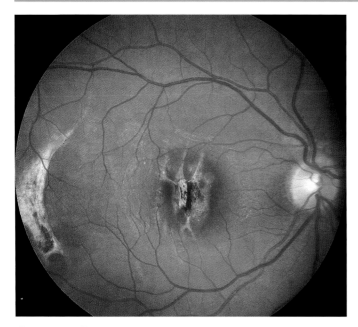

**Figure 3.106** Two old choroidal ruptures, one of which is involving the fovea

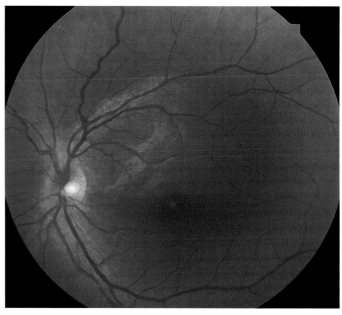

**Figure 3.108** Small yellow foveolar spot in early solar maculopathy

3. **Prognosis** is excellent, with spontaneous resolution without sequelae the usual outcome.

## SOLAR RETINOPATHY

1. **Pathogenesis** – retinal injury caused by photochemical effects of solar radiation as a result of directly or indirectly viewing the sun (eclipse retinopathy).

2. **Presentation** is within 1–4 hours of solar exposure with unilateral or bilateral impairment of central vision, metamorphopsia or central scotomas.

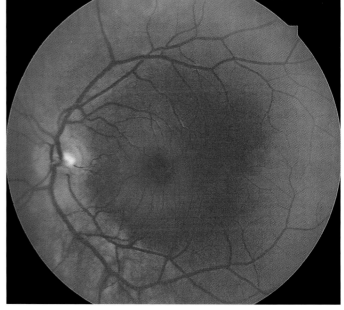

**Figure 3.109** Mild RPE mottling in late solar maculopathy

3. **Signs**

   *a.* *VA* is variable according to the extent of damage.
   *b.* *Fundus*

   - Initially there are small, unilateral or bilateral, yellow foveolar spots with a grey margin (Fig. 3.108).
   - This is followed about 2 weeks later by circumscribed RPE mottling (Fig. 3.109) or a lamellar hole.

4. **Treatment** is not available; systemic steroids have no proven benefit.

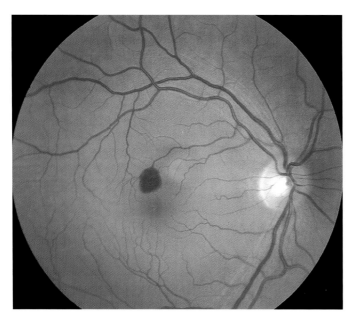

**Figure 3.107** Valsalva retinopathy

**5. Prognosis** is good in most cases, with improvement of VA to normal or near-normal levels within 6 months, although mild symptoms may persist.

## FURTHER READING

Aguilar JP, Green WR. Choroidal rupture: a histopathologic study of 47 cases. *Retina* 1984;4:269–275.

Kempster RC, Green WR, Finkelstein D. Choroidal rupture: clinico-pathologic correlation of an unusual case. *Retina* 1996;16:57–63.

Kohno T, Miki T, Hayashi K. Choroidopathy after blunt trauma to the eye; a fluorescein and indocyanine green angiographic study. *Am J Ophthalmol* 1998; 126:248–260.

Kohno T, Miki T, Shiraki K, et al. Indocyanine green angiographic features of choroidal rupture and choroidal vascular injury after contusion ocular injury. *Am J Ophthalmol* 2000;129:38–46.

Yannuzzi LA, Fisher YL, Krueger A, et al. Solar retinopathy; a photo-biological and geophysical analysis. *Trans Am Ophthalmol Soc* 1987;85:120–128.

# Toxic Retinopathies

## ANTIMALARIALS

Chloroqine (Nivaquine, Avlocor) and hydroxychloroquine (Plaquenil) are quinolone antimalarial drugs which are used in the prophylaxis and treatment of malaria as well as in the treatment of certain rheumatological disorders (e.g. rheumatoid arthritis, juvenile chronic arthritis, systemic lupus erythematosus). The use of chloroquine has also been advocated in the treatment of calcium abnormalities associated with sarcoidosis. Antimalarials are excreted from the body very slowly and are melanotropic drugs that become concentrated in melanin-containing structures of the eye such as the RPE and choroid. The two main ocular side effects of antimalarials are retinotoxicity and corneal deposits. Although uncommon, the retinal changes are potentially serious, but the corneal changes (vortex keratopathy), which are extremely common, are innocuous (Fig. 3.110).

**1. Chloroquine** retinotoxicity is related to the total cumulative dose. The normal daily dose is 250 mg; a cumulative dose of less than 100 g or treatment duration under 1 year is rarely associated with retinal damage. The risk of toxicity increases significantly when the cumulative dose exceeds 300 g (i.e. 250 mg daily for 3 years). However, there have been reports of patients receiving cumulative doses exceeding 1000 g who did not develop retinotoxicity. If possible, chloroquine should be used only if other agents are ineffective.

**2. Hydroxychloroquine** is much safer than chloroquine and if the daily dose does not exceed 400 mg the risk of retinotoxicity is negligible. Physicians should therefore be encouraged to use hydroxychloroquine instead of chloroquine whenever possible.

***Clinical features*** of chloroquine maculopathy can be divided into the following stages:

**1. Premaculopathy** is characterised by normal VA and a scotoma to a red target located between 4° and 9° from fixation. Amsler grid testing may also show a defect. However, the most sensitive test is assessment of colour vision to detect both mild blue–yellow and protan red–green defects. The two most sensitive tests for detecting these defects are the Adams Desaturation-15 test and the American Optical Hardy–Rand–Rittler test. Other colour vision tests such as the Ishihara do not appear to be as sensitive. If the drug is discontinued, visual function usually returns to normal.

**2. Early maculopathy** is the next stage if treatment is not discontinued. It is characterised by a modest reduction of VA (6/9–6/12). Fundus examination shows a subtle 'bull's eye' macular lesion characterised by central foveolar pigmentation surrounded by a depigmented zone of RPE atrophy which is itself encircled by a hyperpigmented ring (Fig. 3.111a). The lesion may be more obvious on FA than on ophthalmoscopy because the RPE atrophy gives rise to an RPE 'window' defect (Fig. 3.111b and c). This stage may progress even if the drug is stopped.

**3. Moderate maculopathy** is characterised by moderate reduction of VA (6/18–6/24) and an obvious 'bull's eye' macular lesion (Fig. 3.112).

**4. Severe maculopathy** is characterised by marked reduction of VA (6/36–6/60) with widespread RPE atrophy surrounding the fovea (Fig. 3.113).

**5. End-stage maculopathy** is characterised by severe reduction of VA and marked atrophy of the RPE with unmasking of the larger choroidal blood vessels (Fig. 3.114). The retinal arterioles may also become attenuated and pigment clumps develop in the peripheral retina.

***Screening*** of patients routinely on hydroxychloroquine is unnecessary. In clinical practice, chloroquine can also be administered safely to patients without the need for repetitive routine examinations by ophthalmologists or the use of complicated tests. Recording of VA and ophthalmoscopy by the prescribing doctor is all that is required. The patient can be given an Amsler grid to use once a week. If symptoms occur

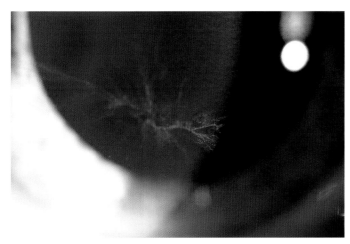

**Figure 3.110** Vortex keratopathy

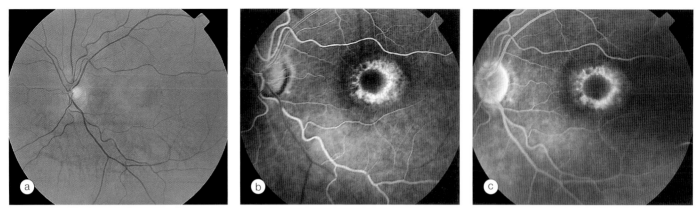

**Figure 3.111** **(a)** Mild chloroquine maculopathy; **(b)** and **(c)** FA shows a ring of hyperfluorescence due to an RPE window defect

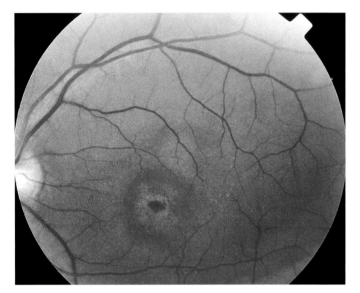

**Figure 3.112** Moderately severe chloroquine maculopathy

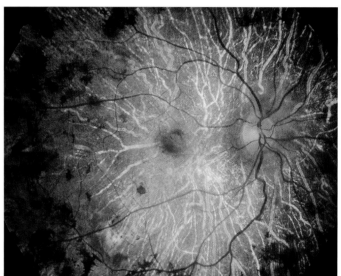

**Figure 3.114** End-stage chloroquine maculopathy

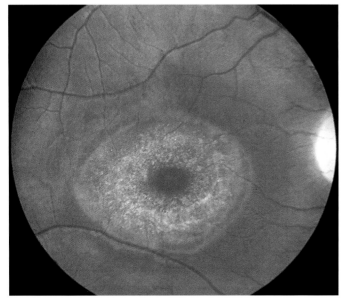

**Figure 3.113** Severe chloroquine maculopathy

or an abnormality is found, then the opinion of an ophthalmologist should be sought. The ophthalmologist can, if necessary, perform more sophisticated tests such as visual fields, macular threshold, colour vision testing as described above, contrast sensitivity, FA and electro-oculography (EOG).

## PHENOTHIAZINES

1. **Thioridazine** (Melleril) is used to treat schizophrenia and related psychoses. The normal daily dose is 150–600 mg. Doses that exceed 800 mg/day for just a few weeks may be sufficient to cause reduced VA and impairment of dark adaptation. The clinical signs of progressive retinotoxicity are as follows:

   - Salt-and-pepper pigmentary disturbance involving the mid-periphery and posterior pole.
   - Plaque-like pigmentation and focal loss of the RPE and choriocapillaris (Fig. 3.115).
   - Diffuse loss of the RPE and choriocapillaris (Fig. 3.116).

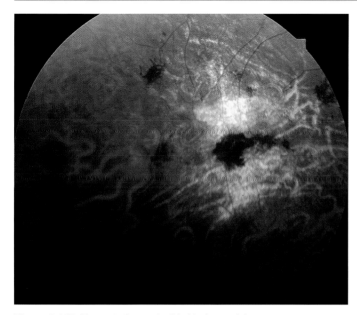

**Figure 3.115** Pigment plaques in thioridazine toxicity

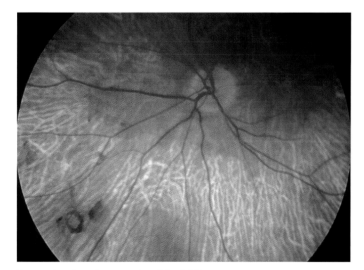

**Figure 3.116** Diffuse atrophy of the RPE and choriocapillaris in severe thioridazine toxicity

2. **Chlorpromazine** (Largactil) is used as a sedative and to treat schizophrenia. The normal daily dose is 75–300 mg. Retinotoxicity may occur if very much larger doses are used over a prolonged period. It is characterised by non-specific pigmentary granularity and clumping. Other, innocuous, ocular side effects include yellowish-brown granules on the anterior lens capsule and corneal endothelial deposits.

## CRYSTALLINE MACULOPATHIES

1. **Tamoxifen** (Nolvodex, Emblon, Noltan and Tamofen) is a specific anti-oestrogen used in the treatment of selected patients with breast carcinoma. It has few systemic side effects and ocular complications are uncommon. The normal daily dose is 20–40 mg. Retinotoxicity may develop in some patients on higher doses and rarely in patients on normal doses. It is characterised by bilateral, yellow, crystalline, ring-like macular deposits (Fig. 3.117). Other rare ocular side effects are vortex keratopathy (see Fig. 3.110) and optic neuritis, which are reversible on cessation of therapy.

2. **Canthaxanthin** is a carotenoid used to enhance sun tanning. If used over prolonged periods of time, it may cause the deposition of bilateral, tiny, glistening, yellow deposits, arranged symmetrically in a doughnut shape at the posterior poles (Fig. 3.118). The deposits are located in the superficial retina and are innocuous.

3. **Methoxyflurate** (Penthrane) is an inhalant general anaesthetic. It is metabolised to oxalic acid, which combines with calcium to form an insoluble salt that is deposited in tissues including the RPE. Prolonged administration may lead to renal failure and secondary hyperoxalosis. It may also result in the formation of innocuous crystals within the retinal vasculature.

4. **Nitroflurantoin** is an antibiotic used in the treatment of urinary tract infections. Retinal changes similar to those seen with canthaxanthin have been reported.

> NB: Other causes of macular crystals include: primary hyperoxaluria, Bietti dystrophy, cystinosis, Sjögren–Larsson syndrome and West African crystalline maculopathy.

## MISCELLANEOUS AGENTS

1. **Interferon retinopathy.** Interferon-alpha is an agent currently used in a variety of systemic conditions, including Kaposi sarcoma, haemangioma in infancy, high-risk cutaneous melanomas, metastatic renal cell carcinoma, leukaemia, lymphoma and chronic hepatitis C. Systemic adverse effects include constitutional symptoms, neutro-

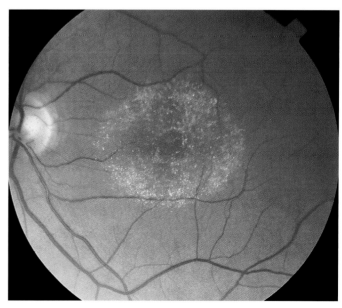

**Figure 3.117** Tamoxifen maculopathy (Courtesy of J. Salmon)

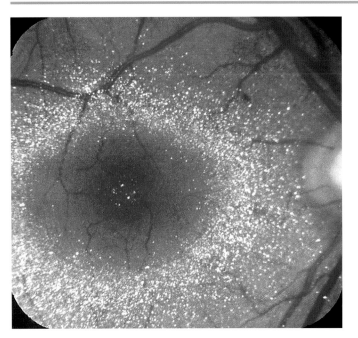

**Figure 3.118** Canthaxanthin maculopathy

penia and thrombocytopenia. Retinopathy characterised by cotton-wool spots and intraretinal haemorrhages may develop in some patients, particularly those on high-dose therapy. The condition usually resolves spontaneously with cessation of therapy and in the majority of patients the visual prognosis is good. Less common ocular side effects include cystoid macular oedema, oculomotor nerve palsy, optic disc oedema, and retinal vein occlusion.

2. **Desferrioxamine** mesylate is an iron chelator used in the treatment of chronic iron overload, to prevent haemosiderosis, in patients with haematological conditions requiring regular transfusion. It is most commonly administered as a slow subcutaneous infusion. Retinopathy is characterised by macular and/or equatorial pigmentary degeneration associated with reduced amplitudes on the electroretinogram (ERG) and reduced EOG light-peak to dark-trough ratios.

3. **Nicotinic acid** (Niacin), a cholesterol-lowering agent, has a number of side effects, including cutaneous flushing, pruritus, nausea and abdominal pain. A small minority of patients develop cystoid maculopathy suggestive of cystoid macular oedema but without leakage on FA. The macular changes cause a mild reduction of VA and occur when doses greater than 1.5 g daily are used, but resolve with discontinuation of the drug.

4. **Gentamicin** may cause severe retinal ischaemia when injected intravitreally for the treatment of bacterial endophthalmitis (Fig. 3.119). Rarely, retinal toxicity may result from periocular injection.

## HIGH-ALTITUDE RETINOPATHY

1. **Systemic features** include progressive severe headache, followed by impaired cortical function and judgement, irrationality, projectile vomiting, diplopia, ataxia and coma. Pulmonary oedema may be rapidly life threatening.

2. **Ocular features,** in chronological order:

   - Mild venous dilatation and a few small retinal haemorrhages.
   - Progression of venous dilatation and large retinal haemorrhages.
   - Severe venous dilatation and multiple large retinal haemorrhages.
   - Venous engorgement, vitreous haemorrhage and papilloedema.

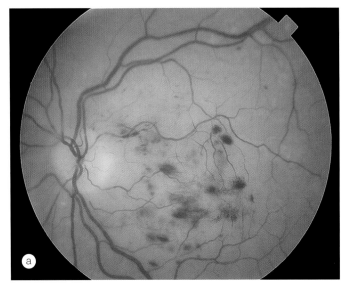
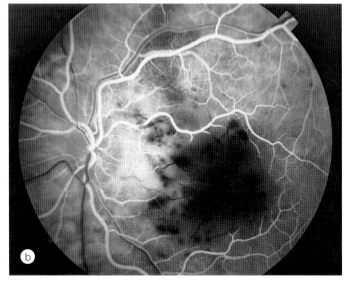

**Figure 3.119** Macular ischaemia following intravitreal gentamicin injection. **(a)** Pallor and haemorrhages at the posterior pole; **(b)** FA shows hypofluorescence due to ischaemia

## FURTHER READING

Block JA. Hydroxychloroquine and retinal safety. *Lancet* 1998; 315:771.

Blyth C, Lane C. Hydroxychloroquine retinopathy: is screening necessary? *BMJ* 1998:916:710–717.

Browning DJ. Hydroxychloroquine and chloroquine retinopathy: screening for drug toxicity. *Am J Ophthalmol* 2002;133:649–656.

Coyle JT. Hydroxychloroquine retinopathy. *Ophthalmology* 2001; 108:243–244.

Esmaeli B, Koller C, Papadopoulos N, et al. Interferon-induced retinopathy in asymptomatic cancer patients. *Ophthalmology* 2001;108:858–860.

Fielder A, Graham E, Jones S, et al. Royal College of Ophthalmologist guidelines: ocular toxicity and hydroxychloroquine. *Eye* 1998; 12:907–909.

Gorin MB, Day R, Costantino JP, et al. Long-term tamoxifen citrate use and potential ocular toxicity. *Am J Ophthalmol* 1998;125: 493–501.

Haimovici R, D'Amico DJ, Gragoudas ES, et al. The expanded clinical spectrum of desferrioxamine retinopathy. *Ophthalmology* 2002;109:164–171.

Hejny C, Sternberg P Jr, Lawson DH, et al. Retinopathy associated with high-dose interferon alpha-2b therapy. *Am J Ophthalmol* 2001;131:782–787.

Noureddin BN, Seoud M, Bashshur Z, et al. Ocular toxicity in low-dose tamoxifen: a prospective study. *Eye* 1999;13:729–733.

Schulman JA, Liang C, Kooragayala LM, et al. Posterior segment complications in patients with hepatitis C treated with interferon and ribavirin. *Ophthalmology* 2003;110:437–442.

Spirin MJ, Warren FA, Guyer DR, et al. Optical coherence tomography findings in nicotinic acid maculopathy. *Am J Ophthalmol* 2003;135:913–914.

Tang R, Shields J, Schiffman J, et al. Retinal changes associated with tamoxifen treatment for breast cancer. *Eye* 1997;11:295–297.

Tokai R, Ikeda T, Miyaura T, et al. Interferon associated retino-pathy and cystoid macular edema. *Arch Ophthalmol* 2001;119: 1077–1079.

Vu LBL, Easterbrook M, Hovis JK. Detection of color vision defects in chloroquine retinopathy. *Ophthalmology* 1999;106:1799–1804.

Wiedman M, Tabin GC. High-altitude retinopathy and altitude illness. *Ophthalmology* 1999;106:1924–1927.

# Cancer-associated Retinopathy

Cancer-associated retinopathy (CAR) is a rare autoimmune photoreceptor destruction in which patients develop visual disturbances in the absence of ocular metastases or involvement of the visual pathways. CAR primarily occurs in patients with small-cell bronchial carcinoma and occasionally with other epithelial tumours. In 50% of cases, CAR is the initial manifestation of the underlying malignancy.

### Diagnosis

1. **Presentation** is with gradual-onset dimming of vision associated with shimmering photopsia, bizarre visual images and night-blindness.

2. **Signs**
   - The fundus may appear normal or show bilateral arteriolar attenuation (Fig. 3.120) and occasionally optic atrophy (Fig. 3.121).

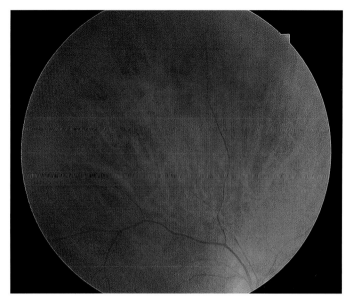

**Figure 3.120** Arteriolar attenuation in cancer-associated retinopathy

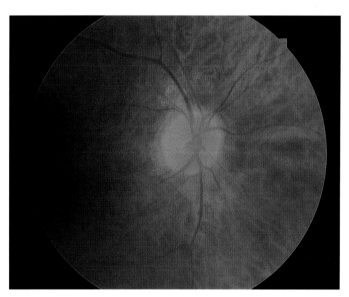

**Figure 3.121** Arteriolar attenuation and mild optic atrophy in cancer-associated retinopathy

   - Other signs include bilateral ring-like scotomas, other visual field defects and dyschromatopsia.

3. **ERG** is subnormal and may become extinct.

***Treatment*** options include systemic steroids, intravenous immunoglobulins and plasmapheresis, but the prognosis is poor.

> **NB:** Melanoma-associated retinopathy (MAR) is a similar condition except that it tends to occur years after treatment of cutaneous melanoma and is usually associated with clinical metastatic disease.

# Chapter 4

# INFLAMMATORY DISEASES

# NON-INFECTIOUS SYSTEMIC DISEASES

## Sarcoidosis

### SYSTEMIC FEATURES

Sarcoidosis is an idiopathic, multisystem, granulomatous inflammatory disorder, more common in patients of African descent than in Caucasians.

### *Presentation*

1. **Acute-onset** sarcoidosis typically occurs during the third decade:

   - Lofgren syndrome is characterised by fever, erythema nodosum (Fig. 4.1), bilateral hilar lymphadenopathy (Fig. 4.2) and frequently arthralgia.

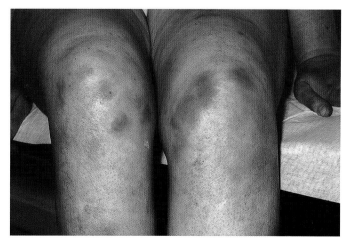

**Figure 4.1** Erythema nodosum

133

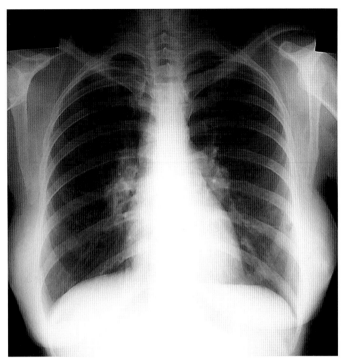

**Figure 4.2** Bilateral hilar lymphadenopathy in acute sarcoidosis

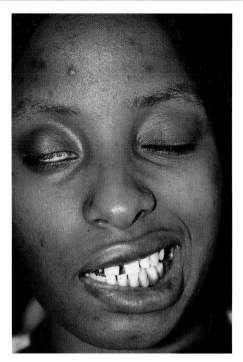

**Figure 4.3** Right facial nerve palsy

- Heerfordt syndrome (uveoparotid fever) is characterised by fever, parotid gland enlargement and uveitis.
- Seventh-nerve palsy (Fig. 4.3) may be associated with other neurological features.

2. **Insidious-onset** sarcoidosis typically occurs during the fifth decade, with fatigue, dyspnoea, and arthralgia.

### Signs

1. **Pulmonary** involvement is present in 90% of patients and varies in severity from asymptomatic bilateral hilar lymphadenopathy to progressive pulmonary fibrosis and bronchiectasis.

2. **Skin** manifestations include erythema nodosum, granulomas (Fig. 4.4) and lupus pernio; the latter is characterised by indurated, purple-blue lesions (Fig. 4.5).

3. **Neurological** features include cranial nerve palsies (particularly facial), meningeal infiltration, and intracranial and intraspinal granulomas.

4. **Other** lesions may involve the reticuloendothelial system, liver, kidneys, bone and heart.

### Diagnostic tests

1. **Chest radiographs** are abnormal in 90% of cases.

2. **Biopsy**

- Of the lungs gives the greatest yield (90%).
- Of the conjunctiva is positive in about 70% of patients in the presence of a visible conjunctival nodule.
- Of lacrimal glands is positive in 25% of un-enlarged and 75% of enlarged glands.

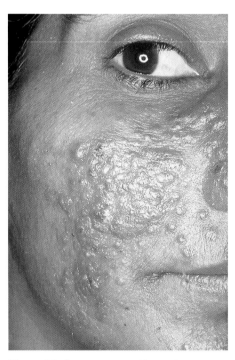

**Figure 4.4** Cutaneous sarcoid granulomas

3. **Serum angiotensin-converting enzyme** (ACE) is elevated in patients with active disease but normal during remissions. The normal serum level in adults is 32.1 +/– 8.5 IU. In children it is higher and diagnostically less useful. In patients with suspected neurosarcoid, ACE can be measured in the cerebrospinal fluid. ACE may also be elevated in other conditions such as tuberculosis, lymphoma and asbestosis.

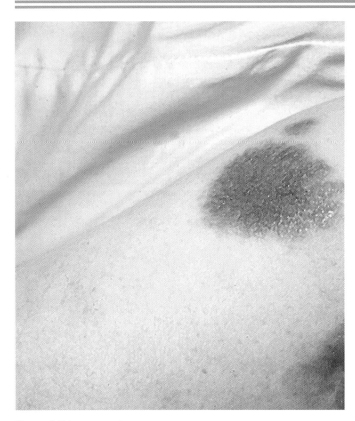

**Figure 4.5** Lupus pernio

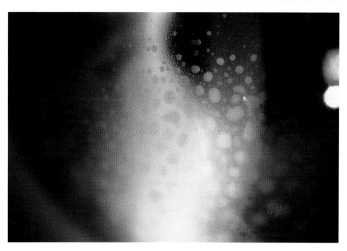

**Figure 4.6** Mutton fat keratic precipitates in sarcoid granulomatous anterior uveitis

4. **Bronchoalveolar lavage** shows a raised proportion of activated T-helper lymphocytes. Sputum examination may also show increased CD4/CD8 ratios.

5. **Pulmonary function tests** reveal a restrictive lung defect with reduced total lung capacity and are very useful for monitoring purposes and indication for systemic therapy.

## OCULAR FEATURES

### Anterior uveitis

1. **Acute** anterior uveitis typically affects patients with acute-onset sarcoid. It can usually be controlled by topical treatment with steroids and mydriatics.

2. **Chronic granulomatous** anterior uveitis typically affects older patients with chronic lung disease. The inflammation is characterised by mutton fat keratic precipitates (Fig. 4.6) and iris nodules (Fig. 4.7). Treatment is initially topical but frequently periocular or systemic steroid administration is required. If severe and longstanding, it may lead to secondary cataract, glaucoma, band keratopathy and cystoid macular oedema (CMO).

**Intermediate uveitis** is relatively uncommon. It is characterised by vitreous inflammation and snowball opacities (Fig. 4.8). Treatment is usually only necessary in case of visual symptoms, usually due to vitreous debris or CMO. Posterior sub-Tenon injection of steroids (Fig. 4.9) is usually the first line of therapy for unilateral or mild bilateral cases. Because some patients with sarcoidosis may not have systemic symptoms, it is important to rule out the possibility in patients with presumed idiopathic intermediate uveitis.

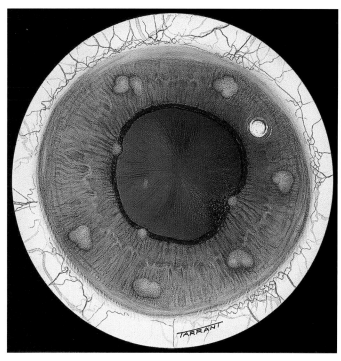

**Figure 4.7** Iris nodules: Koeppe are small and on the pupillary border; Bussaca are larger and more peripheral

**Posterior segment involvement** is seen in about 25% of patients with ocular sarcoid and usually requires systemic steroid therapy. The following lesions may be seen.

1. **Retinal periphlebitis** is characterised by perivenous sheathing (Fig. 4.10), which, if severe, may be associated with perivenous exudates referred to as 'candlewax drippings' (Fig. 4.11). Occasionally, severe periphlebitis may result in branch retinal vein occlusion. Although acute lesions may resolve spontaneously or with the use of systemic steroids, vascular sheathing, once established, usually persists.

2. **Choroidal involvement**

   a. *Choroidal granulomas* may take the following forms:

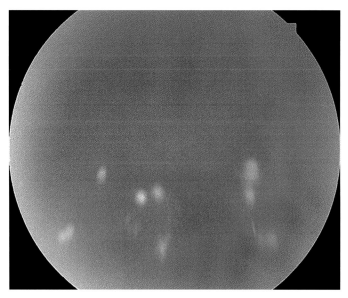

**Figure 4.8** Snowball vitreous opacities in sarcoid intermediate uveitis

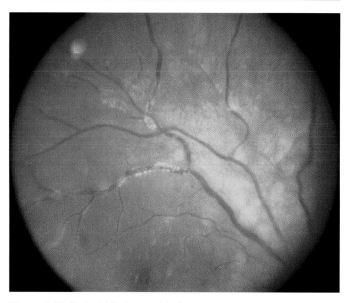

**Figure 4.10** Periphlebitis in sarcoidosis

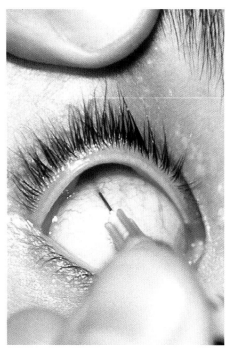

**Figure 4.9** Technique of posterior sub-Tenon steroid injection for intermediate uveitis

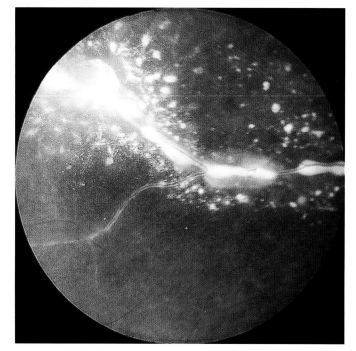

**Figure 4.11** 'Candlewax drippings' in sarcoidosis

- Multiple, small, pale-yellow, infiltrates are common (Fig. 4.12).
- Larger, confluent infiltrates with amoeboid (Fig. 4.13) or geographic outlines are less common (Fig. 4.14).
- Solitary granulomas are uncommon (Fig. 4.15).

b. *Multifocal choroiditis,* which may result in visual loss if associated with secondary choroidal neovascular membranes at the macula.

3. **Retinal granulomas** are small, discrete, yellow lesions (Fig. 4.16).

4. **Preretinal granulomas** are also uncommon and are typically located inferiorly anterior to the equator (Landers sign) (Fig. 4.17).

5. **Peripheral retinal neovascularisation** may occur, and in black patients may be mistaken for proliferative sickle-cell retinopathy (see Chapter 2).

6. **Optic nerve** involvement may take the following forms:

a. *Focal granulomas,* which do not usually affect vision (Fig. 4.18).

b. *Optic neuritis.*

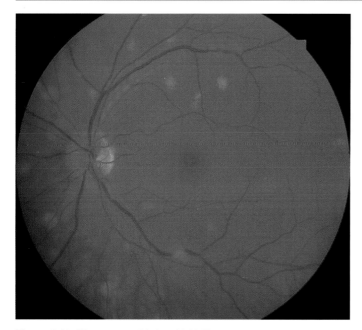

**Figure 4.12** Discrete sarcoid choroidal infiltrates

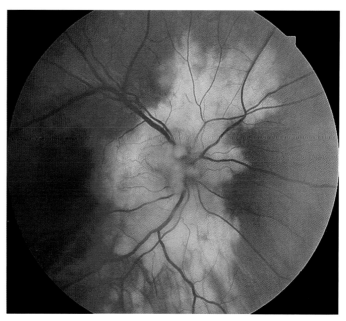

**Figure 4.14** Extensive geographic peripapillary sarcoid infiltration

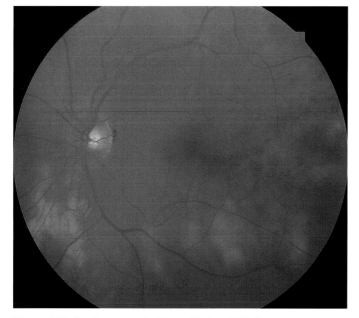

**Figure 4.13** Confluent amoeboid sarcoid choroidal infiltrates

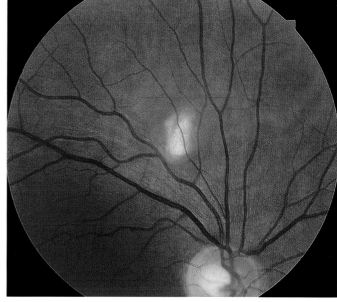

**Figure 4.15** Solitary choroidal sarcoid granuloma

c. *Papilloedema,* which is usually secondary to involvement of the central nervous system (CNS), may occur in the absence of other eye lesions.

d. *Persistent disc oedema* may be seen in association with retinal or vitreous involvement.

## *Differential diagnosis of posterior segment sarcoid*

### 1. Small choroidal lesions

- Multifocal choroiditis with panuveitis.
- Birdshot chorioretinopathy.
- Tuberculosis.

### 2. Large choroidal infiltrates

- Metastatic tumour.
- Large-cell lymphoma.
- Harada disease.
- Serpiginous choroidopathy.

### 3. Periphlebitis

- Tuberculosis.
- Behçet disease.
- Cytomegalovirus retinitis.
- Cat-scratch disease.

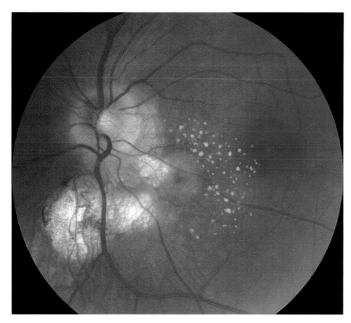

**Figure 4.16** Retinal sarcoid granulomas at the posterior pole and an inferior juxtapapillary chorioretinal scar due to previous choroiditis

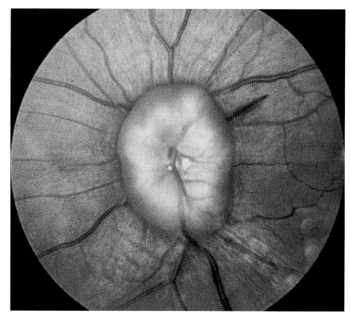

**Figure 4.18** Optic disc sarcoid granuloma (Courtesy of Wilmer Institute)

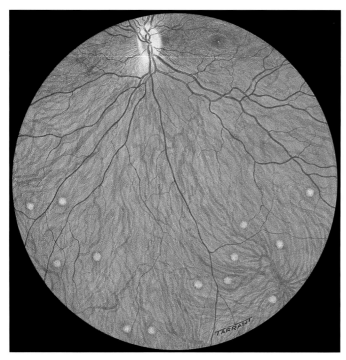

**Figure 4.17** Peripheral preretinal sarcoid granulomas (Landers sign)

## FURTHER READING

Dana M-R, Merayo-Lloves J, Schaumberg DA, et al. Prognosticators for visual outcome in sarcoid uveitis. *Ophthalmology* 1999; 103:1846–1853.

Dev S, McCallum RM, Jaffe GJ. Methotrexate treatment for sarcoid-associated panuveitis. *Ophthalmology* 1999;106:111–118.

Edelsten C, Pearson A, Joyles E, et al. The ocular and systemic prognosis of patients presenting with sarcoid uveitis. *Eye* 1999;13:748–753.

Power WJ, Neves RA, Rodriguez A, et al. The value of combined serum angiotensin-conversion enzyme and gallium scan in the diagnosis of ocular sarcoidosis. *Ophthalmology* 1995;102:2007–2011.

Rothova A. Ocular involvement in sarcoidosis. *Br J Ophthalmol* 2000;84:110–116.

Stavrou P, Linton S, Young DW, et al. Clinical diagnosis of ocular sarcoid. *Eye* 1997;11:365–370.

# Behçet Disease

## SYSTEMIC FEATURES

Behçet disease (BD) is an idiopathic, recurrent, multisystem, inflammatory vasculitis. It typically affects young men from the eastern Mediterranean region and Japan. The disease is strongly associated with human leukocyte antigen (HLA) B51 in different ethnic groups. However, it has not yet been clarified whether the HLA-B51 gene itself is the pathogenic gene related to BD or whether some other gene is in linkage disequilibrium with HLA-B51.

**Presentation** is in the third to fourth decades with localised lesions such as aphthous ulceration.

### Diagnostic criteria

1. **Recurrent oral ulceration** (Figs. 4.19), manifest as minor aphthous ulcers, major aphthous ulcers, or herpetiform lesions that have recurred at least three times in one 12-month period.

2. **Plus two of the following:**

   a. *Recurrent genital ulceration* (Fig. 4.20).
   b. *Eye lesions* (see below).
   c. *Skin lesions* which may be erythema nodosum, pseudo-folliculitis (Fig. 4.21), papulopustular lesions (Fig. 4.22)

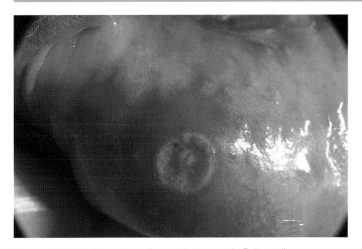

**Figure 4.19** Aphthous ulceration on the tongue in Behçet disease

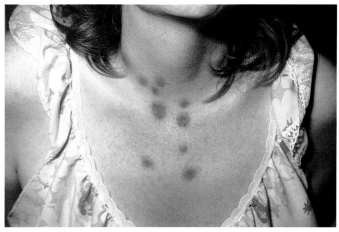

**Figure 4.22** Papulopustular lesions in Behçet disease (Courtesy of B. Noble)

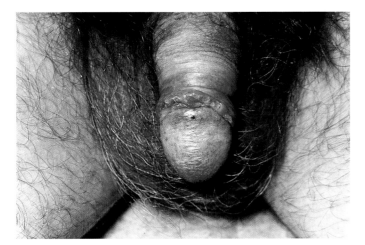

**Figure 4.20** Genital ulceration in Behçet disease

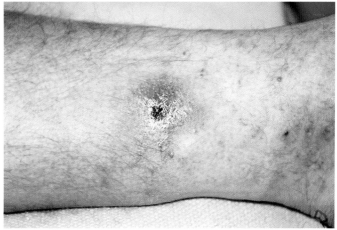

**Figure 4.23** Pustule formation following pricking of the skin (positive pathergy test) (Courtesy of B. Noble)

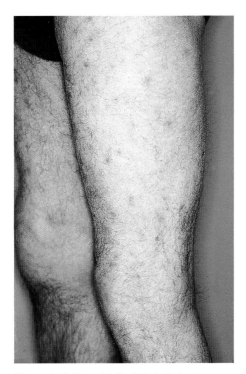

**Figure 4.21** Pseudofolliculosis in Behçet disease (Courtesy of B. Noble)

and acneiform nodules in post-adolescent patients not on corticosteroid treatment.

d. *Positive pathergy test* read at 24–48 hours characterised by the formation of a pustule following a skin prick (Fig. 4.23).

**Other systemic features** include the following:

- Cutaneous hypersensitivity (Fig. 4.24).
- Vasculitis.
- Arthritis involving the knees and ankles, and, occasionally, sacroiliitis.
- Superficial or deep obliterative thrombophlebitis (Fig. 4.25).
- Intestinal ulceration.
- Neurological lesions involving the brain stem or meningoencephalitis.

## OCULAR FEATURES

The following ocular complications occur in up to 95% of men and 70% of women with BD. They are frequently bilateral and usually follow the systemic manifestations of the disease, although occasionally they may be the presenting feature. It is unusual for the systemic and ocular manifestations to develop simultaneously.

### Anterior segment

1. **Acute recurrent anterior uveitis** which may be simultaneously bilateral and frequently associated with a transient mobile hypopyon (Fig. 4.26). It is usually responsive to topical steroids.

2. **Conjunctival ulceration** is rare.

### Posterior segment

1. **Transient retinal infiltrates** may be seen during the acute stage of BD. They are superficial, white, necrotic lesions which heal without scarring (Figs. 4.27).

2. **Retinal vasculitis** may involve both veins (periphlebitis) (Fig. 4.28) and arteries (periarteritis). It is a serious problem because it may result in vascular occlusions and macular

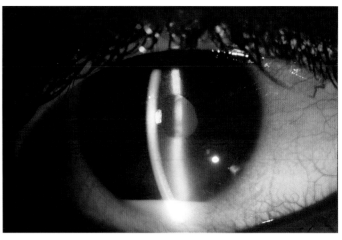

**Figure 4.26** Hypopyon in Behçet disease (Courtesy of B. Noble)

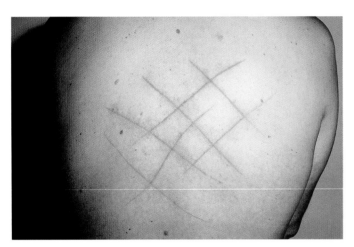

**Figure 4.24** Dermatographism – formation of erythematous lines following stroking of the skin (Courtesy of B. Noble)

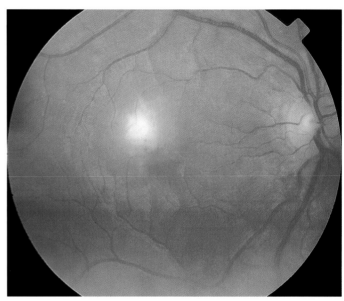

**Figure 4.27** Retinal infiltrate in Behçet disease (Courtesy of B. Noble)

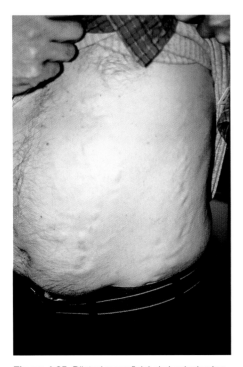

**Figure 4.25** Dilated superficial abdominal veins compensating for deep obliterative thrombophlebitis in Behçet disease (Courtesy of B. Noble)

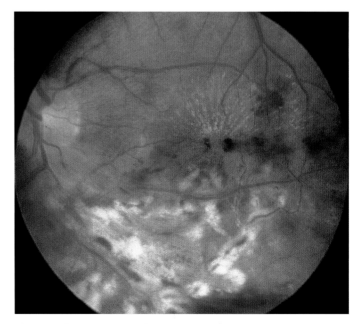

**Figure 4.28** Periphlebitis in Behçet disease (Courtesy of Western Eye Hospital)

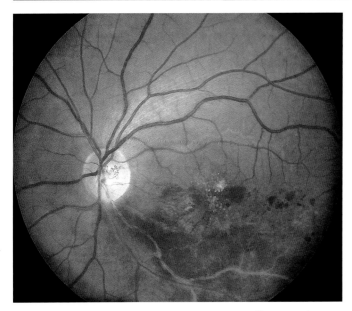

**Figure 4.29** Occlusive periphlebitis in Behçet disease (Courtesy of Western Eye Hospital)

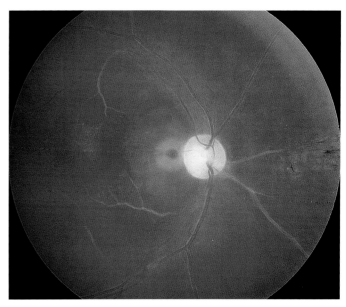

**Figure 4.31** Optic atrophy and vascular sheathing in Behçet disease

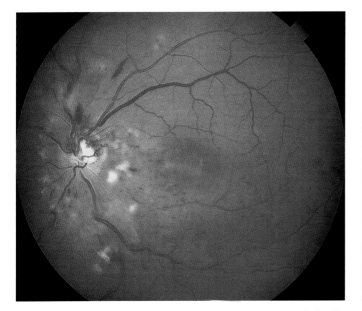

**Figure 4.30** Optic disc vasculitis in Behçet disease (Courtesy of A. Dick)

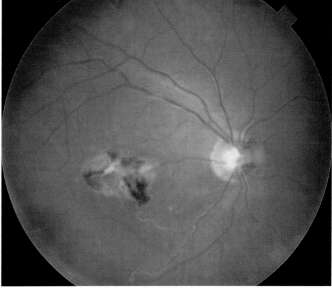

**Figure 4.32** Chorioretinal scar at the macula and old inferotemporal vascular occlusion in Behçet disease (Courtesy of A. Dick)

ischaemia (Fig. 4.29) as well as optic nerve involvement (Fig. 4.30).

3. **Vascular leakage** may give rise to diffuse retinal oedema.

4. **Vitritis,** which may be severe and persistent, is universally present in eyes with active disease.

5. **Prognosis** is guarded and about 20% of involved eyes become blind despite treatment. The end stage of posterior segment involvement is characterised by optic atrophy, vascular attenuation, chronic sheathing (Fig. 4.31) and variable chorioretinal scarring (Fig. 4.32).

***Treatment*** options for posterior uveitis include the following:

1. **Systemic steroids** may shorten the duration of an inflammatory episode but are not effective long term because of poor control and significant side effects. The addition of a steroid-sparing agent is usually required.

2. **Azathioprine** reduces the frequency and severity of attacks. It does not act fast enough in acute disease but it is a good agent for long-term treatment. Close monitoring of bone marrow and liver function is necessary.

3. **Cyclosporine** is an effective and rapidly acting drug but is associated with nephrotoxicity, particularly at doses higher than 5 mg/kg/day, and relapses after cessation often limit its use.

4. **Subcutaneous interferon alpha-2a,** 6 million units daily, is an effective alternative treatment, particularly for the management of mucocutaneous lesions. It may also be effective in the management of ocular disease in patients resistant to high-dose steroids. The main adverse effects include flu-like symptoms, hair loss, itching and depression.

***Differential diagnosis.*** In patients with suggestive ocular findings but lack of classic systemic manifestations, the diagnosis becomes uncertain, especially owing to the lack of definitive laboratory tests. It is therefore important to consider the following conditions.

1. **Recurrent anterior uveitis with hypopyon** may be associated with spondyloarthropathies. However, the uveitis is not usually simultaneously bilateral and the hypopyon is not mobile because it is frequently associated with a fibrinous exudate. In BD, the uveitis is frequently simultaneously bilateral and the hypopyon shifts with gravity as the patient changes head position.

2. **Retinal vasculitis** may be associated with sarcoidosis. However, sarcoid vasculitis involves only veins in a segmental manner and is rarely occlusive. In contrast, BD usually involves both arteries and veins, is diffuse and frequently occlusive.

3. **Retinal infiltrates** similar to those in BD may be seen in viral retinitis such as the acute retinal necrosis syndrome. However, in viral retinitis, the infiltrates eventually coalesce. Multiple retinal infiltrates also occur in idiopathic acute multifocal retinitis. In contrast to BD, the clinical course is favourable, with return to normal vision within 2–4 months of onset.

## FURTHER READING

Demiroglu H, Barista I, Dundar S. Risk factor assessment and prognosis of eye involvement in Behçet disease in Turkey. *Ophthalmology* 1997;104:701–705.

el-Asar AM, al-Momen AK, Alamro SA, et al. Bilateral central retinal vein occlusion in Behçet disease. *Clin Rheumatol* 1996;15:511–513.

Kotter I, Zierhut M, Eckstein AK, et al. Human recombinant interferon alfa-2a for the treatment of Behçet's disease with sight threatening posterior or panuveitis. *Br J Ophthalmol* 2003; 87:423–431.

Mochizuki M, Akduman L, Nussenblatt RB. Behçet disease. In: Pepose JS, Holland GN, Wilhelmus KR, eds. *Ocular immunology and inflammation.* St Louis: Mosby, 1996:663–675.

Sakamoto M, Akazawa K, Nishioka Y, et al. Prognostic factors of vision in patients with Behçet's disease. *Ophthalmology* 1995;102:317–321.

Stanford MR. Behçet's syndrome. New treatments for an old disease [Editorial]. *Br J Ophthalmol* 2003;87:381–382.

Toker E, Kozokoglu H, Acar N. High dose intravenous steroid therapy for severe posterior segment uveitis in Behçet disease. *Br J Ophthalmol* 2002;86:521–523.

# Vogt–Koyanagi–Harada Syndrome

## SYSTEMIC FEATURES

Vogt–Koyanagi–Harada (V-K-H) disease is an idiopathic, multisystem disorder which typically affects Hispanics, Japanese and pigmented individuals. Japanese patients have an increased prevalence of HLA-DR4 and Dw15. In practice, V-K-H can be subdivided into Vogt–Koyanagi disease, characterised mainly by skin changes and anterior uveitis, and Harada disease, in which neurological features and exudative retinal detachments predominate.

### Phases

1. **Prodromal** phase lasting a few days is characterised by neurological and auditory manifestations:

   - Meningitis causing headache and neck stiffness.
   - Encephalopathy is less frequent and may manifest as convulsions, paresis and cranial nerve palsies.
   - Auditory features include tinnitus, vertigo and deafness.

2. **Acute uveitic** phase follows soon thereafter and is characterised by bilateral granulomatous anterior or multifocal posterior uveitis and exudative retinal detachments.

3. **Convalescent** phase follows several weeks later and is characterised by:

   - Localised alopecia, poliosis and vitiligo (Fig. 4.33).
   - Focal depigmented fundus lesions (sunset glow fundus – Fig. 4.34) and depigmented limbal lesions (Sugiura sign).

4. **Chronic-recurrent** phase is characterised by smouldering anterior uveitis with exacerbations.

***Diagnostic criteria*** must include at least three of the following:

1. **Bilateral chronic anterior uveitis.**

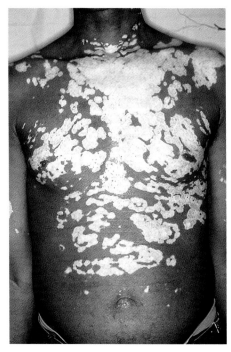

**Figure 4.33** Vitiligo

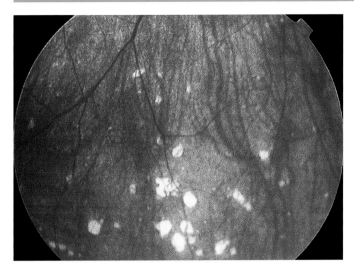

**Figure 4.34** 'Sunset-glow' fundus

2. **Posterior uveitis,** including exudative retinal detachment, disc swelling and 'sunset-glow fundus'.

3. **Neurological features.**

4. **Cutaneous lesions.**

## OCULAR FEATURES

### Signs

1. **Chronic granulomatous anterior uveitis** is characterised by mutton fat keratic precipitates and iris nodules. It runs a protracted course and frequently leads to the formation of posterior synechiae and cataract. Severe anterior uveitis typically occurs in patients with Vogt–Koyanagi syndrome, but mild anterior uveitis may also be seen in patients with Harada disease.

2. **Posterior segment involvement** occurs in patients with Harada disease and is frequently bilateral. In chronological order, the findings are as follows:

- Multifocal choroiditis.
- Multifocal detachments of the sensory retina (Fig. 4.35).
- Exudative retinal detachment.
- Residual lesions consist of atrophy and proliferation of the retinal pigment epithelium (RPE). Choroidal neovascularisation (CNV) may occur in some eyes with RPE changes, particularly when associated with chronic recurrent disease.

***Treatment*** of posterior segment involvement:

1. **Systemic steroids** administered as intravenous pulsed or high-dose oral therapy.

2. **Cyclosporine** may be beneficial in steroid-resistant patients.

> NB: The prognosis depends on early recognition and aggressive control. Late diagnosis or incorrect initial therapy is often associated with a guarded prognosis, with only 50% of patients having a final visual acuity better than 6/12.

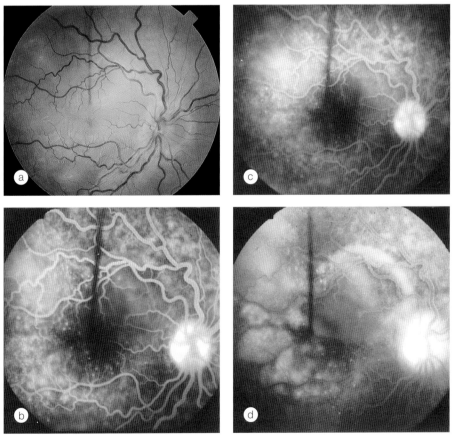

**Figure 4.35** Harada disease. **(a)** Multiple detachment of the sensory retina; **(b)** FA early venous phase shows numerous pin points of hyperfluorescence; **(c)** late venous phase shows diffuse hyperfluorescence; **(d)** late phase shows large hyperfluorescent areas due to pooling of dye under the sensory retina

### *Differential diagnosis of bilateral exudative retinal detachments*

- Metastatic carcinoma to the choroid.
- Uveal effusion syndrome.
- Posterior scleritis.
- Toxaemia of pregnancy.
- Bullous central serous retinopathy.

## FURTHER READING

Kahn M, Pepose JS, Green WR, et al. Immunocytologic findings in a case of Vogt-Koyanagi-Harada syndrome. *Ophthalmology* 1993; 100:1191–1198.

Kohno T, Miki T, Shiraki K, et al. Subtraction ICG angiography in Harada's disease. *Br J Ophthalmol* 1999;83:822–833.

Moorthy RS, Chong LP, Smith RE, et al. Subretinal neovascular membranes in Vogt-Koyanagi-Harada syndrome. *Am J Ophthalmol* 1993;116:164–170.

Moorthy RS, Inomata H, Rao NA. Vogt-Koyanagi-Harada syndrome. *Surv Ophthalmol* 1995;39:265–292.

Perry HD, Font RL. Clinical and histopathologic observations in severe Vogt-Koyanagi-Harada syndrome. *Am J Ophthalmol* 1997;83:242–254.

Rao N. Mechanisms of inflammatory response in sympathetic ophthalmia and VKH syndrome. *Eye* 1997;11:213–216.

Rathinam SR, Namperumalsamy P, Nozik RA, et al. Vogt-Koyanagi-Harada syndrome after cutaneous injury. *Ophthalmology* 1999;106:635–638.

Rubasamen PE, Gass JDM. Vogt-Koyanagi-Harada syndrome: clinical course, therapy, and long-term outcome. *Arch Ophthalmol* 1991; 109:682–687.

# INFESTATIONS

## Toxoplasmosis

### PATHOGENESIS

*Toxoplasma gondii* is an obligate intracellular protozoan which is estimated to infest at least 10% of adults in northern temperate countries and more than half of adults in Mediterranean and tropical countries. The cat is the definitive host of the parasite, and other animals, such as mice, livestock and humans, are intermediate hosts.

1. **Forms of the parasite**

   a. *Sporocyst* (oocyst) which is excreted in cat faeces.
   b. *Bradyzoite* which is encysted in tissues.
   c. *Tachyzoite* (trophozoite) which is the proliferating active form responsible for tissue destruction and inflammation.

2. **Mode of human infection** (Fig. 4.36)

   a. *Ingestion of undercooked* meat (lamb, pork, beef) containing bradyzoites of an intermediate host.
   b. *Ingestion of sporocysts* following accidental contamination of hands when disposing of cat litter trays and then subsequent transfer on to food. Infants may also become infested by eating dirt (pica) containing sporocysts. Water contamination may play an important role in the transmission of the disease in some areas.

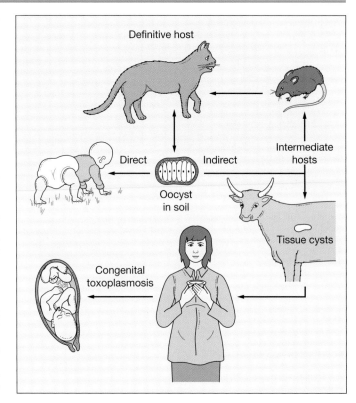

**Figure 4.36** Life cycle of *Toxoplasma gondii*

c. *Transplacental spread* of the parasite (tachyzoite) can occur to the foetus if a pregnant woman becomes infested. The consequences to the foetus will depend on the stage of pregnancy during which the disease is acquired.

### DIAGNOSTIC TESTS

The diagnosis of retinitis caused by toxoplasmosis is based on a compatile fundus lesion and positive serology for toxoplasma antibodies. Any antibody titre is significant because in recurrent ocular toxoplasmosis, no correlation exists between the titre and the activity of retinitis.

1. **Indirect immunofluorescent antibody** tests utilise dead organisms that are exposed to the patient's serum and antihuman globulin labelled with fluorescein. The results are read using a fluorescent microscope.

2. **Haemagglutination** tests involve coating of lysed organisms on to red blood cells which are then exposed to the patient's serum. Positive sera cause the red cells to agglutinate.

3. **Enzyme-linked immunosorbent assay** (ELISA) involves binding of the patient's antibodies to an excess of solid-phase antigen. This complex is then incubated with an enzyme-linked second antibody. Assessment of enzyme activity provides measurement of specific antibody concentration. The test can also be used to detect antibodies in the aqueous, which are more specific than those in the serum.

4. **Aqueous humour PRC** may be useful in immuno-compromised individuals with atypical lesions.

5. **The Sabin–Feldman** dye-test utilises live organisms which are exposed to the patient's serum and complement. The cell membranes are lysed in the presence of specific anti-Toxoplasma IgG; the organisms fail to stain with methylene blue dye.

## SYSTEMIC FEATURES

***Congenital disease*** is transmitted to the foetus through the placenta when a pregnant woman becomes infested. If the mother is infested before pregnancy, the foetus will be unscathed. The severity of involvement of the foetus is dependent on the duration of gestation at the time of maternal infestation. For example, infestation during early pregnancy may result in stillbirth, whereas if it occurs during late pregnancy it may result in convulsions, paralysis, hydrocephalus (Fig. 4.37) and visceral involvement. Intracranial calcification may be seen on plain skull radiographs or CT (Fig. 4.38). However, just as in the acquired form, most cases of congenital systemic toxoplasmosis are subclinical. In these children, bilateral healed chorioretinal scars (Fig. 4.39) may be discovered later in life, either by chance or when the child is found to have defective vision. Infestations occurring towards the end of the second trimester usually result in disease that can be detected at birth, such as macular scars, while infections occurring later in the third trimester may result in normal examinations at birth, but with the appearance of ocular or neurological findings in the future.

***Acquired disease***

1. **In immunocompetent** patients, it may take one of the following forms:

   a. *Subclinical* is the most frequent.
   b. *Lymphadenopathic syndrome,* which is uncommon and self-limiting. It is characterised by cervical lymphadenopathy, fever, malaise and pharyngitis.
   c. *Meningoencephalitis,* which is characterised by convulsions and altered consciousness, occurs in a minority of patients.

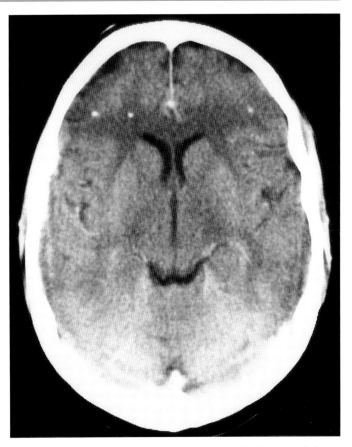

**Figure 4.38** CT scan showing intracerebral calcification in congenital toxoplasmosis

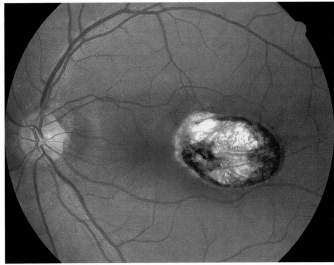

**Figure 4.39** Macular scar in congenital toxoplasmosis

   d. *The exanthematous* form, resembling a rickettsial infection, is the rarest.

2. **In immunocompromised** patients, such as those with acquired immunodeficiency syndrome (AIDS) or organ-graft recipients, systemic infestation may be life threatening. The most common manifestation in AIDS patients is an intracerebral space-occupying lesion which resembles a cerebral abscess on MRI.

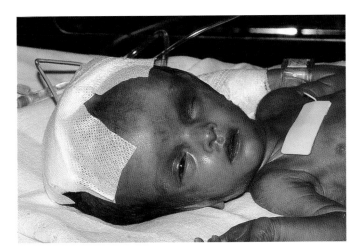

**Figure 4.37** Hydrocephalus and left anophthalmos in congenital toxoplasmosis (Courtesy of M. Szreter)

## TOXOPLASMA RETINITIS

***Clinical features.*** Toxoplasma is the most frequent cause of infectious retinitis in immunocompetent individuals. Although some cases may occur as a result of reactivation of prenatal infestation, the vast majority are acquired postnatally. Recurrent episodes of inflammation are common and occur when the cysts rupture and release hundreds of tachyzoites into normal retinal cells. This usually takes place between the ages of 10 and 35 years (average age 25 years). Active retinitis is usually associated with anterior uveitis, which may be non-granulomatous or granulomatous, and can produce ocular hypertension during the acute stage. It is therefore very important to examine the fundus in all patients with anterior uveitis.

1. **Presentation** is often with unilateral, sudden onset of floaters, visual loss and photophobia.

2. **Focal retinitis**

   - A solitary inflammatory focus near an old pigmented scar ('satellite lesion') associated with overlying vitreous haze (Fig. 4.40) is the most common finding.
   - Very severe vitritis may greatly impair visualisation of the fundus (Fig. 4.41), although the inflammatory focus may still be discernible ('headlight in the fog' appearance) (Fig. 4.42).
   - Associated features include vasculitis and, in some cases, the detached posterior hyaloid face becomes covered by inflammatory precipitates.
   - The fellow eye may show inactive lesions.

3. **Papillitis** (inflammation of the optic nerve head) may be secondary to active retinitis located in the juxtapapillary area (Jensen choroiditis) (Fig. 4.43). Very occasionally, the optic nerve head itself is the primary site of involvement.

4. **Atypical features** that may occur in immunocompromised individuals are characterised by multiple, bilateral, discrete foci (Fig. 4.44) or extensive confluent areas of

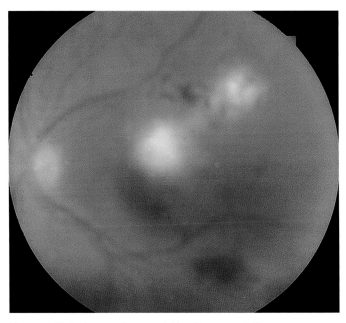

**Figure 4.41** Active toxoplasma retinitis with severe vitritis

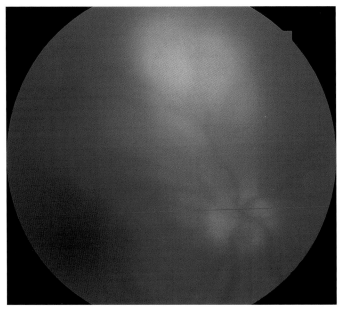

**Figure 4.42** Active toxoplasma retinitis with very severe vitritis giving rise to a 'headlight in the fog' appearance

retinitis. Pre-existing scars are absent, implying that the infestation has been newly acquired or disseminated to the eye from extraocular sites.

***Course and complications.*** The rate of healing is dependent on the virulence of the organism, the competence of the host's immune system and the size of the lesion. In uncompromised hosts, the retinitis heals within 6 to 8 weeks (Fig. 4.45), although symptoms arising from vitreous inflammation take longer to resolve and some vitreous condensation may remain. The inflammatory focus is replaced by a sharply demarcated atrophic scar which will progressively pigment starting from the edges, producing initially a hyperpigmented border (Fig. 4.46). Resolution of anterior uveitis is

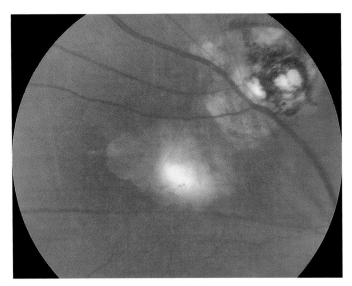

**Figure 4.40** Typical active toxoplasma retinitis

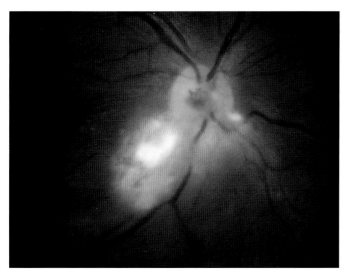

**Figure 4.43** Active juxtapapillary toxoplasma retinitis

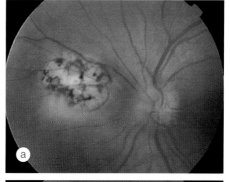

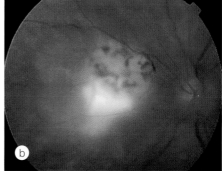

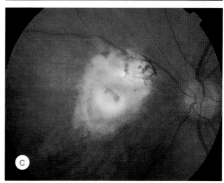

**Figure 4.45** Progression of toxoplasma retinitis. **(a)** At presentation; **(b)** after 2 weeks the area of retinitis is larger; **(c)** after 6 weeks the retinitis is beginning to resolve

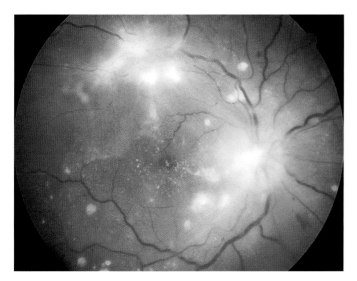

**Figure 4.44** Atypical multiple foci of toxoplasma retinitis in an immunocompromised individual (Courtesy of J. Salmon)

a reliable sign of posterior segment healing. After the first attack, the mean recurrence rate within 3 years is about 50% and the average number of recurrent attacks per patient is 2.7. Nearly one-quarter of eyes develop serious visual loss as a result of the following complications:

- Direct involvement of the fovea (Fig. 4.47), papillomacular bundle, optic nerve head or a major blood vessel.
- Indirect involvement by epiretinal or vitreoretinal traction may result in macular pucker or tractional retinal detachment.
- CNV adjacent to chorioretinal scarring is uncommon.

### Aims of treatment

- To reduce the duration and severity of acute inflammation.
- To reduce the risk of permanent visual loss by reducing the size of the eventual retinochoroidal scar.
- To reduce the risk of recurrences.

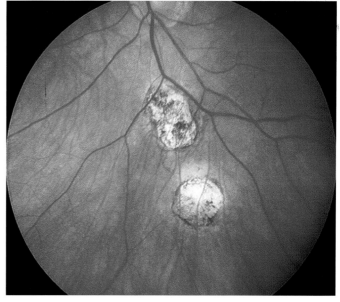

**Figure 4.46** Chorioretinal scars due to previous toxoplasma retinitis

147

***Indications for treatment.*** At present there is lack of evidence that treatment with antibiotics achieves any of the above aims, although adjunctive corticosteroids may diminish the duration and severity of inflammatory symptoms. Despite these reservations, treatment may, however, be considered for the following vision-threatening lesions:

- A lesion threatening or involving the macula, papillomacular bundle (Fig. 4.48), optic nerve head or a major blood vessel.
- Very severe vitritis, because it may subsequently lead to vitreous fibrosis and tractional retinal detachment.
- In immunocompromised patients, all lesions should be treated irrespective of location or severity. Systemic steroids should be avoided in these patients.

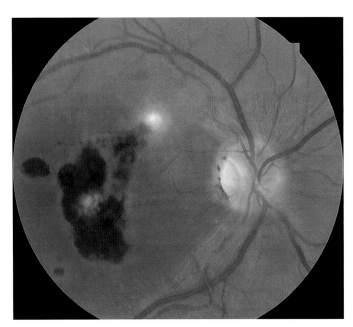

**Figure 4.47** Foveal involvement by a scar with a small focus of active retinitis at its superior edge

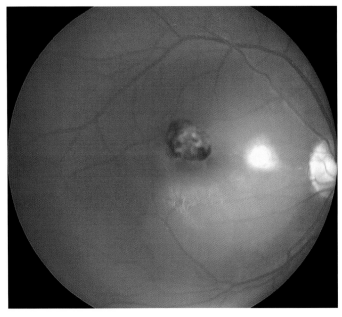

**Figure 4.48** Active retinitis involving the papillomacular bundle and a scar near the fovea

***Therapeutic regimen.*** Currently there is no universally agreed therapeutic regimen. Systemic steroids are recommended in eyes with vision-threatening lesions, particularly if associated with severe vitritis, but not in patients with AIDS. Steroids should never be used without a shield of one or more of the following antiparasitic drugs.

1. **Clindamycin** 300 mg orally four times daily for 3 weeks. However, rarely, if used alone, it may cause a pseudomembranous colitis secondary to clostridial overgrowth. Treatment of colitis is with oral vancomycin 500 mg 6-hourly for 10 days. The risk of colitis is reduced when clindamycin is used together with a sulphonamide that inhibits clostridial overgrowth.

2. **Sulphadiazine.** A loading oral dose of 2 g is followed by 1 g four times daily for 3–4 weeks. Side effects of sulphonamides include renal stones, allergic reactions and Stevens–Johnson syndrome.

3. **Pyrimethamine** (Daraprim) is a strong anti-Toxoplasma agent which may cause thrombocytopenia, leukopenia and folate deficiency. For this reason, weekly blood counts should be done and the drug used only in combination with oral folinic acid 4 mg three times a week (mixed with orange juice) because this counteracts the side effects. The loading dose is 50 mg, followed by 25–50 mg daily for 4 weeks. In AIDS, pyrimethamine is avoided due to possible pre-existing bone marrow suppression and antagonistic effect of zidovudine when the drugs are combined.

4. **Co-trimoxazole** (Septrin) is a combination of trimethoprim (160 mg) and sulphamethoxazole (800 mg). When used in oral doses of 960 mg twice daily for 4–6 weeks, it may be effective alone or in combination with clindamycin. Side effects are similar to those of the sulphonamides.

5. **Atovaquone,** 750 mg three times daily, has been used mainly in the treatment of pneumocystosis and toxoplasmosis in AIDS but is also effective in the treatment of toxoplasma retinitis in immunocompetent individuals. The drug is relatively free of serious side effects but is expensive.

6. **Azithromycin,** 500 mg daily on three successive days, may be an effective alternative for patients who cannot tolerate other drugs.

7. **Combined therapy** with azithromycin and pyrimethamine or azithromycin and sulfadiazine are also both effective, although the former is associated with fewer and less severe side effects.

## FURTHER READING

Bosch-Driessen LEH, Berenscholt TTJM, Ongkosuwito JV, et al. Ocular toxoplasmosis. Clinical features and prognosis in 154 patients. *Ophthalmology* 2002;109:869–878.

Bosch-Driessen LH, Verbraak FD, Suttorp-Schulten MSA, et al. A prospective, randomized trial of pyrimethamine and azithromycin vs pyrimethamine and sulfadiazine for the treatment of ocular toxoplasmosis. *Am J Ophthalmol* 2002;134:34–40.

Bosch-Griessen EH, Rothova A. Recurrent ocular disease in postnatally acquired toxoplasmosis. *Am J Ophthalmol* 1999;128:421–425.

Fardeau C, Romand S, Rao NA, et al. Diagnosis of toxoplasmic retinochoroiditis with atypical clinical features. *Am J Ophthalmol* 2002;134:196–203.

Gilbert RE, Stanford MR. Is ocular toxoplasmosis caused by prenatal or postnatal infection? *Br J Ophthalmol* 2000;84:224–226.

Holland GN, Lewis KG, O'Connor GR. Ocular toxoplasmosis. A 50th anniversary tribute to the contributions of Helenor Campbell Wilder Foerster. *Arch Ophthalmol* 2002;120:1081–1084.

Holland GN, Lewis KG. An update on current practices in the management of ocular toxoplasmosis. *Am J Ophthalmol* 2002;134:102–114.

Holland GN. Reconsidering the pathogenesis of ocular toxoplasmosis. *Am J Ophthalmol* 1999;128:502–505.

Pavesio CE, Lightman S. Toxoplasma gondii and ocular toxoplasmosis: pathogenesis. *Br J Ophthalmol* 1996;80:1099–1107.

Rothova A, Bosch-Driessen EH, van Loon NH, et al. Azithromycin for ocular toxoplasmosis. *Br J Ophthalmol* 1998;82:1306–1308.

Silvera C, Belfort Jr R, Muccioli C, et al. The effect of long-term intermittent trimethoprim/sulfamethoxazole treatment on recurrences of toxoplasma retinochoroiditis. *Am J Ophthalmol* 2002;134:41–46.

Stanford MR, See SE, Jones LV, et al. Antibiotics for toxoplasmic retinochoroiditis. An evidence-based systematic review. *Ophthalmology* 2003;110:926–932.

# Toxocariasis

## PATHOGENESIS

Toxocariasis is caused by infestation with a common intestinal ascarid (roundworm) of dogs, called *Toxocara canis* (Fig. 4.49). About 80% of puppies between the ages of 2 and 6 months are infested with this worm. Human infestation is by accidental ingestion of soil or food contaminated with ova shed in dogs' faeces. Very young children who eat dirt (pica) or are in close contact with puppies are at particular risk of acquiring the disease. In the human intestine, the ova develop into larvae which penetrate the intestinal wall and travel to various organs, such as the liver, lungs, skin, brain and eyes. When the larvae die, they disintegrate and cause an inflammatory reaction followed by granulation. Clinically, human infestation can take one of the following forms:

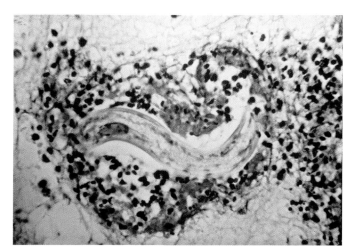

**Figure 4.49** *Toxocara canis*

1. **Visceral larva migrans** (VLM) is caused by severe systemic infection which usually occurs at about the age of 2 years. The clinical features, which vary in severity, include a low-grade fever, hepatosplenomegaly, pneumonitis, convulsions and, rarely, death. The blood shows a leukocytosis and marked eosinophilia.

2. **Ocular toxocariasis** differs markedly from VLM because it involves otherwise healthy individuals who have a normal white cell count with absence of eosinophilia. A history of pica is less common, and the average age at presentation is considerably older (7.5 years) compared with VLM (2 years).

The different presentations are probably related to the parasite load during exposure. In VLM, the infestation is massive, producing a significant immune response responsible for the clinical findings. In ocular toxocariasis, fewer organisms are involved, and because they are not recognised by the immune system, they can freely migrate throughout the body and eventually reach the eye.

## DIAGNOSTIC TESTS

1. **ELISA** can be used to determine the level of serum antibodies to *Toxocara canis*. When ocular toxocariasis is suspected, exact ELISA titres should be requested, including testing of undiluted serum. Any positive titre is consistent with, but not necessarily diagnostic of, toxocariasis. Consequently, it must be interpreted in conjunction with the clinical findings. A positive titre does not therefore exclude the possibility of retinoblastoma.

2. **Ultrasonography** may be useful both in establishing the diagnosis in eyes with hazy media and in excluding other causes of leukocoria.

## OCULAR FEATURES

### Chronic endophthalmitis

1. **Presentation** is between the ages of 2 and 9 years with leukocoria (Fig. 4.50), strabismus or unilateral visual loss.

2. **Signs**

   - Anterior uveitis and vitritis.
   - In some cases, there may be a peripheral granuloma.
   - The peripheral retina and pars plana may be covered by a dense greyish-white exudate, similar to the 'snow-banking' seen in pars planitis (Fig. 4.51).

3. **Treatment**

   - Systemic or periocular steroids may be helpful in some cases.
   - Vitreoretinal surgery may be beneficial in some eyes with tractional retinal detachment.

4. **Prognosis** in most cases is very poor and some eyes eventually require enucleation. The main causes of visual loss are:

   - Tractional retinal detachment secondary to contraction of vitreoretinal membranes.

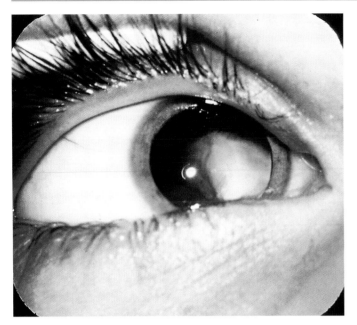

**Figure 4.50** Toxocara endophthalmitis causing leukocoria

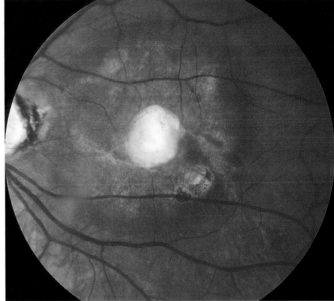

**Figure 4.52** Posterior pole toxocara granuloma

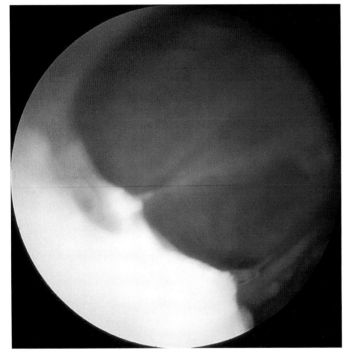

**Figure 4.51** Peripheral exudation and vitreoretinal traction bands in toxocara endophthalmitis (Courtesy of S. Lightman)

- Ocular hypotony and phthisis bulbi caused by separation of the ciliary body from the sclera, brought about by contraction of a cyclitic membrane.
- Cataract.

### Posterior pole granuloma

1. **Presentation** is typically with unilateral visual impairment between the ages of 6 and 14 years.

2. **Signs**

   - Anterior uveitis and vitritis are absent.

- Round, yellow-white, solid granuloma which varies between one to two disc-diameters in diameter, usually located at the posterior pole (Fig. 4.52) or near the disc (Fig. 4.53). The lesion is usually stationary and the extent of visual loss is dependent on its location.
- Associated findings include vitreoretinal bands (Fig. 4.54), distortion of blood vessels (Fig. 4.55), and occasionally the granuloma is surrounded by yellow hard exudates (Fig. 4.56).

3. **Complications,** which are rare, include retinal detachment (Fig. 4.57) and subretinal haemorrhage.

### PERIPHERAL GRANULOMA

1. **Presentation** is usually during adolescence or adult life as a result of visual impairment from distortion of the macula or retinal detachment. In uncomplicated cases, the lesion may remain undetected throughout life.

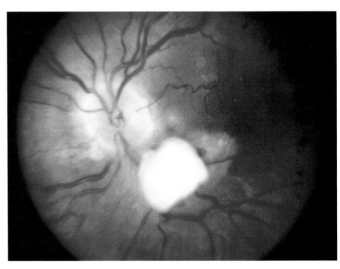

**Figure 4.53** Juxtapapillary toxocara granuloma

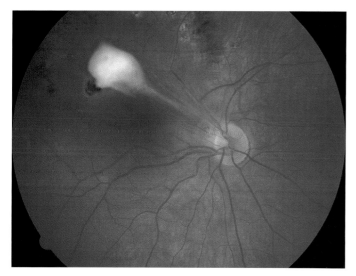

**Figure 4.54** Vitreoretinal band associated with a toxocara granuloma

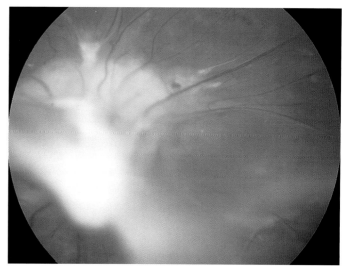

**Figure 4.57** Toxocara granuloma and a tractional retinal detachment

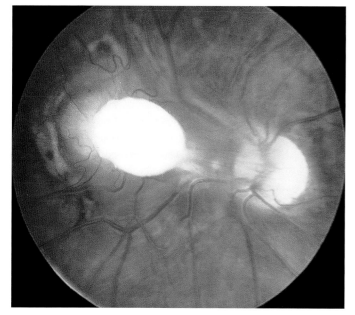

**Figure 4.55** Vascular distortion associated with a toxocara granuloma

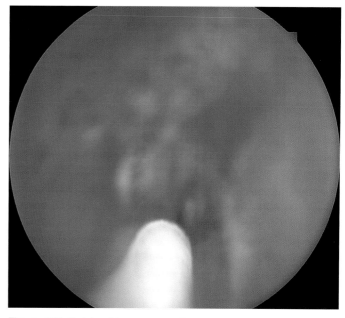

**Figure 4.58** Peripheral toxocara granuloma

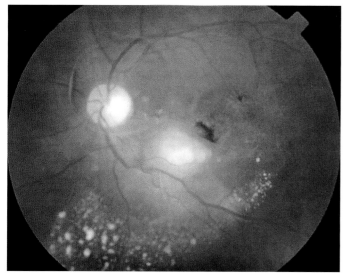

**Figure 4.56** Toxocara granuloma associated with hard exudates

## 2. Signs

- Absence of anterior uveitis and vitritis.
- A white hemispherical granuloma located at, or anterior to, the equator in any quadrant of the fundus (Fig. 4.58).
- Vitreous bands frequently extend from the lesion to the posterior fundus and on contracting may give rise to 'dragging' of the disc and straightening of blood vessels (Fig. 4.59).

## 3. Complications in severe cases are the following:

- Macular heterotopia caused by contraction of the bands connecting the granuloma with the optic nerve head.
- Retinal detachment caused by contraction of vitreoretinal bands. In some cases, vitreoretinal surgery may be successful in reattaching the retina.

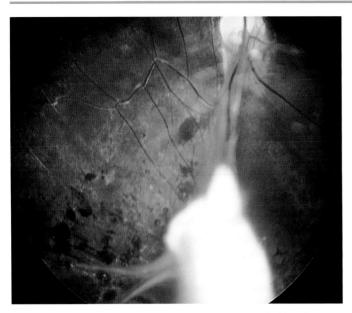

**Figure 4.59** Peripheral toxocara granuloma with vitreoretinal bands 'dragging' the disc (Courtesy of K. Rahman)

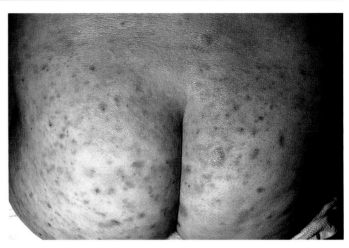

**Figure 4.60** Acute skin lesions in onchocerciasis

## FURTHER READING

Dinning WJ, Gillespie SH, Cooling RJ, et al. Toxocariasis: a practical approach to management of ocular disease. *Eye* 1988;2:580–582.

Sharkey JA, McKay PS. Ocular toxocariasis in a patient with repeatedly negative ELISA titre to Toxoplasma canis. *Br J Ophthalmol* 1993; 77:253–254.

Shields JA. Ocular toxocariasis: a review. *Surv Ophthalmol* 1984; 28:361–381.

Small KW, McCuen BW, deJuan E, et al. Surgical management of retinal traction caused by toxocariasis. *Am J Ophthalmol* 1989; 108:10–14.

Wan WL, Cano MR, Pince KJ, et al. Echographic characteristics of ocular toxocariasis. *Ophthalmology* 1991;98:28–32.

# Onchocerciasis

## PATHOGENESIS

Onchocerciasis is caused by the filarial parasite *Onchocerca volvulus* which is transmitted by the bite of a blackfly (Simulium) and results in the migration of millions of tiny worms (microfilariae) throughout the body. The disease is endemic in areas of Africa and Central and South America, and is the world's second leading cause of blindness. Because onchocerciasis tends to occur near rivers and streams, ocular involvement is referred to as 'river blindness'. The diagnosis depends on seeing micrifilariae in the skin or eye, or finding a nodule containing adult worms. It appears that *Wolbachia*, a symbiotic bacterium, is essential for the fertility of the nematode hosts and the endotoxin-like products of *Wolbachia* act as the major inflammatory stimulus in the eye.

## SYSTEMIC FEATURES

1. **Signs**

   a. *Acute skin lesions* consist of numerous small, discrete pruritic papules usually involving the buttocks (Fig. 4.60) and extremities. Chronic lesions are characterised by thickening and hyperpigmentation, most frequently involving the lower limbs.

   b. *Subcutaneous nodules* consisting of encapsulated worms develop over bony prominences and the head. A common site for small nodules is just behind the ear. Occasionally, the lymph nodes become grossly enlarged, resulting in chronic lymphatic obstruction and lymphoedema.

2. **Treatment** is with ivermectin 12 mg given as an annual single dose. Although it acts rapidly to reduce the number of skin microfilariae, it depletes them for only a few months, after which microfilariae reappear at levels of 20% or more of pre-treatment numbers within 1 year, which is sufficient for transmission to continue.

> **NB: New therapies are being developed targeting Wolbachia.**

## OCULAR FEATURES

1. **The aqueous** may contain live microfilariae. Anterior uveitis may result in pear-shaped pupillary distortion, secondary glaucoma and cataract formation.

2. **Punctate keratitis** is characterised by fluffy, snowflake opacities in the superficial stroma, consisting of cellular infiltrates around dead microfilariae. The keratitis is frequently asymptomatic and resolves spontaneously.

3. **Sclerosing keratitis** is characterised by progressive stromal opacification and pannus formation.

4. **Chorioretinitis** is usually bilateral and predominantly involves the posterior fundus. The severity of involvement varies from atrophy and clumping of the RPE to widespread chorioretinal atrophy (Fig. 4.61).

5. **Treatment** of chorioretinitis is with ivermectin 12 mg every 6 months. Anterior uveitis requires topical steroids.

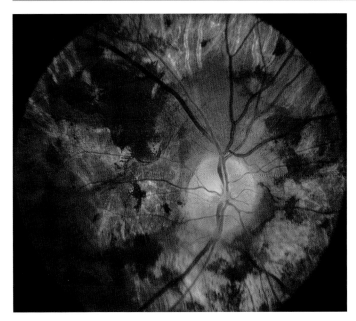

**Figure 4.61** Old chorioretinitis due to onchocerciasis

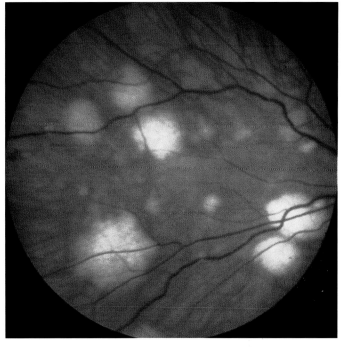

**Figure 4.62** Choroidal pneumocystosis (Courtesy of S. Mitchell)

## Choroidal Pneumocystosis

1. **Pathogenesis.** *Pneumocystis carinii,* an opportunistic protozoan parasite, is a major cause of morbidity and mortality in AIDS. The presence of choroidal involvement can be an important sign of extrapulmonary systemic dissemination. Most patients with choroiditis have received inhaled pentamidine as prophylaxis against *Pneumocystis carinii* pneumonia, because systemic prophylaxis protects against choroiditis, while aerosolised pentamidine protects only the lungs, allowing the organisms to disseminate throughout the body. The presence of choroiditis implies a grave prognosis for life.

2. **Signs**

   - Variable number of flat, yellow, round, choroidal lesions (Fig. 4.62) which are frequently bilateral and not associated with vitritis.
   - Even when the fovea is involved, there is little, if any, impairment of visual acuity.

3. **Treatment** with intravenous trimethoprim, sulphamethoxazole or parenteral pentamidine causes resolution of the lesions within several weeks (Fig. 4.63).

## Diffuse Unilateral Subacute Neuroretinitis

1. **Pathogenesis.** Diffuse unilateral subacute neuroretinitis (DUSN) is an inflammatory disease characterised by a motile subretinal nematode that typically causes monocular visual loss in an otherwise healthy individual. DUSN is caused by at least two unidentified nematodes of different size.

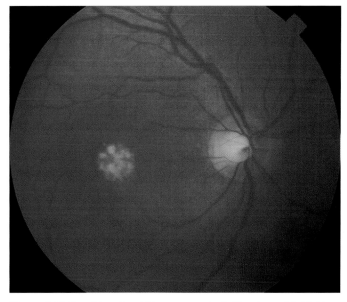

**Figure 4.63** Resolving choroidal pneumocystosis (Courtesy of A. Dick)

2. **Signs,** in chronological order:

   - Papillitis, retinal vasculitis and recurrent crops of evanescent grey-white outer retinal lesions.
   - Optic atrophy, retinal vascular attenuation and diffuse RPE degeneration.

3. **Treatment** involves direct laser photocoagulation of the subretinal nematode.

### FURTHER READING

Cialdini AP, Cunha de Souza E, Avila MP. The first South American case of diffuse unilateral subacute neuroretinitis caused by a large nematode. *Arch Ophthalmol* 1999;117:1431–1432.

Gass JDM, Gilbert WR Jr, Guerry RK, et al. Diffuse unilateral subacute neuroretinitis. *Ophthalmology* 1978;85:521–545.

Moraes LR, Cialdini AP, Avia MP, et al. Identifying live nematodes in diffuse unilateral subacute neuroretinitis by using the scanning laser ophthalmoscope. *Arch Ophthalmol* 2002;120:135–138.

## Ophthalmomyiasis Interna

1. **Pathogenesis.** Ophthalmomyiasis is invasion of the eye or adnexa by larvae of flies, often by the rodent botfly larva (maggot) of the *Cuterebra* and *Hypoderma* species. The larvae usually gain access to the posterior segment from the conjunctival fornices through the peripheral sclera and choroid.

2. **Signs**

   - The larvae travel in the subretinal space, leaving characteristic grey-white tracks in the RPE; these later become depigmented streaks dotted with focal pigment proliferation, which may involve the fovea and cause visual impairment. The larvae may also penetrate the vitreous.
   - Death of the larvae may result in intraocular inflammation.

3. **Treatment** involves photocoagulation of subretinal larvae and surgical removal of vitreous larvae.

## Cysticercosis

1. **Pathogenesis.** Cysticercosis refers to a parasitic infestation by *Cysticercus cellulosae*, the larval form of the pork tapeworm *Taenia solium*. Pigs are the intermediate hosts and humans are the definitive hosts, acquiring the disease by ingesting cysts of *T. solium* from contaminated pork, vegetables or water. As a consequence, humans develop the adult parasite in the intestine, a condition called taeniasis. Cysticercosis occurs after ingestion of eggs which are eliminated in the faeces, or by retrograde peristaltic movements; after penetrating the intestinal wall, the embryo invades the bloodstream and can lodge in various organs, including the eye. The intraocular location may involve the anterior chamber (Fig. 4.64), choroid, subretinal space (Fig. 4.65) and vitreous. Posterior segment ocular involvement occurs in about 10% of cases. The larvae enter the subretinal space, presumably through the posterior ciliary arteries, and can also pass into the vitreous. The larvae release toxins that incite an intense inflammatory reaction, which may ultimately lead to blindness within 3–5 years. The subconjunctival location is the most frequent one for the extraocular form (90%), followed by the orbit (7%) and lids (3%).

2. **Diagnosis**

   - Visualisation of the cyst with a scolex.
   - A history of exposure to an endemic area or consumption of uncooked pork is also supportive.
   - Ultrasonography and MRI may also be helpful.

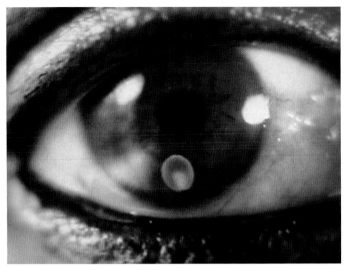

**Figure 4.64** Anterior chamber cysticercosis (Courtesy of A. Pearson)

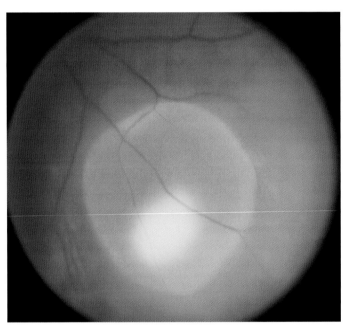

**Figure 4.65** Subretinal cysticercus (Courtesy of J. D. M. Gass, from *Stereoscopic Atlas of Macular Diseases*, Mosby, 1997)

3. **Treatment** involves surgical removal of the larvae. Subretinal cysts may be removed trans-sclerally and intra-vitreal cysts transvitreally.

### FURTHER READING

Sharma T, Sinha S, Shah N, et al. Intraocular cysticercosis: clinical characteristics and visual outcome after vitreoretinal surgery. *Ophthalmology* 2003;110:996–1004.

# VIRAL INFECTIONS

## Acquired Immunodeficiency Syndrome

### PATHOGENESIS

AIDS is caused by the human immunodeficiency virus (HIV), which is predominantly transmitted by sexual intercourse and occasionally by contaminated blood or needles. On a worldwide basis, heterosexual intercourse is the predominant mode of transmission; in the western world, however, AIDS is commonly transmitted by homosexual contact. Transmission may also occur transplacentally or via breast milk. Infection with HIV is typically followed by a latent period, after which develop the clinical manifestations of AIDS. HIV targets CD4+ (helper) T-lymphocytes, which are vital to the initiation of the immune response to pathogens. A steady decline in the absolute number of CD4+ T-lymphocytes therefore occurs, resulting in progressive immune deficiency, particularly cell-mediated immunity. Regular estimation of the CD4+ T count is therefore a useful measure of disease progression. Apart from immunodeficiency, HIV also has the property of mediating direct damage to the CNS.

## SYSTEMIC FEATURES

### 1. Presentation

a. *Acute seroconversion illness.* HIV infection is sometimes followed a few weeks later by constitutional symptoms such as fever, headache, malaise and a maculopapular rash, associated with generalised lymphadenopathy, soon after which anti-HIV antibodies appear.

b. *An asymptomatic phase,* often lasting many years, then follows, during which steady depletion of CD4+ T-lymphocytes occurs.

c. *Symptomatic HIV infection* (AIDS) then follows, characterised by immunosuppression with opportunistic infections, neoplasms and tissue damage directly due to HIV infection.

### 2. Opportunistic infections in AIDS include:

a. *Protozoan.* Toxoplasma, cryptosporidium, microsporidium and *Pneumocystis carinii* (Fig. 4.66).

b. *Viral.* Cytomegalovirus (CMV), herpes simplex and zoster, molluscum contagiosum and Epstein-Barr.

c. *Fungal.* Cryptococcus, candida (Fig. 4.67) and histoplasma.

d. *Bacterial. Mycobacterium tuberculosis, Mycobacterium avium-intracellulare,* staphylococci, streptococci, Haemophilus and *Bartonella henselae.*

### 3. Tumours include Kaposi sarcoma (Figs. 4.68), non-Hodgkin B-cell lymphoma, and squamous cell carcinoma of the conjunctiva (in Africa), cervix and anus.

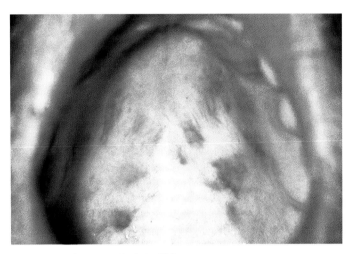

**Figure 4.67** Oral candidiasis in AIDS

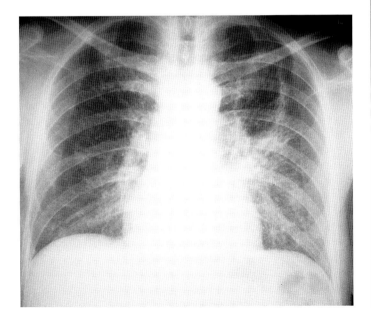

**Figure 4.66** *Pneumocystis carinii* pneumonia in AIDS

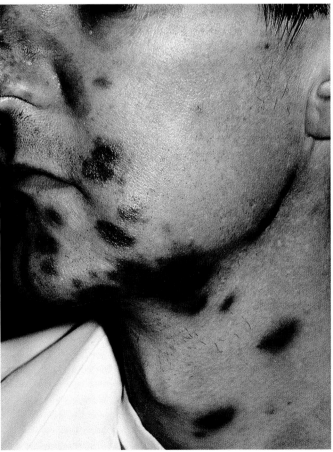

**Figure 4.68** Kaposi sarcoma in AIDS

**4. Other manifestations** include HIV wasting syndrome, encephalopathy and progressive multifocal leuko-encephalopathy.

## DIAGNOSTIC TESTS

Serological testing for HIV infection should be performed only with informed consent after proper counseling, due to the profound implications of a positive result. HIV is confirmed most commonly by the demonstration of anti-HIV antibodies in the serum, by the ELISA and Western blot tests. 'Seroconversion' may take 3 months or longer to occur following exposure to the virus, sometimes necessitating serial testing in individuals at high risk. Subsequent to the establishment of HIV positivity, CD4+ T-lymphocyte counts are measured every 3 months. A CD4+ T-lymphocyte count <200/mm³ implies a high risk of HIV-related disease. AIDS is diagnosed when an HIV-positive subject develops one or more of a defined list of indicator diseases (Table 4.1).

## TREATMENT

Although there is no cure for AIDS, the progression of disease can be slowed by a number of drugs. The aim of treatment is to reduce the plasma viral load. Ideally, therapy should be commenced before the development of irreversible damage to the immune system.

1. **Indications** for commencement of anti-HIV therapy include:

   - Symptomatic HIV disease.
   - CD4+ T-lymphocyte count <300/mm³.

---

- Rapidly falling CD4+ T-lymphocyte count.
- Viral load >10,000/ml of plasma.

2. **Drug treatment** is with 'highly active antiretroviral therapy' (HAART), which involves two nucleoside reverse transcriptase inhibitors with either a non-nucleoside reverse transcriptase inhibitor or one or two protease inhibitors.

   a. *Nucleoside reverse transcriptase inhibitors* include zidovudine, lamivudine and zalcitabine.

   b. *Protease inhibitors* include amprenavir, indinavir and nelfinadir.

   c. *Non-nucleoside reverse transcriptase inhibitors* include efavirenz and nevirapine.

> **NB: Antiretroviral therapy is continuously evolving and should therefore be left to a trained physician.**

## OPHTHALMIC FEATURES

1. **Eyelids:** blepharitis, Kaposi sarcoma, multiple molluscum lesions and severe herpes zoster ophthalmicus.

2. **Orbital:** cellulitis, usually from contiguous sinus infection, and B-cell lymphoma.

3. **Anterior segment**

   - Conjunctival Kaposi sarcoma, squamous cell carcinoma and microangiopathy.
   - Keratitis due to microsporidium, herpes simplex and herpes zoster.
   - Keratoconjunctivitis sicca.
   - Anterior uveitis (usually secondary to systemic drug toxicity: rifabutin, cidofovir).

4. **Posterior segment**

   - HIV retinopathy.
   - CMV retinitis.
   - Progressive outer retinal necrosis.
   - Toxoplasmosis, frequently atypical.
   - Choroidal cryptococcosis.
   - Choroidal pneumocystosis.
   - B-cell intraocular lymphoma.

## CYTOMEGALOVIRUS RETINITIS

In the pre-HAART era, CMV (Fig. 4.69) retinitis was much more common, affecting 25% of patients with AIDS. Its appearance usually signifies severe immunosuppression, although on rare occasions it is the initial manifestation of the disease.

### Signs

1. **Indolent** CMV retinitis is characterised by a mild granular opacification without vasculitis which often starts in the periphery (Fig. 4.70) and progresses slowly (Fig. 4.71).

2. **Fulminating** retinitis is characterised by the following:

   - Mild vitritis.
   - Vasculitis with perivascular sheathing (Fig. 4.72) and opacification (Fig. 4.73).

---

**Table 4.1** AIDS-defining diagnoses (1993 Classification, Europe)

- Candidiasis of bronchi, trachea, lungs or oesophagus
- Cervical carcinoma, invasive
- Coccidioidomycosis, disseminated or extrapulmonary
- Cryptococcus, extrapulmonary
- Cryptosporidiosis, with diarrhoea for >1 month
- Cytomegalovirus disease other than in liver, spleen or lymph nodes
- Encephalopathy, HIV-related
- Herpes simplex ulcers for 1 month or bronchitis, pneumonitis or oesophagitis
- Histoplasmosis, disseminated or extrapulmonary
- Isosporiasis, with diarrhoea for >1 month
- Kaposi sarcoma
- Lymphoid interstitial pneumonitis
- *Mycobacterium avium* complex or *M. kansasii*, disseminated or extrapulmonary
- *Mycobacterium tuberculosis*
- Mycobacterium, other species or unidentified species, disseminated or extrapulmonary
- *Pneumocystis carinii* pneumonia
- Pneumonia, recurrent
- Progressive multifocal leukoencephalopathy
- Salmonella (non-typhoid) septicaemia, recurrent
- Toxoplasmosis of brain
- Wasting syndrome due to HIV (weight loss >10% baseline with no other identified cause)

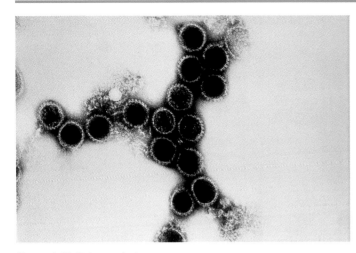

**Figure 4.69** Cytomegalovirus

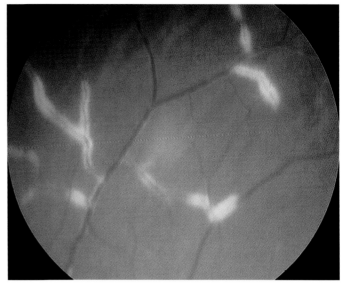

**Figure 4.72** Vasculitis in CMV retinitis

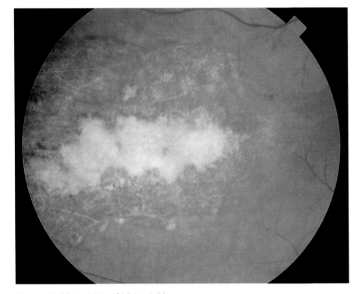

**Figure 4.70** Indolent CMV retinitis

- Dense, white, well-demarcated, geographical area of confluent opacification (Fig. 4.74).
- Retinal haemorrhages may develop either within the area of retinitis or along its leading edge (Fig. 4.75).
- 'Brushfire-like' extension along the course of the retinal blood vessels (Figs. 4.76, 4.77 and 4.78a); FA shows corresponding hypofluorescence in areas of retinal necrosis (Fig. 4.78b).
- Without treatment, the entire retina becomes involved within a few months (Fig. 4.79).

3. **Regression** is characterised by fewer haemorrhages and less opacification, followed by diffuse atrophy and mild pigmentary changes (Fig. 4.80).

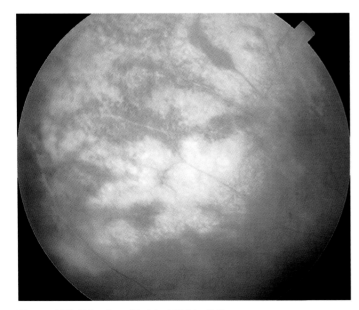

**Figure 4.71** Extension of indolent CMV retinitis

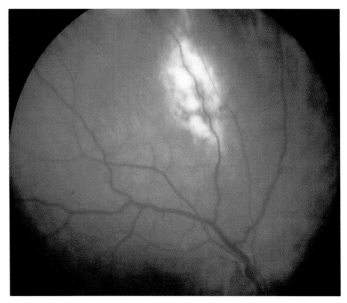

**Figure 4.73** Early fulminating CMV retinitis

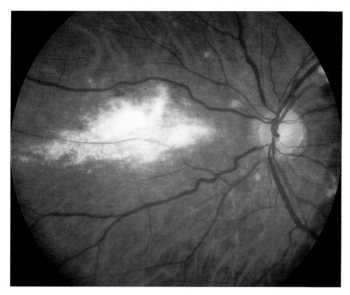

**Figure 4.74** Confluent retinal opacification in fulminating CMV retinitis

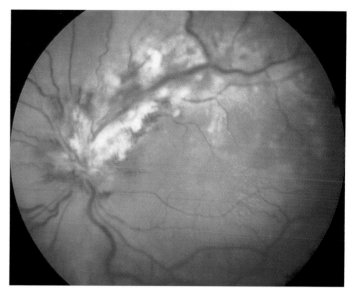

**Figure 4.76** Paravascular spread of fulminating CMV retinitis

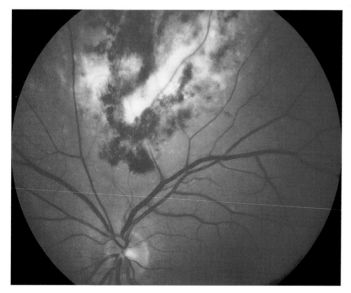

**Figure 4.75** Fulminating CMV retinitis with haemorrhages

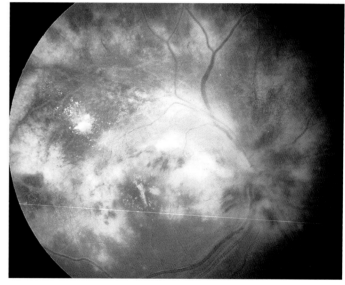

**Figure 4.77** Severe fulminating CMV with severe optic nerve involvement

### 4. Complications

a. *Macular* complications include necrosis, epiretinal membrane formation and hard exudates.

b. *Other* complications include retinal detachment associated with retinal atrophy (Fig. 4.81) and multiple posterior breaks, and consecutive optic atrophy.

***Treatment*** with the following drugs may be used as monotherapy or in combination.

1. **Ganciclovir** is initially given intravenously (induction) 5 mg/kg every 12 hours for 2–3 weeks, then 5 mg/kg every 24 hours. Patients with stable retinitis may be treated with oral ganciclovir 300–450 mg daily for prophylaxis and maintenance. Ganciclovir is effective in 80% of patients but 50% subsequently relapse and require reinduction of therapy. The drug carries a high risk of bone marrow suppression, which often forces interruption of treatment. Ganciclovir can also be administered as a pro-drug (valaganciclovir) with improved gastrointestinal absorption and as effective as intravenous therapy for treatment and prophylaxis.

2. **Intravenous foscarnet,** unlike ganciclovir, also improves life expectancy. The initial dose is 60 mg/kg every 8 hours for 2–3 weeks and then 90–120 mg/kg every 24 hours. Its side effects include nephrotoxicity, electrolyte disturbances and seizures. Foscarnet can also be given intravitreally (2.4 mg in 0.1 ml).

3. **Intravitreal ganciclovir** in the form of injections (2.0–2.5 mg in 0.1 ml) or slow-release devices (Vitrasert – appears to be as effective as intravenous therapy. The duration of the implant is 8 months. However, it fails to protect the fellow

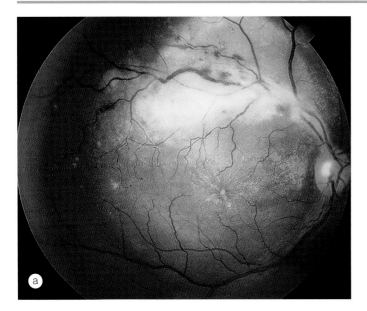

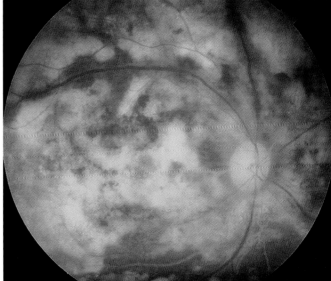

**Figure 4.79** End-stage CMV retinitis

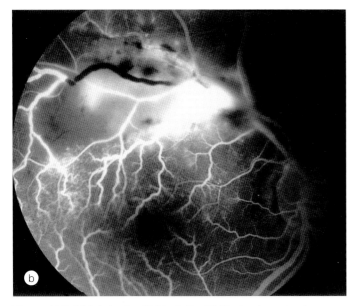

**Figure 4.78 (a)** Fulminating CMV retinitis; **(b)** FA showing extensive hypofluorescence due to ischaemia

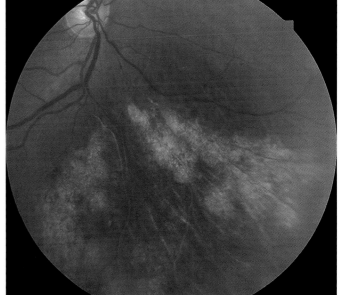

**Figure 4.80** Regressing CMV retinitis

eye from retinitis. Complications of intravitreal therapy include vitreous haemorrhage, retinal detachment and endophthalmitis, and cataract if the implant touches the lens (Fig. 4.82).

4. **Intravenous cidofovir,** 5 mg/kg once weekly for 2 weeks and then every 2 weeks, may be used where other agents are unsuitable. It must be administered in combination with probenecid. Side effects include nephrotoxicity and neutropenia. It can also cause anterior uveitis, usually after several infusions. Cidofovir can also be given intravitreally (15–20 μg in 0.1 ml) but is more toxic than ganciclovir and may cause severe inflammation.

5. **Intravitreal fomivirsen** is the latest drug which has a different mechanism of action from that of other agents. Adverse effects include anterior uveitis, vitritis, cataract and, rarely, retinopathy.

6. **Retinal detachment surgery** often requires vitrectomy and silicone oil to tamponade multiple holes in atrophic retina.

### Prognosis

● Without treatment, the eye becomes blind within 6 weeks to 6 months.
● With treatment, there is a 95% response with decrease in size of the lesions. However, 100% relapse within 2 weeks when treatment is discontinued and there is a 50% relapse rate within 6 months in patients on maintenance therapy.

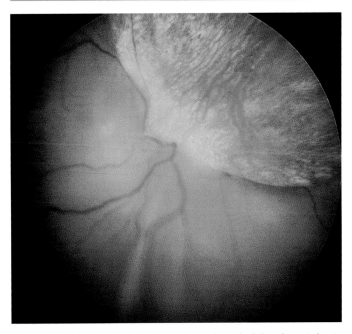

**Figure 4.81** Inferior retinal atrophy and superior retinal detachment due to CMV retinitis (Courtesy of S. Mitchell)

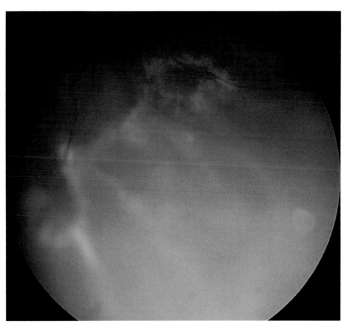

**Figure 4.83** Early progressive outer retinal necrosis (Courtesy of S. Mitchell)

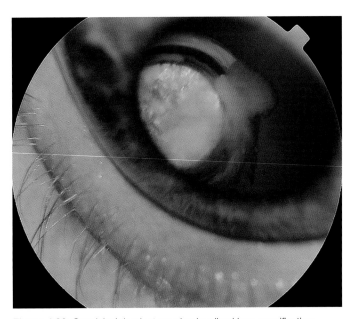

**Figure 4.82** Ganciclovir implant causing localised lens opacification

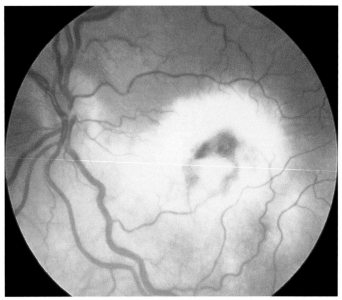

**Figure 4.84** Advanced progressive outer retinal necrosis with macular involvement (Courtesy of S. Lightman)

## PROGRESSIVE OUTER RETINAL NECROSIS

1. **Pathogenesis.** Progressive outer retinal necrosis (PORN) is a rare but devastating necrotising retinitis caused by varicella zoster virus, which behaves more aggressively in patients with profound immunosuppression.

2. **Presentation** is with rapidly progressive visual loss, which is initially unilateral in 75% of cases.

3. **Signs,** in chronological order:

   ● Multifocal, yellow-white, retinal infiltrates with minimal vitritis (Fig. 4.83).

   ● Rapid confluence, full-thickness retinal necrosis and early macular involvement (Fig. 4.84).

   ● Anterior segment inflammation is usually minimal.

4. **Investigations.** Specific PCR-based diagnostic assay for varicella zoster virus DNA may be performed on vitreous samples to confirm the diagnosis.

5. **Treatment** with intravenous ganciclovir, alone or in combination with foscarnet, is often disappointing and most patients become blind in both eyes within a few weeks as a result macular necrosis or retinal detachment. In addition, 50% are dead 5 months after the diagnosis. The

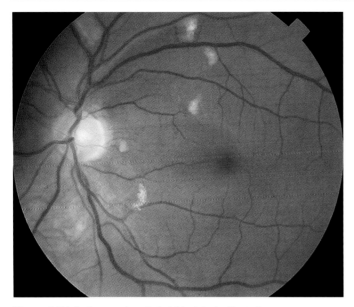

**Figure 4.85** Cotton-wool spots in HIV-related retinopathy

results of vitreoretinal surgery for retinal detachment are disappointing, although silicone oil tamponade and relaxing retinotomies may salvage ambulatory vision in a few cases.

## HIV-RELATED RETINOPATHY

Retinal microangiopathy develops in up to 70% of patients with AIDS and is associated with a declining CD4+ count. It is characterised by cotton-wool spots (Fig. 4.85) which may be associated with retinal haemorrhages and capillary abnormalities. The lesions may be mistaken for early CMV retinitis. However, in contrast to CMV retinitis, the cotton-wool spots are usually asymptomatic and almost invariably disappear spontaneously after several weeks. Postulated causes of the microangiopathy include immune complex deposition, HIV infection of the retinal vascular endothelium, haemorheological abnormalities and abnormal retinal haemodynamics.

## FURTHER READING

Belfort R Jr. The ophthalmologist and the global impact of the AIDS epidemic. LV Edward Jackson Memorial Lecture. *Am J Ophthalmol* 2000;129:1–8.

Cunningham ET Jr, Levinson RD, Jampol LM, et al. Ischaemic maculopathy in patients with acquired immunodeficiency syndrome. *Am J Ophthalmol* 2001;132:727–733.

Goldberg DE, Wang H, Azen SP, et al. Long term visual outcome of patients with cytomegalovirus retinitis treated with highly active antiretroviral therapy. *Br J Ophthalmol* 2003;87:853–855.

Holland GN. Treatment options for cytomegalovirus retinitis. A time for reassessment. *Arch Ophthalmol* 1999;117:1549–1550.

Holland GN. New issues in the management of patients with AIDS-related cytomegalovirus retinitis [Commentary]. *Arch Ophthalmol* 2000;118:704–706.

Jabs DA, Griffiths PD. Fomivirsen for treatment of cytomegalovirus retinitis [Editorial]. *Am J Ophthalmol* 2002;133;552–556.

Jabs DA, Martin BK, Forman MS, et al. Cytomegalovirus resistance to ganciclovir and clinical outcomes of patients with cytomegalovirus retinitis. *Am J Ophthalmol* 2003;135:26–34.

Kashiwase M, Sata T, Yamauchi Y, et al. Progressive outer retinal necrosis caused by herpes simplex virus type 1 in a patient with acquired immunodeficiency syndrome. *Ophthalmology* 2000; 107:790–794.

Kempen JH, Jabs DA, Wilson LA, et al. Risk of visual loss in patients with cytomegalovirus retinitis and the acquired immunodeficiency syndrome. *Arch Ophthalmol* 2003;121:466–476.

Kempen JH, Martin BK, Wu AW, et al. The effect of cytomegalovirus retinitis on the quality of life of patients with AIDS in the era of highly active antiretroviral therapy. *Ophthalmology* 2003; 110:987–995.

Macdonald JC, Karavellas MP, Torriani FJ, et al. High active antiretroviral therapy-related immune recovery in AIDS patients with cytomegalovirus retinitis. *Ophthalmology* 2000;107:877–883.

Mitchell SM, Membrey WL, Youle MS, et al. Cytomegalovirus retinitis after initiation of highly active antiretroviral therapy: a 2 year prospective study. *Br J Ophthalmol* 1999;83:652–655.

Pavcsio CE, Mitchell SM, Barton K, et al. Progressive outer retinal necrosis syndrome (PORN) in AIDS patients: a different appearance of varicella-zoster retinitis. *Eye* 1995;9:271–276.

Roth DB, Feuer WJ, Blenke AJ, et al. Treatment of cytomegalovirus retinitis with the ganciclovir implant. *Am J Ophthalmol* 1999; 127:276–282.

Sarrafizadeh R, Weinberg DV, Huang C-F. An analysis of lesion size and location in newly diagnosed cytomegalovirus retinitis. *Ophthalmology* 2002;109:119–125.

The Vitravene Study Group. A randomized controlled clinical trial of intravenous fomivirsen for treatment of newly diagnosed peripheral cytomegalovirus retinitis in patients with AIDS. *Am J Ophthalmol* 2002;133:467–474.

The Vitravene Study Group. Randomized dose-comparison studies of intravenous fomivirsen for treatment of cytomegalovirus retinitis that has reactivated or is persistently active despite other therapies in patients with AIDS. *Am J Ophthalmol* 2002;133: 475–483.

The Vitravene Study Group. Safety of intravenous fomivirsen for treatment of cytomegalovirus retinitis in patients with AIDS. *Am J Ophthalmol* 2002;133:484–498.

# Acute Retinal Necrosis

***Pathogenesis.*** Acute retinal necrosis (ARN) is a rare but devastating necrotising retinitis which typically affects otherwise healthy individuals of all ages. ARN is a biphasic disease which tends to be caused by herpes simplex in younger patients and herpes zoster in older individuals. Males are more frequently affected than females by a 2:1 ratio. Since the introduction of antiviral therapy, ARN is unilateral in two-thirds of cases.

## *Diagnosis*

1. **Presentation** is initially unilateral and varies according to severity. Some patients develop severe visual impairment over a few days associated with pain, whereas others have an insidious onset with mild visual symptoms such as floaters.

2. **Signs,** in chronological order:

   - Anterior granulomatous uveitis is universal and unless the fundus is examined the diagnosis may be missed.
   - Vitritis is universal (Fig. 4.86).
   - Peripheral retinal periarteritis associated with multifocal, deep, yellow-white, retinal infiltrates (Fig. 4.87).
   - Gradual confluence of lesions associated with full-thickness retinal necrosis (Fig. 4.88).

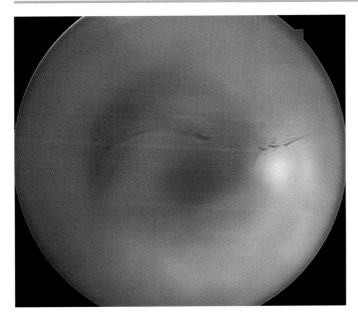

**Figure 4.86** Vitritis in acute retinal necrosis

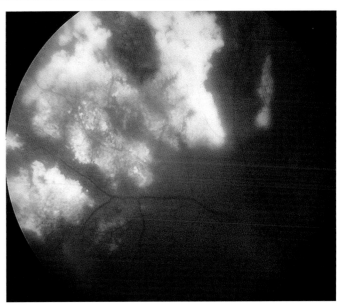

**Figure 4.88** Advanced retinal infiltration in acute retinal necrosis

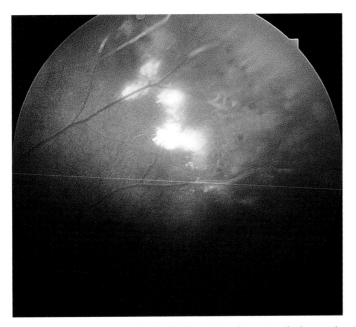

**Figure 4.87** Periarteritis and retinal infiltrates in early acute retinal necrosis

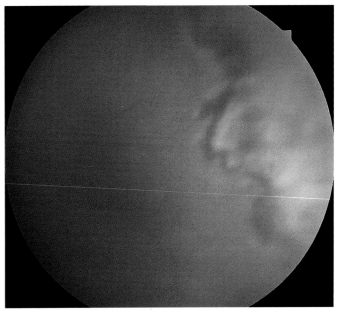

**Figure 4.89** Resolved acute retinal necrosis with a hyperpigmented border

- The posterior pole is usually spared, so visual acuity may remain good despite severe surrounding necrosis, but optic neuropathy may occur early and cause visual loss.
- Other signs include disc oedema, choroidal thickening and retinal haemorrhages.

***Course.*** The acute lesions resolve within 6–12 weeks, leaving behind a transparent and necrotic retina with hyperpigmented borders (Fig. 4.89). Unless the patient received appropriate treatment, the second eye becomes involved in 30% of patients, usually within 2 months, although in some patients the interval may be much longer.

## *Treatment*

1. **Systemic acyclovir,** initially given intravenously (10 mg/kg every 8 hours) for 10 days and then orally for 6–12 weeks, may hasten resolution of the acute lesions and reduce the risk of second eye involvement, but it does not prevent retinal detachment. Recurrences may occur in some patients and long-term therapy may be required.

2. **Systemic steroid** therapy may be started 24 hours after initiation of antiviral therapy in severe cases, especially those with optic neuropathy.

3. **Vitreoretinal surgery** involving silicone oil tamponade is often successful in repairing retinal detachment.

***Prognosis*** is relatively poor, with 60% of patients having a final visual acuity of less than 6/60. The following are the main vision-threatening complications:

1. **Rhegmatogenous retinal detachment,** which develops as a result of the formation of retinal holes at the margin of uninvolved and involved zones.

2. **Tractional retinal detachment** caused by secondary condensation and fibrosis of the vitreous base is less common.

3. **Ischaemic optic neuropathy** caused by thrombotic arteriolar occlusion and infiltration of the optic nerve by inflammatory cells.

4. **Retinal vein occlusion** secondary to periphlebitis.

### Differential diagnosis

1. **Behçet disease** is also characterised by panuveitis, retinitis and necrotising periarteritis. However, the onset and course are more chronic, systemic symptoms are present and the anterior uveitis is non-granulomatous.

2. **CMV retinitis** is also characterised by retinitis and vasculitis. However, the onset is more gradual and vitritis is mild or absent.

3. **Progressive outer retinal necrosis** is also a severe necrotising retinitis. However, it occurs only in AIDS, has a more rapid course and there is no intraocular inflammation.

## FURTHER READING

Crapotta JA, Freeman WR, Feldman RM, et al. Visual outcome in acute retinal necrosis. *Retina* 1993;13:208–213.

Duker JS, Blumenkranz MS. Diagnosis and management of the acute retinal necrosis (ARN) syndrome. *Surv Ophthalmol* 1991; 35:327–343.

Duker JS, Nielsen JC, Eagle RC Jr, et al. Rapidly progressive acute retinal necrosis secondary to herpes simplex virus type 1. *Ophthalmology* 1990;97:1638–1643.

Ganatra JB, Chandler D, Santos C, et al. Viral causes of the acute retinal necrosis syndrome. *Am J Ophthalmol* 2000;129:166–172.

Holland GN. Standard diagnostic criteria for the acute retinal necrosis syndrome. *Am J Ophthalmol* 1994;117:663–666.

# Congenital Rubella

Rubella (German measles) is usually a benign febrile exanthema. Congenital rubella results from transplacental transmission of virus to the foetus from an infected mother, usually during the first trimester of pregnancy. This may lead to serious chronic foetal infection and malformations. It appears that the risk to the foetus is closely related to the stage of gestation at the time of maternal infection. Foetal infection is about 50% during the first 8 weeks, 33% between weeks 9 and 12, and about 10% between weeks 13 and 24. Each of the various organs affected has its own period of susceptibility to the infection, after which no gross malformations are produced. Systemic complications of maternal rubella include: spontaneous abortion, stillbirth, congenital heart malformations, deafness, microcephaly, mental handicap, hypotonia, hepatosplenomegaly, thrombocytopenic purpura, pneumonitis, myocarditis and metaphyseal bone lesions.

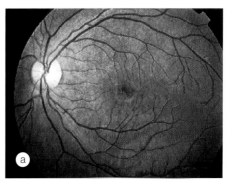

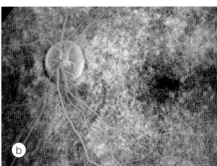

**Figure 4.90 (a)** Rubella retinopathy; **(b)** FA (see text)

***Retinal involvement*** is the most common ocular complication, but the exact incidence is unknown because cataracts frequently impair visualisation of the fundus. Retinopathy may involve one or both eyes.

1. **Signs**

   ● 'Salt and pepper' pigmentary disturbance, most often involving the posterior pole and most marked at the macula (Fig. 4.90a); fluorescein angiography (FA) shows corresponding hypofluorescent spots (Fig. 4.90b).

   ● The optic nerve head and retinal blood vessels are usually normal.

2. **Prognosis** is usually good and visual acuity may be normal or slightly impaired. A small percentage of eyes develop CNV.

### Other ocular manifestations

1. **Cataract** affects about 15% of infants.

2. **Microphthalmos** affects 10–20% of cases and may be associated with cataract, optic nerve abnormalities and glaucoma.

3. **Glaucoma** develops in about 10% of eyes, usually during the neonatal period. It may or may not be associated with cataract. When occurring in a microphthalmic eye, the raised intraocular pressure could enlarge the cornea to normal size. When occurring in a normal-size eye, the cornea may become larger than normal (buphthalmos). Corneal haze resulting from corneal oedema is also an important feature of glaucoma.

4. **Miscellaneous** manifestations, which are less common, are corneal haze, iritis, iris atrophy and extreme refractive errors. Pendular nystagmus and strabismus may develop as a consequence of the various ocular abnormalities.

## FURTHER READING

Yoser SL, Forster DJ, Rao NA. Systemic viral infections and their retinal and choroidal manifestations. *Surv Ophthalmol* 1993;37:313–352.

# BACTERIAL INFECTIONS

## Tuberculosis

Tuberculosis (TB) is a chronic granulomatous infection caused by the tubercule bacillus, either bovine (*Mycobacterium bovis*) or human (*Mycobacterium tuberculosis*). The former is acquired by drinking milk from infected cattle and the latter by 'droplet infection'. Immunocompromised patients carry an increased risk of TB.

## SYSTEMIC FEATURES

### Stages

1. **Primary TB** occurs in subjects not previously exposed to the bacillus. It is characterised by the 'primary complex' in the chest (Ghon focus + regional lymphadenopathy), which causes few if any symptoms and usually heals spontaneously.

2. **Post-primary TB** is the result of re-infection or recrudescence of a primary lesion, usually in a patient with impaired

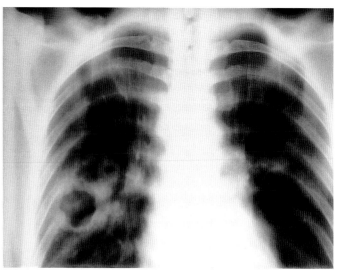

**Figure 4.92** Chest radiograph showing tuberculous cavitation in the right lung

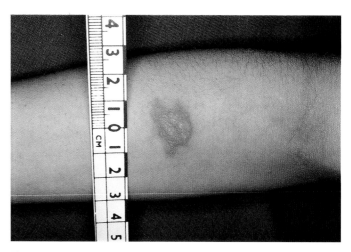

**Figure 4.93** Positive BCG test

immunity. Clinical features include erythema nodosum, fibrocaseous pulmonary lesions and lymph node involvement (Fig. 4.91). Haematogenous spread (miliary TB) may involve internal organs and bones.

### Diagnostic tests

1. **Sputum examination** for acid-fast bacilli.

2. **Chest radiographs** (Fig. 4.92).

3. **Tuberculin testing** may be useful in the diagnosis of extra-thoracic TB. A negative result usually excludes TB, but may also occur in the setting of advanced consumptive disease. A weakly positive result does not necessarily distinguish between previous exposure and active disease. This is because most individuals have already received Bacille Calmette-Guerin (BCG) and will therefore exhibit a hypersensitivity response. A strongly positive result characterised by induration of more than 10 mm (Fig. 4.93) is usually indicative of active disease.

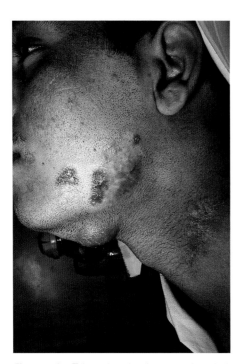

**Figure 4.91** Tuberculous involvement of cervical lymph glands

4. **Anticord factor antibody** is a new test for ocular TB.

***Treatment*** is initially with at least three drugs (isoniazid, rifampicin, pyrazinamide or ethambutol) and then with isoniazid and rifampicin. Quadruple therapy is sometimes necessary in resistant cases, more frequently seen in highly endemic areas such as India.

## TUBERCULOUS UVEITIS

This is rare in the developed world. However, it may occur without systemic signs of TB, rendering definitive diagnosis difficult. The diagnosis of tuberculous uveitis is therefore often presumptive, based on indirect evidence such as intractable uveitis unresponsive to steroid therapy, a positive history of contact, a positive skin test and negative findings for other causes of uveitis.

### Clinical features

1. **Chronic anterior uveitis,** usually granulomatous, but occasionally non-granulomatous, is the most frequent feature.

2. **Choroiditis** may be focal or multifocal.

3. **A large solitary choroidal granuloma** (Fig. 4.94), which may be mistaken for a choroidal tumour, is rare.

4. **Periphlebitis** (Fig. 4.95) may lead to peripheral retinal capillary closure and neovascularisation, very similar to that seen in Eales disease.

> NB: Periphlebitis is usually bilateral and represents a manifestation of hypersensitivity to the bacillus, while choroidal involvement is usually unilateral and reflects direct infection.

***Treatment*** is that of the systemic disease. Topical steroids are also used for anterior uveitis but systemic steroids are absolutely contraindicated.

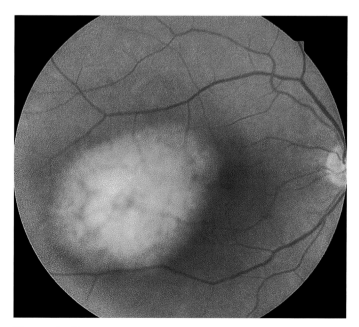

**Figure 4.94** Tuberculous choroidal granuloma

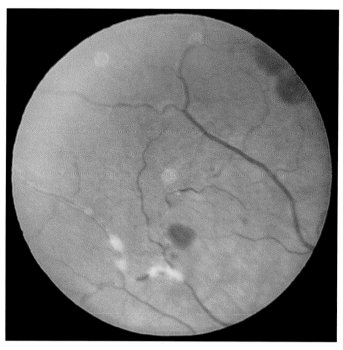

**Figure 4.95** Mild tuberculous periphlebitis (Courtesy of K. Bibby)

## FURTHER READING

Helm CJ, Holland GN. Ocular tuberculosis. *Surv Ophthalmol* 1993;38:229–256.

Morimura Y, Okada AA, Kawahara S, et al. Tuberculin skin testing in uveitis patients and treatment of presumed intraocular tuberculosis. *Ophthalmology* 2002;109:851–857.

# Syphilis

Syphilis is a sexually transmitted infection caused by the spirochaete *Treponema pallidum.*

## SYSTEMIC FEATURES

### Stages

1. **Primary** syphilis occurs after an incubation period commonly lasting 2–4 weeks and is characterised by a painless ulcer (chancre) at the site of inoculation (usually genitalia) and associated regional lymphadenopathy.

2. **Secondary** syphilis occurs usually 6–8 weeks after the chancre and is characterised by the following:

   - Generalised lymphadenopathy with mild or absent constitutional symptoms.
   - Symmetrical maculopapular rash on the trunk (Fig. 4.96), palms and soles.
   - Condylomata lata in the anal region.
   - Mucous patches in the mouth, pharynx and genitalia, consisting of painless greyish-white circular erosions ('snail-track ulcers').
   - Meningitis, nephritis and hepatitis may occur.

3. **Latent** syphilis follows resolution of secondary syphilis, may last for years and can be detected only by serological tests

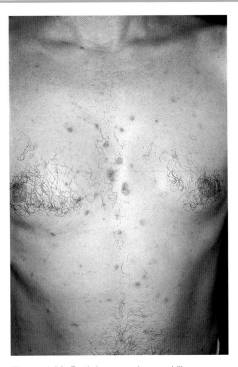

**Figure 4.96** Rash in secondary syphilis

4. **Tertiary** syphilis occurs in about 40% of untreated cases and is characterised by:

- Cardiovascular manifestations: aortitis with aneurysm formation and aortic regurgitation.
- Neurosyphilis: tabes dorsalis, Charcot joints and general paralysis of the insane.
- Gummata in various organs.

### Diagnostic tests

1. **VDRL** (Venereal Disease Research Laboratory). The titres reflect disease activity. It becomes positive during the primary stage and may become negative if treatment is given early.

2. **FTA-ABS** (fluorescent treponemal antibody absorption) is specific for treponema antibodies but is not titratable; it never becomes negative ('serologic scar').

3. **MHA-TP** (microhaemagglutination assay with *Treponema pallidum* antigen) is specific for treponema antibodies but may be negative in early primary syphilis.

**Treatment** is with procaine penicillin (10 days in primary and secondary syphilis; 4 weeks in tertiary syphilis); alternatives in penicillin-allergic patients include doxycycline, tetracycline and erythromycin.

## SYPHILITIC UVEITIS

This is uncommon and there are no pathognomonic signs. Eye involvement typically occurs during the secondary and tertiary stages, although occasionally it may be seen during primary syphilis. The disease must therefore be suspected in any case of intraocular inflammation resistant to conventional therapy.

### Clinical features

1. **Anterior uveitis** occurs in about 4% of patients with secondary syphilis and is bilateral in 50%. The inflammation is usually acute and, unless appropriately treated, becomes chronic. In some cases, iridocyclitis is first associated with dilated iris capillaries (roseolae – Fig. 4.97), which may develop into more localised papules and subsequently into larger yellowish nodules. Various types of post-inflammatory iris atrophy may ensue.

2. **Posterior uveitis** may take several forms.

    a. *Multifocal choroiditis*, which, on healing, appears as focal areas of chorioretinal atrophy associated with hyperpigmentation (Fig. 4.98). Occasionally, extensive pigmentary changes with perivascular bone spicules, similar to those seen in retinitis pigmentosa, may be associated with night blindness and a ring scotoma.

    b. *Focal chorioretinitis* is less common and frequently bilateral. It is characterised by an inflammatory focus near the disc or at the macula.

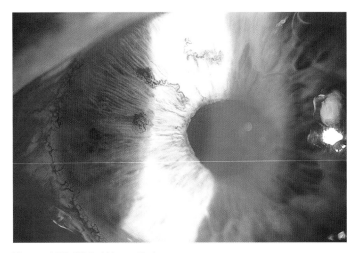

**Figure 4.97** Dilated iris capillaries

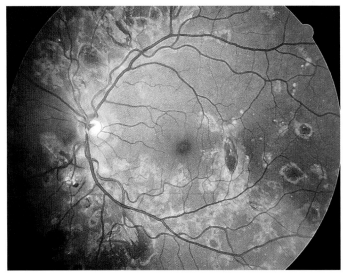

**Figure 4.98** Old syphilitic multifocal choroiditis (Courtesy of J. Salmon)

c. *Neuroretinitis* (Fig. 4.99) may give rise to secondary optic atrophy and replacement of retinal vessels by white strands (Fig. 4.100).

d. *Acute posterior placoid chorioretinitis.*

e. *Periphlebitis,* which may be associated with central retinal vein occlusion.

**Treatment** with conventional doses of penicillin is inadequate; the therapeutic regimen is the same as for neurosyphilis (which should be ruled out by lumbar puncture). One of the following regimens may be used:

1. **Intravenous aqueous penicillin** G 12–24 mega units (MU) daily for 10–15 days.

2. **Intramuscular procaine penicillin** 2.4 MU daily, supplemented with oral probenecid (2 g daily), for 10–15 days.

3. **Oral amoxycillin** 3 g twice daily for 28 days.

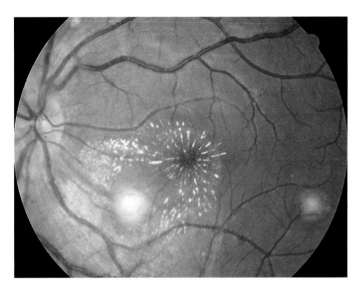

**Figure 4.99** Active syphilitic neuroretinitis (Courtesy of J. Salmon)

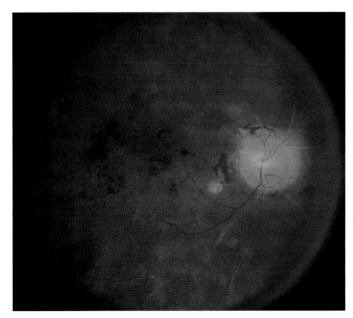

**Figure 4.100** End-stage syphilitic neuroretinitis

---

> **NB:** Penicillin-allergic patients can be treated with oral tetracycline or erythromycin 500 mg four times daily for 30 days.

## FURTHER READING

Gass JDM, Braunstein RA, Chenoweth RG. Acute syphilitic posterior placoid chorioretinitis. *Ophthalmology* 1990;97:1288–1297.

# Metastatic Endophthalmitis

***Pathogenesis.*** Metastatic (endogenous) bacterial endophthalmitis is much less common than post-surgical. Its treatment is less well established and visual results are often disappointing. Both eyes are involved in about 25% of cases. The infection is caused by haematogenous spread of bacteria from a site of infection in the body or from contaminated intravenous catheters or needles. Potential causes include septic arthritis, urinary tract infection, endocarditis, liver abscess and infected skin wounds. Often the primary site of infection is occult. The most frequent pathogen is Bacillus cereus, although a wide variety of organisms have been implicated, including Proprionibacterium acnes and streptococci. The infecting organisms enter the uveal or retinal circulations and lodge in capillaries, where they establish a septic focus. Subsequently they break through into the aqueous and vitreous. Immunocompromised patients are particularly susceptible to rapid involvement of the vitreous.

### Clinical features

1. **Anterior**

   a. *Focal* infection is characterised by discrete iris nodules or plaques and anterior uveitis of variable severity.

   b. *Diffuse* infection manifests as very severe fibrinous anterior uveitis (Fig. 4.101).

2. **Posterior**

   a. *Focal* infection is characterised by white or yellow infiltrates (Fig. 4.102) and vitreous haze. The visual prognosis is usually good.

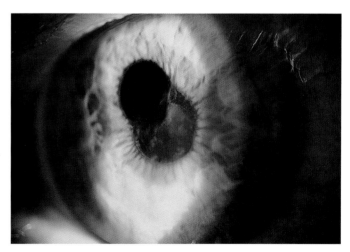

**Figure 4.101** Diffuse anterior uveitis in metastatic endophthalmitis

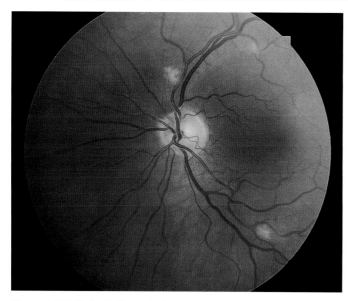

**Figure 4.102** Retinal infiltrates in focal endogenous endophthalmitis

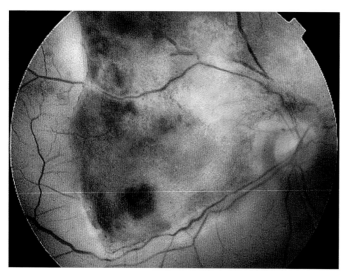

**Figure 4.103** Retinal necrosis in diffuse endogenous endophthalmitis

b. *Diffuse* infection is characterised by severe involvement of the retina and vitreous, which may result in retinal necrosis (Fig. 4.103) and vitreous abscess formation. The visual prognosis is poor.

### Investigations

1. **Systemic.** Blood and urine cultures should be obtained in all patients. If appropriate, cultures from other sites should also be obtained depending on the clinical features (e.g. cerebrospinal fluid, skin wounds, joints and abscesses).

2. **Ocular.** Aqueous samples should be obtained in patients with anterior infection, and vitreous samples in cases of diffuse posterior involvement.

### Treatment

1. **Intravenous** antibiotic therapy is the same as that for any other life-threatening generalised systemic infection. The choice of antibiotic is based on culture and sensitivity results, and should continue for 2–3 weeks. Patients without an evident source of infection should be treated with a combination of ceftazidime 1 g every 12 hours and vancomycin 1 g every 12 hours.

2. **Intravitreal** antibiotics should be used in posterior diffuse infection and in posterior focal infection that has not responded to 2 days' treatment with systemic therapy.

### FURTHER READING
Okada A, Johnson P, Liles C, et al. Endogenous bacterial endophthalmitis. *Ophthalmology* 1994;101:832–838.

## Whipple Disease

Whipple disease is a rare, chronic, bacterial infection with *Tropheryma whippelii* that primarily involves the gastro-intestinal tract and its lymphatic drainage in middle-aged individuals.

### Clinical features

1. **Extraintestinal manifestations** include primarily the CNS, lungs, heart, joints and eyes.

2. **Diagnostic tests**
   - Jejunal biopsy, which shows the typical PAS-positive 'foamy' macrophages.
   - PCR on vitreous samples in patients with ocular involvement.

3. **Ocular involvement** may be in the form of vitritis, retinitis, retinal haemorrhages, cotton-wool spots, multifocal choroiditis, papilloedema, optic atrophy and keratitis.

4. **Neuro-ophthalmological** findings may include ophthalmoplegia, supranuclear gaze palsy, nystagmus, myoclonus and ptosis.

**Treatment** is with antibiotics such as trimethoprim–sulphamethoxazole and tetracycline.

### FURTHER READING
Avila MP, Jalkh AE, Feldman E, et al. Manifestations of Whipple's disease in the posterior segment of the eye. *Arch Ophthalmol* 1984;102:384–390.

Chan RY, Yannuzzi LA, Foster CS. Ocular Whipple's disease. Earlier definitive diagnosis. *Ophthalmology* 2001;108:2225–2231.

## Nocardia Endophthalmitis

***Pathogenesis.*** *Nocardia asteroides*, a Gram-positive, aerobic bacterium, is a cause of opportunistic infections in immunocompromised patients, particularly those with lymphomas, long-term pulmonary disease and long-term systemic steroid therapy. The organism is usually inhaled and may cause localised or systemic disease with a predilection for the brain and soft tissues, with suppurative necrosis and abscess formation. Ocular involvement, however, is rare.

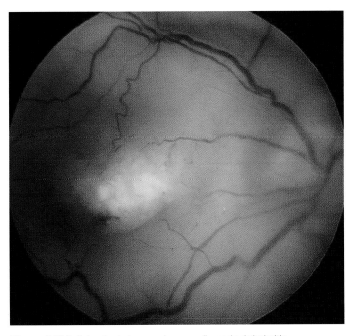

**Figure 4.104** Subretinal abscess in nocardia endophthalmitis

### Diagnosis

1. **Presentation** is with floaters, decreased vision and photophobia.

2. **Signs**

   - Anterior uveitis and vitritis.
   - Chorioretinitis with subretinal abscess (Fig. 4.104) formation is the hallmark.

***Treatment*** with intravitreal amikacin and imipenem and intravenous ceftriaxone may be effective; however, the prognosis is poor.

### FURTHER READING

Davitt B, Gehers K, Bowers T. Endogenous *Nocardia* endophthalmitis. *Retina* 1998;18:71–73.
Ng EWM, Zimmer-Galler IE, Green WR. Endogenous *Nocardia asteroides* endophthalmitis. *Arch Ophthalmol* 2002;120: 210–212.

# FUNGAL INFECTIONS

## Histoplasmosis

### PATHOGENESIS

Histoplasmosis is a fungal infection caused by *Histoplasma capsulatum*. The disease is acquired by inhalation and the organisms pass via the bloodstream to the spleen, liver and, on occasion, the choroid, setting up multiple foci of granulomatous inflammation. In the vast majority of patients, the fungaemia is innocuous and asymptomatic, because the organisms disappear after a few weeks. A small minority of patients develop severe, disseminated systemic histoplasmosis. Although ocular histoplasmosis has never been reported in patients with active, systemic histoplasmosis, eye disease has an increased prevalence in areas where histoplasmosis is endemic, such as the Mississippi– Missouri river valley.

> **NB: Organisms have never been isolated from the eyes, hence the name Presumed Ocular Histoplasmosis Syndrome (POHS).**

### DIAGNOSTIC TESTS

1. **Histoplasma skin testing,** although positive in about 90% of patients with ocular involvement, it is now seldom performed, and should be avoided in patients with macular lesions due to the potential risk of reactivation and visual loss.

2. **Complement fixation** tests are of limited value because they usually become negative several years after the original infection.

3. **Radiographs** may occasionally show old calcified granulomata in the lungs and spleen.

4. **Tissue typing** of patients with ocular disease, particularly if associated with maculopathy, shows an increased prevalence of HLA-B7.

### OCULAR HISTOPLASMOSIS

***Asymptomatic lesions*** are bilateral in 60% of cases.

1. **Absence of intraocular inflammation.**

2. **Atrophic 'histo spots'** consist of roundish, slightly irregular, yellowish-white lesions about 200 $\mu$m in diameter. Small pigment clumps may be present within or at the margins of the scars, although some spots are not associated with pigmentation. The lesions are scattered in the mid-retinal periphery (Fig. 4.105) and the posterior pole (Fig. 4.106).

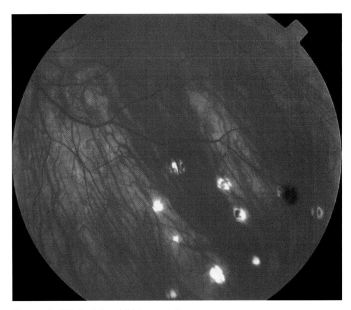

**Figure 4.105** Peripheral 'histo spots'

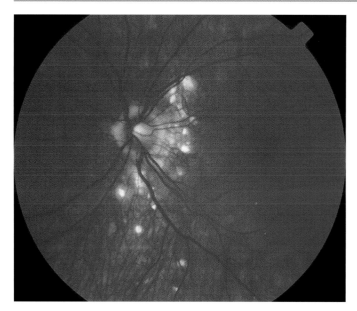

**Figure 4.106** Central 'histo spots'

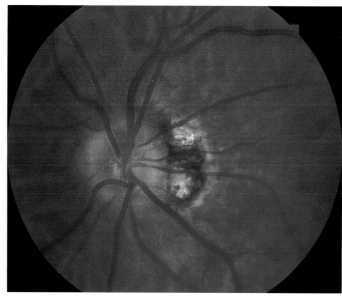

**Figure 4.108** Focal juxtapapillary atrophy in ocular histoplasmosis

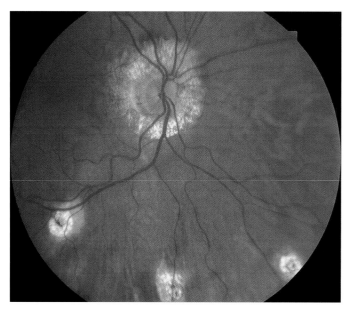

**Figure 4.107** Circumferential juxtapapillary atrophy and 'histo spots'

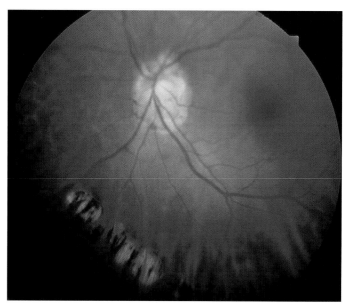

**Figure 4.109** Linear streaks of chorioretinal atrophy in ocular histoplasmosis

3. **Juxtapapillary atrophy** may be diffuse or focal or a combination of both.

   a. *Circumferential* choroidal atrophy extends up to half a disc diameter beyond the disc margin (Fig. 4.107).

   b. *Focal* lesions are less common and are irregular and punched out, resembling the peripheral spots (Fig. 4.108).

4. **Linear streaks** of chorioretinal atrophy are seen in the fundus periphery (Fig. 4.109).

### *Exudative maculopathy*

1. **CNV** is a late manifestation which usually develops between the ages of 20 and 45 years in about 5% of eyes. In most cases, CNV is associated with an old macular 'histo spot',

although occasionally it develops within a peripapillary lesion. Very rarely, the CNV occurs in the absence of a pre-existing scar.

2. **The clinical course** of maculopathy follows one of the following patterns:

   ● The CNV may initially leak fluid and give rise to metamorphopsia, blurring of central vision and a scotoma. Careful slit-lamp biomicroscopy with a fundus contact lens shows that the macula is elevated by serous fluid and an underlying focal yellow-white or grey lesion. In 12% of eyes, the subretinal fluid absorbs spontaneously and visual symptoms regress.

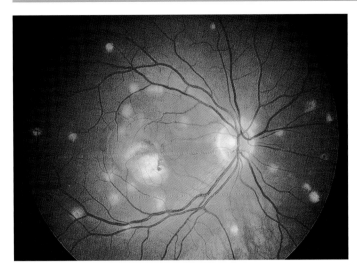

**Figure 4.110** Ocular histoplasmosis with numerous 'histo spots' and a disciform scar at the macula due to previous CNV

- A dark green-black ring frequently develops on the surface of the yellow-white lesion and bleeding occurs into the sub-sensory retinal space, causing a marked drop in visual acuity. In a few eyes, the subretinal haemorrhage resolves and visual acuity improves.
- In some eyes, the initial CNV remains active for about 2 years, giving rise to repeated haemorrhages. This finally causes a profound and permanent impairment of central vision, resulting from the development of a fibrous disciform scar at the fovea (Fig. 4.110). Patients with maculopathy in one eye and an asymptomatic atrophic macular scar in the other are likely to develop a disciform lesion in the second eye. They should therefore test themselves every day with an Amsler grid to detect early metamorphopsia because without treatment 60% of eyes with CNV have a final visual acuity of less than 6/60.

### 3. Treatment of CNV

a. *Laser photocoagulation* is at present the treatment of choice. Pre-treatment FA is vital in evaluating the extent and location of CNV (Fig. 4.111).
b. *Surgical removal* of subfoveal CMV may be indicated in selected cases.

### FURTHER READING

Fine SL, Wood WJ, Singerman LJ, et al. Laser treatment for subfoveal neovascular membranes in ocular histoplasmosis syndrome: results of a pilot randomized clinical trial. *Arch Ophthalmol* 1993;111:19–20.

Macular Photocoagulation Study Group. Five-year follow-up of fellow eyes in individuals with ocular histoplasmosis and unilateral extrafoveal or juxtafoveal choroidal neovascularization. *Arch Ophthalmol* 1996;114:677–688.

## Candidiasis

***Pathogenesis.*** Candida albicans, a yeast-like fungus, is a frequent commensal of the human skin, mouth, gastrointestinal tract and vagina. Candidiasis is an opportunistic infection in which the organism acquires pathogenic properties. Candidaemia, which may result in ocular involvement, occurs in two main groups of patients.

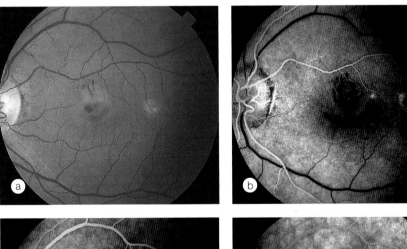

**Figure 4.111** CNV in ocular histoplasmosis. **(a)** Foveal oedema and haemorrhage; **(b)** FA arterial phase shows lacy hyperfluorescence at the fovea; **(c)** the venous phase shows increasing hyperfluorescence; **(d)** the late phase shows intense hyperfluorescence due to leakage. There is also an area of increasing hyperfluorescence temporal to the fovea due to an RPE window defect corresponding to a 'histo spot'

1. **Drug addicts** may become infected through the use of non-sterile needles and syringes, or by the use of heroin diluted with lemon juice, which is ideal because of its low pH and is usually contaminated by *Candida,* which can be found on the lemon skin. Frequently, however, there is no obvious evidence of disseminated candidiasis and blood and urine cultures are negative for *Candida* species. In this group, the diagnosis may be missed unless the skin is carefully examined for evidence of injection site scars.

2. **Patients with long-term indwelling catheters** used for haemodialysis or intravenous nutrition following extensive bowel surgery, are at increased risk.

### Diagnosis

1. **Presentation** is with gradual unilateral blurring of vision and floaters.

2. **Signs,** in chronological order:

   ● Choroiditis (Fig. 4.112).
   ● Multifocal retinitis manifest as small, round, white, slightly elevated lesions with indistinct borders (Fig. 4.113).
   ● Vitreous involvement characterised by floating white 'cotton-ball' colonies (Fig. 4.114 and Fig. 4.115).
   ● Chronic endophthalmitis characterised by severe vitreous infiltration.

3. **The course** is chronic and may result in the development of retinal necrosis and retinal detachment, often associated with proliferative vitreoretinopathy.

4. **Investigations** involving vitreous biopsy and smears and cultures may be required to confirm the diagnosis and test the sensitivity of the organisms to antifungal agents.

### Treatment

1. **Systemic** treatment is with a combination of oral 5-fluorocytosine (flucytosine) 150 mg/kg daily and fluconazole 200–400 mg daily for 3 weeks. Alternative therapy in

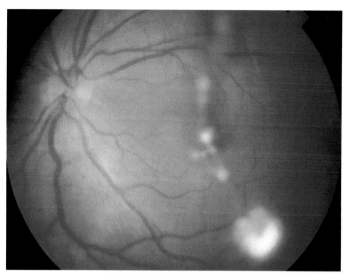

**Figure 4.113** Multifocal retinitis with early vitreous involvement in ocular candidiasis

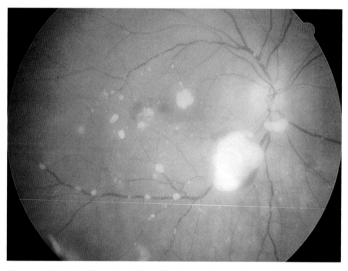

**Figure 4.114** Multifocal retinitis with vitreous 'cotton-balls' (Courtesy of J. Salmon)

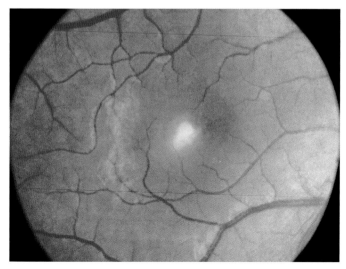

**Figure 4.112** Focal choroiditis in ocular candidiasis

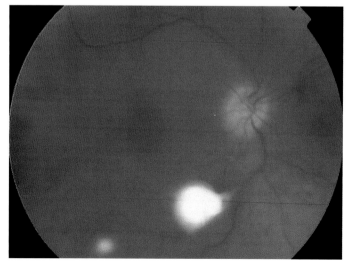

**Figure 4.115** Vitreous 'cotton balls' and vitritis

resistant cases is intravenous amphotericin B in 5% dextrose, given over a period of several days until a cumulative dose of 200 mg has been reached. The initial daily dose is 5 mg and after a few days this can be increased to 20 mg.

> NB: Steroids are contraindicated in fungal infections.

2. **Pars plana vitrectomy** is indicated when there is vitreous involvement and for moderate–severe endophthalmitis, with combined intravitreal injection of 5 µg of amphotericin B.

***Differential diagnosis*** includes Aspergillosis which is typically associated with drug-induced immunosuppression following organ transplantation or valvular heart surgery and carries a high mortality rate from cerebral and cardiac complications. Ocular involvement is characterised by extensive areas of choroiditis but less vitritis than in candidiasis. Vitreous cultures are usually negative.

### FURTHER READING

Chignell AH. Endogenous candidiasis. *J R Soc Med* 1992;85:721–724.

Graham DA, Kinyoun JL, George DP. Endogenous *Aspergillus* endophthalmitis after lung transplantation. *Am J Ophthalmol* 1995;119:107–109.

Luttrull JK, Wan WL, Kubak BM, et al. Treatment of ocular fungal infections with oral fluconazole. *Am J Ophthalmol* 1995; 119:477–481.

Rao NA, Hidayat AA. Endogenous mycotic endophthalmitis: variations in clinical and histopathologic changes in candidiasis compared with aspergillosis. *Am J Ophthalmol* 2001;132:244–251.

Weishar PD, Flynn HW Jr, Murray TG, et al. Endogenous *Aspergillus* endophthalmitis. Clinical features and treatment outcomes. *Ophthalmology* 1998;105:57–65.

## Cryptococcosis

*Cryptococccus neoformans* frequently infects the CNS in patients with AIDS, although clinical ocular involvement is rare. When it does occur, it usually follows systemic disease, most commonly meningitis.

1. **Signs,** in chronological order:

   - Asymptomatic multifocal choroiditis (Fig. 4.116).
   - Retinitis, which is rare, is characterised by small, glistening spheres at the vitreoretinal interface.
   - Optic nerve involvement is usually manifest as papilloedema due to raised intracranial pressure, but direct optic nerve involvement may result in rapid visual loss.

2. **Treatment** of sight-threatening lesions is with intravenous amphotericin B. Endophthalmitis may require pars plana vitrectomy and intravitreal amphotericin.

### FURTHER READING

Sheu SJ, Chen YC, Kuo NW, et al. Endogenous cryptococcal endophthalmitis. *Ophthalmology* 1998;105:377–381.

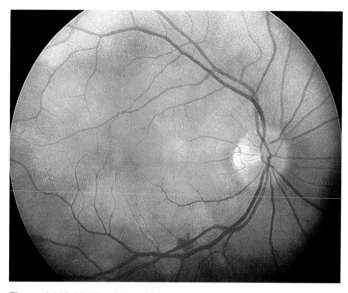

**Figure 4.116** Multifocal choroiditis in cryptococcosis (Courtesy of S. Mitchell)

# IDIOPATHIC MULTIFOCAL WHITE DOT SYNDROMES

## Acute Posterior Multifocal Placoid Pigment Epitheliopathy

Acute posterior multifocal placoid pigment epitheliopathy (APMPPE) is an uncommon, idiopathic, usually bilateral, self-limiting condition which typically affects healthy young adults. In about one-third of patients, APMPPE follows a flu-like illness and a few may also develop erythema nodosum. It is thought that in some cases APMPPE may be the initial manifestation of a CNS vasculitis. The condition affects both sexes equally and there is an association with HLA-B7 and HLA-DR2.

### *Diagnosis*

1. **Presentation** is with subacute visual impairment and paracentral scotomas. Within a few days, the fellow eye also becomes affected.

2. **Signs**

   - Multiple, large, cream-coloured or grayish-white, subretinal plaque-like lesions of variable size (Fig. 4.117 and see Fig. 4.119a).
   - The lesions typically begin at the posterior pole and then extend to involve the post-equatorial fundus.
   - Mild vitritis in 50% of cases.
   - Occasional findings include anterior uveitis, disc oedema and periphlebitis.
   - After a few weeks, lesions fade, leaving variable residual multifocal areas of depigmentation and clumping of the RPE (Fig. 4.118).

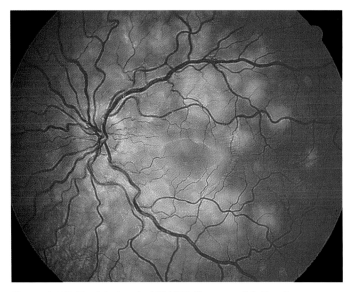

**Figure 4.117** Fresh lesions in APMPPE (Courtesy of C. Barry)

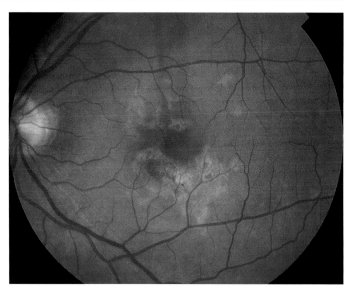

**Figure 4.118** Residual lesions of APMPPE

- New lesions may appear during resolution of the early lesions and it is not uncommon to find lesions at different stages of evolution.
- Recurrences can also occur later in life.

3. **FA** of active lesions shows early dense hypofluorescence due to non-perfusion of the choriocapillaris (Fig. 4.119b) and late hyperfluorescence due to staining (Fig. 4.119c).

**Treatment.** Although there is no evidence that systemic steroids change the natural course of the disease, some ophthalmologists still recommend steroid therapy for patients with macular involvement and poor vision. Some patients require treatment of cerebral vasculitis.

**Prognosis** is usually good and the majority of patients slowly recover visual acuity to normal or near-normal, although this may take up to 6 months. Occasionally, paracentral scotomas associated with healed lesions lead to annoying symptoms despite good visual acuity. CNV is a very rare late complication.

### Differential diagnosis

1. **Serpiginous choroidopathy.** The early lesions may resemble APMPPE but it occurs in an older age group, runs a recurrent course, and has a poor prognosis.

2. **Multiple evanescent white dot syndrome** also causes subacute visual loss in healthy young adults and has a good prognosis. However, the lesions are smaller and unilateral.

3. **Harada disease** is characterised by diffuse choroidal infiltrates during the acute stage and similar residual RPE changes during the inactive stage. However, it typically affects specific ethnic groups and is characterised by exudative retinal detachment.

### FURTHER READING

Damato BE, Nanjiani M, Foulds WS. Acute posterior multifocal placoid pigment epitheliopathy. A follow-up study. *Trans Ophthalmol Soc UK* 1983;103:517–522.

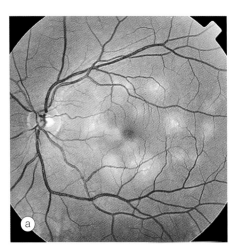
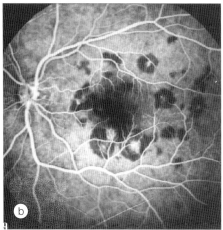
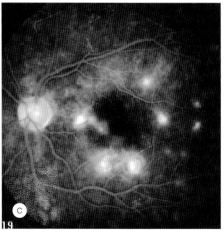

**Figure 4.119 (a)** APMPPE; **(b)** FA venous phase showing hypofluorescence; **(c)** late phase showing hyperfluorescence

Jones NP. Acute posterior multifocal placoid pigment epitheliopathy. *Br J Ophthalmol* 1995;79:384–389.

Kersten DH, Lessell S, Carlow TJ. Acute posterior multifocal placoid pigment epitheliopathy and late-onset meningoencephalitis. *Ophthalmology* 1987;94:393–396.

# Serpiginous Choroidopathy

Serpiginous choroidopathy is a rare, idiopathic, progressive inflammatory chorioretinopathy which typically affects patients between the fourth and sixth decades of life. The disease is usually bilateral but the extent of involvement is frequently asymmetrical. Both sexes are equally affected.

## Diagnosis

1. **Presentation** is with unilateral blurring of central vision or metamorphopsia as a result of macular involvement. After a variable period of time, the fellow eye is also affected, although it is not uncommon to find evidence of inactive asymptomatic disease in the fellow eye at the time of presentation.

2. **Signs**

   - Active lesions consist of grey-white to yellow-white subretinal lesions with hazy borders which typically start around the optic disc (Fig. 4.120b) and then gradually spread outwards in a snake-like manner along the major vascular arcades and towards the macula (Fig. 4.120c and 4.120d). Rarely, the initial lesion involves the macula.
   - Vitritis is usually minimal and is present in about 30% of eyes, and a mild anterior uveitis may also be present in some cases.

3. **Investigations**

   a. *FA* of active lesions shows early hypofluorescence due to non-perfusion (Fig. 4.121b) and late hyperfluorescence due to staining (Fig. 4.121c and 4.121d).

   b. *Electro-oculogram (EOG)* is decreased.

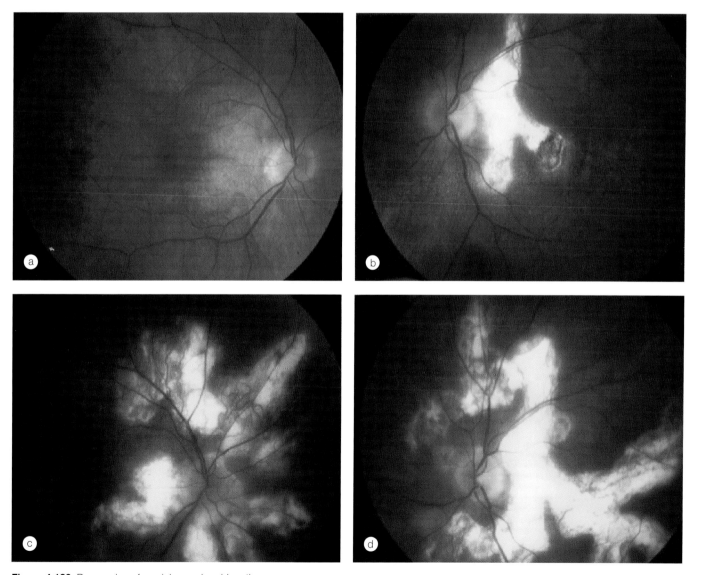

**Figure 4.120** Progression of serpiginous choroidopathy:
1. At presentation. **(a)** The right eye is normal, **(b)** the left shows serpiginous choroidopathy
2. Four years later. **(c)** The right eye shows advanced serpiginous choroidopathy, **(d)** the left eye shows marked progression of the disease

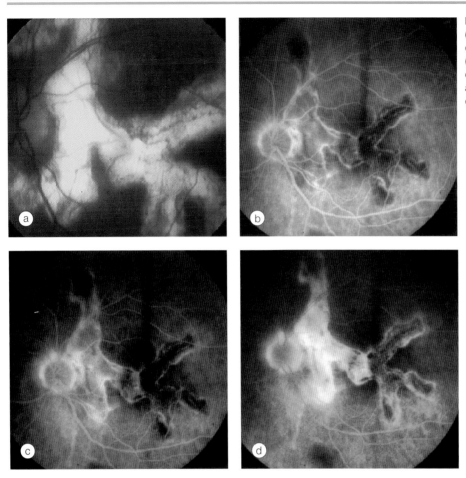

**Figure 4.121** **(a)** Serpiginous choroidopathy; **(b)** FA venous phase shows hypofluorescence of the lesion with a hyperfluorescent outline; **(c)** & **(d)** late phases show hyperfluorescence of part of the lesion near the disc due to staining, and persistent hypofluorescence of the remainder due to blockage

***Course.*** This lasts many years in an episodic and recurrent fashion and it is not uncommon for disease activity to recur after several months of remission. Recurrences are characterised by yellow-grey extensions at the level of the choriocapillaris, contiguous or as satellites to existing areas of chorioretinal atrophy. Inactive lesions are characterised by scalloped, atrophic, 'punched-out' areas of choroidal atrophy associated with RPE changes (Fig. 4.122).

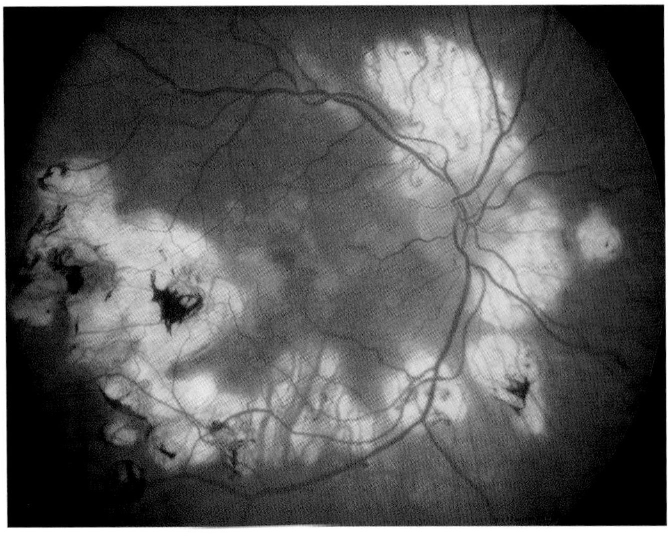

***Treatment.*** Currently there is no definitive treatment strategy for serpiginous choroidopathy. Treatment options include triple therapy with a combination of systemic steroids, azathioprine and cyclosporine, although a recent report has suggested that early monotherapy with cyclosporine may be adequate.

***Prognosis*** is generally poor. Visual loss caused by involvement of the fovea occurs in about 50% of cases. It is usually profound and permanent. Some eyes develop CNV associated with an old scar, which may be amenable to laser photocoagulation. Subretinal fibrosis is a rare late complication.

## FURTHER READING

Araujo AAQ, Wells AP, Dick AD, et al. Early treatment with cyclosporin in serpiginous choroidopathy maintains remission and good visual outcome. *Br J Ophthalmol* 2000;84:979–982.

Hooper PL, Kaplan HJ. Triple agent immunosuppression in serpiginous choroiditis. *Ophthalmology* 1991;98:944–952.

Mansour AM, Jampol LM, Packo KH, et al. Macular serpiginous choroidopathy. *Retina* 1988;8:125–131.

Secchi AG, Tognon MS, Maselli C. Cyclosporine-A in the treatment of serpiginous choroiditis. *Int Ophthalmol* 1990;14:395–399.

Wu JS, Lewis H, Fine SL, et al. Clinicopathologic findings in a patient with serpiginous choroidopathy and treated choroidal neovascularization. *Retina* 1989;9:292–301.

**Figure 4.122** Inactive serpiginous choroidopathy

# Birdshot Retinochoroidopathy

Birdshot retinochoroidopathy is an uncommon, bilateral, chronic inflammatory disease of the retina and choroid which typically affects middle-aged individuals. About 90% of patients are positive for HLA-A29.

## Diagnosis

1. **Presentation** is with painless impairment of central vision associated with nyctalopia, and with vitreous floaters. Disturbances of colour vision are also common. The severity of visual disturbance is frequently out of proportion to the measured visual acuity, indicating diffuse retinal dysfunction.

2. **Signs** are usually bilateral but may be asymmetrical.

    a. *Diffuse vitritis* without snowbanking but little if any anterior uveitis.
    b. *Acute lesions* consist of distinctive, subretinal, poorly defined, cream-coloured, small (100–300 $\mu$m) ovoid spots distributed in one of the following four patterns:

    - Involving the macula (Fig. 4.123) and mid-periphery (Fig. 4.124).
    - With relative macular sparing (Fig. 4.125).
    - With macular predominance.
    - Asymmetrical, with predominance of lesions in the inferonasal fundus and relative macular sparing.

> **NB: These lesions may not be present at presentation of symptoms and may take several years to appear.**

3. **Investigations**

    a. *FA* during the active stage may be useful in demonstrating the presence of CMO and CNV. Initially, the lesions may remain silent throughout the angiogram if they do not affect the RPE. Thus, more lesions may be seen clinically than angiographically. Later there may be staining of the lesions as the RPE becomes affected (Fig. 4.126b).
    b. *Indocyanine green (ICG) angiography* is more useful than FA and shows early hypofluorescence and late hyperfluorescence.
    c. *Electroretinography (ERG)* is normal in early disease, but, with time, the rod and cone b-wave amplitudes and oscillatory potentials become decreased.

> **NB: The need for early therapy is based on ERG findings (see below).**

**Course** is chronic, with exacerbations and remissions over several years. With some time, the lesions may become confluent. Inactive lesions consist of well-delineated, white atrophic spots (Fig. 4.127).

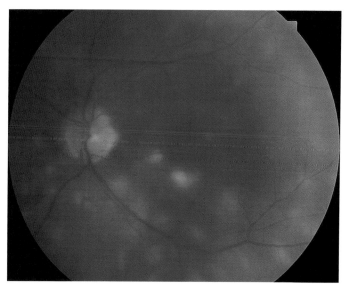

**Figure 4.123** Birdshot chorioretinopathy with macular involvement

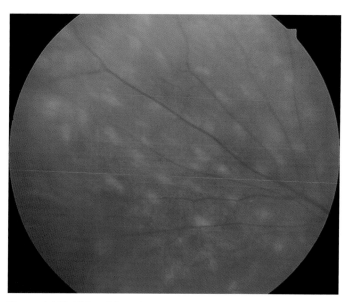

**Figure 4.124** Mid-peripheral lesions in birdshot chorioretinopathy

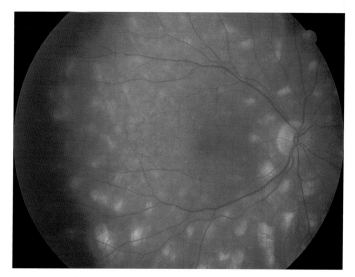

**Figure 4.125** Birdshot chorioretinopathy with macular sparing

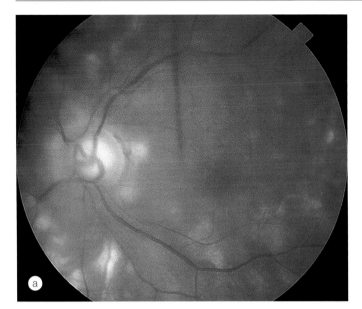

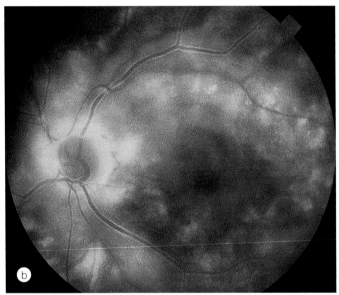

**Figure 4.126** **(a)** Active birdshot chorioretinopathy; **(b)** FA shows hyperfluorescence due to staining

### Treatment

Although there is currently no definitive treatment, the following may be considered.

1. **Steroids,** both periocular and systemic, may be effective if given early in patients with abnormal EOG but normal visual acuity.

2. **Cyclosporine** has been shown to be superior to steroids in uncontrolled studies and may prove to be the treatment of choice for chronic disease.

**Prognosis** is guarded. About 20% of patients have a self-limited course and maintain normal visual acuity. The remainder have variable impairment of visual acuity in one or both eyes as a result of one or more of the following complications:

- CMO and optic atrophy are the most common causes of visual loss, occurring in over 50% of cases.

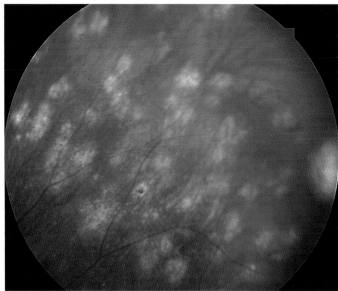

**Figure 4.127** Inactive birdshot chorioretinopathy

- Epiretinal membrane formation, which may progress to macular pucker, is the next most common, affecting about 10% of patients.
- Serous macular detachment.
- CNV, which eventually develops in 6% of patients.

## Punctate Inner Choroidopathy

Punctate inner choroidopathy (PIC) is an uncommon, idiopathic disease which typically affects young myopic women. Both eyes are frequently involved but not simultaneously.

### Diagnosis

1. **Presentation** is with blurring of central vision or paracentral scotomas, which may be associated with photopsia.

2. **Signs**

- Absent or minimal intraocular inflammation.
- Small, yellow-white spots with fuzzy borders at the level of the inner choroid. The lesions are all of the same age, range in diameter from 100 to 300 $\mu$m, and principally involve the posterior pole (Figs. 4.128 and 4.129). Plentiful lesions occasionally may be associated with an overlying serous sensory retinal detachment.

3. **Investigations**

   a. *FA* shows early hyperfluorescence and late staining (Fig. 4.130b and 4.130c); hyperfluorescence may also be seen in the presence of CNV (Fig. 4.131c and 4.131d).
   b. *ERG* is normal.

4. **Course**

- After a few weeks, the acute lesions resolve, to leave behind sharply demarcated atrophic scars which, with time, become pigmented and may enlarge (Fig. 4.132).
- CNV develops from scars in about 25% of cases and may result in loss of central vision if the fovea is involved.

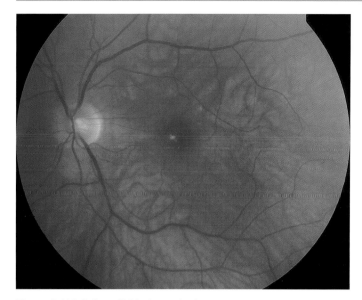

**Figure 4.128** Solitary PIC lesion at the fovea

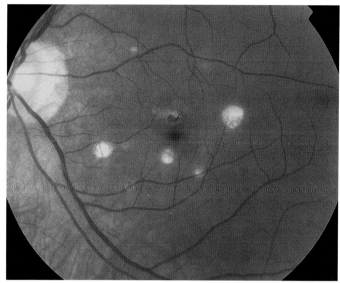

**Figure 4.129** Multiple PIC lesions (Courtesy of Moorfields Eye Hospital)

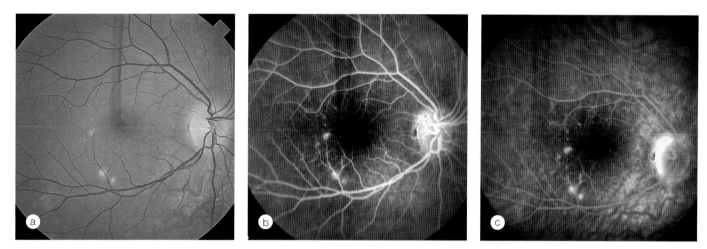

**Figure 4.130** **(a)** Uncomplicated PIC; **(b)** FA venous phase shows punctate hyperfluorescence; **(c)** late phase shows staining

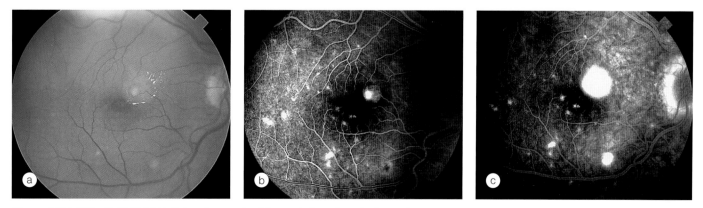

**Figure 4.131** PIC with CNV. **(a)** Multiple yellow spots at the posterior pole and a larger dot superotemporal to the fovea surrounded by small hard exudates; **(b)** FA arteriovenous phase shows multiple pin-point areas of hyperfluorescence and a larger hyperfluorescent dot superotemporal to the fovea; **(c)** late phase shows increase in intensity and area of hyperfluorescence due to leakage from CNV

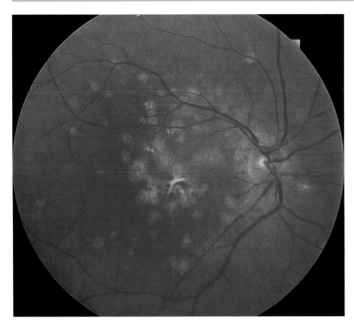

**Figure 4.132** Inactive PIC

- After a variable period of time, the fellow eye frequently becomes similarly involved.

**Treatment.** Eyes with extrafoveal CNV may benefit from laser photocoagulation, particularly if there is evidence of progression and threat to the fovea. Systemic steroid therapy in patients with subfoveal CNV may reduce subretinal vascular leakage and stabilise vision. Photodynamic therapy or surgical excision of subfoveal CNV may be appropriate in selected cases.

**Prognosis** is guarded because central vision may become compromised by either foveal involvement by a lesion (see Fig. 4.128) or the development of CNV, which usually occurs within the first year of presentation (see Fig. 4.131). Subfoveal CNV may undergo spontaneous involution, with or without recovery of central vision. Small, well-defined subfoveal areas of CNV carry a reasonable prognosis and many patients retain a visual acuity of 6/18 or better.

### Differential diagnosis

1. **Multifocal choroiditis and panuveitis** is characterised by similar lesions when they affect the posterior pole and CNV. However, it is associated with intraocular inflammation and involvement of the peripheral fundus.

2. **Ocular histoplasmosis** is characterised by punched-out chorioretinal scars, CNV and absence of intraocular inflammation. However, there is also peripapillary atrophy as well as linear peripheral streaks and peripheral lesions.

3. **Myopic maculopathy** may have similar macular changes, CNV and absence of intraocular inflammation. However, the severity of myopia is greater and other degenerative changes are present.

### FURTHER READING

Brueggeman RM, Noffke AS, Jampol LM. Resolution of punctate inner choroidopathy lesions with oral prednisone therapy. *Arch Ophthalmol* 2002;120:996.

Eldlam B, Sener C. Punctate inner choriodopathy and its differential diagnosis. *Ann Ophthalmol* 1991;23:153–158.

Olsen TW, Capone A Jr, Sternberg P Jr, et al. Subfoveal choroidal neovascularization in punctate inner choroidopathy. Surgical management and pathologic findings. *Ophthalmology* 1996; 103:2061–2069.

## Multifocal Choroiditis with Panuveitis

Multifocal choroiditis with panuveitis is an uncommon, usually bilateral, recurrent choroidal inflammatory disease. Although the exact aetiology is unknown, it has been suggested that Epstein-Barr virus infection may be responsible. The disease typically occurs during the fourth decade of life and affects females more commonly than males by a 3:1 ratio.

### Diagnosis

1. **Presentation** is usually with blurring of central vision, which may be associated with vitreous floaters and photopsia.

2. **Signs**

   - Vitritis of variable severity is universal and anterior uveitis is present in 50% of cases.
   - Bilateral, multiple (up to several hundred), discrete, round or ovoid, yellowish-grey lesions located at the level of the RPE and choriocapillaris. The lesions range in diameter from 50 to 350 $\mu$m and involve the posterior pole (Fig. 4.133) and/or periphery and may be arranged in clumps or linear streaks (Schlagel lines). Occasionally, in older patients, the lesions are confined to the periphery.
   - Mild disc oedema may occasionally be present and the blind spot enlarged.

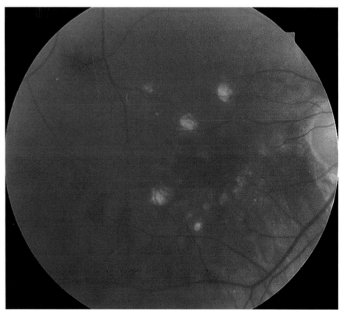

**Figure 4.133** Active multifocal choroiditis

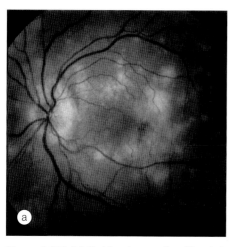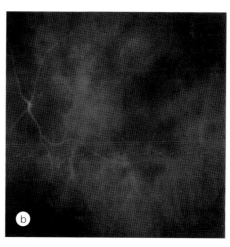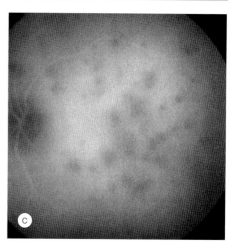

**Figure 4.134** **(a)** Red-free image of multifocal choroiditis; **(b)** and **(c)** ICG show hypofluorescence of the lesions throughout the angiogram

### 3. Investigations

   *a. FA* of active lesions shows early hypofluorescence and late hyperfluorescence due to staining. Old inactive lesions show early hyperfluorescence which subsequently fades during the late phase.

   *b. ICG* shows hypofluorescence (Fig. 4.134).

   *c. ERG* is often abnormal without recovery.

   *d. Visual fields* may be constricted.

**4. Course** is prolonged and may last many months with the development of new lesions and recurrent inflammatory episodes. Inactive lesions have sharp 'punched-out' margins and pigmented borders (Fig. 4.135).

***Treatment*** with immunosuppressive agents (e.g. cyclosporine, azathioprine, methotrexate), with or without adjunctive steroids, appears to be most effective, but monotherapy with steroids is disappointing. Eyes with CNV may require laser photocoagulation (Fig. 4.136), which should be performed under steroid cover.

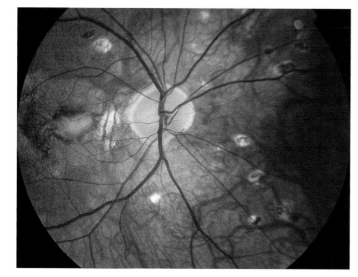

**Figure 4.135** Inactive multifocal choroiditis

***Prognosis*** is variable because the disease has a wide spectrum, varying between those with few lesions and short periods of activity to patients with progressive scarring and visual loss due to one or more of the following:

- Direct involvement of the fovea, although some patients may have an apparently normal fovea and yet have very poor visual acuity.
- CNV, which develops in 50% of cases from an old scar.
- Diffuse subretinal fibrosis (Fig. 4.137), which is uncommon but serious.
- CMO.

### FURTHER READING

Ben Ezra D, Forrester JV. Fundal white dots: the spectrum of a similar pathological process. *Br J Ophthalmol* 1995;79:856–860.

Brown J, Folk JC, Reddy CV, et al. Visual prognosis of multifocal choroiditis, punctate inner choroidopathy, and diffuse subretinal fibrosis syndrome. *Ophthalmology* 1996;103:1100–1105.

Dunlop AAS, Cree IA, Hague S, et al. Multifocal choroiditis. Clinicopathologic correlation. *Arch Ophthalmol* 1998;116:801–803.

Lardenoye CWTA, Van der Lelij A, de Loos WS, et al. Peripheral multifocal choroiditis. A distinct clinical entity? *Ophthalmology* 1997;104:1820–1826.

Michel SS, Ekong A, Baltatzis S, et al. Multifocal choroiditis and panuveitis. Immunomodulatory therapy. *Ophthalmology* 2002; 109:378–383.

Parnell J, Jampol LM, Yannuzzi LA, et al. Differentiation between presumed ocular histoplasmosis syndrome and multifocal choroiditis with panuveitis based on morphology of photographic fundus lesions and fluorescein angiography. *Arch Ophthalmol* 2002;119:208–212.

## Multiple Evanescent White Dot Syndrome

Multiple evanescent white dot syndrome (MEWDS) is an uncommon, idiopathic, self-limiting, multifocal inflammatory disease which typically affects healthy young individuals, particularly females. The condition is usually unilateral and

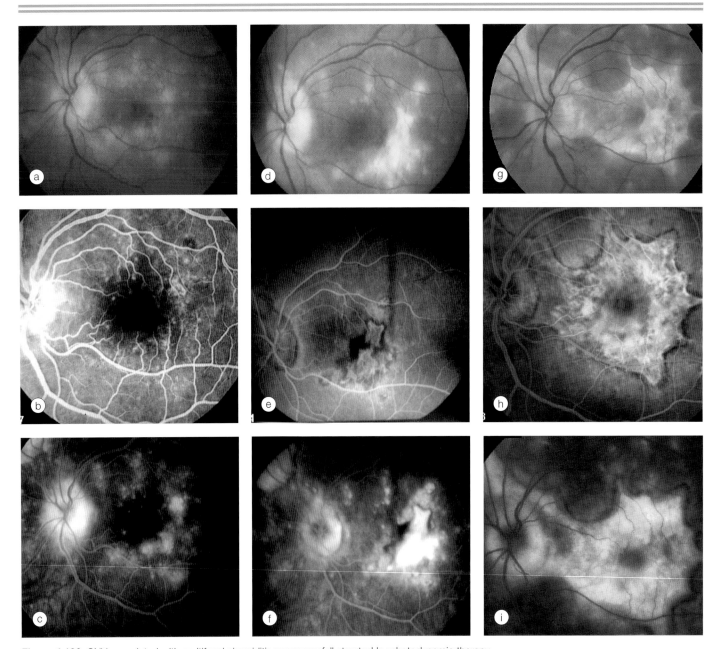

**Figure 4.136** CNV associated with multifocal choroiditis unsuccessfully treated by photodynamic therapy
1. At presentation. **(a)** Multiple, deep, cream-coloured lesions at the posterior pole and surrounding a swollen optic disc; **(b)** FA venous phase shows multiple pin-point hyperfluorescent spots; **(c)** late phase shows more diffuse hyperfluorescence of the lesions and hyperfluorescence of the disc
2. Four months later. **(d)** Coalescence of lesions inferotemporal to the fovea; **(e)** FA venous phase shows hyperfluorescence due to extensive choroidal neovascularisation; **(f)** late phase shows increase in intensity and size of hyperfluorescence due to leakage
3. Nine months after a course of systemic steroids and three sessions of photodynamic therapy. **(g)** Chorioretinal scarring extending from the disc to the macula and superonasal to the disc; **(h)** FA venous phase shows hyperfluorescence of the scar; **(i)** late phase shows increase in intensity but not in area of hyperfluorescence due to staining

may be preceded by a viral-like illness. Although uncommon, it is important to be aware of MEWDS because the subtle signs may be overlooked and a misdiagnosis made of a more serious disorder such as retrobulbar neuritis with its possible implications.

1. **Presentation** is with sudden-onset decreased vision or paracentral scotomas, which may be associated with photopsia typically affecting the temporal visual field.

## 2. Signs

- Numerous, very small, white dots at the level of the deep retina and RPE, involving the posterior pole but sparing the fovea (Fig. 4.138a).
- The fovea has a granular appearance which renders the foveal reflex abnormal or absent.
- Mild vitritis and vasculitis.

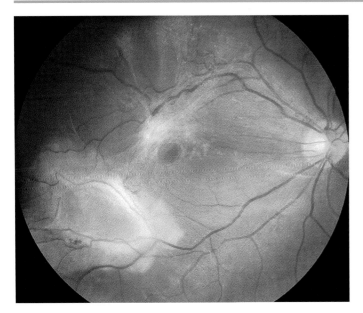

**Figure 4.137** Diffuse subretinal fibrosis

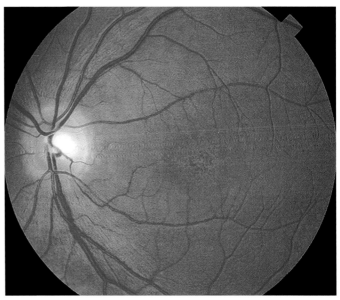

**Figure 4.139** Residual foveal granularity following resolution of acute MEWDS

- Optic disc oedema and enlargement of the physiological blind spot, which can also be explained on the basis of peripapillary non-perfusion.

3. **Investigations**

   a. *FA* of active lesions shows a normal early phase (Fig. 4.138b). The late phase shows a wreath-like pattern of hyperfluorescence corresponding, to some extent, to the white dots seen clinically (Fig. 4.138c).

   b. *ERG* shows a decrease in a-wave amplitude, which returns to a normal pattern within a few weeks.

4. **Course.** Over several weeks to months, central vision returns to normal or near-normal levels while there is progressive fading of the white dots and disc oedema. However, the fovea retains its abnormal appearance (Fig. 4.139) and the enlarged blind spot may take a long time to diminish in size. Persistent photopsia may also be seen. Relapses occur in about 10% of cases and a very small minority of eyes develop chorioretinal scarring or CNV.

**FURTHER READING**

Barile GR, Reppucci VS, Schiff WM, et al. Circumpapillary chorioretinopathy in multiple evanescent white dot syndrome. *Retina* 1997;17:75–77.

Borruat FX, Auer CA, Piguet B. Choroidopathy in multiple evanescent white dot syndrome. *Arch Ophthalmol* 1995;113:1569–1570.

Ie D, Glaser BM, Murphy RP, et al. Indocyanine green angiography in multiple evanescent white dot syndrome. *Am J Ophthalmol* 1994;117:7–12.

# Acute Idiopathic Blind Spot Enlargement Syndrome

This is a rare condition affecting the peripapillary retina which seems to exclusively affect women. MEWDS shares clinical features and perhaps represents a different form of the same disease.

1. **Presentation** is between the third and sixth decades of life with photopsia and decreased vision, which may be

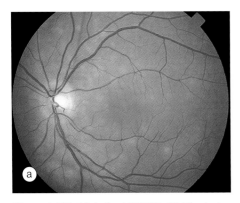
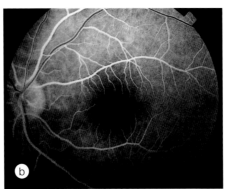
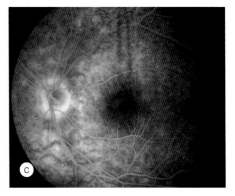

**Figure 4.138 (a)** Active MEWDS; **(b)** FA arteriovenous phase is normal; **(c)** venous phase shows hyperfluorescence of the disc and lesions

misdiagnosed as migraine or optic neuritis. Occasionally, photopsia may precede visual loss by several weeks.

## 2. Signs

- Visual acuity may be normal or reduced.
- Afferent pupillary defect may be present.
- Blind spot enlargement with steep margins but variable size is universal.
- Mild disc swelling or hyperaemia with peripapillary subretinal pigmentary changes occurs in 50% of cases.

## 3. FA may show late staining of the optic nerve head.

## 4. Course. Visual acuity improves spontaneously but blind spot enlargement may persist. Recurrence may occur in the same or fellow eye.

### FURTHER READING

Singh K, de Frank MP, Shults WT, et al. Acute idiopathic blind spot enlargement – a spectrum of disease. *Ophthalmology* 1991; 98:497–502.

Volpe NJ, Rizzo JF III, Lessell S. Acute idiopathic blind spot enlargement syndrome. A review of 27 new cases. *Arch Ophthalmol* 2001;119:59–63.

Watzke RC, Shults WT. Clinical features and natural history of the acute idiopathic enlarged blind spot syndrome. *Ophthalmology* 2002;109:1326–1335.

# Acute Retinal Pigment Epitheliitis

Acute retinal pigment epitheliitis is a rare, idiopathic, self-limiting inflammatory condition of the macular RPE. It typically affects otherwise healthy young adults, and, although there is no treatment, the visual prognosis is excellent. The condition is unilateral in 75% of cases.

## 1. Presentation is with sudden-onset impairment of central vision, which may be associated with metamorphopsia.

## 2. Signs

- Absence of intraocular inflammation.
- The fovea shows a blunted reflex with discrete clusters of a few, subtle, small, brown or grey spots at the level of the RPE, which may be surrounded by hypopigmented yellow halos (Fig. 4.140a).

## 3. Investigations

a. FA shows small hyperfluorescent dots with hypofluorescent centres ('honeycomb' appearance) without leakage (Fig. 4.140b).

b. EOG is decreased.

## 4. Course lasts 6–12 weeks during which the acute fundus lesions resolve and visual acuity returns to normal. Innocuous residual pigment clumping at the fovea may remain. Recurrences may occur but are uncommon.

### FURTHER READING

Deutman AF. Acute retinal pigment epitheliitis. *Am J Ophthalmol* 1974;78:571–578.

Friedman MW. Bilateral recurrent acute retinal pigment epitheliitis. *Am J Ophthalmol* 1975;79:567–570.

Luttrull JK. Acute retinal pigment epitheliitis. *Am J Ophthalmol* 1997;123:127–129.

Prost M. Long-term observations of patients with acute retinal pigment epitheliitis. *Ophthalmologica* 1989;199:84–89.

# Acute Zonular Outer Retinopathies

The acute zonal outer retinopathies (AZOR) are a group of very rare, idiopathic syndromes characterised by acute onset

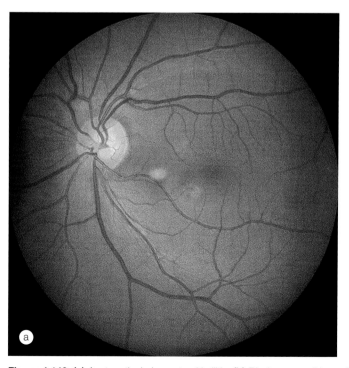

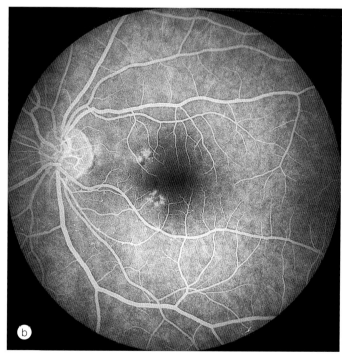

**Figure 4.140 (a)** Acute retinal pigment epitheliitis; **(b)** FA shows small hyperfluorescent dots with hypofluorescent centres (Courtesy of M. Prost)

of loss of one or more zones of visual field caused by damage to the retinal receptor elements. During the acute stage these syndromes can be subclassified on the basis of ophthalmoscopic and FA characteristics into two types: (a) those with primary retinal receptor damage and (b) those with combined retinal receptor and RPE involvement (see below). Although AZOR is a rare condition, it is important to be aware of its existence, to save the patient inappropriate and unrewarding medical and neurological investigations.

## CLASSIFICATION

### 1. Primary retinal receptor involvement

*a. Absence of fundus and FA changes*

- Acute zonal occult outer retinopathy.
- AZOR, occult + multifocal chorioretinal lesions.
- AZOR, occult annular type: white ring.

*b. Fundus changes corresponding to zones of visual field loss*

- AZOR, overt retinal type: white retina without FA changes.

### 2. Combined retinal receptor and RPE involvement

*a. Presence of fundus and FA changes*

- AZOR, overt combined retinal and RPE.
- AZOR, overt annular type: white or yellow orange ring.

## ACUTE ZONAL OCCULT OUTER RETINOPATHY

Because acute zonal occult outer retinopathy (AZOOR) is the most common of the AZOR syndromes, it will be discussed in more detail. The condition typically affects healthy, young, frequently myopic women, some of whom have an antecedent viral-like illness, and is bilateral in 50% of cases. Even though the predilection for AZOOR to affect young and middle-aged women, and its association with one or more autoimmune diseases, may suggest that the affected patients have a predisposition for autoimmune disease, other factors such as the asymmetric nature of retinal involvement, the infrequency of improvement after administration of corticosteroids, and the absence of circulating retinal antibodies, suggest that AZOOR is probably not primarily an autoimmune disease. The acute loss of one or more zones of visual field, which is associated with photopsia in almost 90% of patients with AZOOR, is probably caused by a disorder affecting primarily the retinal photoreceptors.

**1. Presentation** is with acute visual loss affecting one or more zones, which is frequently associated with photopsia. The temporal field is frequently involved but the central field is usually spared.

**2. Signs,** in chronological order:

- Normal fundus.
- Several weeks later, there may be mild vitritis, attenuation of retinal vessels in the affected zone and, occasionally, periphlebitis.
- The zones may enlarge, or less frequently they remain the same or improve.
- In 50% of cases, visual field loss stabilises within 4–6 months.

- Late findings include mild RPE mottling and bone-spicule pigmentary changes (Fig. 4.141) in 50% of cases; in the remainder, the fundus appearance remains normal.

**3. Investigations**

*a. FA* is helpful in detecting early alteration and redistribution of melanin within the RPE cells.
*b. ERG* amplitudes in the affected area are abnormal.

**4. Prognosis** is relatively good, with a final visual acuity of 6/12 in at least one eye in 85% of cases.

> **NB:** It is important to obtain peripheral and central visual fields because large peripheral zones of visual field loss may go undetected if only the central fields are tested.

## FURTHER READING

Arai M, Nao-I N, Sawada A, et al. Multifocal electroretinogram indicates visual field loss in acute zonal occult outer retinopathy. *Am J Ophthalmol* 1998;126:446–449.

Fekrat S, Wilkinson CP, Chang B, et al. Acute annular outer retinopathy: report of four cases. *Am J Ophthalmol* 2000;130:636–644.

Gass JDM. The acute zonal outer retinopathies [Editorial]. *Am J Ophthalmol* 2000;130:655–657.

Gass JDM, Agarwal A, Scott IU. Acute zonal occult outer retinopathy: a long-term follow-up study. *Am J Ophthalmol* 2002; 134:329–339.

Gass JDM, Stern C. Acute annular outer retinopathy as a variant of acute zonular occult outer retinopathy. *Am J Ophthalmol* 1995;119:330–334.

Jacobson SG, Morales DS, Sun XK, et al. Pattern of retinal dysfunction in acute zonal occult outer retinopathy. *Ophthalmology* 1995;102:1187–1198.

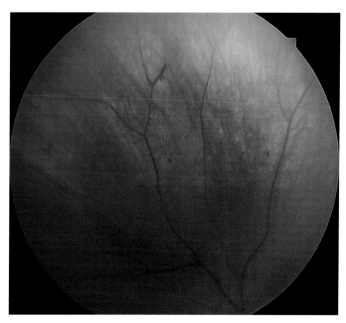

**Figure 4.141** Subtle RPE mottling and bone-corpuscle pigmentation in AZOOR

# MISCELLANEOUS DISORDERS

## Acute Macular Neuroretinopathy

Acute macular neuroretinopathy is a rare idiopathic condition that typically affects healthy females between the second and fourth decades of life. The disease may affect one or both eyes and may be preceded by a flu-like illness. Although there is no treatment, the condition is self-limited and may produce temporary or permanent visual impairment.

1. **Presentation** is with sudden decrease of visual acuity and paracentral scotomas.

2. **Signs**

   - Absence of intraocular inflammation.
   - Darkish, brown-red, wedge-shaped lesions in a flower petal arrangement around the centre of the macula (Fig. 4.142); the reddish appearance is due to loss of retinal outer receptor elements which produce outer retinal thinning.

3. **Investigations**

   a. *FA* is usually normal.
   b. *ERG* is normal.
   c. *Amsler grid* and visual fields reveal remarkable correspondence of the lesions with the shape and location of the scotomas.

4. **Course** lasts several months with gradual improvement in visual symptoms and fading but not complete resolution of the fundus lesions for many years; recurrences are uncommon.

### FURTHER READING
Bos PJM, Deutman AF. Acute macular neuroretinopathy. *Am J Ophthalmol* 1975;80:573–584.

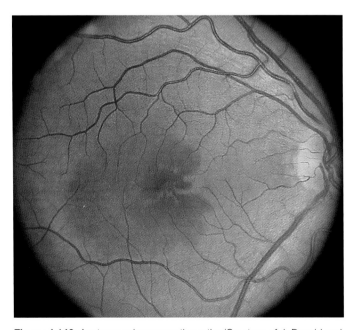

**Figure 4.142** Acute macular neuroretinopathy (Courtesy of J. Donald and M. Gass, from *Stereoscopic Atlas of Macular Disease*, Mosby, 1997)

Gandorfer A, Ulbig MW. Scanning laser ophthalmoscope findings in acute macular neuroretinopathy. *Am J Ophthalmol* 2002; 133:413–415.

## Acute Idiopathic Maculopathy

Acute idiopathic maculopathy is a very rare inflammatory condition which typically affects young adults. The condition is most frequently unilateral and may be preceded by a flu-like illness.

1. **Presentation** is with a unilateral sudden and severe loss of vision.

2. **Signs**

   - Wedge-shaped detachment of the sensory retina at the macula with an irregular outline (Fig. 4.143a).
   - Smaller, greyish, subretinal thickening at the level of the RPE beneath the sensory detachment is frequently present.
   - Iritis and papillitis may be present.

3. **FA** in the early venous phase shows minimal subretinal hypofluorescence and hyperfluorescence beneath the sensory retinal detachment (Fig. 4.143b). The mid-venous phases show two levels of hyperfluorescence, one from staining of the subretinal thickening at the level of the RPE, and the second from pooling of dye within the subretinal space (Fig. 4.143c). The late phase shows complete staining of the overlying sensory retinal detachment (Fig. 4.143d).

4. **Course** is short, with complete resolution of the exudative changes and nearly complete recovery of vision. Innocuous residual RPE atrophic changes which may have a 'bull's-eye' pattern remain. A few patients may subsequently develop CNV.

### FURTHER READING
Freund, KB, Yannuzzi LA, Barile GR, et al. The expanding clinical spectrum of unilateral acute idiopathic maculopathy. *Arch Ophthalmol* 1996;114:555–559.
Yannuzzi LA, Jampol LM, Rabb MF, et al. Unilateral acute idiopathic maculopathy. *Arch Ophthalmol* 1991;109:1411–1416.

## Acute Multifocal Retinitis

Acute multifocal retinitis is a very rare idiopathic condition that typically affects healthy, young to middle-aged adults. It may be preceded by a flu-like illness. The condition is frequently bilateral.

1. **Presentation** is with sudden onset of mild visual loss.

2. **Signs**

   - Several, white, retinal infiltrates of variable size (Fig. 4.144).
   - Mild vitritis and disc oedema are frequent.
   - A macular star is occasionally present.

3. **FA** shows early hypofluorescence due to blockage, with late staining of the lesions.

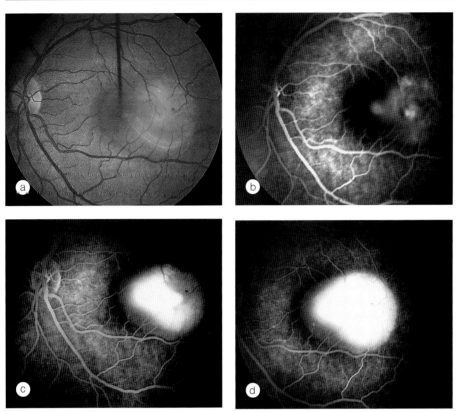

**Figure 4.143** Acute idiopathic maculopathy (see text)

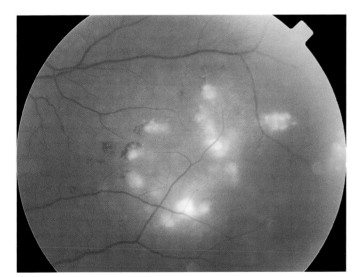

**Figure 4.144** Acute multifocal retinitis

## Progressive Subretinal Fibrosis and Uveitis Syndrome

The progressive subretinal fibrosis and uveitis syndrome is a rare, idiopathic, bilateral condition which typically affects healthy young adult females.

1. **Presentation** is with gradual unilateral blurring of vision although both eyes are usually eventually involved.

4. **Course** lasts 2–4 months with resolution of the fundus lesions and return of visual acuity to normal, with little or no residual fundus changes. Small retinal branch artery occlusions may occur in a minority of cases.

### FURTHER READING

Cunningham ET Jr, Schatz H, McDonald HR, et al. Acute multifocal retinitis. *Am J Ophthalmol* 1997;123:347–357.
Foster RE, Gutman FA, Myers SM, et al. Acute multifocal inner retinitis. *Am J Ophthalmol* 1991;111:673–681.
Golstein BG, Pavan PR. Retinal infiltrates in six patients with an associated viral syndrome. *Retina* 1985;5:144–150.

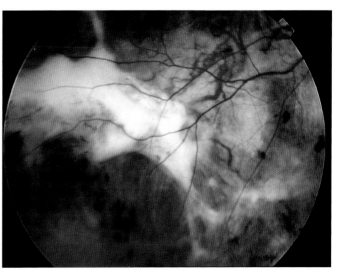

**Figure 4.145** Advanced stage of subretinal fibrosis and uveitis syndrome

**2. Signs**

- Yellow, indistinct subretinal lesions which coalesce into dirty-yellow mounds.
- Vitritis.

**3. ERG** is decreased.

**4. Course** is chronic, with expansion of the lesions to involve most of the fundus. The prognosis is poor because of subretinal opaque bands and RPE changes at the macula (Fig. 4.145).

**5. Treatment** with immunosuppressive agents may be beneficial in certain cases. Systemic steroids are usually not effective, although there are anecdotal reports that they may protect the fellow eye.

### FURTHER READING

Palestine AG, Nussenblatt RB, Chan CC, et al. Histopathology of the subretinal fibrosis and uveitis syndrome. *Ophthalmology* 1985;92:838–844.

Palestine AG, Nussenblatt RB, Parver LM, et al. Progressive subretinal fibriosis and uveitis. *Br J Ophthalmol* 1984;68:667–673.

# Solitary Idiopathic Choroiditis

Solitary idiopathic choroiditis is a distinct clinical entity that may give rise to diagnostic problems as it may simulate other pathology, particularly amelanotic tumours.

**1. Presentation** is often in the fourth decade, with mild visual loss and floaters.

**2. Signs**

- A postequatorial, dull-yellow, choroidal lesion with an ill-defined margin and localised subretinal fluid (Fig. 4.146).
- Associated yellow exudation is common and may assume a stellate configuration in the foveal area, often separate from the main lesion.
- Vitritis is present in one-third of cases.
- Occasional features include retinal vascular dilatation and focal retinal haemorrhages.

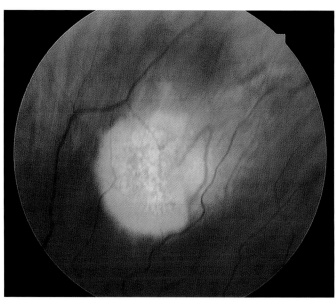

**Figure 4.146** Solitary idiopathic choroiditis

**3. FA** of active lesions shows early hypofluorescence and intense late hyperfluorescence due to staining.

**4. Course** is chronic. As the inflammation resolves, the lesion develops a better-defined margin with resolution of subretinal fluid and exudation.

**5. Treatment.** Lesions with active inflammation respond well to systemic steroids. Most inactive lesions either remain stable or resolve without treatment.

**6. Differential diagnosis**

- *a. Solitary choroidal granuloma* due to sarcoidosis, tuberculosis and toxocariasis.
- *b. Amelanotic tumour* such as amelanotic melanoma, metastasis, circumscribed choroidal haemangioma and choroidal osteoma.

# Chapter 5

# FUNDUS DYSTROPHIES

# RETINAL DYSTROPHIES

## Retinitis Pigmentosa

Retinitis pigmentosa (RP), perhaps more appropriately termed pigmentary retinal dystrophy because of absence of inflammation, is a diffuse retinal dystrophy, initially predominantly affecting the rod photoreceptor cells with subsequent degeneration of cones. Its prevalence is 1:5000.

### INHERITANCE
The age of onset, rate of progression, eventual visual loss and associated ocular features are frequently related to the mode of inheritance. RP may occur as an isolated sporadic disorder, or be inherited as an autosomal dominant (AD), autosomal recessive (AR) or X-linked (XL) trait. Many cases are due to mutation of the rhodopsin gene. RP may also be associated with certain systemic disorders which are usually AR.

- Isolated, without any family history, is common.
- AD is also common and has the best prognosis.
- AR is less common and has an intermediate prognosis.
- XL is the least common but most severe. Female carriers may have normal fundi or exhibit a golden-metallic reflex at the macula (Fig. 5.1) with atrophic and pigmentary peripheral irregularities.

### DIAGNOSIS
The diagnostic criteria for RP comprise bilateral involvement, loss of peripheral vision and progressive loss of predominantly rod photoreceptor function. The classic clinical triad of RP is (a) *arteriolar attenuation*, (b) *retinal bone-spicule pigmentation* and (c) *waxy disc pallor*.

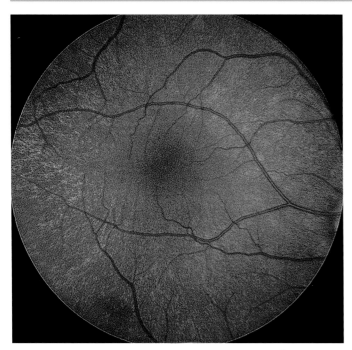

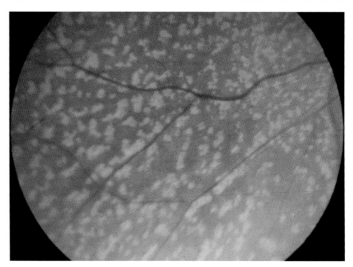

**Figure 5.3** Retinitis punctata albescens

**Figure 5.1** Scintillating golden reflex at the macula in a carrier of X-linked RP

**Presentation** is with nyctalopia, often during the third decade, but may be sooner depending on the pedigree.

**Signs,** in chronological order:

- Arteriolar narrowing, fine dust-like intraretinal pigmentation and loss of retinal pigment epithelium (RPE), an appearance previously referred to as RP *sine pigmento* (Fig. 5.2).
- A minority of patients have scattered white dots, most numerous at the equator; this is referred to as *retinitis punctata albescens* (Fig. 5.3).

- Mid-peripheral, coarse, perivascular 'bone-spicule' pigmentary changes (Fig. 5.4) which gradually increase in density and spread anteriorly and posteriorly (Fig. 5.5 and 5.6).
- Tessellated fundus appearance, due to RPE atrophy and unmasking of large choroidal vessels, severe arteriolar attenuation and waxy disc pallor (Fig. 5.7).
- The macula may show atrophy (see Fig. 5.6), cello-phane formation and cystoid oedema; the latter may respond to systemic acetazolamide.

### Investigations

1. **Electroretinography (ERG)** shows reduced scotopic rod and combined responses during the early stages of the disease in which fundus changes are minimal (Fig. 5.8);

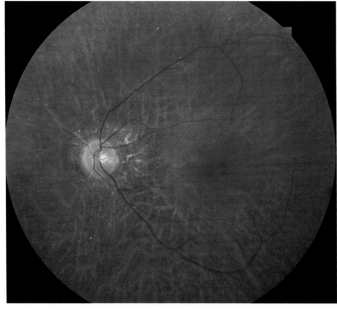

**Figure 5.2** RP with vascular attenuation and minimal pigmentary changes

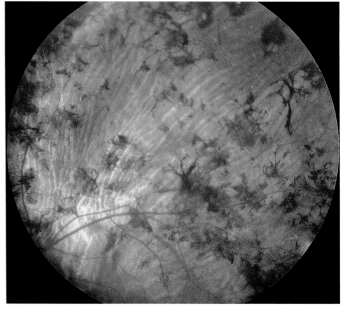

**Figure 5.4** 'Bone-spicule' pigmentary changes in RP

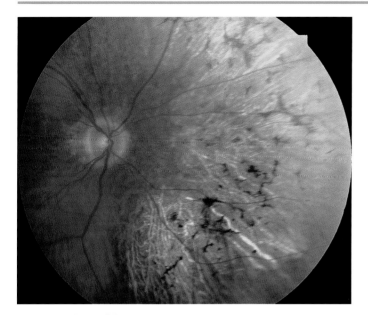

**Figure 5.5** Severe RP

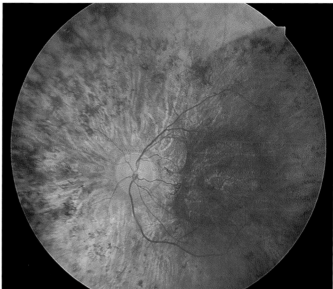

**Figure 5.7** Advanced RP with unmasking of choroidal vessels

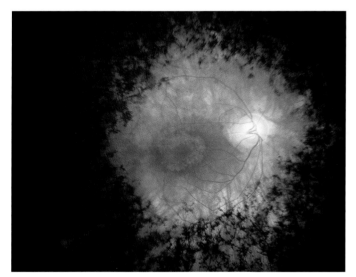

**Figure 5.6** Very severe RP with atrophic maculopathy

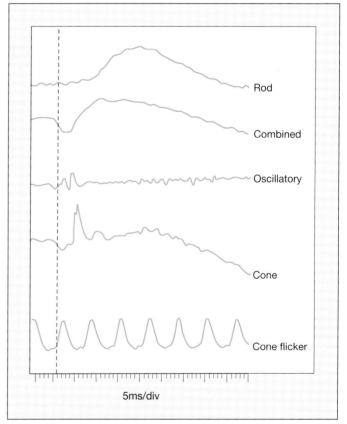

**Figure 5.8** ERG in RP (see text)

later, photopic responses become reduced and eventually the ERG becomes extinguished.

2. **Electro-oculography (EOG)** is subnormal with an absence of the light rise.

3. **Dark adaptometry (DA)** is prolonged and may be useful in early cases where the diagnosis is uncertain.

4. **Colour vision (CV)** is normal.

5. **Visual fields (VF)** are useful in monitoring disease progress. Perimetry classically demonstrates an annular mid-peripheral scotoma (Fig. 5.9a), which expands both peripherally and centrally. It ultimately leaves a tiny island of central vision (Fig. 5.9b) which may eventually be extinguished. Perimetry is useful in monitoring the progression of disease.

6. **Fundus fluorescein angiography (FA)** is not required to make the diagnosis, but when performed shows diffuse hyperfluorescence due to window defects and discrete areas of hypofluorescence corresponding to masking by pigment (Fig. 5.10).

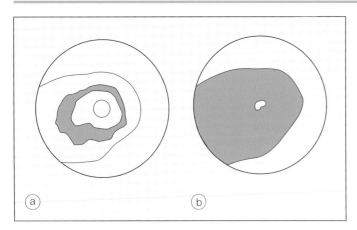

**Figure 5.9** Progression of visual field loss in RP. **(a)** Ring scotoma; **(b)** small residual central island of vision

## PROGNOSIS

The long-term prognosis is often poor, with eventual loss of central vision due to direct involvement of the fovea by RP itself or maculopathy. Daily administration of supplemental vitamin A, if instituted early, may possibly retard progression of RP, but because of lack of definite evidence of efficacy it is not routinely prescribed. The overall prognosis is as follows:

- About 25% of patients maintain good visual acuity and are able to read throughout their working lives, despite an extinguished ERG and 2–3° central field.
- Under the age of 20 years, most patients have a visual acuity better than 6/60.
- By the age of 50 years, an appreciable number have a visual acuity less than 6/60.

## OCULAR ASSOCIATIONS

Regular follow-up of patients with RP is essential to detect other vision-threatening complications, some of which may be amenable to treatment.

1. **Posterior subcapsular cataracts** (Fig. 5.11) are common in all forms of RP; surgery is often beneficial.

2. **Open-angle glaucoma** occurs in 3% of cases.

3. **Myopia** is frequent.

4. **Keratoconus** (Fig. 5.12) is uncommon.

5. **Vitreous changes,** which are common, consist of posterior vitreous detachment and, occasionally, intermediate uveitis.

6. **Optic disc drusen** occur more frequently in patients with RP (Fig. 5.13) than in normals.

## DIFFERENTIAL DIAGNOSIS

1. **End-stage chloroquine retinopathy** is also characterised by bilateral diffuse loss of RPE with unmasking of choroidal vessels and arteriolar attenuation. However, the pigmentary changes do not have a perivascular 'bone cor-puscle' configuration, and the optic atrophy is not waxy.

2. **End-stage syphilitic neuroretinitis** is also characterised by gross restriction of visual fields, vascular attenuation and pigmentary changes. However, nyctalopia is mild, involvement is asymmetrical and choroidal unmasking is mild or absent.

3. **Cancer-related retinopathy** is also characterised by nyctalopia, restriction of peripheral visual field, arteriolar attenuation and extinguished ERG. However, the clinical course is more rapid and pigmentary changes are mild or absent.

## SYSTEMIC ASSOCIATIONS

***Bassen–Kornzweig syndrome*** is an AR disease caused by deficiency in beta-lipoprotein, resulting in intestinal malabsorption.

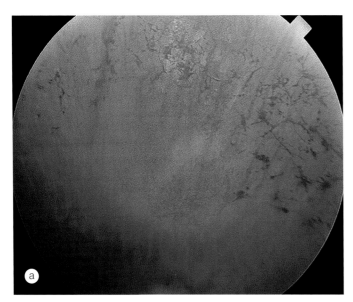
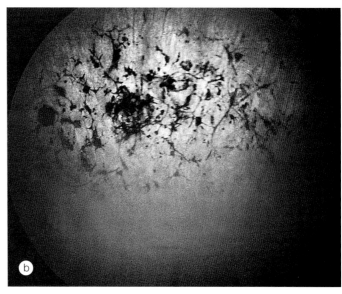

**Figure 5.10 (a)** RP; **(b)** FA shows diffuse hyperfluorescence due to window defects and focal hypofluorescence due to masking by pigment

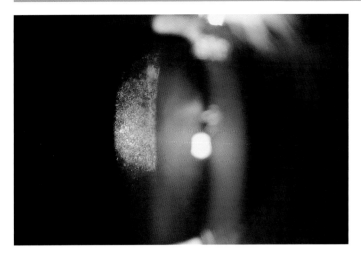

**Figure 5.11** Posterior subcapsular cataract

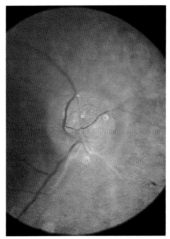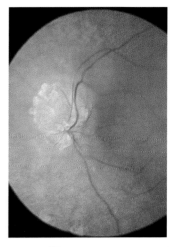

**Figure 5.13** Optic disc drusen associated with RP

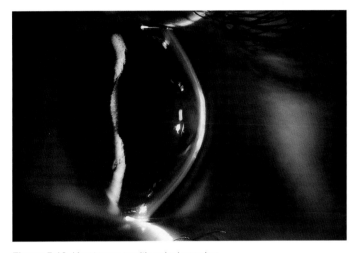

**Figure 5.12** Keratoconus with apical scarring

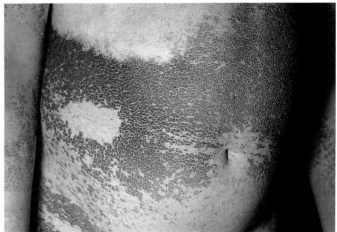

**Figure 5.14** Ichthyosis

1. **Signs.** Spinocerebellar ataxia, ptosis and progressive external ophthalmoplegia.

2. **Diagnostic tests.** The blood film shows acanthocytosis.

3. **RP** develops towards the end of the first decade; the pigment clumps are often larger than in classic RP and are not confined to the equatorial region. Peripheral white dots are also common.

4. **Treatment** with vitamin E, if instituted early, may be beneficial for neurological disability.

***Refsum disease*** (heredopathia atactica polyneuritiformis) is an AR inborn error of metabolism in which deficiency of phytanic acid 2-hydroxylase results in the accumulation of phytanic acid in the blood and body tissues.

1. **Clinical features** include polyneuropathy, cerebellar ataxia, deafness, anosmia, cardiomyopathy and ichthyosis (Fig. 5.14).

2. **Diagnostic tests.** Lumbar puncture shows elevated cerebrospinal fluid (CSF) protein in the absence of pleocytosis (cytoalbuminous inversion).

3. **RP** develops in the second decade and is characterised by generalised 'salt-and-pepper' changes.

4. **Other ocular features** include cataract, miosis and prominent corneal nerves.

5. **Treatment,** initially with plasmapheresis and later with a phytanic-acid-free diet, may prevent progression of both systemic and retinal involvement.

***Usher syndrome*** is a distressing AR condition which accounts for about 5% of all cases of profound deafness in children, and is responsible for about half of all cases of combined deafness and blindness. RP develops before puberty.

***Kearns–Sayre*** syndrome is a mitochondrial cytopathy associated with mitochondrial DNA deletions.

1. **Presentation** is in the first to second decades with an insidious onset of bilateral and symmetrical ptosis (Fig. 5.15a) and limitation of ocular movements in all directions of gaze (progressive external ophthalmoplegia – Fig. 5.15b).

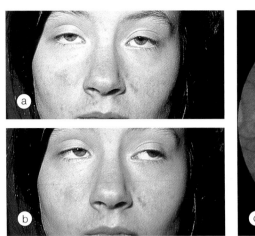
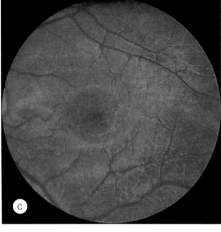
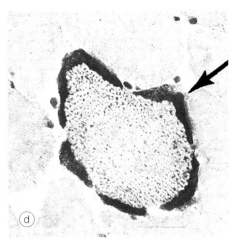

**Figure 5.15** Kearns–Sayre syndrome. **(a)** Symmetrical ptosis; **(b)** external ophthalmoplegia; **(c)** RP; **(d)** histology shows ragged-red muscle fibres (arrow) (Courtesy of Wilmer Institute)

2. **Signs** include ataxia, cardiac conduction defects, fatigue and proximal muscle weakness, deafness, diabetes and short stature.

3. **Diagnostic tests.** Lumbar puncture shows increased CSF protein concentration (>1 g/l) and ECG demonstrates cardiac conduction defects.

4. **RP** is characterised by coarse pigment clumping which principally affects the central fundus (Fig. 5.15c).

***Bardet–Biedl syndrome*** is an AR disorder.

1. **Signs** include obesity, brachydactyly and polydactyly (Fig. 5.16), dental anomalies, hypogenitalism and renal disease. The syndrome is also associated with mental handicap, cardiac disease and hypertension. There is, however, considerable variation in the clinical picture. Intelligence can be nearly normal and polydactyly absent in some patients. Overlap with Laurence-Moon syndrome and Alström syndrome has also been observed.

2. **RP** is severe and almost 75% of patients are blind by the age of 20 years. Some patients develop a bull's-eye maculopathy.

***Friedreich ataxia*** is usually an AR condition.

1. **Signs** include childhood spinocerebellar ataxia, dysarthria, cardiomyopathy, deafness and diabetes.

2. **RP** is common.

## ATYPICAL RP

1. **Sector RP** is characterised by involvement of one quadrant (usually nasal – Fig. 5.17) or one half (usually inferior). Progression is slow and many cases remain stationary.

2. **Pericentral RP** in which the pigmentary abnormalities emanate from near the disc and extend along the temporal arcades and nasally.

3. **RP with exudative vasculopathy** is characterised by a Coats disease-like appearance with lipid deposition in the peripheral retina and exudative retinal detachment.

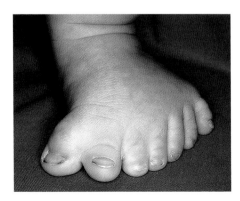

**Figure 5.16** Polydactyly

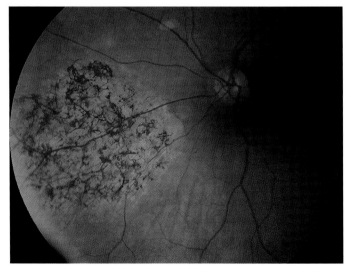

**Figure 5.17** Sector RP

## FURTHER READING

Bessant DAR, Holder GE, Fitzke FW, et al. Phenotype of retinitis pigmentosa associated with the Ser50Thr mutation in the *NRL* gene. *Arch Ophthalmol* 2003; 121:793–802.

Bird AC. Photoreceptor dystrophies. *Am J Ophthalmol* 1995;119: 543–562.

Chong NH, Bird AC. Management of inherited outer retinal dystrophies: present and future. *Br J Ophthalmol* 1999;83:120–122.

DeAngelis MM, Jonna JL, Sandberg MA, et al. Novel mutations in the *NRL* gene and associated clinical findings in patients with dominant retinitis pigmentosa. *Arch Ophthalmol* 2002;120: 369–375.

Garcia-Arumi J, Martinez V, Sararols L, et al. Vitreoretinal surgery for cystoid macular edema associated with retinitis pigmentosa. *Ophthalmology* 2003;110:1164–1169.

Riise R, Tornqvist K, Wright AF, et al. The phenotype in Norwegian patients with Bardet-Biedl syndrome with mutations in the *BBS4* gene. *Arch Ophthalmol* 2002;120:1364–1367.

van Soest S, Westerveld A, de Jong PT, et al. Retinitis pigmentosa: defined from a molecular point of view. *Surv Ophthalmol* 1999; 43:321–334.

# Progressive Cone Dystrophy

Progressive cone dystrophy comprises a heterogeneous group of rare disorders. Patients with pure cone dystrophy initially have only cone dysfunction. Those with cone–rod dystrophy have an associated but less severe rod dysfunction. However, in many patients with initially pure cone dysfunction, the rod system subsequently becomes affected; the term 'cone–rod dystrophy' is therefore more appropriate.

## Diagnosis

1. **Inheritance.** Most cases are sporadic; of the remainder, the most frequent inheritance pattern is AD, but the condition may also be AR or XL.

2. **Presentation** is in the first to second decades with gradual bilateral impairment of central and colour vision, which may later be associated with photophobia and fine pendular nystagmus.

3. **Signs,** in chronological order:

   - The fovea may be normal or exhibit non-specific granularity.
   - Bull's-eye maculopathy (Fig. 5.18) is classically described but is not universal.
   - Progressive RPE atrophy at the macula with eventual geographic atrophy (Fig. 5.19).
   - Mid-peripheral, 'bone-spicule' pigmentation (Fig. 5.20), arteriolar attenuation and temporal disc pallor may develop.

4. **Investigations**

   a. *ERG.* Photopic is abnormal or non-recordable; flicker fusion frequency is reduced; rod responses are preserved until late (Fig. 5.21).

   b. *EOG* is normal to subnormal.

   c. *DA.* The cone segment is abnormal; the rod segment is initially normal but may become subnormal later.

   d. *CV* shows a severe deuteran-tritan defect out of proportion to visual acuity.

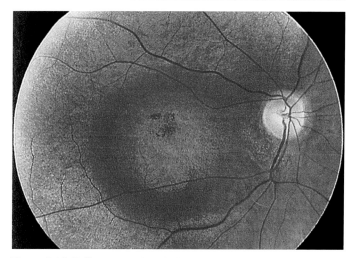

**Figure 5.18** Bull's-eye maculopathy in cone dystrophy

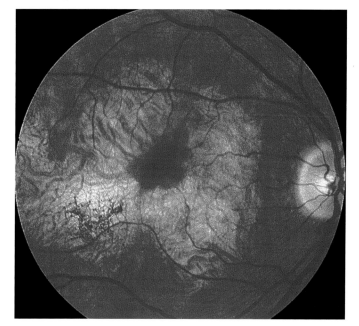

**Figure 5.19** Atrophic maculopathy in cone dystrophy

   e. *FA* of bull's-eye maculopathy shows a round hyperfluorescent window defect with a hypofluorescent centre (Fig. 5.22).

**Prognosis** depends on the severity of rod involvement; minimal involvement has a better prognosis, at least in the intermediate term.

### Other causes of bull's-eye macula

1. **In adults**

   - Chloroquine maculopathy.
   - Advanced Stargardt disease.
   - Fenestrated sheen macular dystrophy.
   - Benign concentric annular macular dystrophy.
   - Clofazimine retinopathy.

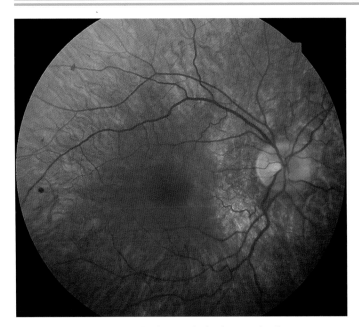

**Figure 5.20** Mild, perivascular bone-spicule pigmentation in cone dystrophy

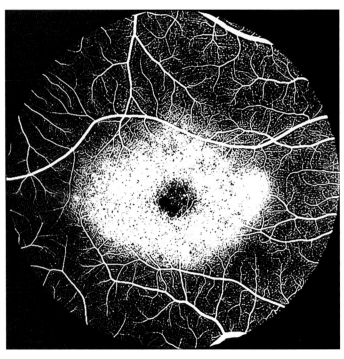

**Figure 5.22** FA in cone dystrophy showing a 'bull's-eye' pattern due to a window defect

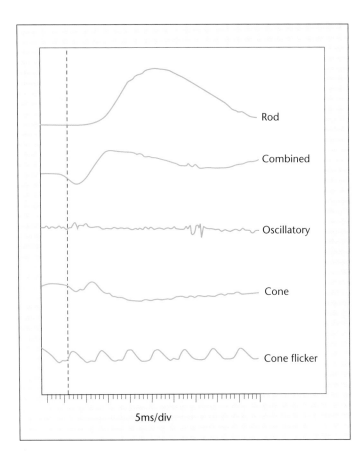

**Figure 5.21** ERG in cone dystrophy (see text)

### 2. In children

- Bardet–Biedl syndrome.
- Hallervorden–Spatz syndrome.
- Leber congenital amaurosis.

- Lipofuscinosis.
- AD cerebellar ataxia.

### FURTHER READING

Fishman GA, Stone EM, Eliason DA, et al. ABCA4 gene sequence variations in patients with autosomal recessive cone-rod dystrophy. *Arch Ophthalmol* 2003;121:851–855.

MM Kurz-Levin, Halfyard AS, Bunce C, et al. Clinical variations in assessment of bull's-eye maculopathy. *Arch Ophthalmol* 2002;120:567–575.

# Albinism

Albinism is a genetically determined, heterogeneous group of disorders of melanin synthesis in which either the eyes alone (ocular albinism) or the eyes, skin and hair (oculocutaneous albinism) may be affected. The latter may be either tyrosinase-positive or tyrosinase-negative. The different mutations are thought to act through a common pathway involving reduced melanin synthesis in the eye during development. Tyrosinase activity is assessed by using the hair bulb incubation test, which is reliable only after 5 years of age.

### OCULOCUTANEOUS ALBINISM

***Tyrosinase-negative*** (complete) albinos are incapable of synthesising melanin and have blond hair and very pale skin (Fig. 5.23) throughout life, with lack of melanin pigment in all ocular structures. They also have an increased susceptibility to skin neoplasia.

1. **Inheritance** is usually AR with the gene locus on 15p11–q13.

2. **Signs**

   *a. Visual acuity* is usually <6/60 due to foveal hypoplasia.

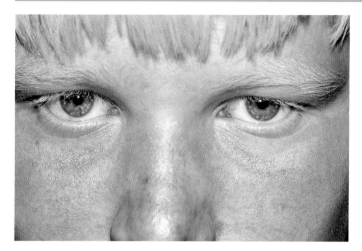

**Figure 5.23** Fair skin and blond hair in tyrosinase-negative oculocutaneous albinism

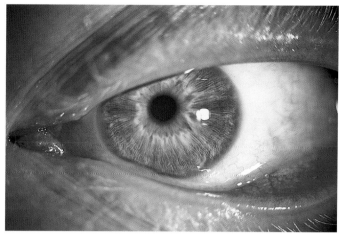

**Figure 5.25** 'Pink-eye' appearance in tyrosinase-negative oculocutaneous albinism

b. *Nystagmus* is usually pendular and horizontal. It usually increases in bright illumination and tends to lessen in severity with age.

c. *The iris* is diaphanous and translucent (Fig. 5.24), giving rise to a 'pink-eyed' appearance (Fig. 5.25).

d. *The fundus* shows lack of pigment with conspicuously large choroidal vessels, foveal hypoplasia with absence of the foveal pit and lack of vessels forming the perimacular arcades, and, occasionally, optic nerve hypoplasia (Fig. 5.26).

e. *The optic chiasm* has fewer uncrossed nerve fibres than normal so that the majority of fibres from each eye cross to the contralateral hemisphere. This can be demonstrated by visual evoked potential (VEP), which shows predominance in the response to monocular stimulation.

f. *Other features* commonly seen include refractive errors, squint and absence of stereopsis.

**Tyrosinase-positive** (incomplete) albinos synthesise variable amounts of melanin. The hair, which may be white, yellow or red, darkens with age. Skin colour is very pale at birth but usually darkens by 2 years of age.

1. **Inheritance** is usually AR with the gene locus on 15p11–q13.

2. **Signs**

   a. *Visual acuity* is usually impaired due to foveal hypoplasia.
   b. *The iris* may be blue or dark brown with variable translucency (Fig. 5.27).
   c. *The fundus* shows variable hypopigmentation (Fig. 5.28).

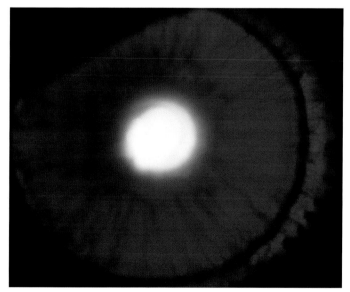

**Figure 5.24** Marked iris transillumination in tyrosinase-negative oculocutaneous albinism

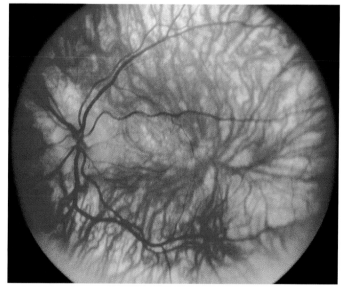

**Figure 5.26** Severe fundus hypopigmentation in tyrosinase-negative oculocutaneous albinism (Courtesy of K. Nischal)

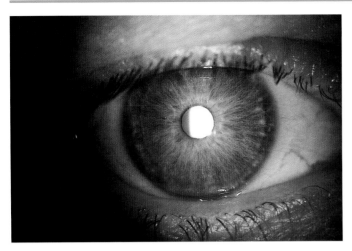

**Figure 5.27** Partial iris transillumination in tyrosinase-positive oculocutaneous albinism

### *Associated syndromes*

**1. Chediak–Higashi syndrome**

- Inheritance is AR with the gene locus on 1q43.
- Mild oculocutaneous albinism.
- Leukocytic abnormalities resulting in recurrent pyogenic infections and an early demise.

**2. Hermansky–Pudlak syndrome** is a lysosomal storage disease of the reticuloendothelial system.

- Inheritance is AR with the gene locus on 15p11–q13.
- Mild oculocutaneous albinism.
- Platelet dysfunction resulting in early bruising.

## OCULAR ALBINISM

Involvement is predominantly ocular with normal skin and hair, although, occasionally, hypopigmented skin macules may be seen.

**1. Inheritance** is usually XL and occasionally AR with the gene locus on Xp22.2–22.3.

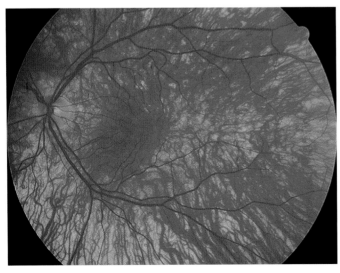

**Figure 5.28** Moderate fundus hypopigmentation in tyrosinase-positive oculocutaneous albinism (Courtesy of C. Barry)

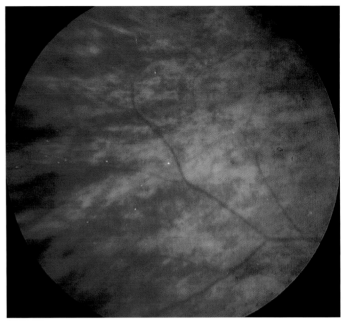

**Figure 5.29** Peripheral pigmentary changes in a carrier of ocular albinism

**2. Female carriers** are asymptomatic although they may show partial iris translucency, macular stippling and mid-peripheral scattered areas of depigmentation and granularity (Fig. 5.29).

**3. Affected males** manifest hypopigmented irides and fundi.

## FURTHER READING

Carden SM, Boissy RE, Schoettker PJ, et al. Albinism: modern molecular diagnosis. *Br J Ophthalmol* 1998;82:189–195.

Dorey SE, Neveu MM, Burton LC, et al. The clinical features of albinism and their correlation with visual evoked potential. *Br J Ophthalmol* 2003;87:767–772.

Guillery RW. Why do albinos and other hypopigmented mutants lack normal binocular vision, and what else is abnormal in their central visual pathways? *Eye* 1996;10:217–221.

Kinnear PE, Jay B, Witkop CL Jr. Albinism. *Surv Ophthalmol* 1985; 30:75–101.

Russell-Eggitt I, Kriss A, Taylor D. Albinism in childhood. *Br J Ophthalmol* 1990;74:136–140.

Summers C, King RA. Ophthalmic features of minimal pigment oculocutaneous albinism. *Ophthalmology* 1994;101:906–914.

# Stargardt Disease and Fundus Flavimaculatus

Stargardt disease (juvenile macular dystrophy) and fundus flavimaculatus are regarded as variants of the same disease despite presenting at different times and carrying different prognoses.

## STARGARDT DISEASE

Stargardt disease is the most common form of juvenile-onset macular dystrophy.

### *Diagnosis*

**1. Inheritance** is AR with the gene *ABCA4* on 1p21–22.

2. **Presentation** is in the first or second decade with bilateral, gradual impairment of central vision which may be out of proportion to the macular changes so that the child may be suspected of malingering.

3. **Signs** in chronological order:

  ● The fovea may be normal or show non-specific mottling (Fig. 5.30).
  ● Oval, 'snail-slime' or 'beaten-bronze' foveal appearance, which may be surrounded by yellow-white flecks (Fig. 5.31).
  ● Geographic atrophy which may have a bull's-eye configuration (Fig. 5.32).

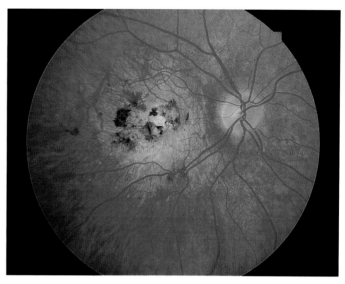

**Figure 5.32** End-stage Stargardt macular dystrophy

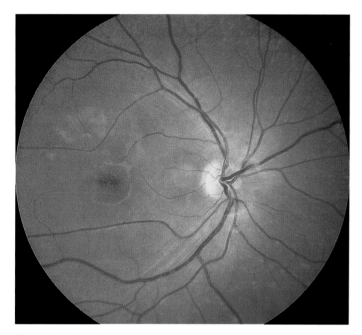

**Figure 5.30** Early Stargardt macular dystrophy

4. **Investigations**

  a. *ERG.* Photopic is normal to subnormal; scotopic is normal.
  b. *EOG* is subnormal in advanced cases.
  c. *CV* shows deuteran-tritan defects.
  d. *FA* is characterised by the absence of normal background fluorescence – a 'dark choroid' effect due to lipofuscin deposits in the RPE; this enhances the prominence of the retinal circulation. Eyes with geographic atrophy show a window defect at the macula (Fig. 5.33).

**Prognosis** is poor; once visual acuity drops below 6/12 it tends to decrease rapidly and stabilise at about 6/60.

## FUNDUS FLAVIMACULATUS

### Diagnosis

1. **Inheritance** is AR.

2. **Presentation** is in adult life, although, in the absence of macular involvement, the condition may be asymptomatic and discovered by chance.

3. **Signs,** in chronological order:

  ● Bilateral, ill-defined, yellow-white flecks, at the level of the RPE, scattered throughout the posterior pole and mid-periphery but sparing the peripapillary area (Fig. 5.34).
  ● The flecks may be round, oval, linear, semilunar or pisciform (fish-tail-like).
  ● The fundus has a vermilion colour in about 50% of cases.
  ● New lesions develop as older ones become ill-defined and softer.
  ● Geographic atrophy develops in some cases (Figs. 5.35 and 5.36).

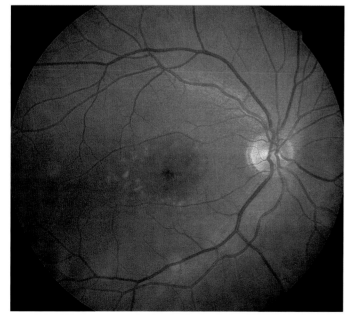

**Figure 5.31** Stargardt macular dystrophy with surrounding flecks

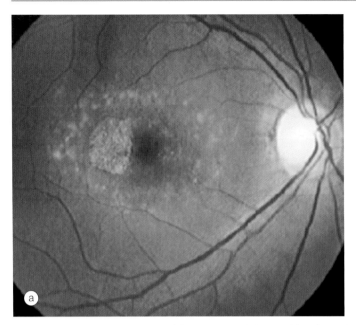 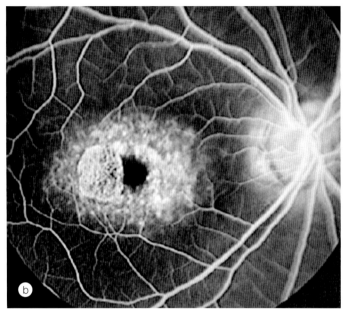

**Figure 5.33 (a)** Stargardt disease; **(b)** FA shows a dark choroid and macular hyperfluorescence due to a window defect

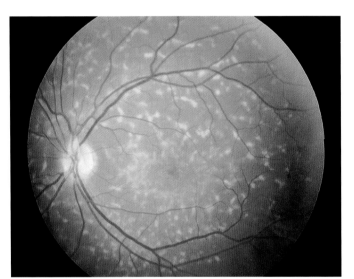

**Figure 5.34** Fundus flavimaculatus

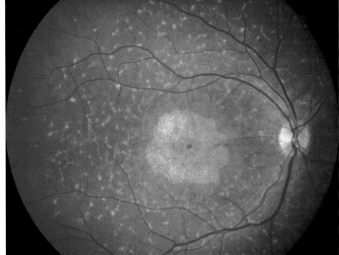

**Figure 5.36** Fundus flavimaculatus with geographic atrophy

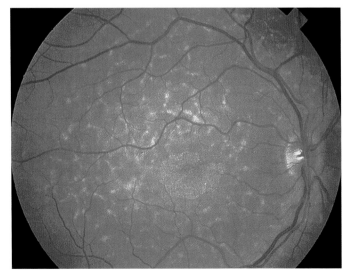

**Figure 5.35** Fundus flavimaculatus with early atrophic maculopathy

### 4. Investigations

   *a. ERG.* Photopic is normal to subnormal; scotopic is normal.

   *b. EOG* is subnormal.

   *c. CV* is normal.

   *d. FA* shows a generalised 'dark choroid'. Fresh flecks show early hypofluorescence due to blockage and late hyperfluorescence due to staining; old flecks show RPE window defects (Fig. 5.37).

***Prognosis*** is relatively good and patients may remain asymptomatic for many years unless one of the flecks involves the foveola or geographic atrophy develops.

***Differential diagnosis*** of retinal flecks includes dominant drusen, fundus albipunctatus, early North Carolina macular dystrophy and benign fleck retina.

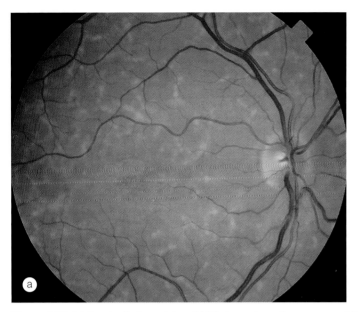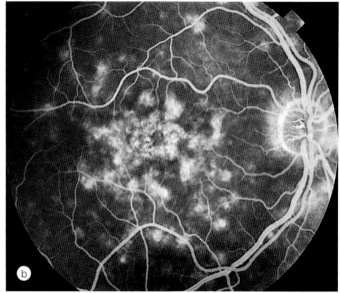

**Figure 5.37 (a)** Fundus flavimaculatus; **(b)** FA shows hyperfluorescence of the flecks

## FURTHER READING

Armstrong JD, Meyer D, Xu S, et al. Long-term follow-up of Stargardt's disease and fundus flavimaculatus. *Ophthalmology* 1998;105: 448–457.

Lois N, Holder GE, Bunce C, et al. Phenotypic subtypes of Stargardt macular dystrophy–fundus flavimaculatus. *Arch Ophthalmol* 2001;119:359–369.

Rotenstreich Y, Fishman GA, Anderson RJ. Visual acuity loss and clinical observations in a large series of patients with Stargardt disease. *Ophthalmology* 2003;110:1151–1158.

## Juvenile Best Macular Dystrophy

Juvenile Best disease (vitelliform dystrophy) is a rare condition which evolves gradually through five stages.

### *Diagnosis*

1. **Inheritance** is AD with variable penetrance and expressivity with the gene locus on 11q13.

2. **Signs,** in chronological order:

   a. *Stage 0* (pre-vitelliform) is characterised by a subnormal EOG in an asymptomatic child with a normal fundus appearance.

   b. *Stage 1* is characterised by pigment mottling at the macula.

   c. *Stage 2* (vitelliform), which develops in the first to second decades, is characterised by a round egg-yolk ('sunny side up') macular lesion consisting of accu-mulation of lipo-fuscin within the RPE (Fig. 5.38a); FA shows corresponding hypofluorescence due to blockage (Fig. 5.38b). Visual acuity may be normal or slightly decreased.

   d. *Stage 3* (pseudo-hypopyon) may occur when part of the lesion becomes absorbed (Fig. 5.39). Occasionally, the whole lesion becomes absorbed with little effect on vision.

   e. *Stage 4* (vitelliruptive) in which the egg yolk begins to break up ('scrambled egg') (Fig. 5.40) and visual acuity drops.

3. **Investigations**

   a. *ERG* is normal.

   b. *EOG* is severely subnormal during all stages and in carriers with normal fundi.

   c. *CV* defects are proportional to the degree of visual loss.

***Prognosis*** is reasonably good until the fifth decade, after which visual acuity declines and some patients become legally blind due to macular scarring, choroidal neovascularisation (CNV), geographic atrophy or hole formation which may lead to retinal detachment.

## Multifocal Vitelliform Disease

Rarely, multifocal vitelliform lesions (Fig. 5.41) may be seen in the absence of Best disease and without a family history and with a normal EOG. The condition may develop acutely in adult life and give rise to diagnostic difficulties.

## Familial Drusen

Familial drusen (Doyne honeycomb choroiditis, malattia leventinese) is thought to represent an early manifestation of age-related macular degeneration.

1. **Inheritance** is AD with full penetrance but variable expressivity. The gene *EFEMP1* is on 2p16–21.

2. **Signs and prognosis**

   a. *Mild disease* is characterised by a few small, discrete, hard drusen confined to the macula (Fig. 5.42). The

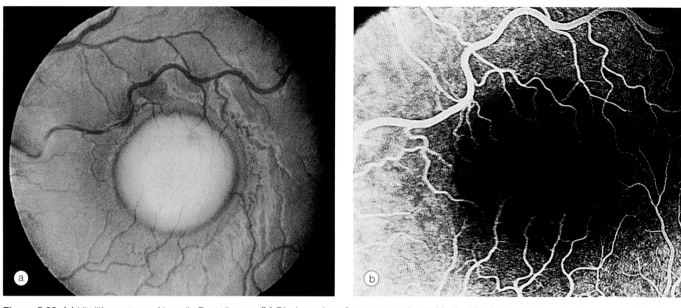

**Figure 5.38 (a)** Vitelliform stage of juvenile Best disease; **(b)** FA shows hypofluorescence due to blocked background choroidal fluorescence (Courtesy of Wilmer Institute)

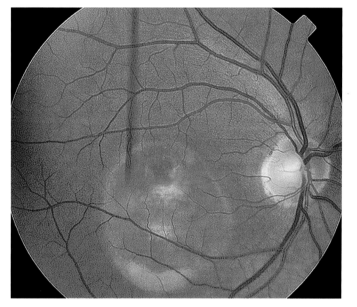

**Figure 5.39** Pseudo-hypopyon stage of juvenile Best disease

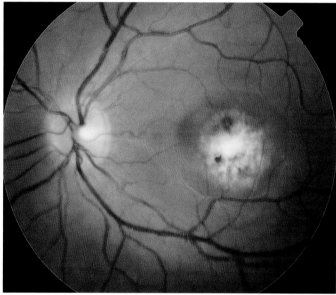

**Figure 5.40** Vitelliruptive ('scrambled egg') stage of juvenile Best disease

lesions typically appear in the third decade and are innocuous.

b. *Moderate disease* is characterised by large, soft drusen at the posterior pole and peripapillary region (Fig. 5.43). The lesions appear after the third decade and are associated with normal or mild impairment of visual acuity.

c. *Advanced disease* is uncommon and presents after the fifth decade with CNV or geographic atrophy.

d. *Malattia leventinese* shares phenotypic overlap with familial drusen. It is characterised by numerous, small, elongated, basal laminar drusen with a spoke-like or radial distribution centered on the fovea and peripapillary area (Fig. 5.44). Most patients are asymptomatic until the fourth or fifth decades, when they may develop CNV or geographic atrophy (Fig. 5.45).

### 3. Investigations

a. *ERG* is normal.

b. *EOG* is subnormal in patients with advanced disease.

c. *FA* shows well-defined hyperfluorescent spots due to window defects, which are more extensive on FA (Fig. 5.46) than on clinical examination.

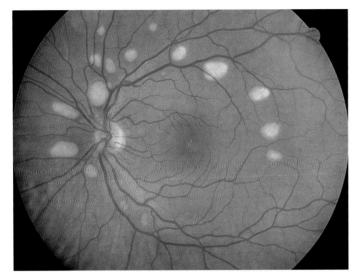

**Figure 5.41** Multifocal vitelliform disease (Courtesy of C. Barry)

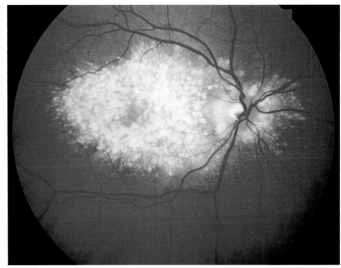

**Figure 5.44** Malattia leventinese (Courtesy of Moorfields Eye Hospital)

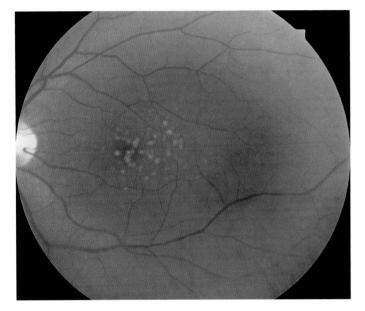

**Figure 5.42** Mild familial dominant drusen

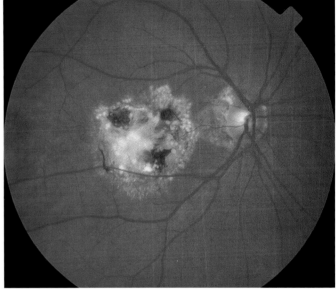

**Figure 5.45** Atrophic maculopathy in malattia leventinese (Courtesy of Moorfields Eye Hospital)

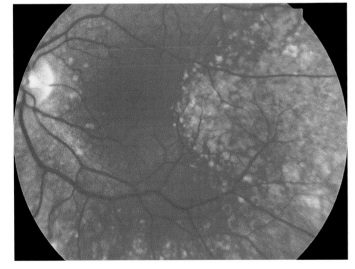

**Figure 5.43** Moderately advanced familial dominant drusen

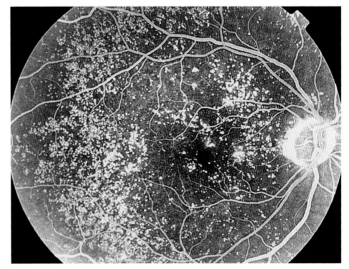

**Figure 5.46** FA in familial dominant drusen, showing numerous well-defined hyperfluorescent spots due to window defects

## FURTHER READING

Dantas MA, Slakter JS, Negrao S, et al. Photodynamic therapy with verteporfin in malattia leventinese. *Ophthalmology* 2002;109: 296–301.

Heon E, Piguet B, Munier F, et al. Linkage of autosomal dominant radial drusen (malattia leventinese) to chromosome 2p16-21. *Arch Ophthalmol* 1996;114:193–198.

Holz FG, Owens SL, Marks J, et al. Ultrastructural findings in autosomal dominant drusen. *Arch Ophthalmol* 1997;115: 788–792.

Piquet B, Haimovici R, Bird AC. Dominantly inherited drusen represent more than one disorder: a historical review. *Eye* 1995;9:34–41.

# Leber Congenital Amaurosis

Leber congenital amaurosis is the name ascribed to a group of inherited retinal dystrophies representing the commonest genetic cause of visual impairment in infants and children. It carries a very poor prognosis.

### Diagnosis

1. **Inheritance** is AR with the gene locus on 17p.

2. **Presentation** is with blindness at birth or shortly thereafter, associated with roving eye movements.

3. **Signs**

   - The pupillary light reflexes are absent or diminished.
   - The fundi may be initially normal despite very poor vision. The most common findings are patches of peripheral chorioretinal atrophy and granularity (Fig. 5.47).
   - Other findings include disc oedema, salt-and-pepper changes (Fig. 5.48), diffuse white spots, macular coloboma and bull's-eye maculopathy.

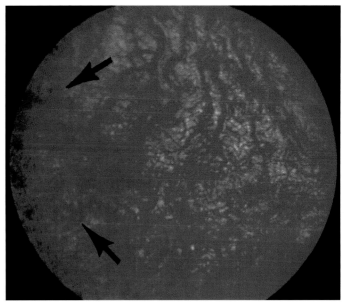

**Figure 5.48** Salt-and-pepper fundus changes in Leber congenital amaurosis (Courtesy of Wilmer Institute)

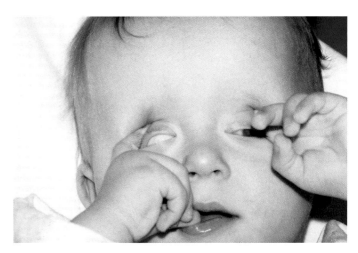

**Figure 5.49** Oculodigital syndrome (Courtesy of M. Szreter)

   - Optic disc pallor and arteriolar attenuation develop concurrently with the retinal changes.
   - Oculodigital syndrome in which constant rubbing of the eyes by the child causes enophthalmos as a result of resorption of orbital fat (Fig. 5.49).

4. **Ocular associations** include strabismus, hypermetropia, keratoconus, keratoglobus and cataract.

5. **ERG** is usually non-recordable even in early cases with normal fundi.

*Systemic associations* include mental handicap, deafness, epilepsy, central nervous system (CNS) and renal anomalies, skeletal malformations and endocrine dysfunction.

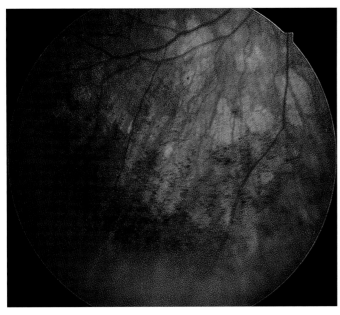

**Figure 5.47** Peripheral chorioretinal atrophy and granularity in Leber congenital amaurosis

## FURTHER READING

Heher KL, Traboulsi EI, Maumenee IH. The natural history of Leber's congenital amaurosis. *Ophthalmology* 1992;99:241–251.

Lotery AJ, Jacobson SG, Fishman GA, et al. Mutations in the CRB1 gene cause Leber's congenital amaurosis. *Arch Ophthalmol* 2001; 119:415–420.

Mohamed MD, Topping NC, Jafir H, et al. Progression of phenotype in Leber's congenital amaurosis with a mutation of the LCA5 locus. *Br J Ophthalmol* 2003;87:473–475.

# Sorsby Pseudo-inflammatory Macular Dystrophy

Sorsby pseudo-inflammatory macular dystrophy, also referred to as hereditary haemorrhagic macular dystrophy, is a very rare but serious condition.

### Diagnosis

1. **Inheritance** is AD with full penetrance, with the gene *TIMP3* on 22q12.1–13.2.

2. **Presentation** is in the fifth decade with bilateral exudative maculopathy.

3. **Signs,** in chronological order:

   - Yellow-white, confluent, drusen-like deposits along the arcades, nasal to the disc and mid-periphery (Fig. 5.50).
   - Exudative maculopathy secondary to CNV (Fig. 5.51) and subretinal scarring (Fig. 5.52) may occur in the fourth to fifth decades.
   - Peripheral chorioretinal atrophy may occur by the seventh decade and result in loss of ambulatory vision.

4. **Investigations**

   a. *ERG* is initially normal but may be subnormal in late disease.

   b. *EOG* is normal.

**Prognosis** is universally poor.

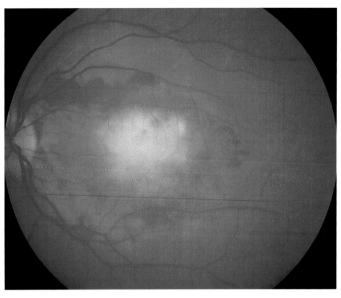

**Figure 5.51** Exudative maculopathy in Sorsby pseudo-inflammatory macular dystrophy

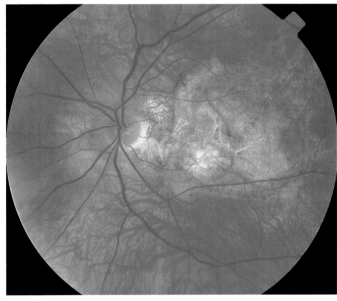

**Figure 5.52** Subretinal scarring in end-stage Sorsby pseudo-inflammatory macular dystrophy

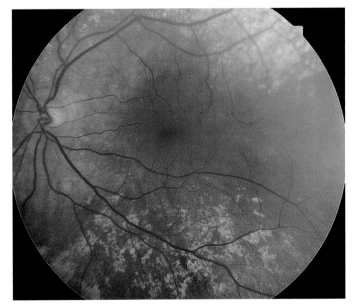

**Figure 5.50** Early Sorsby pseudo-inflammatory macular dystrophy with confluent flecks along the arcades

## FURTHER READING

Jacobson SG, Cideciyan AV, Bennett J, et al. Novel mutation in the *TIMP3* gene causes Sorsby fundus dystrophy. *Arch Ophthalmol* 2002;120:376–379.

# North Carolina Macular Dystrophy

North Carolina macular dystrophy is a very rare non-progressive condition. It was first described in families living in the mountains of North Carolina and subsequently in many unrelated families in other parts of the world.

1. **Inheritance** is AD with complete penetrance but highly variable expressivity, with the gene *MCDR1* on 6q14–16.2.

2. **Grading and prognosis**

   a. *Grade 1* is characterised by yellow-white, drusen-like peripheral (Fig. 5.53) and macular deposits which develop during the first decade and may remain asymptomatic throughout life.

   b. *Grade 2* is characterised by deep, confluent macular deposits (Fig. 5.54). The long-term visual prognosis is guarded because some patients develop exudative maculopathy (Fig. 5.55) and subretinal scarring (Fig. 5.56).

   c. *Grade 3* is characterised by coloboma-like atrophic macular lesions (Fig. 5.57) associated with variable impairment of visual acuity.

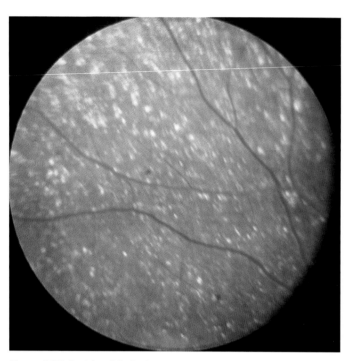

**Figure 5.53** Peripheral flecks in grade 1 North Carolina macular dystrophy (Courtesy of P. Morse)

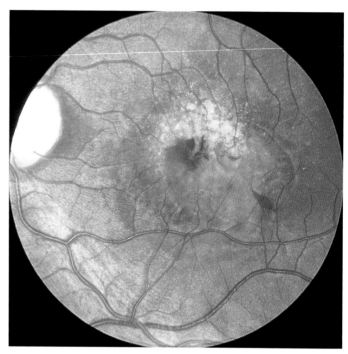

**Figure 5.55** Exudative maculopathy in North Carolina macular dystrophy (Courtesy of P. Morse)

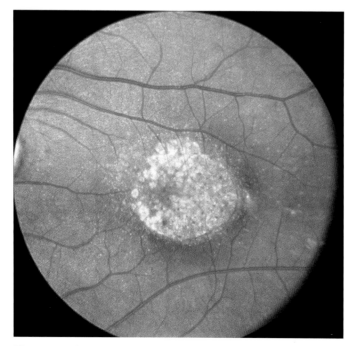

**Figure 5.54** Grade 2 North Carolina macular dystrophy (Courtesy of P. Morse)

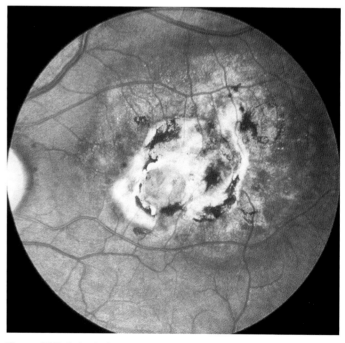

**Figure 5.56** Subretinal scarring in North Carolina macular dystrophy

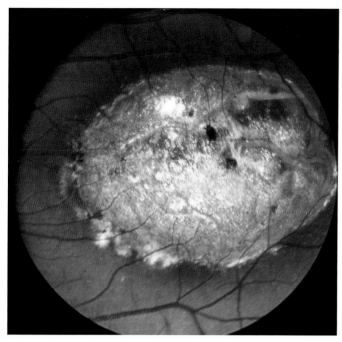

**Figure 5.57** Coloboma-like macular lesion in grade 3 North Carolina macular dystrophy (Courtesy of P. Morse)

### 3. Investigations

   *a.* *ERG* is normal.

   *b.* *EOG* is normal.

   *c.* *FA* in grades 1 and 2 shows transmission defects and late staining.

### FURTHER READING

Francis PJ, Johnson S, Edmunds B, et al. Genetic linkage analysis of a novel syndrome comprising North Carolina-like macular dystrophy and progressive sensorineural hearing loss. *Br J Ophthalmol* 2003; 87:893–898.

Pauleikhoff D, Sauer CG, Muller CR, et al. Clinical and genetic evidence for North Carolina macular dystrophy in a German family. *Am J Ophthalmol* 1997; 124:412–415.

Reichel MB, Kelsell RE, Fan J, et al. Phenotype of British North Carolina macular dystrophy family linked to chromosome 6q. *Br J Ophthalmol* 1998;82:1162–1168.

Voo I, Glasgow BJ, Flannery J, et al. North Carolina macular dystrophy: clinico-pathologic correlation. *Am J Ophthalmol* 2001;132:933–935.

## Pattern Dystrophies

### ADULT-ONSET FOVEOMACULAR VITELLIFORM DYSTROPHY

In contrast to juvenile Best disease, the foveal lesions are smaller, present later and do not demonstrate similar evolutionary changes.

### *Diagnosis*

1. **Inheritance** is AD with the gene locus on 6p21.

2. **Presentation** is in the fourth to sixth decades with mild-to-moderate decrease of visual acuity and, sometimes, metamorphopsia, although often the condition is discovered by chance.

### 3. Signs

  ● Bilateral, symmetrical, round or oval, slightly elevated, yellowish subfoveal deposits, about one-third of a disc diameter in size, often centered by a pigmented spot (Fig. 5.58a).

  ● Associated macular drusen may be seen in some cases.

### 4. Investigations

   *a.* *ERG* is normal.

   *b.* *EOG* may be subnormal.

   *c.* *CV* shows a mild tritan defect.

   *d.* *FA* shows early central hypofluorescence surrounded by a small irregular hyperfluorescent ring (Fig. 5.58b); the late phase shows persistent central hypofluorescence.

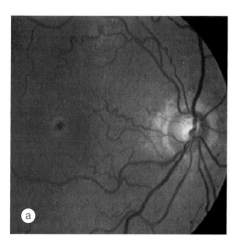
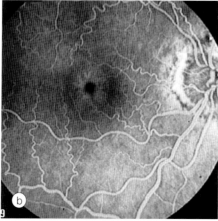
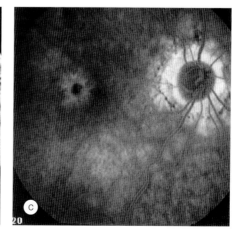

**Figure 5.58** **(a)** Adult-onset foveomacular vitelliform dystrophy; **(b)** & **(c)** FA shows central hypofluorescence with a hyperfluorescent halo

*Prognosis* is good in the majority of cases although some eyes may develop visual loss due to progressive foveal thinning and the possible evolution to a full-thickness macular hole.

## BUTTERFLY-SHAPED MACULAR DYSTROPHY

Butterfly dystrophy is a rare and relatively innocuous condition.

### Diagnosis

1. **Inheritance** is probably AD.

2. **Presentation** is in the second to third decades, usually by chance and occasionally with mild impairment of central vision.

3. **Signs**

   - Yellow pigment at the fovea arranged in a triradiate manner (Fig. 5.59).
   - Peripheral pigmentary stippling may be present.
   - Atrophic maculopathy may develop with time.

4. **Investigations**

   a. *ERG* is normal.
   b. *EOG* may be subnormal.

*Prognosis* is good in the majority of patients.

## RETICULAR DYSTROPHY OF THE RPE

### Diagnosis

1. **Inheritance** is AR or AD.

2. **Presentation** is in the third decade with mild impairment of central vision.

3. **Signs**

   - Coarse, net-like lesion at the posterior pole.
   - With time the lesions may fade and atrophic maculopathy ensue.

4. **Investigations**

   a. *ERG* is normal.

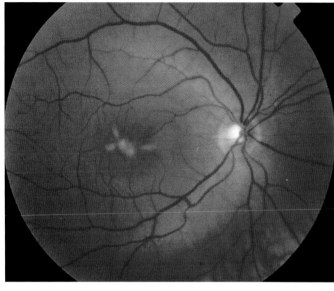

**Figure 5.59** Butterfly dystrophy

b. *EOG* may be subnormal.

*Prognosis* is usually good.

## MULTIFOCAL PATTERN DYSTROPHY SIMULATING FUNDUS FLAVIMACULATUS

### Diagnosis

1. **Inheritance** is AD.

2. **Presentation** is in the fourth decade with mild impairment of central vision.

3. **Signs** – multiple, widely scattered, irregular, yellow lesions that may be similar to those seen in fundus flavimaculatus (Fig. 5.60a).

4. **Investigations**

   a. *ERG* is normal.

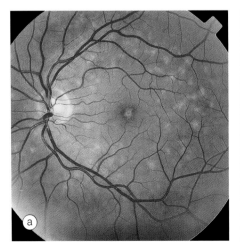
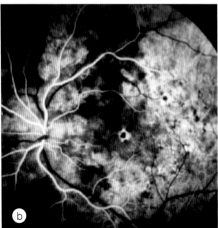
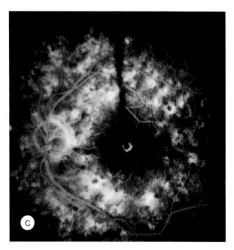

**Figure 5.60 (a)** Multifocal pattern dystrophy simulating fundus flavimaculatus; **(b)** & **(c)** FA shows hyperfluorescence of flecks but the choroid is not dark

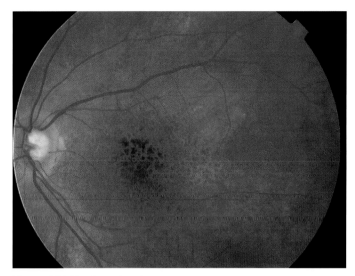

**Figure 5.61** Fundus pulverulentus

b. *EOG* may be subnormal.

c. *FA* shows hyperfluorescence of flecks but the choroid is not dark (Fig. 5.60b and 5.60c).

***Prognosis*** is good.

## FUNDUS PULVERULENTUS

1. **Inheritance** is AD.

2. **Signs** – coarse pigmentary mottling at the macula (Fig. 5.61).

3. **Prognosis** is excellent.

## FURTHER READING

Benhamou N, Souied EH, Zolf R, et al. Adult-onset foveomacular vitelliform dystrophy: a study of optical coherence tomography. *Am J Ophthalmol* 2003;135:362–367.

Brecher R, Bird AC. Adult vitelliform macular dystrophy. *Eye* 1990; 4:210–215.

Pierro L, Tremolada G, Introini U, et al. Optical coherence tomography in adult-onset foveomacular vitelliform dystrophy. *Am J Ophthalmol* 2002;134:675–680.

Saito W, Yamamoto S, Hayashi M, et al. Morphological and functional analysis of adult onset vitelliform macular dystrophy. *Br J Ophthalmol* 2003;87:758–762.

Zhang K, Garibaldi DC, Li Y, et al. Butterfly-shaped pattern dystrophy. *Arch Ophthalmol* 2002;119:485–490.

## Dominant Macular Oedema

Dominant cystoid macular oedema is an extremely rare but serious condition.

### Diagnosis

1. **Inheritance** is AD with the gene locus on 7q.

2. **Presentation** is in the first to second decades with gradual impairment of central vision.

3. **Signs** – bilateral cystoid macular oedema.

### 4. Investigations

a. *ERG* is normal.

b. *EOG* is normal to subnormal.

c. *FA* shows a flower-petal pattern of leakage at the fovea (see Fig. 3.73).

***Prognosis*** is poor because the oedema does not respond to treatment with systemic acetazolamide and geographic atrophy inevitably ensues.

## Bietti Crystalline Dystrophy

Bietti crystalline dystrophy is characterised by deposition of crystals in the retina and the superficial peripheral cornea.

### Diagnosis

1. **Inheritance** is usually AR and occasionally AD or XL.

2. **Presentation** is in the third decade with slowly progressive visual loss.

3. **Signs,** in chronological order:

   - Numerous, fine, glistening, yellow-white crystals scattered throughout the posterior fundus (Fig. 5.62).
   - Localised atrophy of the RPE and choriocapillaris at the macula.
   - Diffuse atrophy of the choriocapillaris with a decrease in size and number of the crystals.
   - Gradual confluence and expansion of the atrophic areas into the retinal periphery; normal optic nerves and retinal vasculature.

### 4. Investigations

a. *ERG* is subnormal.

b. *EOG* is subnormal.

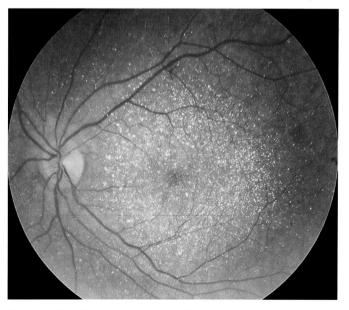

**Figure 5.62** Bietti crystalline dystrophy (Courtesy of J. Salmon)

*Prognosis* is variable because the rate of disease progression differs in individual cases.

## FURTHER READING

Chan WM, Pang CP, Leung ATS, et al. Bietti crystalline retinopathy affecting all 3 male siblings in a family. *Arch Ophthalmol* 2000; 118:129–131.

Usui T, Tanimoto N, Takagi M, et al. Rod and cone a-waves in three cases of Bietti crystalline chorioretinal dystrophy. *Am J Ophthalmol* 2001;132:395–402.

# Alport Syndrome

Alport syndrome is a rare abnormality of glomerular basement membrane caused by mutations in several different genes, all of which encode particular forms of type IV collagen, a major component of basement membrane. It is characterised by chronic renal failure, often associated with sensorineural deafness.

## Diagnosis

1. **Inheritance** is XL dominant.

2. **Signs**

   - Scattered, yellowish, punctate flecks in the perimacular area, sparing the fovea, with normal visual acuity (Fig. 5.63).
   - Larger flecks, some of which may become confluent, in the periphery (Fig. 5.64).

3. **ERG** is normal.

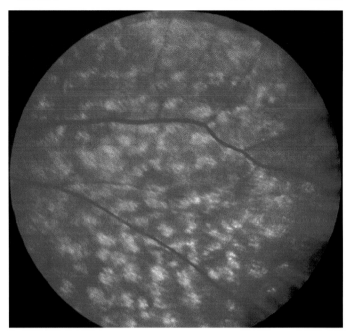

**Figure 5.64** Peripheral flecks in Alport syndrome (Courtesy of J. Govan)

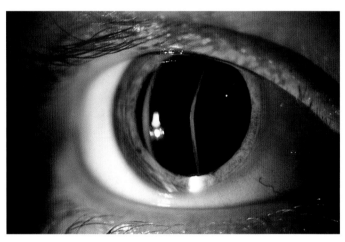

**Figure 5.65** Anterior lenticonus

4. **Ocular associations** are anterior lenticonus (Fig. 5.65) and, occasionally, posterior polymorphous corneal dystrophy.

*Prognosis* for vision is excellent.

# Benign Familial Flecked Retina

Benign familial flecked retina is a very rare disorder which is asymptomatic and therefore usually discovered by chance.

## Diagnosis

1. **Inheritance** is AR.

2. **Signs** – widespread, discrete, yellow-white flecks of variable shapes which spare the fovea (Fig. 5.66) and extend to the far periphery (Fig. 5.67).

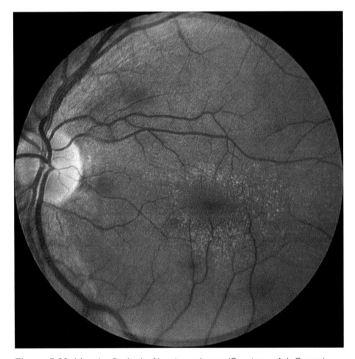

**Figure 5.63** Macular flecks in Alport syndrome (Courtesy of J. Govan)

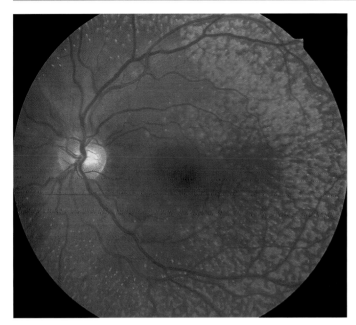

**Figure 5.66** Central lesions which spare the fovea in benign familial fleck retina

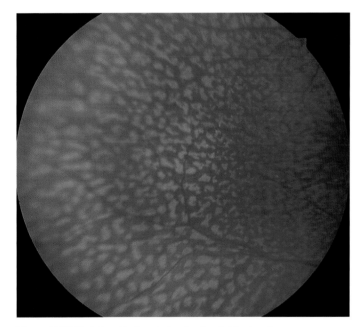

**Figure 5.67** Peripheral lesions in benign familial fleck retina

3. **ERG** is normal.

***Prognosis*** is excellent.

# Occult Macular Dystrophy

This very rare inherited condition may give rise to diagnostic problems in patients with unexplained loss of central vision, particularly in the presence of coincident ocular conditions.

## *Diagnosis*

1. **Presentation** is at any time between the third and seventh decades with bilateral progressive loss of visual acuity.

2. **Signs** – the fundi are normal.

3. **Investigations**

   a. *ERG:* full-field is normal but focal cone ERG and multifocal ERG are abnormal.
   b. *FA* is normal.
   c. *Optical coherence tomography* shows decreased foveal thickness.

***Prognosis*** is poor.

## FURTHER READING
Kondo M, Ito Y, Ueno S, et al. Foveal thinness in occult macular dystrophy. *Am J Ophthalmol* 2003;135:725–728.
Miyake Y, Horiguchi M, Tomita N, et al. Occult macular dystrophy. *Am J Ophthalmol* 1996;122:644–653.

# Enhanced S-cone Syndrome

## *Diagnosis*

1. **Inheritance** is AR.

2. **Presentation** is with nyctalopia in childhood.

3. **Signs**

   - Abnormal maculae, often showing cystoid changes.
   - Pigmentary changes along the vascular arcades.

4. **ERG.** Cone ERG to short wavelength stimuli is enhanced (hence the name enhanced S-cone syndrome). Cone ERG to long and middle wavelengths are reduced. The rod ERG is non-recordable.

***Prognosis*** is guarded because some eyes develop CNV.

## FURTHER READING
Marmor MF, Jacobson SG, Foerster MH, et al. Diagnostic clinical findings of a new syndrome with night blindness, maculopathy, and enhanced S cone sensitivity. *Am J Ophthalmol* 1990;110:124–134.

# Late-onset Retinal Degeneration

## *Diagnosis*

1. **Inheritance** is AD.

2. **Presentation** is with nyctalopia in the sixth decade. This is followed by progressive loss of central and peripheral vision over ensuing decades.

3. **Signs,** in chronological order

   - Normal fundus.
   - Clusters of fine yellow-white dots in the mid-periphery.
   - Pigmentary retinopathy and chorioretinal atrophy (Fig. 5.68).

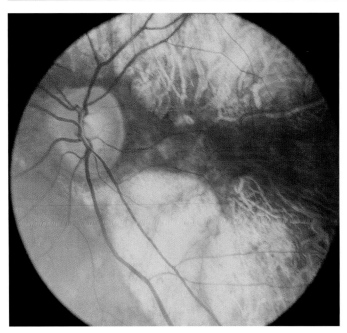

**Figure 5.68** Chorioretinal atrophy in late-onset retinal degeneration

- Atrophic maculopathy and optic atrophy.

4. **ERG** is initially normal. End-stage disease shows only reduced amplitude.

***Prognosis*** is very poor.

## FURTHER READING

Milam AH, Curcio CA, Cideciyan AV, et al. Dominant late-onset retinal degeneration with regional variation of sub-epithelial pigment epithelial deposits, retinal function and photoreceptor degeneration. *Ophthalmology* 2000;107:2256–2266.

## Fenestrated Sheen Maculopathy

### *Diagnosis*

1. **Inheritance** is AD.

2. **Presentation** is in the third decade.

3. **Signs,** in chronological order:

- Yellowish refractile sheen with red fenestrations in the sensory retina at the macula, with normal visual acuity. The sheen is deep to the retinal vessels but superficial to the RPE.
- Enlarging annular hypopigmentation at the level of the RPE gives rise to a 'bull's-eye' appearance.

4. **Investigations**

   *a. ERG* may be mildly subnormal.
   *b. FA* shows an annular window defect but no leakage.

***Prognosis*** is fairly good.

# Familial Internal Limiting Membrane Dystrophy

### *Diagnosis*

1. **Inheritance** is AD.

2. **Presentation** is in the third to fourth decades with visual loss.

3. **Signs** – glistening inner retinal surface throughout the posterior pole (Fig. 5.69).

4. **Investigations**

   *a. ERG* shows a selective diminution of the b-wave.
   *b. FA* shows diffuse retinal capillary permeability alterations.

***Prognosis*** is poor, with visual loss occurring by the sixth decade due to the development of retinoschisis, retinal oedema and retinal folds.

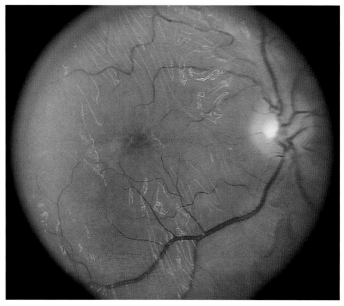

**Figure 5.69** Familial internal limiting membrane dystrophy (Courtesy of J.D.M. Gass, from *Stereoscopic Atlas of Macular Diseases*, Mosby, 1997)

## FURTHER READING

Polk TD, Gass DM, Green WR, et al. Familial internal limiting membrane dystrophy. A new sheen retinal dystrophy. *Arch Ophthalmol* 1997;115:878–885.

## Sjögren–Larsson Syndrome

This is a neurocutaneous disorder characterised by congenital ichthyosis (Fig. 5.70), spasticity, convulsions and mental retardation, with reduced life expectancy. The basic metabolic defect is deficient activity of fatty aldehyde dehydrogenase.

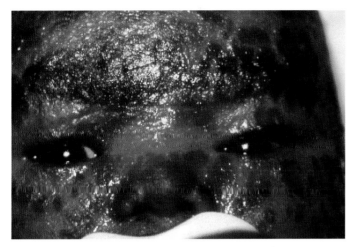

**Figure 5.70** Congenital ichthyosis (Courtesy of K. Nischal)

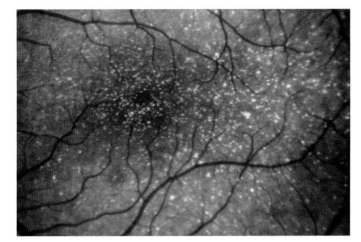

**Figure 5.71** Macular deposits in Sjögren–Larsson syndrome

**1. Inheritance** is AR.

**2. Presentation** is with photophobia and poor vision.

**3. Signs**

- Bilateral, glistening, yellow-white crystalline deposits at the macula which appear during the first 2 years of life (Fig. 5.71) and become more numerous with time.
- The presence of the macular lesions is thought to be a cardinal and perhaps pathognomonic sign of the syndrome.

**4. Investigations**

- a. ERG is normal.
- b. VEP is abnormal.
- c. FA shows mottled hyperfluorescence of the RPE without leakage.

## FURTHER READING

Willemsen MAAP, Cruysberg JRM, Rotteveel JJ, et al. Juvenile macular dystrophy associated with deficient activity of fatty aldehyde dehydrogenase in Sjogren-Larsson syndrome. *Am J Ophthalmol* 2000;130:782–789.

# Benign Concentric Annular Macular Dystrophy

### Diagnosis

**1. Inheritance** is AD.

**2. Presentation** is in adult life with very mild impairment of central vision.

**3. Signs**

- Bull's-eye maculopathy (Fig. 5.72a).
- Slight vascular attenuation but a normal disc.

**4. Investigations**

- a. ERG is normal or slightly subnormal.
- b. EOG may be subnormal.
- c. CV may be slightly–moderately impaired.
- d. VF shows a paracentral ring scotoma.
- e. FA shows an annular RPE window defect (Fig. 5.72b and 5.72c).

***Prognosis*** is good in the majority or cases although a minority develop progressive loss of visual acuity and nyctalopia.

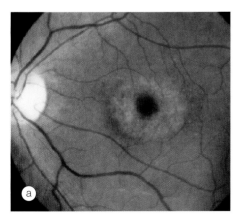
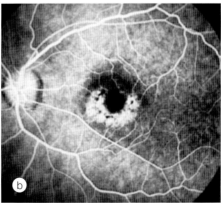
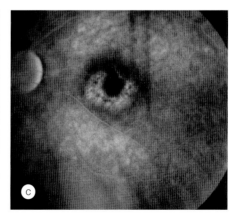

**Figure 5.72 (a)** Benign concentric annular macular dystrophy; **(b)** & **(c)** FA shows central hypofluorescence with incomplete surrounding hyperfluorescence

# Congenital Stationary Night Blindness

## WITH A NORMAL FUNDUS

1. **AD congenital nyctalopia** (Nougaret type) is characterised by a slightly impaired cone ERG and subnormal rod ERG function.

2. **AD stationary nyctalopia without myopia** (Riggs type) is characterised by a normal cone ERG.

3. **AR or XL congenital nyctalopia with myopia** (Schubert–Bornschein type).

## WITH AN ABNORMAL FUNDUS

1. **Oguchi disease** is an AR condition characterised by a 2- to 12-hour delay in attaining normal dark-adapted rod thresholds. There is an accompanying change in fundus colour from golden brown in the light-adapted state (Fig. 5.73a) to a normal colour in the dark-adapted state (Fig. 5.73b) – Mizuo phenomenon.

2. **Fundus albipunctatus** is an AR condition characterised by a multitude of tiny yellow-white spots at the posterior pole, sparing the fovea (Fig. 5.74), and extending to the periphery. The retinal blood vessels, optic disc, peripheral fields and visual acuity remain normal. The ERG and EOG may be abnormal when tested routinely but revert to normal on prolonged dark adaptation.

## FURTHER READING

Dryja TP. Molecular genetics of Oguchi disease, fundus albipunctatus, and other forms of stationary night blindness: LVII Edward Jackson Memorial Lecture. *Am J Ophthalmol* 2000;130:547–563.

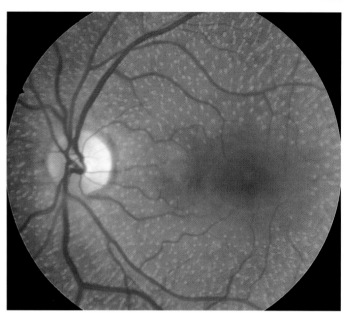

**Figure 5.74** Fundus albipunctatus

# Congenital Monochromatism

## COMPLETE ROD MONOCHROMATISM

1. **Inheritance** is AR.

2. **Signs**

   - Visual acuity is 6/60.
   - Macula usually appears normal but may be hypoplastic.
   - Congenital nystagmus and photophobia.

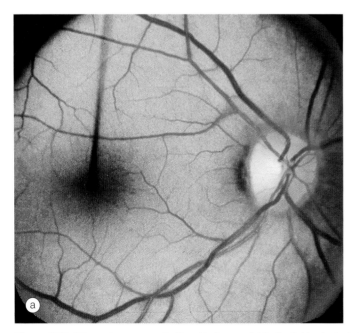

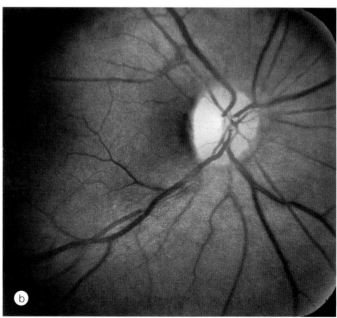

**Figure 5.73** Mizuo phenomenon in Oguchi disease. **(a)** In the light-adapted state; **(b)** in the dark-adapted state (Courtesy of J.D.M. Gass, from *Stereoscopic Atlas of Macular Diseases*, Mosby, 1997)

## 3. Investigations

    *a.* *ERG.* Photopic abnormal; scotopic may be subnormal; flicker fusion <30 Hz.

    *b.* *CV* is totally absent; all colours appear as shades of grey.

## INCOMPLETE ROD MONOCHROMATISM

### 1. Inheritance is AR or XL.

### 2. Signs

- Visual acuity is 6/12–6/24.
- Macula is usually normal.
- Nystagmus and photophobia may be present.

### 3. Investigations

    *a.* *ERG.* Abnormal photopic but normal scotopic.

    *b.* *CV.* Some colour vision may be present.

## CONE MONOCHROMATISM

### 1. Inheritance is uncertain.

### 2. Signs

- Visual acuity is 6/6–6/9.
- Normal macula.
- Nystagmus and photophobia are absent.

### 3. Investigations

    *a.* *ERG* is normal.

    *b.* *CV* is totally absent.

# Cherry-red Spot at Macula

***Ocular features.*** The cherry-red spot at the macula (Fig. 5.75) is a clinical sign seen in the context of thickening and loss of transparency of the retina at the posterior pole. The fovea, being the thinnest part of the retina and devoid of ganglion cells, retains relative transparency, allowing persistent transmission of the underlying highly vascular choroidal hue.

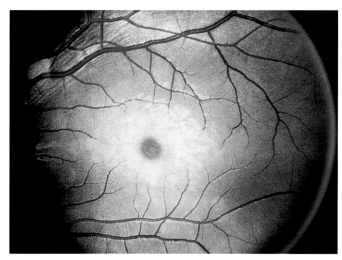

**Figure 5.75** Cherry-red spot at the macula

This striking retinal lesion, commonly seen in occlusion of the central retinal artery, is additionally a feature of a rare group of inherited metabolic diseases, the sphingolipidoses, characterised by the progressive intracellular accretion of excessive quantities of certain glycolipids and phospholipids in various tissues of the body, including the retina. The lipids accumulate in the ganglion cell layer of the retina, giving the retina a white appearance. As ganglion cells are absent at the foveola, this area retains relative transparency and contrasts with the surrounding opaque retina. With the passage of time, the ganglion cells die and the spot becomes less evident. The late stage of the disease is characterised by degeneration of the retinal nerve fibre layer and consecutive optic atrophy.

### Systemic associations

1. **Tay–Sachs disease** (GM$_2$ gangliosidosis type 1), also known as infantile amaurotic familial idiocy, is an AR disease with an onset during the first year of life, usually ending in death before the age of 2 years. It typically affects European Jews and is characterised by progressive neurological disease and eventual blindness. A cherry-red spot is present in about 90% of cases.

2. **Niemann–Pick disease** is divided on a clinical and chemical basis into the following four groups:

       *a.* *Group A* with severe early CNS deterioration.

       *b.* *Group B* with normal CNS function.

       *c.* *Group C* with moderate CNS involvement and a slow course.

       *d.* *Group D* with a late onset and eventual severe CNS involvement.

   The incidence of a cherry-red spot is lower than in Tay–Sachs disease.

3. **Sandhoff disease** (GM$_2$ gangliosidosis type 2) is almost identical to Tay–Sachs disease.

4. **Generalised gangliosidosis** (GM$_1$ gangliosidosis type 1) is characterised by hypoactivity, oedema of the face and extremities, and skeletal anomalies from birth.

5. **Sialidosis types 1 and 2** (cherry-red spot myoclonus syndrome) are characterised by myoclonic jerks, pain in the limbs and unsteadiness. A cherry-red spot may be the initial finding.

# VITREORETINOPATHIES

## Congenital Retinoschisis

Congenital retinoschisis is characterised by bilateral maculo-pathy, with associated peripheral retinoschisis in 50% of patients. The basic defect is in the Müller cells, causing splitting of the retinal nerve fibre layer from the rest of the sensory retina. This differs from acquired (senile) retinoschisis, in which splitting occurs at the outer plexiform layer.

### Diagnosis

1. **Inheritance** is XL with the implicated gene designated *RS1*.

2. **Presentation** is between the ages of 5 and 10 years with reading difficulties due to maculopathy. Less frequently the disease presents in infancy with squint or nystagmus associated with advanced peripheral retinoschisis, often with vitreous haemorrhage.

3. **Foveal schisis** is characterised by tiny cystoid spaces with a 'bicycle-wheel' pattern of radial striae (Fig. 5.76) more apparent when examined under red-free light. Over time, the radial folds become less evident, leaving a blunted foveal reflex (see Fig. 5.80a).

4. **Peripheral schisis** predominantly involves the inferotemporal quadrant. It does not extend but may undergo the following secondary changes:

   - The inner layer, which consists only of the internal limiting membrane and the retinal nerve fibre layer, may develop oval defects (Fig. 5.77).
   - In extreme cases, the defects coalesce, leaving only retinal blood vessels floating in the vitreous ('vitreous veils') (Fig. 5.78).
   - Other signs include perivascular sheathing, a golden glistening of the peripheral retina, nasal dragging of retinal vessels, retinal flecks, subretinal exudates and neovascularisation.

5. **Complications** include vitreous and intra-schisis haemorrhage, and retinal detachment.

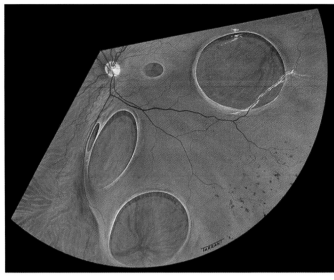

**Figure 5.77** Inner leaf defects in congenital retinoschisis

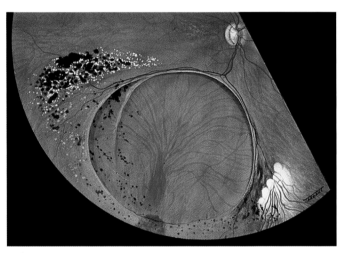

**Figure 5.78** Coalescent inner leaf defects in congenital retinoschisis

6. **Investigations**

   a. *ERG* is normal in eyes with isolated maculopathy. Eyes with peripheral schisis show a characteristic selective decrease in amplitude of the b-wave as compared with the a-wave on scotopic and photopic testing (Fig. 5.79).
   b. *EOG* is normal in eyes with isolated maculopathy but subnormal in eyes with advanced peripheral lesions.
   c. *CV* shows tritan defect.
   d. *FA* of maculopathy may show mild window defects but no leakage (Fig. 5.80b).
   e. *VF* in eyes with peripheral schisis show corresponding absolute defects.

**Prognosis** is poor due to progressive maculopathy. Visual acuity deteriorates during the first two decades and may then remain stable until the fifth or sixth decades, when it further deteriorates. Patients with peripheral schisis may have sudden visual loss at any time, due to haemorrhage or retinal detachment.

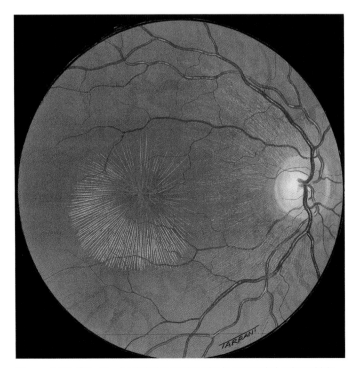

**Figure 5.76** 'Bicycle wheel-like' maculopathy in congenital retinoschisis

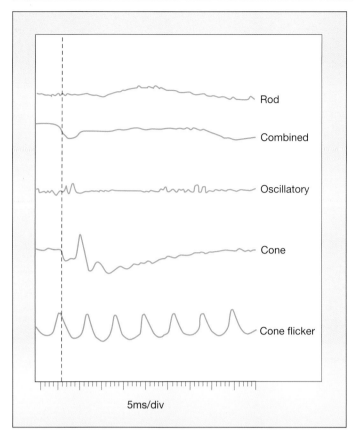

**Figure 5.79** ERG in congenital retinoschisis (see text)

5ms/div

Rod
Combined
Oscillatory
Cone
Cone flicker

## FURTHER READING

Arden GB, Gorin MB, Polkingholme PJ, et al. Detection of the carrier state of X-linked retinoschisis. *Am J Ophthalmol* 1988; 105:590–595.

George ND, Yates JR, Moore AT. X-linked retinoschisis. *Br J Ophthalmol* 1995;79:697–702.

George ND, Yates JR, Moore AT. Clinical features in affected males with X-linked retinoschisis. *Arch Ophthalmol* 1996;114:274–280.

# Stickler Syndrome

Stickler syndrome (hereditary arthro-ophthalmopathy) is a disorder of collagen connective tissue, resulting in abnormal vitreous, myopia, and a variable degree of orofacial abnormality, deafness and arthropathy. Inheritance is AD with complete penetrance but variable expressivity. Stickler syndrome is the commonest inherited cause of retinal detachment in children.

## *Classification*

1. **Type 1** results from mutations in the *COL2A1* gene and accounts for approximately 60% of cases. These subjects have the classic ocular and systemic features as originally described by Stickler.

2. **Type 2** is caused by mutations in the *COL11A1* gene. These subjects have congenital non-progressive high myopia, sensorineural deafness, and other features of Stickler syndrome type 1.

3. **Type 3** is caused by mutation in the *COL11A2* gene. These subjects have the typical systemic features, but no ocular manifestations.

## *Ocular features*

1. **Signs**

   - An optically empty central vitreous cavity due to liquefaction and syneresis (contraction) associated with circumferential, equatorial, membranes extending a short way into the vitreous cavity (Fig. 5.81).
   - Radial lattice-like degeneration associated with RPE hyperplasia, vascular sheathing and sclerosis (Fig. 5.82).

2. **Complications.** Retinal detachment, often bilateral, develops in approximately 30% in the first decade of life, often as a result of multiple or giant tears (Fig. 5.83).

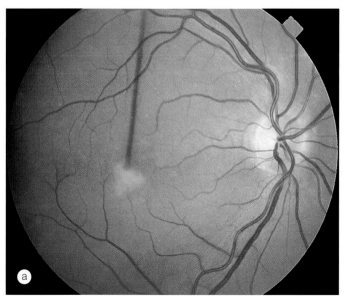
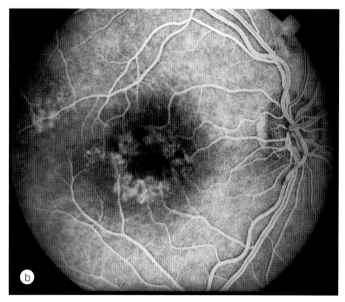

**Figure 5.80 (a)** Late-stage maculopathy in congenital retinoschisis; **(b)** FA shows window defects

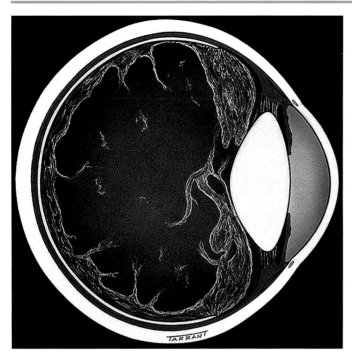

**Figure 5.81** Vitreous changes in Stickler syndrome

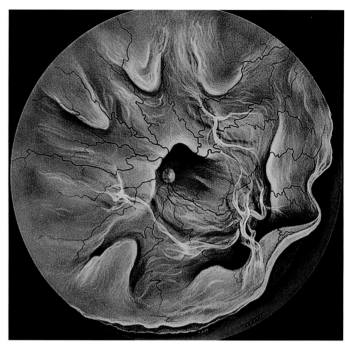

**Figure 5.83** Total retinal detachment due to a giant tear

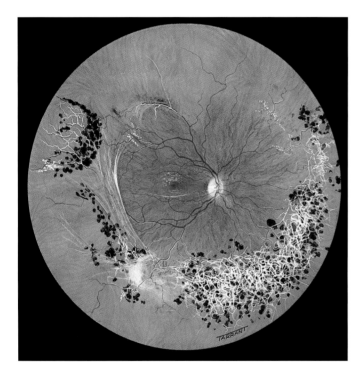

**Figure 5.82** Radial lattice degeneration and pigmentary changes in Stickler syndrome

### 3. Associations

a. *Early-onset, myopia,* often severe (Fig. 5.84) but rarely progressive, is present in about 80% of cases. The remainder of patients may be either emmetropic or hypermetropic.

b. *Presenile cataract* characterised by frequently non-progressive peripheral cortical 'wedge' or 'fleck' opacities is very common.

c. *Ectopia lentis* in about 10%.

d. *Glaucoma,* which may be associated with a congenital angle anomaly characterised by prominent iris processes and hypoplasia of the iris root with anterior stromal iris defects, is uncommon.

### Systemic features

1. **Facial** anomalies include a fat nasal bridge and maxillary hypoplasia.

2. **Skeletal** involvement includes a marfanoid habitus, arachnodactyly, arthropathy and joint hyperextensibility.

3. **Robin sequence** is characterised by micrognathia, small tongue, cleft soft palate and high-arched palate.

4. **Deafness.**

5. **Mitral valve prolapse.**

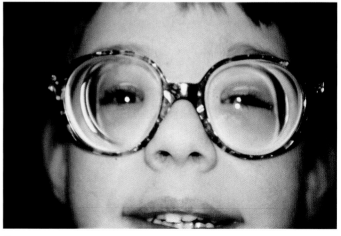

**Figure 5.84** High myopia in Stickler syndrome (Courtesy of K. Nischal)

## FURTHER READING

Donoso LA, Edwards AO, Frost AT, et al. Identification of a stop codon mutation in exon 2 of the collagen 2A1 in a large Stickler syndrome family. *Am J Ophthalmol* 2002;134:720–727.

Parke DW II. Stickler syndrome: clinical care and molecular genetics [Editorial]. *Am J Ophthalmol* 2002;134:746–748.

Snead MP. Hereditary vitreopathy. *Eye* 1996;10:653–663.

Vu CD, Brown J Jr, Korkko J, et al. Posterior chorioretinal atrophy and vitreous phenotype in a family with Stickler syndrome from mutation in the COL2A1 gene. *Ophthalmology* 2003;110:70–77.

# Wagner Syndrome

1. **Inheritance** is AD with the gene locus on 5q13–14.

2. **Signs**

   - Low myopia (–3.00 or less).
   - Vitreous liquefaction with complete absence of normal scaffolding.
   - Preretinal, equatorial, avascular greyish-white membranes.
   - Progressive chorioretinal atrophy.

3. **Complications**

   *a.* *Cortical cataracts* develop during the fourth decade.

   *b.* *Retinal detachment* occurs in about 50% of patients older than 45 years of age.

## FURTHER READING

Brown DM, Graemiger RA, Hergersberg M, et al, Genetic linkage of Wagner disease and erosive vitreoretinopathy to chromosome 5q13-14. *Arch Ophthalmol* 1995;113:671–675.

Graemiger RA, Niemyer G, Schneeberger SA, et al. Wagner vitreo-retinal degeneration. Follow-up of the original pedigree. *Ophthalmology* 1995;102:1830–1839.

# Marshall Syndrome

1. **Inheritance** is AD.

2. **Ocular signs**

   - Myopia ranging from mild to very severe.
   - Fluid vitreous.
   - Occasionally, ectopia lentis.

3. **Systemic signs**

   - Lack of sweating is very common.
   - Micrognathia.
   - Absence of the nasal bone, producing a short nose with a very flat nasal bridge (Fig. 5.85).
   - Anteverted nares and a long philtrum.

# Favre–Goldmann Syndrome

Favre–Goldmann syndrome manifests features of retinoschisis and pigmentary retinopathy.

1. **Inheritance** is AR.

2. **Presentation** is in childhood with nyctalopia.

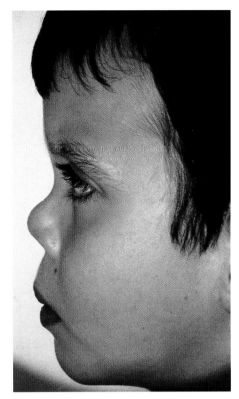

**Figure 5.85** Short nose and flat nasal bridge in Marshall syndrome

3. **Signs**

   - Vitreous syneresis but the cavity is not optically 'empty'.
   - Retinal lesions are similar to congenital retinoschisis.
   - The macula is diffusely thickened.
   - Atypical peripheral pigmentary dystrophy and white, arborescent retinal vessels (Fig. 5.86).
   - Arteriolar attenuation and waxy disc pallor.

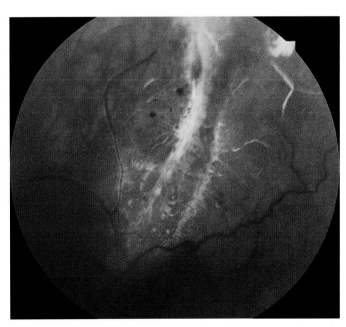

**Figure 5.86** Peripheral vascular lesions in Favre–Goldmann syndrome

4. **ERG** is subnormal and some patients demonstrate relatively enhanced S-cone function identical to that found in the enhanced S-cone syndrome.

5. **Prognosis** is poor.

# Familial Exudative Vitreoretinopathy

Familial exudative vitreoretinopathy (Criswick–Schepens syndrome) is a slowly progressive condition characterised by an avascular temporal retinal periphery, similar to that seen in retinopathy of prematurity but not associated with low birth weight and prematurity.

1. **Inheritance** is AD and rarely XL recessive with high penetrance and variable expressivity.

2. **Presentation** is in late childhood.

3. **Signs,** in chronological order

   - Vitreous degeneration (Fig. 5.87) and peripheral vitreoretinal attachments associated with areas of 'white without pressure'.
   - Peripheral vascular tortuosity and telangiectasis (Fig. 5.88).
   - Fibrovascular proliferation and vitreoretinal traction resulting in ridge formation (Fig. 5.89), vascular straightening, localised retinal detachment and temporal dragging of the macula and disc (Fig. 5.90).

4. **Complications** include tractional retinal detachment, massive subretinal exudation, band keratopathy, cataract and glaucoma.

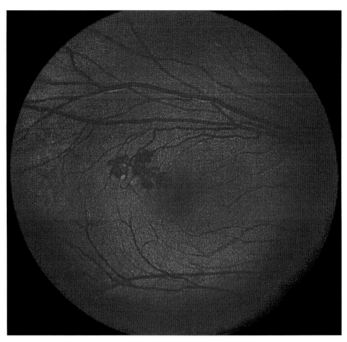

**Figure 5.88** Peripheral telangiectasis in familial exudative vitreoretinopathy

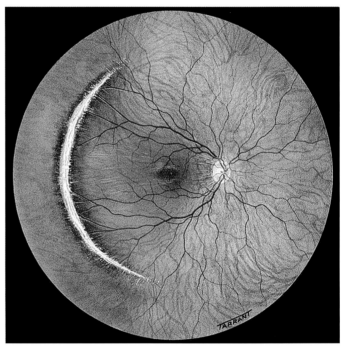

**Figure 5.89** Fibrovascular ridge in familial exudative vitreoretinopathy

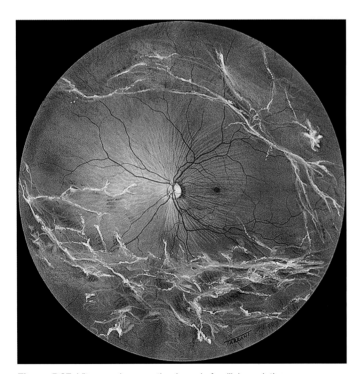

**Figure 5.87** Vitreous degeneration in early familial exudative vitreoretinopathy

5. **Investigations**

   a. *ERG* is normal.
   b. *FA* shows peripheral retinal non-perfusion and highlights straightening of blood vessels (Fig. 5.91).

6. **Prognosis** is poor although in some cases peripheral retinal laser photocoagulation or cryotherapy may be beneficial. Vitreoretinal surgery for retinal detachment, whilst difficult, may be successful in selected cases.

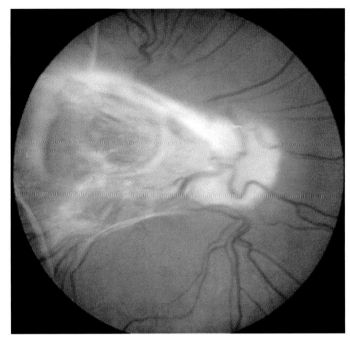

**Figure 5.90** 'Dragging' of the disc and macula in familial exudative vitreoretinopathy

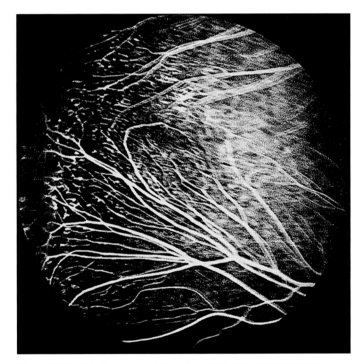

**Figure 5.91** FA in familial exudative vitreoretinopathy shows abrupt termination of peripheral retinal vessels

## Erosive Vitreoretinopathy

1. **Inheritance** is AD with the gene locus on 5q13–14.

2. **Presentation** is in early childhood.

3. **Signs**

- Vitreous syneresis and multiple foci of vitreoretinal traction.
- Thinning of the RPE and progressive choroidal atrophy which may eventually involve the macula.
- Attenuation of retinal vessels and occasionally bone-spicule pigmentary changes.

4. **Complications** – retinal detachment in 70%, often bilateral and associated with giant tears.

5. **ERG** is subnormal.

6. **Prognosis** is guarded because retinal detachment may be difficult to treat.

### FURTHER READING
Brown DM, Kimura AE, Weingeist TA, et al. Erosive vitreo-retino-pathy. A new clinical entity. *Ophthalmology* 1994;101: 694–704.

## Dominant Neovascular Inflammatory Vitreoretinopathy

1. **Inheritance** is AD.

2. **Presentation** is in the second to third decades with vitreous floaters.

3. **Signs**

- Uveitis.
- Pigmentary retinal degeneration.
- Peripheral vascular closure and neovascularisation.

4. **Complications** include vitreous haemorrhage, tractional retinal detachment and cystoid macular oedema.

5. **ERG** shows selective loss of b-wave amplitude.

6. **Prognosis** is guarded. Peripheral retinal photocoagulation and vitreous surgery may be required to preserve vision.

## Dominant Vitreoretinochoroidopathy

1. **Inheritance** is AD.

2. **Presentation** is in adult life if symptomatic, but frequently the condition is discovered by chance.

3. **Signs**

- An encircling band of pigmentary disturbance between the ora serrata and equator, with a sharply defined posterior border.
- Within the band there is arteriolar attenuation, neovascularisation, punctate white opacities and, later, chorioretinal atrophy.

4. **Complications,** which are uncommon, include cystoid macular oedema and, occasionally, vitreous haemorrhage.

5. **ERG** is subnormal.

6. **Prognosis** is good.

## Snowflake Degeneration

1. **Inheritance** is AD.

2. **Signs,** in chronological order (Fig. 5.92):

   - Stage 1 – extensive areas of 'white-without-pressure' in patients under the age of 15 years.
   - Stage 2 – snowflake-like, yellow-white spots in areas of 'white-with-pressure' in patients aged between 15 and 25 years.
   - Stage 3 – vascular sheathing and pigmentation posterior to the area of snowflake degeneration in patients aged between 25 and 50 years.
   - Stage 4 – increased pigmentation, gross vascular attenuation, areas of chorioretinal atrophy and less apparent snowflakes in patients over the age of 60 years. The macula and disc remain normal.

3. **Associations** include myopia, vitreous fibrillary degeneration and liquefaction.

4. **Complications** include retinal break formation, retinal detachment and presenile cataract.

5. **ERG** shows low scotopic b-wave amplitude.

6. **Prognosis** is usually good.

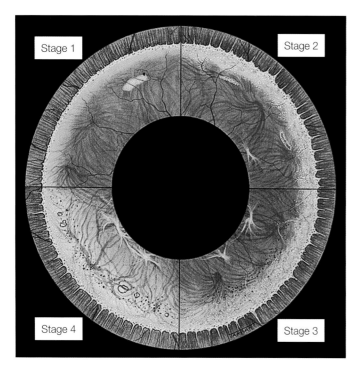

**Figure 5.92** Snowflake degeneration

# CHOROIDAL DYSTROPHIES

## Choroideremia

Choroideremia is a progressive, diffuse degeneration of the choroid, RPE and retinal photoreceptors.

**Inheritance** is XL recessive with the gene locus on Xq21. This has the following implications:

- All daughters of affected fathers will be carriers.
- Half of the sons of female carriers will develop the disease.
- Half of the daughters of female carriers will also be carriers.
- An affected male cannot transmit the gene to his sons.

> **NB:** Female carriers show mild, usually innocuous, patchy peripheral atrophy and mottling of the RPE (Figure 5.93). However, visual acuity, peripheral fields and ERG are normal.

### Diagnosis

1. **Presentation** is in the first decade with nyctalopia.

2. **Signs,** in chronological order

   - Mid-peripheral pigmentary stippling and patches of choroidal and RPE atrophy (Fig. 5.94).
   - Diffuse atrophy of the choriocapillaris and RPE with preservation of the intermediate and large choroidal vessels (Fig. 5.95).
   - Atrophy of intermediate and large choroidal vessels, rendering visible the underlying sclera. Numerous elongated crystals may be seen along the unaffected RPE.
   - Only remnants of choroidal vasculature apparent at the macula, far peripheral retina and near the optic discs (Fig. 5.96).
   - In contrast to primary retinal dystrophies, the fovea is spared until late (Fig. 5.97a) and the optic disc and retinal blood vessels remain relatively normal.

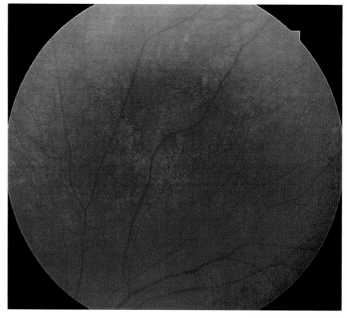

**Figure 5.93** Peripheral changes in a carrier of choroideremia

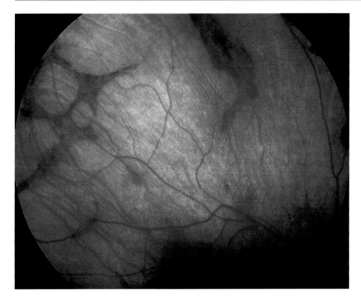

**Figure 5.94** Mid-peripheral changes in choroideremia (Courtesy of K. Jordan)

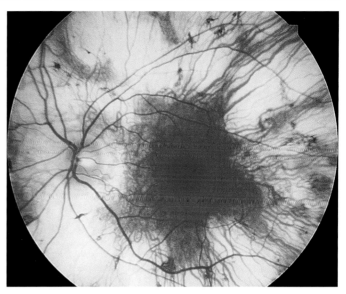

**Figure 5.96** Very advanced choroideremia (Courtesy of K. Nischal)

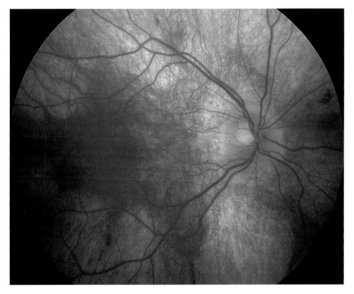

**Figure 5.95** Diffuse changes in choroideremia (Courtesy of K. Jordan)

### 3. Investigations

a. *ERG*. Scotopic is non-recordable; photopic is severely subnormal.

b. *EOG* is subnormal.

c. *FA* of the intermediate stage of choroideremia shows filling of the retinal and large choroidal vessels but not of the choriocapillaris. There is also hypofluorescence corresponding to the intact fovea and a surrounding area of hyperfluorescence due to a window defect (Fig. 5.97b).

d. *VF* shows restriction with progression from annular scotomas to concentric defects and eventual involvement of fixation.

**Prognosis** is very poor. Although most patients retain useful vision until the sixth decade, very severe visual loss occurs thereafter.

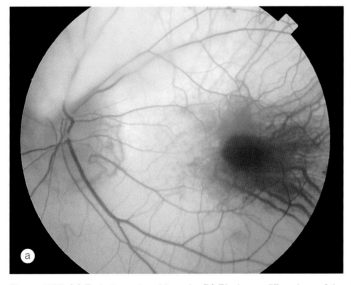

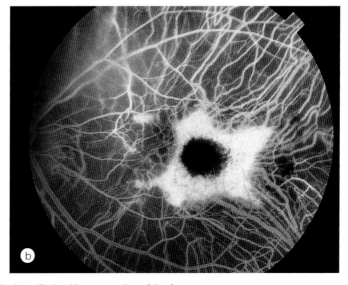

**Figure 5.97 (a)** End-stage choroideremia; **(b)** FA shows diffuse loss of the choriocapillaris with preservation of the fovea

223

## FURTHER READING

Flynn Roberts M, Fishman GA, Roberts DK, et al. Retrospective, longitudinal, and cross sectional study of visual acuity impairment in choroideremia. *Br J Ophthalmol* 2002;86:658–662.

# Gyrate Atrophy

## *Diagnosis*

1. **Inheritance** is AR.

2. **Metabolic defect** – mutations of the gene encoding the main ornithine degradation enzyme, ornithine aminotransferase. Deficiency of the enzyme leads to elevated ornithine levels in the plasma, urine, CSF and aqueous humour.

3. **Presentation** is in the first decade with axial myopia and reduction of peripheral vision, often associated with nyctalopia.

4. **Signs,** in chronological order

   - Peripheral patches of chorioretinal atrophy (Fig. 5.98) and vitreous degeneration.
   - Increase in size and number of the lesions with coalescence forming a scalloped posterior border (Fig. 5.99).
   - Gradual peripheral and central spread, sparing the fovea (Fig. 5.100) until late.
   - Extreme attenuation of retinal blood vessels.

5. **Investigations**

   a. *ERG* is abnormal and later extinguished.
   b. *EOG* is subnormal in late disease.
   c. *FA* shows the sharp contrast between normal and atrophic areas (Fig. 5.101b).

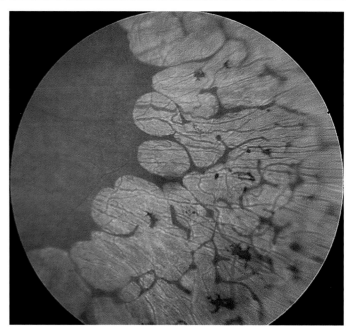

**Figure 5.99** Coalescence of lesions in gyrate atrophy

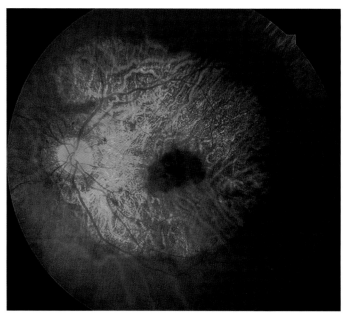

**Figure 5.100** Advanced gyrate atrophy with preservation of the fovea

***Treatment.*** There are two clinically different subtypes of gyrate atrophy based on response to pyridoxine (vitamin B6), which may normalise plasma and urinary ornithine levels. Patients responsive to vitamin B6 generally have a less severe and more slowly progressive clinical course than those who are not. Reduction in ornithine levels with an arginine-restricted diet is also beneficial.

***Prognosis*** is generally poor, with legal blindness occurring in the fourth to sixth decades from geographic atrophy, although vision may fail earlier due to cataract, cystoid macular oedema or epiretinal membrane formation.

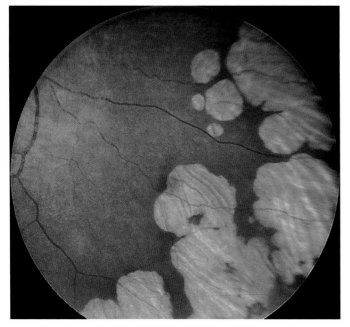

**Figure 5.98** Peripheral patches of gyrate atrophy

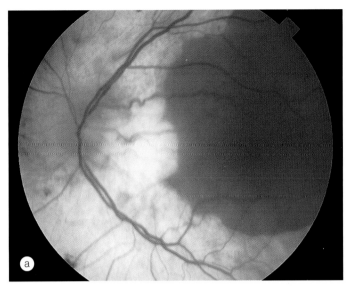

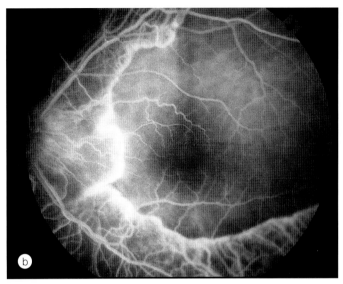

**Figure 5.101** **(a)** Gyrate atrophy; **(b)** FA shows a hyperfluorescent line demarcating normal from involved areas

## FURTHER READING
Kaiser-Kupfer MI, Caruso RC, Valle D. Gyrate atrophy of the retina and choroid. *Arch Ophthalmol* 1991;109:1539–1548.

Kaiser-Kupfer MI, Caruso RC, Valle D. Gyrate atrophy of the choroid and retina. Further experience with long-term reduction of ornithine levels in children. *Arch Ophthalmol* 2002;120: 146–153.

Vannas-Sulonen, Silipa K, Vannas I, et al. Gyrate atrophy of the retina and choroid. *Ophthalmology* 1985;92:1719–1727.

# Central Areolar Choroidal Dystrophy

## *Diagnosis*

1. **Inheritance** is AD with the implicated gene locus on 17p, although sporadic cases have been described.

2. **Presentation** is in the third to fourth decades with gradual impairment of central vision.

3. **Signs,** in chronological order

   - Non-specific foveal granularity.
   - Circumscribed RPE atrophy and loss of the choriocapillaris at the macula (Fig. 5.102).
   - Slowly expanding geographic atrophy within which the larger choroidal vessels are prominent (Fig. 5.103).

4. **Investigations**

   *a.* *ERG* is normal.
   *b.* *EOG* is normal.

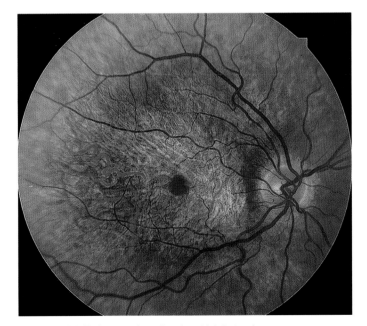

**Figure 5.102** Early central areolar choroidal dystrophy

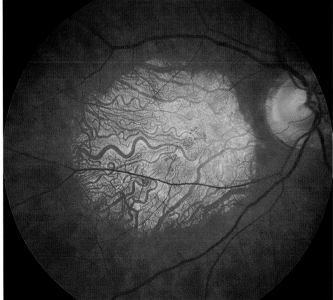

**Figure 5.103** Late central areolar choroidal dystrophy

**Prognosis** is poor, with severe visual loss occurring by the sixth to seventh decades.

## FURTHER READING

Hoyng CB, Heutink T, Testers L, et al. Autosomal dominant central areolar choroidal dystrophy caused by a mutation in codon 142 in the peripherin/RDS gene. *Am J Ophthalmol* 1996;121:623–629.

## Diffuse Choroidal Atrophy

### Diagnosis

1. **Inheritance** is AD.

2. **Presentation** is in the fourth to fifth decades with impairment of central vision or nyctalopia.

3. **Signs,** in chronological order:

   - Peripapillary and pericentral atrophy of the RPE and choriocapillaris.
   - Gradual enlargement until the entire fundus is affected (Fig. 5.104).
   - Atrophy of most of the larger choroidal vessels with scleral exposure (Fig. 5.105).
   - The retinal vessels may be normal or slightly constricted.

4. **ERG** is subnormal.

**Prognosis** is poor because of early macular involvement.

## Helicoid Peripapillary Chorioretinal Dystrophy

### Diagnosis

1. **Inheritance** is AD.

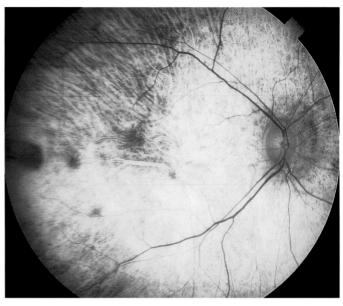

**Figure 5.105** End-stage diffuse choroidal atrophy

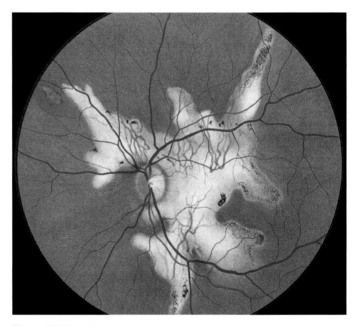

**Figure 5.106** Helicoid chorioretinal degeneration

2. **Presentation** is in childhood.

3. **Signs**

   - Slowly-enlarging, well-defined strips of chorioretinal atrophy radiating from the optic nerve head (Fig. 5.106).
   - Separate, peripheral, circular lesions may be present.

4. **ERG** ranges from normal to severely abnormal.

**Prognosis** is variable as severe disease may be seen in the young and mild disease in the elderly.

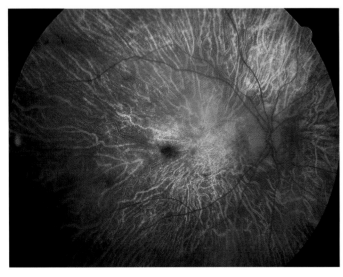

**Figure 5.104** Diffuse choroidal atrophy

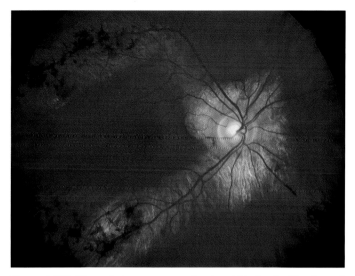

**Figure 5.107** Pigmented paravenous retinochoroidal atrophy (Courtesy of C. Barry)

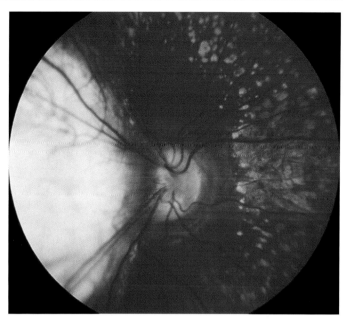

**Figure 5.108** Progressive bifocal chorioretinal atrophy (Courtesy of Moorfields Eye Hospital)

# Pigmented Paravenous Retinochoroidal Atrophy

## *Diagnosis*

1. **Inheritance** is uncertain although AD, AR, XL and even Y-linked transmissions have been proposed.

2. **Presentation** is often by chance because the condition is usually asymptomatic.

3. **Signs**

   - Bilateral, paravenous zones of chorioretinal atrophy associated with bone-spicule pigmentation (Fig. 5.107).
   - Cystoid macular oedema is rare.

4. **ERG** is usually normal.

*Prognosis* is excellent.

## FURTHER READING

Noble KG, Carr RE. Pigmented paravenous chorioretinal atrophy. Am J Ophthalmol 1983;96:338–344.

# Progressive Bifocal Chorioretinal Atrophy

## *Diagnosis*

1. **Inheritance** is AD with the gene locus on 6q.

2. **Presentation** is at birth.

3. **Signs,** in chronological order

   - A focus of chorioretinal atrophy temporal to the disc which extends in all directions.
   - A similar lesion develops nasally.
   - The end result manifests two discrete areas of chorioretinal atrophy separated by a normal segment (Fig. 5.108).

*Prognosis* is poor because macular involvement is inevitable.

## FURTHER READING

Godley BF, Tiffin PA, Evans K, et al. Clinical features of progressive bifocal atrophy: a retinal dystrophy linked to chromosome 6q. *Ophthalmology* 1996;103:893–898.

# RETINAL DETACHMENT

## Introduction

### APPLIED ANATOMY

**The pars plana** starts 1 mm from the limbus and extends posteriorly for about 6mm. The first 2 mm consists of the pars plicata and the remaining 4 mm comprises the flattened pars plana. In order not to endanger the lens or retina, the ideal location for pars plana surgical incision is 3.5 mm from the limbus.

**The ora serrata** forms the junction between the retina and ciliary body (Fig. 6.1). Externally the ora corresponds to the spiral of Tillaux, a theoretical circumferential line con-necting the insertions of the rectus muscles, which are located 5.5 mm (medial rectus), 6.5 mm (inferior rectus), 6.9 mm (lateral rectus) and 7.7 mm (superior rectus) posterior to the limbus (Fig. 6.2). The ora serrata has teeth-like extensions of retina onto the pars plana (dentate processes) which are more marked nasally than temporally and can have extreme variations in contour. Oral bays are the scalloped edges of the pars plana epithelium in between the dentate processes (Fig. 6.3). Microcystoid degeneration is a normal finding involving the perioral retina, characterised by tiny vesicles with indistinct boundaries which make the retina appear thickened and less transparent (Fig. 6.4). At the ora, fusion of the sensory retina with the retinal pigment epithelium (RPE) and choroid limits forward extension of subretinal fluid (SRF). However, because there is no equivalent adhesion between the choroid and sclera, choroidal detach-ments invariably progress anteriorly to involve the ciliary body (ciliochoroidal detachment). The following develop-mental variations may occasionally have clinical significance:

1. **A meridional fold** is a small radial fold of thickened retinal tissue in line with a dentate process, usually located in the superonasal quadrant (Fig. 6.5a). A fold may

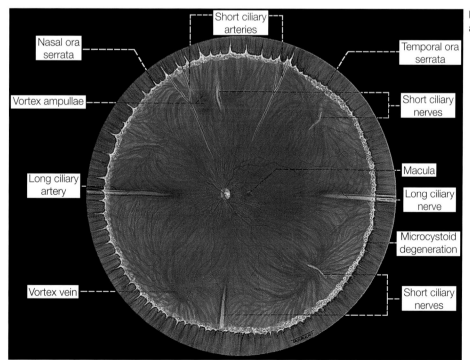

**Figure 6.1** The ora serrata and normal anatomical landmarks

Short ciliary arteries

Nasal ora serrata

Temporal ora serrata

Vortex ampullae

Short ciliary nerves

Macula

Long ciliary artery

Long ciliary nerve

Microcystoid degeneration

Vortex vein

Short ciliary nerves

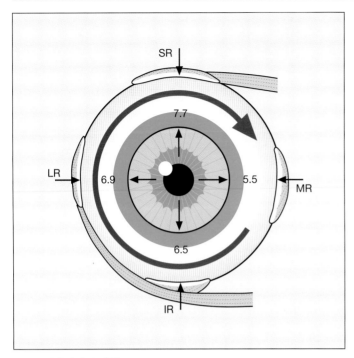

**Figure 6.2** Spiral of Tillaux

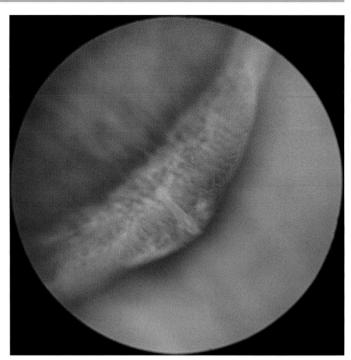

**Figure 6.4** Peripheral microcystoid degeneration (Courtesy of N.E. Byer, from *The Peripheral Retina in Profile, a Stereoscopic Atlas*, Criterion Press, Torrance, California, 1982)

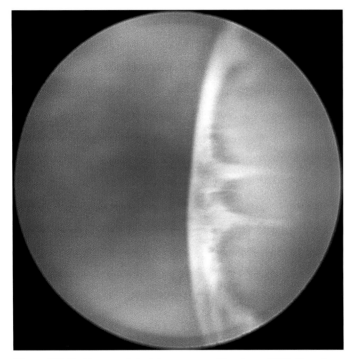

**Figure 6.3** Oral bays and dentate processes (Courtesy of N.E. Byer, from *The Peripheral Retina in Profile, a Stereoscopic Atlas*, Criterion Press, Torrance, California, 1982)

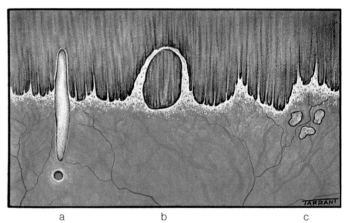

**Figure 6.5** Normal variants of the ora serrata. **(a)** Meridional fold with a small hole at its base; **(b)** enclosed oral bay; **(c)** granular tissue

occasionally exhibit a small retinal hole at its apex. A meridional complex is a configuration in which a dentate process, usually with a meridional fold, is aligned with a ciliary process.

2. **An enclosed oral bay** is a small island of pars plana surrounded by retina as a result of meeting of two adjacent dentate processes (Fig. 6.5b). It should not be mistaken for a retinal hole because it is located anterior to the ora serrata.

3. **Granular tissue** characterised by multiple, white opacities within the vitreous base can sometimes be mistaken for small peripheral opercula (Fig. 6.5c).

4. **Oral pearls** are glistening white lesions usually located on a dentate process which occur in approximately 20% of adult eyes (Fig. 6.6). Histologically, they are similar to drusen and have no clinical significance.

5. **Pars plana cysts** are located between the non-pigmented and pigmented epithelium of the pars plana, and are most frequently sited temporally (Fig. 6.7). Rarely, they may have a turbid appearance in patients with dysproteinaemias (e.g. multiple myeloma), due to the accumulation of abnormal proteins within the cysts.

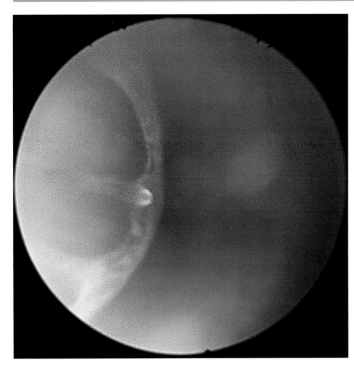

Figure 6.6 Oral pearl (Courtesy of N.E. Byer, from *The Peripheral Retina in Profile, a Stereoscopic Atlas*, Criterion Press, Torrance, California, 1982)

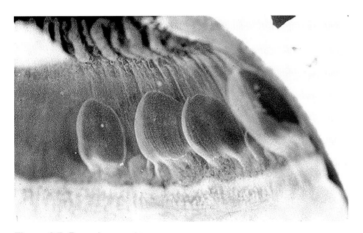

Figure 6.7 Pars plana cysts

**The vitreous base** is a 3–4 mm wide zone straddling the ora serrata (Fig. 6.8). An incision through the mid-part of the pars plana will usually be located anterior to the vitreous base. The cortical vitreous is strongly adherent at the vitreous base, so that following acute posterior vitreous detachment (PVD) the posterior hyaloid face remains attached to the posterior border of the vitreous base. If a blunt-ended instrument is introduced into the eye through the vitreous base, it may exert traction and give rise to a peripheral retinal tear. Pre-existing retinal holes within the vitreous base do not lead to retinal detachment (RD). Severe blunt trauma may cause an avulsion of the vitreous base with tearing of the non-pigmented epithelium of the pars plana along its anterior border and of the retina along its posterior border. Posterior tongue-like extensions and isolated islands of dense cortical vitreous associated with abnormally strong vitreoretinal adhesions may become sites of retinal tears in eyes with acute

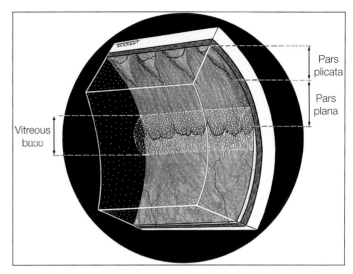

Figure 6.8 Anatomy of the vitreous base

PVD. Vitreous base excavations are ovoid depressions with sharp margins involving the inner one-third of the retina.

### Vitreous adhesions

1. **Normal.** The peripheral cortical vitreous is loosely attached to the internal limiting membrane (ILM) of the sensory retina. Stronger adhesions occur at the following sites:

   ● Vitreous base, where they are very strong (see above).
   ● Around the optic nerve head, where they are fairly strong.
   ● Around the fovea, where they are fairly weak.
   ● Along peripheral blood vessels, where they are usually weak.

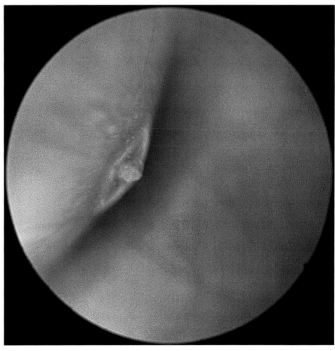

Figure 6.9 Cystic retinal tuft (Courtesy of N.E. Byer, from *The Peripheral Retina in Profile, a Stereoscopic Atlas*, Criterion Press, Torrance, California, 1982)

2. **Abnormal** adhesions, at the following sites, may be associated with retinal tear formation as a result of dynamic vitreoretinal traction associated with acute PVD.

- Posterior border of islands of lattice degeneration.
- Congenital cystic retinal tufts are white, ovoid, small, discrete, sharply circumscribed inward projections of post-oral sensory retina associated with vitreous condensations (Fig. 6.9). The base of a tuft may show pigmentary changes. It has been estimated that 10% of RDs are caused by retinal tears in areas of cystic retinal tufts.
- Congenital zonular traction tufts consist of thickened zonules displaced posteriorly towards the anterior retina, resulting in an anterior projection of the retina which may rarely be associated with retinal break formation.
- Retinal pigment clumps.
- Peripheral paravascular condensations.
- Vitreous base anomalies such as tongue-like extensions and posterior islands.
- 'White-without-pressure' (see below).

## DEFINITIONS

*Retinal detachment* is the separation of the neuroretina (NR) from the RPE, caused by a breakdown of the forces that attach the NR to the RPE. This results in the accumulation of SRF in the potential space between the NR and RPE. The main types of RD are:

1. **Rhegmatogenous** (*rhegma* – break) occurs secondarily to a full-thickness defect in the NR, which permits fluid derived from liquefied vitreous to gain access to the subretinal space.

2. **Tractional,** in which the NR is pulled away from the RPE by contracting vitreoretinal membranes in the absence of a retinal break.

3. **Exudative** (serous, secondary) is caused by neither a break nor traction; the SRF is derived from fluid in the vessels of the NR, or the choroid, or both.

4. **Combined tractional–rhegmatogenous,** as the name implies, is the result of a combination of a retinal break and retinal traction. The retinal break, which is mostly located near a fibrous or fibrovascular proliferation, is usually secondary to traction, which is the major component of the RD in these cases.

*Vitreoretinal traction* is a force exerted on the retina by structures originating in the vitreous and may be dynamic or static.

1. **Dynamic** traction is induced by eye movements and exerts a centripetal force towards the vitreous cavity. It plays an important role in the pathogenesis of retinal tears and rhegmatogenous RD.

2. **Static** traction is independent of ocular movements. It plays an important role in the pathogenesis of tractional RD and proliferative vitreoretinopathy.

> **NB:** The difference between the two is crucial in understanding the pathogenesis of the various types of RD.

*Posterior vitreous detachment* is a separation of the cortical vitreous from the ILM posterior to the vitreous base. PVD can be classified according to the following characteristics:

1. **Onset**

   a. *Acute* PVD is by far the most common. It develops suddenly and may become complete soon after onset.

   b. *Chronic* PVD develops gradually and may take weeks or months to become complete.

2. **Extent**

   a. *Complete* PVD, in which the entire vitreous cortex detaches up to the posterior margin of the vitreous base.

   b. *Incomplete* PVD, in which residual vitreoretinal attachments remain posterior to the vitreous base.

> **NB:** Rhegmatogenous RD is usually associated with acute PVD; tractional RD is associated with chronic, incomplete PVD; and exudative RD is unrelated to the presence of PVD.

*Retinal breaks* are full-thickness defects in the NR which can be classified according to (a) *pathogenesis*, (b) *morphology* and (c) *location*.

1. **Pathogenesis**

   a. *Tears* are caused by dynamic vitreoretinal traction. They have a predilection for the upper fundus (temporal more than nasal).

   b. *Holes* are caused by chronic atrophy of the NR and may be round or oval. They have a predilec-tion for the temporal fundus (upper more than lower) and are less likely to progress to RD than are tears.

2. **Morphology**

   a. *U-tears,* also described as horseshoe, flap or arrowhead, consist of a flap, the apex of which is pulled anteriorly by the vitreous, the base remaining attached to the retina (Fig. 6.10a). The actual tear consists of two anterior extensions (horns) running forward from the apex.

   b. *Incomplete U-tears,* which may be linear (Fig. 6.10b), L-shaped (Fig. 6.10c) or J-shaped, are often paravascular.

   c. *Operculated tears,* in which the flap is completely torn away from the retina by detached vitreous gel (Fig. 6.10d).

   d. *Dialyses* are circumferential tears along the ora serrata with the vitreous gel attached to their posterior margins (Fig. 6.10e).

   e. *Giant tears* involve 90° or more of the circumference of the globe (Fig. 6.11). They are a variant of U-shaped tears with the vitreous gel attached to the anterior margin of the break. Giant tears are most frequently located in the immediate post-oral retina or, less commonly, at the equator.

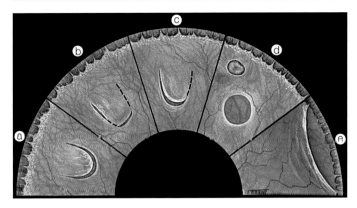

**Figure 6.10** Retinal tears. **(a)** Complete U-tear; **(b)** linear tears; **(c)** L-shaped tear; **(d)** operculated tear; **(e)** dialysis

### 3. Location

  a. *Oral* breaks are located within the vitreous base.
  b. *Post-oral* breaks are located between the posterior border of the vitreous base and the equator.
  c. *Equatorial* breaks are near the equator.
  d. *Post-equatorial* breaks are behind the equator.
  e. *Macular* breaks (invariably holes) are at the fovea.

## HOW TO FIND THE PRIMARY RETINAL BREAK

The primary break is defined as the one responsible for the RD. A secondary break is not responsible for the RD because it is either present before the development of RD or forms after RD has occurred. Finding the primary break is of paramount importance and aided by the following considerations.

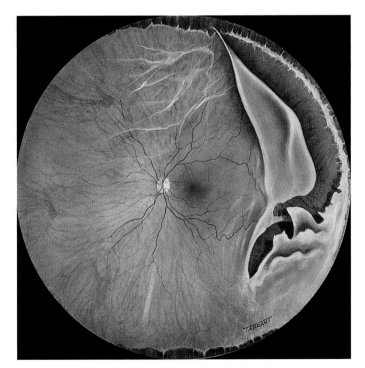

**Figure 6.11** Giant retinal tear

***Quadrantic distribution*** of breaks in eyes with RD is approximately as follows:

● 60% in the upper temporal quadrant.
● 15% in the upper nasal quadrant.
● 15% in the lower temporal quadrant.
● 10% in the lower nasal quadrant.

> **NB:** The upper temporal quadrant is therefore by far the most common site for retinal break formation and should be examined in great detail if a retinal break cannot be detected initially. It should also be remembered that about 50% of eyes with RD have more than one break, and in most cases these are located within 90° of each other.

***Configuration of SRF*** is of relevance because SRF spreads in a gravitational fashion, and its shape is governed by anatomical limits (ora serrata and optic nerve) and the location of the primary retinal break. If the primary break is located superiorly, the SRF first spreads inferiorly on the same side as the break and then spreads superiorly on the opposite side of the fundus. The likely location of the primary retinal break can therefore be predicted by studying the shape of the RD.

● A shallow inferior RD in which the SRF is slightly higher on the temporal side points to a primary break located inferiorly on that side (Fig. 6.12a).
● A primary break located at 6 o'clock will cause an inferior RD with equal fluid levels (Fig. 6.12b).
● In a bullous inferior RD, the primary break usually lies above the horizontal meridian (Fig. 6.12c).
● If the primary break is located in the upper nasal quadrant, the SRF will revolve around the optic disc and then rise on the temporal side until it is level with the primary break (Fig. 6.12d).
● A subtotal RD with a superior wedge of attached retina points to a primary break located in the periphery nearest its highest border (Fig. 6.12e).
● When the SRF crosses the vertical midline above, the primary break is near to 12 o'clock, the lower edge of the RD corresponding to the side of the break (Fig. 6.12f).

> **NB:** The above points are important because they prevent treatment of a secondary break whilst overlooking the primary break. It is therefore essential to ensure that the shape of the RD corresponds to the location of the primary retinal break.

### History

Although the quadrantic location of light flashes is of no value in predicting the location of the primary break, the quadrant in which the visual field detect first appears may be of considerable value. For example, if the field defect started in the upper nasal quadrant, the primary break is probably located in the lower temporal quadrant.

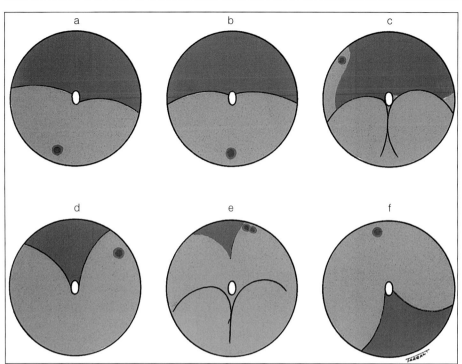

**Figure 6.12** Distribution of subretinal fluid in relation to the location of the primary retinal break (see text)

# Pathogenesis

## *Rhegmatogenous retinal detachment*

Rhegmatogenous RD affects about 1 in 10 000 of the population each year and both eyes may eventually be involved in about 10% of cases. It is characterised by the presence of a retinal break held open by vitreoretinal traction which allows accumulation of liquefied vitreous under the NR, separating it from the RPE. The retinal breaks responsible for RD are caused by interplay between dynamic vitreoretinal traction and an underlying weakness in the peripheral retina, referred to as predisposing degeneration.

> **NB:** Even if a retinal break is present, RD will not occur if the vitreous is not at least partially liquefied and if the necessary traction is not present.

### DYNAMIC VITREORETINAL TRACTION

Synchysis is a liquefaction of the vitreous gel caused by alterations of its micromolecular structure (Fig. 6.13a). Some eyes with synchysis develop a hole in the posterior hyaloid membrane and fluid from within the centre of the vitreous cavity passes through this defect into the newly formed retrohyaloid space. This process forcibly detaches the posterior vitreous surface from the ILM of the NR as far as the posterior border of the vitreous base. The remaining solid vitreous gel collapses inferiorly and the retrohyaloid space is occupied entirely by synchytic fluid. This process is called acute rhegmatogenous PVD with collapse and will be referred to as acute PVD henceforth.

### COMPLICATIONS OF ACUTE PVD

Following PVD, the NR is no longer protected by the stable vitreous cortex, and can be directly affected by dynamic vitreoretinal tractional forces. The vision-threatening complications of acute PVD are dependent on the strength and extent of pre-existing vitreoretinal adhesions.

1. **No complications** occur in most eyes because vitreoretinal attachments are weak, so that the vitreous cortex detaches completely without sequelae (Fig. 6.13b).

2. **Retinal tears** develop in 10–15% of eyes as a result of transmission of traction at sites of abnormally strong vitreoretinal adhesions, as previously described (Fig. 6.13c). Although tears usually develop at the time of PVD, very occasionally they may be delayed by several weeks or even months. Tears associated with acute PVD are usually symptomatic, U-shaped, located in the upper fundus and frequently associated with vitreous haemorrhage resulting from rupture of a peripheral retinal blood vessel (Fig. 6.14). After the tear has formed, the retrohyaloid fluid has direct access to the subretinal space.

3. **Avulsion of a peripheral blood vessel** resulting in vitreous haemorrhage in the absence of retinal tear formation is rare (see Fig. 6.13d).

### PREDISPOSING PERIPHERAL RETINAL DEGENERATIONS

About 60% of all breaks develop in areas of the peripheral retina that shows specific changes. These lesions may be associated with a spontaneous breakdown of pathologically thin retinal tissue to cause a retinal hole, or they may predispose to retinal tear formation in eyes with acute PVD. Retinal holes are round or oval in shape. They are usually smaller than tears and carry a lower risk of RD.

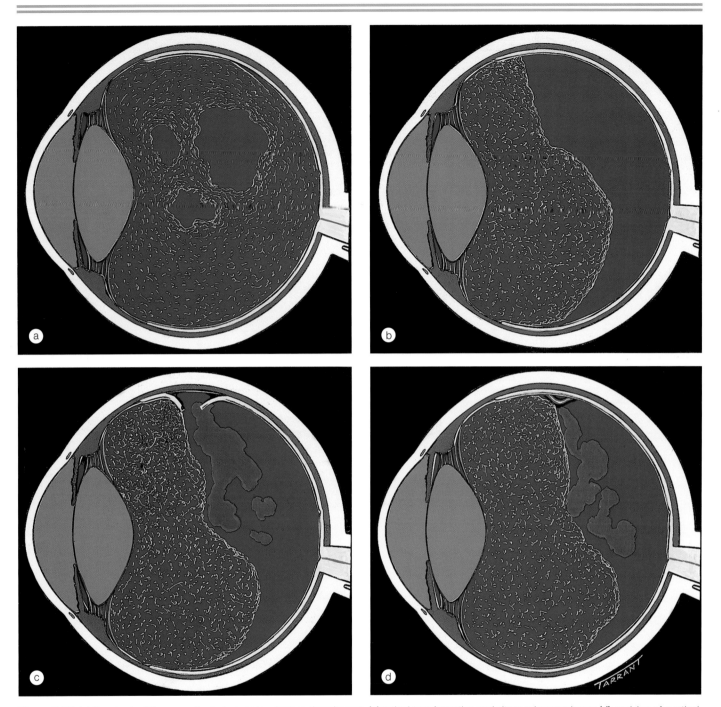

**Figure 6.13** **(a)** Synchysis; **(b)** uncomplicated posterior vitreous detachment; **(c)** retinal tear formation and vitreous haemorrhage; **(d)** avulsion of a retinal blood vessel and vitreous haemorrhage

### *Lattice degeneration*

1. **Prevalence.** Lattice degeneration is present in about 8% of the general population. It probably develops early in life, with a peak incidence during the second and third decades. It is therefore not related to very advanced age. Although lattice may be familial, it shows no sexual predilection. It is found more commonly in moderate myopes and is the most important degeneration directly related to RD. Lattice is present in about 40% of eyes with RD and is an important cause of RD in young myopes.

2. **Pathology.** Lattice degeneration is characterised by discontinuity of the ILM with variable atrophy of the underlying NR. The vitreous overlying an area of lattice is synchytic but the vitreous attachments around the margin of the lesion are exaggerated (Fig. 6.15).

3. **Clinical features**

   a. *Typical lattice*

      ● Sharply demarcated, spindle-shaped areas of retinal thinning, most frequently located between the equa-

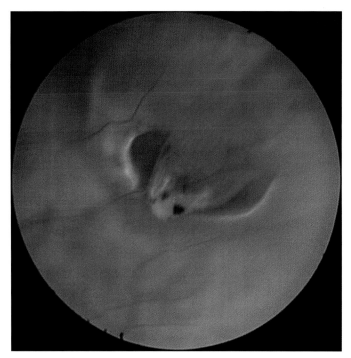

**Figure 6.14** Superior U-shaped tear associated with acute posterior vitreous detachment (Courtesy of N.E. Byer, from *The Peripheral Retina in Profile, a Stereoscopic Atlas*, Criterion Press, Torrance, California, 1982)

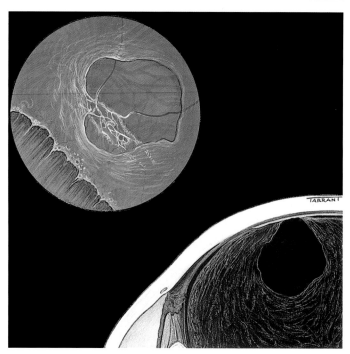

**Figure 6.15** Vitreous changes associated with lattice degeneration

tor and the posterior border of the vitreous base (Fig. 6.16).

- The condition is usually bilateral and more frequently located in the temporal than the nasal half of the fundus, and superiorly rather than inferiorly.
- The islands of lattice may form two, three or even four circumferentially orientated rows.
- A characteristic feature is an arborising network of white lines within the islands, which may be associated with hyperplasia of the RPE (Fig. 6.17).
- Some lattice lesions may be associated with 'snowflakes' (remnants of degenerate Müller cells) (Fig. 6.18) and 'white-with-pressure' (see below).
- Small holes within the lattice lesions are common and usually innocuous (Figs. 6.19 and 6.20d).

b. *Atypical lattice* is characterised by radially orientated lesions continuous with peripheral blood vessels, which may extend posterior to the equator (Figs. 6.20a and 6.21). It is frequently seen in patients with Stickler syndrome and occasionally in those with Marfan syndrome and Ehlers–Danlos syndrome, all of which are associated with an increased risk of RD.

## 4. Complications

a. *No complications* are encountered in most patients, even in the presence of small holes which are frequently found within islands of lattice.
b. *RD associated with tractional tears* may occur in eyes with acute PVD. The tears typically develop along the posterior edge of an island of lattice as a result of dynamic traction at the site of an exaggerated vitreoretinal attach-

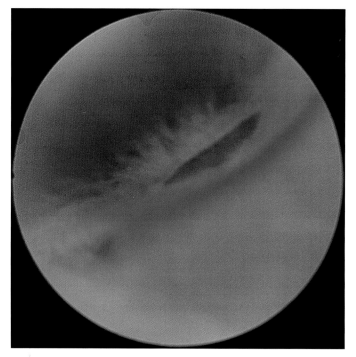

**Figure 6.16** Lattice degeneration forming a shallow crater (Courtesy of N.E. Byer, from *The Peripheral Retina in Profile, a Stereoscopic Atlas*, Criterion Press, Torrance, California, 1982)

ment (see Fig. 6.20c). Occasionally, a small island of lattice is present on the flap of a retinal tear (see Fig. 6.20b). Tears typically occur in myopes over the age of 50 years; the SRF progresses more rapidly than in RDs caused by small round holes. Tears associated with atypical radial lattice are usually longer and more posterior, and hence may be more difficult to close (Fig. 6.22).

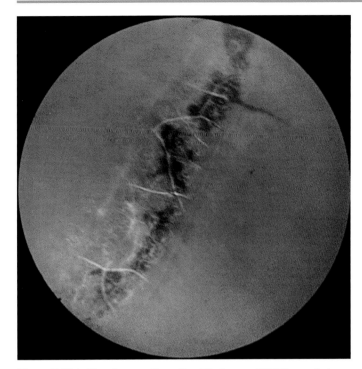

**Figure 6.17** Lattice degeneration with white lines and RPE hyperplasia

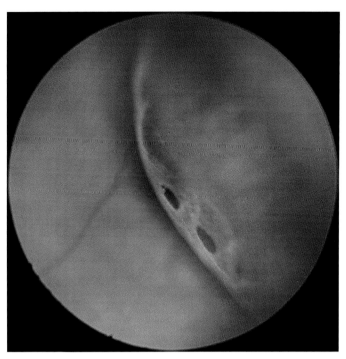

**Figure 6.19** Holes within lattice degeneration (Courtesy of N.E. Byer MD, from *The Peripheral Retina in Profile, a Stereoscopic Atlas*, Criterion Press, Torrance, California, 1982)

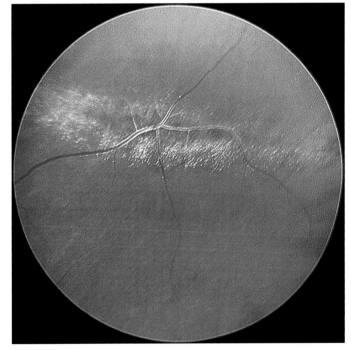

**Figure 6.18** Lattice degeneration with snowflakes (Courtesy of N.E. Byer, from *The Peripheral Retina in Profile, a Stereoscopic Atlas*, Criterion Press, Torrance, California, 1982)

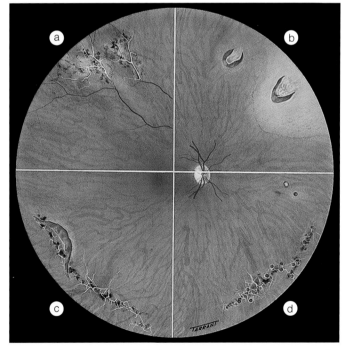

**Figure 6.20 (a)** Atypical radial lattice degeneration; **(b)** lattice degeneration on the flap of a U-tear; **(c)** tractional tear along the posterior margin of lattice degeneration; **(d)** small round holes in lattice degeneration

c. *RD associated with atrophic holes* may occasionally occur, particularly in young myopes. In these patients, the RD may not be preceded by symptoms of acute PVD (photopsia and floaters) and the SRF usually spreads slowly.

**Snailtrack degeneration** is characterised by sharply demarcated bands of tightly packed 'snowflakes' which give the peripheral retina a white frost-like appearance (Fig. 6.23). They are usually longer than islands of lattice and may be associated with overlying vitreous liquefaction. However,

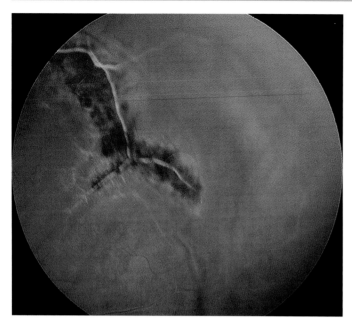

**Figure 6.21** Atypical radial lattice degeneration in Stickler syndrome

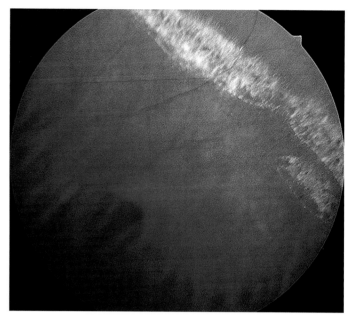

**Figure 6.23** Islands of snailtrack degeneration

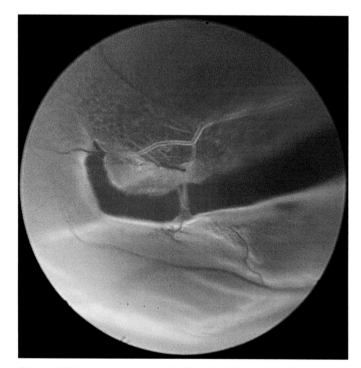

**Figure 6.22** Large tear associated with lattice degeneration (Courtesy of N.E. Byer, from *The Peripheral Retina in Profile, a Stereoscopic Atlas*, Criterion Press, Torrance, California, 1982)

marked vitreous traction at the posterior border of the lesions is seldom present, so that tractional U-tears rarely occur. Round holes within the snailtracks occasionally result in RD.

### Degenerative retinoschisis

1. **Prevalence.** Degenerative retinoschisis is present in about 5% of the population over the age of 20 years and is particularly prevalent in hypermetropes (70% of patients are hypermetropic). Frequently, both eyes are involved.

2. **Pathology.** There is coalescence of cystic lesions as a result of degeneration of neuroretinal and glial supporting elements within areas of peripheral cystoid degeneration. This eventually results in separation or splitting of the NR into an inner (vitreous) layer and an outer (choroidal) layer with severing of neurons and complete loss of visual function in the affected area.

   a. *In typical* retinoschisis, the split is in the outer plexiform layer.
   b. *In reticular* retinoschisis, which is less common, splitting occurs at the level of the nerve fibre layer.

3. **Clinical features**

   ● Early retinoschisis usually involves the extreme inferotemporal periphery of both fundi, appearing as an exaggeration of microcystoid degeneration with a smooth elevation of the retina (Fig. 6.24). The lesion may progress circumferentially until it has involved the entire fundus periphery.
   ● The typical form usually remains anterior to the equator although the reticular type may spread beyond the equator (Fig. 6.25).
   ● The surface of the inner layer may show 'snowflakes' as well as sheathing or 'silver-wiring' of blood vessels, and the schisis cavity may be bridged by rows of torn grey-white tissue (Fig. 6.26).
   ● The outer layer has a 'beaten-metal' appearance (Fig. 6.27) and shows the phenomenon of 'white-with-pressure' (see below).

**NB: Unlike RD, retinoschisis is relatively immobile.**

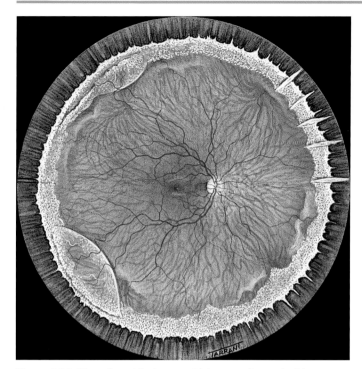

**Figure 6.24** Circumferential microcystoid degeneration and mild degenerative retinoschisis in the inferotemporal and superotemporal quadrants

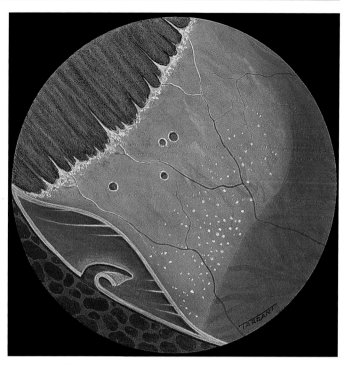

**Figure 6.26** Degenerative retinoschisis with holes in both layers; snowflakes and 'silver-wiring' of blood vessels on the inner layer; the cavity is bridged by torn grey-white tissue

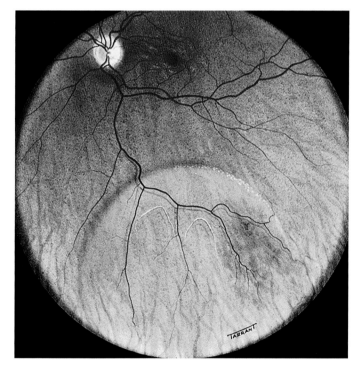

**Figure 6.25** Reticular degenerative retinoschisis with inner layer breaks extending beyond the equator

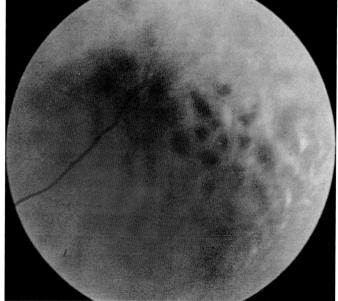

**Figure 6.27** 'Beaten-metal' appearance on the outer layer of degenerative retinoschisis

### 4. Complications

a. *No complications* occur in most cases and the condition is asymptomatic and innocuous.

b. *Breaks* may develop in the reticular type. Inner layer breaks are small and round, whilst the less common outer layer breaks are usually larger, with rolled edges and located behind the equator (Fig. 6.28). Eyes with only inner layer breaks do not develop RD as there is no communication with the subretinal space.

c. *RD* may occasionally develop in eyes with breaks in both layers (Fig. 6.29a), especially in the presence of PVD. Eyes with only outer layer breaks do not as a rule develop RD because the fluid within the schisis cavity is viscous and does not pass readily into the subretinal

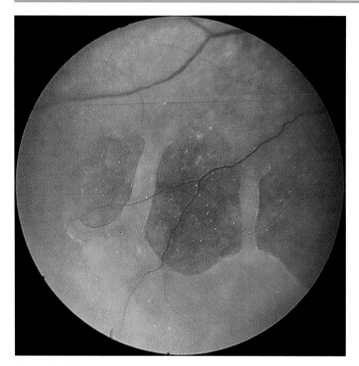

**Figure 6.28** Degenerative retinoschisis with snowflakes and outer layer breaks (Courtesy of N.E. Byer, from *The Peripheral Retina in Profile, a Stereoscopic Atlas*, Criterion Press, Torrance, California, 1982)

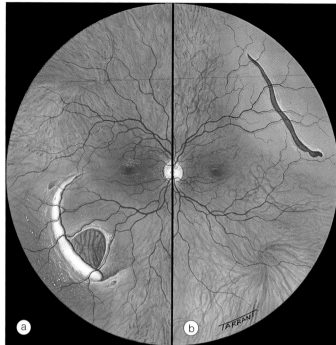

**Figure 6.29** Degenerative retinoschisis. **(a)** Large breaks in both layers; **(b)** linear break in the outer layer associated with a localised retinal detachment

space. However, occasionally the schisis fluid loses its viscosity and passes through the break into the sub-retinal space, giving rise to a localised detachment of the outer retinal layer which is usually confined to the area of retinoschisis (Fig. 6.29b). The detachment is almost always asymptomatic, infrequently progressive and rarely requires treatment.

d.  *Vitreous haemorrhage* is uncommon.

### 'White-with-pressure' and 'white-without-pressure'

a.  *'White-with-pressure'* is a translucent grey appearance of the retina, induced by indenting the sclera (Fig. 6.30). Each area has a fixed configuration which does not change when the scleral indenter is moved to an adjacent area. It is frequently seen in normal eyes and may be observed along the posterior border of islands of lattice degeneration, snailtrack degeneration and outer layer of acquired retinoschisis

b.  *'White-without-pressure'* has the same appearance but is present without scleral indentation. On cursory examination, a normal area of retina surrounded by white-without-pressure may be mistaken for a flat retinal hole, and the appearance can be quite dramatic in heavily pigmented fundi (Fig. 6.31a). Giant tears occasionally develop along the posterior border of white-without-pressure (Fig. 6.31b). For this reason, if white-*without*-pressure is found in the fellow eye of a patient with a spontaneous giant retinal tear, prophylactic therapy may be considered.

### Diffuse chorioretinal atrophy is characterised by choroidal depigmentation and thinning of the overlying retina in the

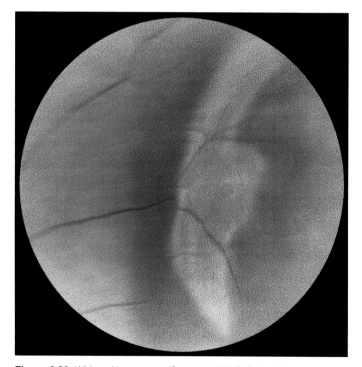

**Figure 6.30** White-with-pressure (Courtesy of N.E. Byer, from *The Peripheral Retina in Profile, a Stereoscopic Atlas*, Criterion Press, Torrance, California, 1982)

equatorial area of highly myopic eyes. Retinal holes developing in the atrophic retina may lead to RD. Because of lack of contrast between the depigmented choroid and NR, small holes may be very difficult to visualise without the help of slit-lamp biomicroscopy.

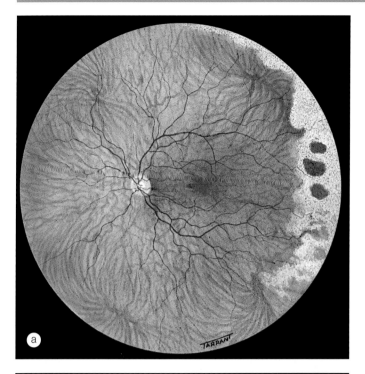

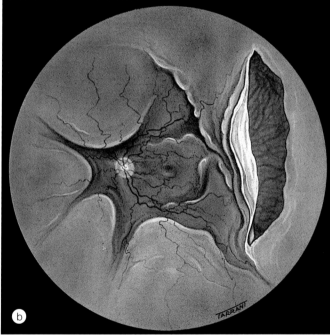

**Figure 6.31 (a)** White-without-pressure with pseudoholes; **(b)** total retinal detachment due to a giant tear

## SIGNIFICANCE OF MYOPIA

Although myopes make up 10% of the general population, over 40% of all RDs occur in myopic eyes; the higher the refractive error, the greater is the risk of RD. The following interrelated factors predispose a myopic eye to RD:

1. **Lattice degeneration** is more common in moderate myopes and may give rise to either tears or atrophic holes.

2. **Snailtrack degeneration** is common in myopic eyes and may be associated with atrophic holes.

3. **Diffuse chorioretinal atrophy** may give rise to small round holes in highly myopic eyes.

4. **Macular holes** may give rise to RD in highly myopic eyes, particularly those with a posterior staphyloma.

5. **Vitreous degeneration and PVD** are more common.

6. **Vitreous loss during cataract surgery,** particularly if inappropriately managed, is associated with an increased risk of subsequent RD, particularly in myopic eyes.

7. **Laser posterior capsulotomy** is associated with an increased risk of RD.

## SIGNIFICANCE OF TRAUMA

Trauma is responsible for about 10% of all cases of RD and is the most common cause in children, particularly boys. A great variety of breaks may develop in traumatised eyes, either at the time of impact or subsequently.

1. **Penetrating injuries** of the posterior segment carry a high risk of RD, particularly if there is vitreous incarceration at the site of penetration, which subsequently leads to vitreoretinal traction (Fig. 6.32).

2. **Severe blunt trauma** causes a compression of the antero-posterior diameter of the globe and a simultaneous expansion at the equatorial plane (Fig. 6.33). The relatively inelastic vitreous gel causes traction along the posterior aspect of the vitreous base, with tearing of the retina, to form a dialysis (Fig. 6.34). In some cases, the vitreous base becomes avulsed, giving rise to a 'bucket-handle' appearance, which comprises a strip of ciliary epithelium, ora serrata and the immediate post-oral retina into which basal vitreous gel remains inserted (Fig. 6.35). Traumatic dialyses occur most frequently in the superonasal (Fig. 6.36) and inferotemporal quadrants. Although they occur at the time of injury, they may not result in RD, as the vitreous gel is healthy in young individuals, although prophylactic treatment is recommended (Fig. 6.37). In cases that do detach, the RD may not develop until several months later, and progression is slow. Other less common post-

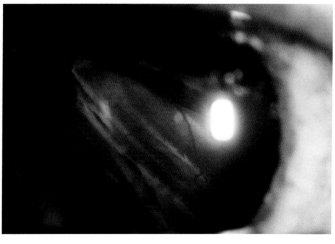

**Figure 6.32** Retrolental fibrous proliferation following penetrating trauma

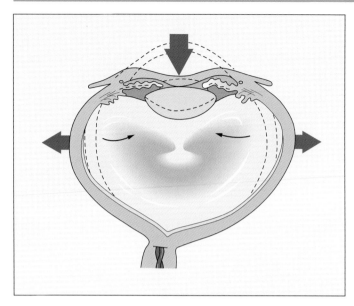

**Figure 6.33** Pathogenesis of ocular damage by blunt trauma

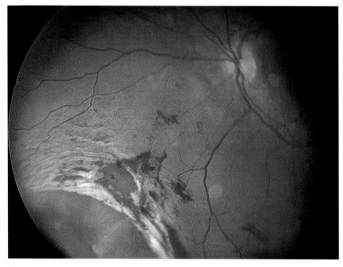

**Figure 6.34** Traumatic retinal dialysis and haemorrhage (Courtesy of Wilmer Institute)

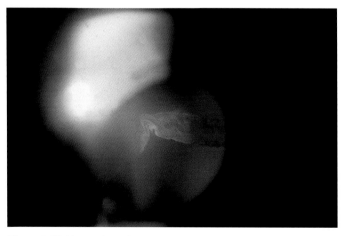

**Figure 6.35** Traumatic avulsion of the vitreous base (Courtesy of P. Rosen)

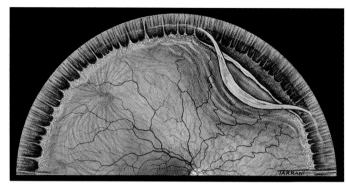

**Figure 6.36** Traumatic retinal dialysis with vitreous base avulsion and localised subretinal fluid

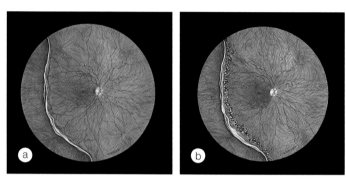

**Figure 6.37 (a)** Large traumatic retinal dialysis; **(b)** several weeks after prophylactic laser photocoagulation

contusive breaks are macular and equatorial holes. The latter often occur at the site of scleral impact (direct retinal injury). In extreme cases, there is complete disruption of the retina and the choroid, with subsequent overgrowth of fibrous tissue (chorioretinitis sclopetaria).

# Tractional retinal detachment

The main causes of tractional RD are (a) *proliferative diabetic retinopathy*, (b) *retinopathy of prematurity*, (c) *proliferative sickle cell retinopathy* and (d) *penetrating posterior segment trauma*.

## DIABETIC TRACTIONAL RETINAL DETACHMENT

***Pathogenesis of PVD.*** Tractional RD is a devastating complication of proliferative diabetic retinopathy. It is caused by progressive contraction of fibrovascular membranes over large areas of vitreoretinal adhesion. In contrast to acute PVD in eyes with rhegmatogenous RD, PVD in diabetic eyes is gradual and frequently incomplete. It is thought to be caused by leakage of plasma constituents into the vitreous gel from a fibrovascular network adherent to the posterior vitreous surface. Owing to the strong adhesions of the cortical vitreous to areas of fibrovascular proliferation, PVD is usually incomplete. In the very rare event of a complete PVD, the new blood vessels are avulsed and RD does not develop.

***Vitreoretinal traction.*** The following three main types of static vitreoretinal traction are recognised.

1. **Tangential** traction is caused by the contraction of epiretinal fibrovascular membranes with puckering of the retina and distortion of retinal blood vessels (Fig. 6.38).

2. **Anteroposterior** traction is caused by the contraction of fibrovascular membranes extending from the posterior retina, usually in association with the major arcades, to the vitreous base anteriorly (Fig. 6.39).

3. **Bridging** (trampoline) traction is the result of contraction of fibrovascular membranes which stretch from one part of the posterior retina to another or between the vascular arcades. This tends to pull the two involved points together and may be responsible for the formation of stress lines as well as displacement of the macula towards the disc or elsewhere depending on the direction of traction (Fig. 6.40). Occasionally, vitreoretinal traction causes tractional retinoschisis rather than RD. In some eyes, incomplete avulsion of a portion of fibrovascular membrane gives rise to a retinal tear (usually small and posterior to the equator). When this happens, the characteristic shape of a tractional RD assumes the configuration of a rhegmatogenous RD and is referred to as a combined tractional–rhegmatogenous RD.

## TRAUMATIC TRACTIONAL RETINAL DETACHMENT

Traumatic tractional RD is the result of vitreous incarceration in the wound and the presence of blood within the vitreous gel, which acts as a stimulus to fibroblastic proliferation along the planes of incarcerated vitreous. The contraction of such anterior epiretinal membranes leads to a shortening and a rolling effect on the peripheral retina in the region of the vitreous base and eventually to an anterior tractional RD (Fig. 6.41). A retinal break may develop several weeks later, leading to a sudden extension of SRF and

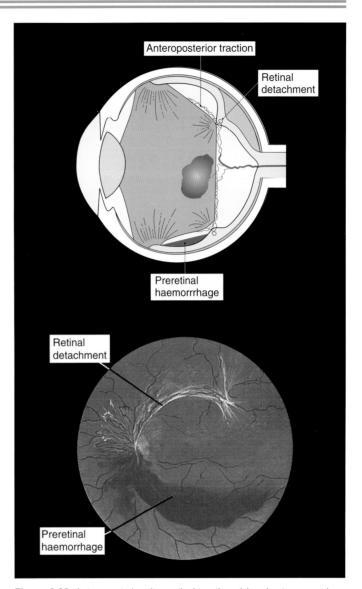

**Figure 6.39** Anteroposterior vitreoretinal traction giving rise to a superior retinal detachment

consequent visual loss. As a rule, therefore, in penetrating trauma the traction is mainly anterior, whereas in diabetes it is mainly posterior.

## *Exudative retinal detachment*

Exudative RD is characterised by the accumulation of SRF in the absence of retinal breaks or traction. It may occur in a variety of vascular, inflammatory or neoplastic diseases involving the NR, RPE and choroid in which fluid leaks outside the vessels and accumulates under the retina. As long as the RPE is able to pump the leaking fluid into the choroidal circulation, no fluid accumulates in the subretinal space and RD does not occur. However, when the normal RPE pump is overwhelmed, or if the RPE activity is decreased, then fluid starts to accumulate in the subretinal space.

### *Causes*

1. **Choroidal tumours** such as melanomas, haemangiomas and metastases.

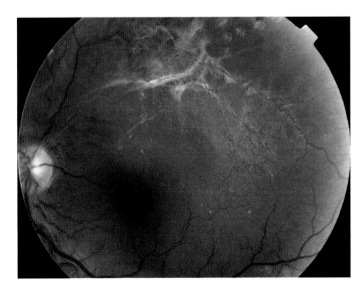

**Figure 6.38** Tangential vitreoretinal traction causing vascular distortion

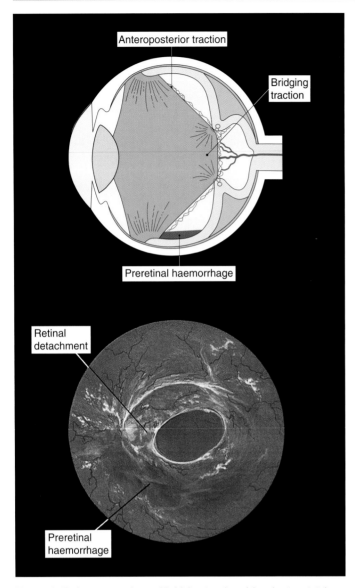

**Figure 6.40** Anteroposterior and bridging traction giving rise to a total retinal detachment

---

**NB: It is important always to consider that exudative RD is caused by an intraocular tumour until proved otherwise.**

---

2. **Inflammation** such as Harada disease and posterior scleritis.

3. **Bullous central serous retinopathy** is a rare cause.

4. **Iatrogenic** causes include retinal detachment surgery and panretinal photocoagulation.

5. **Subretinal neovascularisation,** which may leak and give rise to extensive subretinal accumulation of fluid at the posterior pole.

6. **Hypertensive choroidopathy,** which may occur in toxaemia of pregnancy, is a very rare cause.

7. **Idiopathic** such as the uveal effusion syndrome (see below).

***Treatment*** depends on the cause. Some resolve spontaneously (postoperative), whilst others are treated with systemic

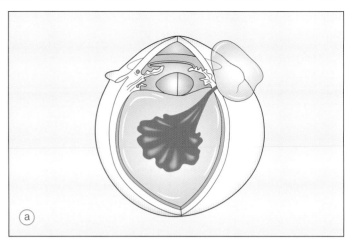

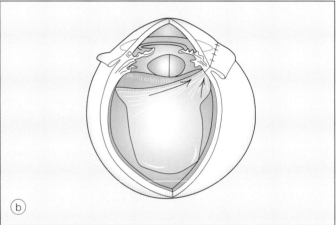

**Figure 6.41 (a)** Penetrating injury resulting in vitreous prolapse and intraocular haemorrhage; **(b)** subsequent proliferation and vitreoretinal traction resulting in retinal detachment (Courtesy of Wilmer Institute)

corticosteroids (Harada disease and posterior scleritis). In some eyes with central serous choroidopathy, the leak in the RPE can sometimes be sealed by argon laser photocoagulation.

# Clinical Features

## *Rhegmatogenous retinal detachment*

### SYMPTOMS

The classic premonitory symptoms reported in about 60% of patients with spontaneous rhegmatogenous RD are flashing lights and vitreous floaters caused by acute PVD with collapse. After a variable period of time, the patient notices a relative peripheral visual field defect, which may progress to involve central vision.

***Photopsia*** is a subjective sensation perceived as a flash of light. In eyes with acute PVD, it is probably caused by traction at sites of vitreoretinal adhesion. The cessation of photopsia is the result of either separation of the adhesion or complete tearing away of a piece of retina (operculum). In eyes with PVD, the photopsia may be induced by eye movements and is more noticeable in dim illumination. It tends to be projected into the patient's temporal peripheral visual field and has no lateralising value. Photopsia caused by vitreo-retinal traction should be differentiated from migraine.

*Floaters* are moving vitreous opacities which are perceived when they cast shadows on the retina. Vitreous opacities in eyes with acute PVD are of the following three types:

1. **Weiss ring** is a solitary floater consisting of the detached annular attachment of vitreous to the margin of the optic disc (see Fig. 1.9).

2. **Cobwebs** are caused by condensation of collagen fibres within the collapsed vitreous cortex.

3. **A sudden shower** of minute red-coloured or dark spots usually indicates vitreous haemorrhage secondary to tearing of a peripheral retinal blood vessel. Although vitreous haemorrhage associated with acute PVD is usually sparse, due to the small calibre of peripheral retinal vessels, occasionally a severe bleed may impair visualisation of the fundus.

*A visual field defect* is perceived as a 'black curtain'. In some patients it may not be present on waking in the morning, due to spontaneous absorption of SRF while lying inactive overnight, only to reappear later in the day. A lower field defect is usually appreciated more quickly by the patient than is an upper field defect. The quadrant of the visual field in which the field defect first appears is useful in predicting the location of the primary retinal break (which will be in the opposite quadrant). Loss of central vision may be due either to involvement of the fovea by SRF or, less frequently, to obstruction of the visual axis by a large upper bullous RD.

## GENERAL SIGNS

1. **Marcus Gunn pupil** (relative afferent pupillary defect) is present in eyes with extensive RDs irrespective of the type.

2. **The intraocular pressure** is usually lower by about 5 mmHg compared with the normal eye. If the intraocular pressure is extremely low, an associated choroidal detachment may be present. If a patient with known pre-existing primary open-angle glaucoma develops a sudden drop of intraocular pressure, the possibility of RD should be excluded. Conversely, if an eye with an extensive RD has normal intraocular pressure, the presence of primary open-angle glaucoma, which coexists with RD in about 5% of patients, should be suspected.

3. **A mild iritis** is very common. Occasionally it may be severe enough to cause posterior synechiae. In these cases, the underlying RD may be overlooked and the poor visual acuity incorrectly ascribed to some other cause.

4. **'Tobacco dust'** is seen in the anterior vitreous (Fig. 6.42 and see Fig. 1.10).

5. **Retinal breaks** appear as discontinuities in the retinal surface. They are usually red because of the colour contrast between the sensory retina and underlying choroid. However, in eyes with hypopigmented choroid (as in high myopia), the colour contrast is decreased and small breaks may be overlooked unless careful slit-lamp and indirect ophthalmoscopy examination is performed.

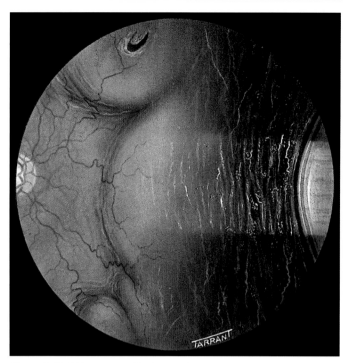

**Figure 6.42** 'Tobacco dust' in the anterior vitreous associated with an extensive retinal detachment caused by a superior U-tear

6. **Retinal signs** depend on the duration of RD and the presence or absence of proliferative vitreoretinopathy (PVR), as described next.

## FRESH RETINAL DETACHMENT

1. **The RD** has a convex configuration and a slightly opaque and corrugated appearance as a result of intraretinal oedema. There is loss of the underlying choroidal pattern and retinal blood vessels appear darker than in flat retina, so the colour contrast between venules and arterioles is less apparent (Fig. 6.43). The detached retina undulates freely with ocular movements (Fig. 6.44).

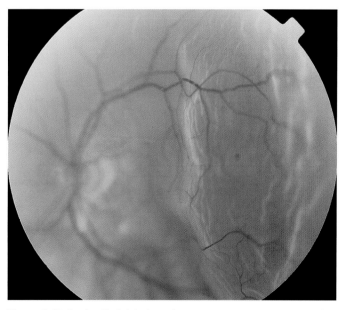

**Figure 6.43** Fresh retinal detachment

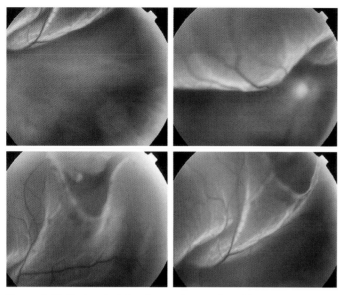

**Figure 6.44** Fresh retinal detachment due to a large U-tear with mobile subretinal fluid

2. **SRF** extends up to the ora serrata except in the rare cases caused by a macular hole in which the SRF is initially confined to the posterior pole.

> **NB:** Because of the thinness of the retina at the fovea, a pseudo-hole is frequently seen if the posterior pole is detached. This should not be mistaken for a true macular hole which may give rise to RD in highly myopic eyes or following blunt ocular trauma.

## LONGSTANDING RETINAL DETACHMENT

The following are the main features of a longstanding rhegmatogenous RD (Fig. 6.45).

1. **Retinal thinning** secondary to atrophy is a characteristic finding which must not be mistaken for retinoschisis.

2. **Secondary intraretinal cysts** may develop if the RD has been present for about 1 year (Fig. 6.46). They tend to disappear after retinal reattachment.

3. **Subretinal demarcation lines** (high water marks) caused by proliferation of RPE cells at the junction of flat and detached retina are common and take about 3 months to develop. They are initially pigmented (Fig. 6.47) and then tend to lose their pigment (Fig. 6.48). Demarcation lines are convex with respect to the ora serrata, and, although they represent sites of increased adhesion, they do not invariably limit spread of SRF.

## PROLIFERATIVE VITREORETINOPATHY

***Pathogenesis.*** PVR is characterised by proliferation of membranes on the inner retinal surface (epiretinal membranes), on the posterior surface of the detached hyaloid and occasionally also on the outer retinal surface (subretinal membranes). These membranes are thought to be caused by the proliferation and metaplasia of cells derived from the RPE

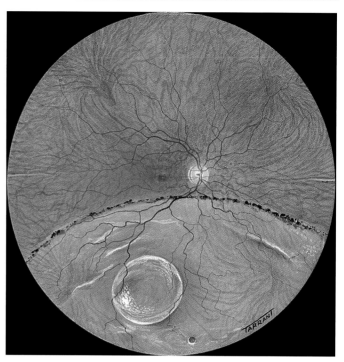

**Figure 6.45** Longstanding inferior retinal detachment associated with a secondary intraretinal cyst and a pigmented demarcation line

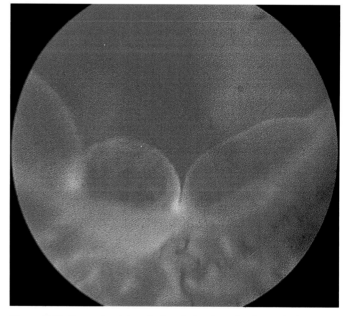

**Figure 6.46** Secondary intraretinal cysts in a longstanding retinal detachment

and retinal glia. The more advanced stages of PVR are usually seen following failed retinal detachment repair. The two commonest causes of surgical failure are severe PVR leading to the re-opening or creation of retinal breaks, and missed or inadequately closed retinal breaks leading to PVR.

***Signs.*** The main features are retinal folds and rigidity so that retinal mobility induced by eye movements or scleral indentation is decreased according to severity. Classification is as follows, although it should be emphasised that progression from one stage to the next is not inevitable.

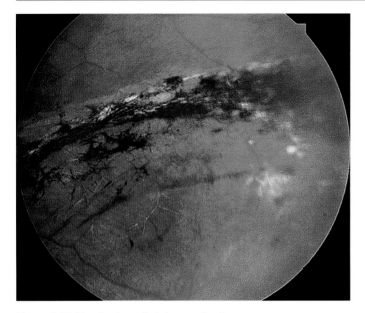

**Figure 6.47** Heavily pigmented demarcation line

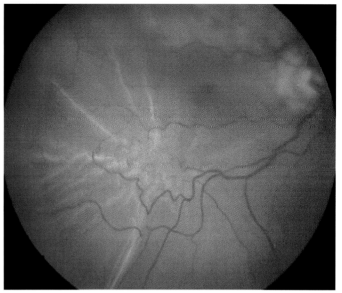

**Figure 6.49** Retinal wrinkling and vascular distortion in grade B PVR

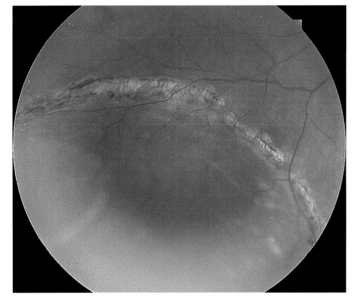

**Figure 6.48** Lightly pigmented demarcation line

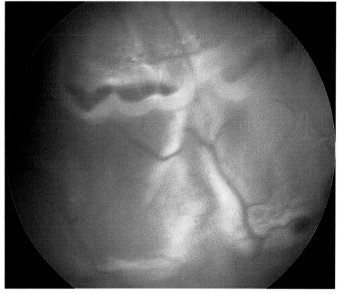

**Figure 6.50** Retinal tears with rolled edges in grade B PVR

1. **Grade A** (minimal) PVR is characterised by diffuse vitreous haze and 'tobacco dust'. There may also be pigmented cells on the inferior surface of the retina. Although these findings occur in many eyes with RD, they are particularly severe in eyes with early PVR.

2. **Grade B** (moderate) PVR is characterised by wrinkling of the inner retinal surface, tortuosity of blood vessels (Fig. 6.49), retinal stiffness, decreased mobility of vitreous gel, and rolled and irregular edges of retinal breaks (Fig. 6.50). The epiretinal membranes responsible for these findings cannot be identified by indirect ophthalmoscopy.

3. **Grade C** (marked) PVR is characterised by full-thickness rigid retinal folds with heavy vitreous condensation and

strands. It can be either anterior (A) or posterior (P), the approximate dividing line being the equator of the globe. The severity of proliferation in each area is expressed by the number of clock hours of retina involved (1–12) although proliferations need not be contiguous. The type of contraction is further described as:

- Focal (type 1) (Fig. 6.51).
- Diffuse (type 2) (Fig. 6.52).
- Subretinal (type 3) (Fig. 6.53).
- Circumferential (type 4).
- Anterior displacement (type 5).

4. **Grade C-P** is therefore subdivided into the following three types:

- Focal contraction with starfolds posterior to the vitreous base (type 1).
- Diffuse contraction with confluent starfolds (type 2).
- Subretinal proliferation (type 3).

5. **Grade C-A** is subdivided as follows:

- Subretinal proliferation (type 3).
- Circumferential contraction along posterior border of vitreous base (type 4).
- Vitreous base is pulled anteriorly by proliferative tissue (type 5).

## SUBSEQUENT COURSE OF UNTREATED RD

1. **Progression** occurs in most cases. The RD becomes total and eventually gives rise to secondary cataract, chronic

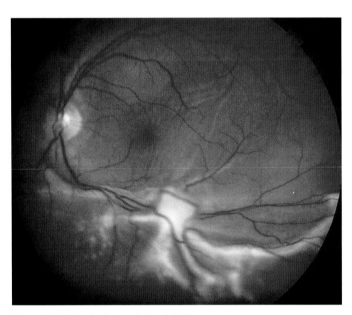

**Figure 6.51** Grade C type 1 (focal) PVR

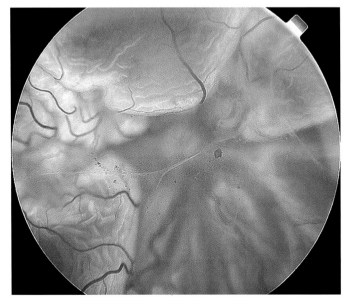

**Figure 6.52** Grade C type 2 (diffuse) PVR

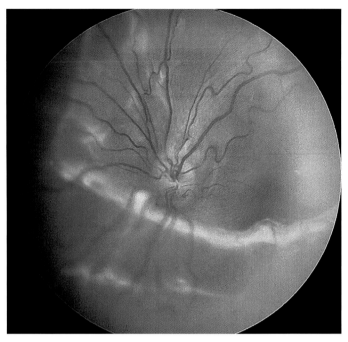

**Figure 6.53** Grade C type 3 (subretinal) PVR

uveitis, rubeosis iridis, hypotony and eventually phthisis bulbi.

2. **Non-progression** occurs in a minority of cases. The RD may remain stationary for many years, or indefinitely, in association with the formation of demarcation lines.

3. **Regression** is very rare but a small RD may reattach spontaneously, particularly if the patient is subjected to prolonged bed rest.

## Tractional retinal detachment

**Symptoms.** Photopsia and floaters are usually absent because vitreo-retinal traction develops insidiously and is not associated with acute PVD. The visual field defect usually progresses slowly and may become stationary for months or even years.

### Signs

1. **The RD** has a concave configuration and breaks are absent (Fig. 6.54). Retinal mobility is severely reduced and shifting fluid is absent.

2. **SRF** is less than in a rhegmatogenous RD and seldom extends to the ora serrata. The highest elevation of the retina occurs at sites of vitreoretinal traction.

3. **PVD** is present but incomplete.

NB: If a tractional RD develops a break, it assumes the characteristics of a rhegmatogenous RD and progresses more quickly (combined tractional–rhegmatogenous RD) (Figure 6.55).

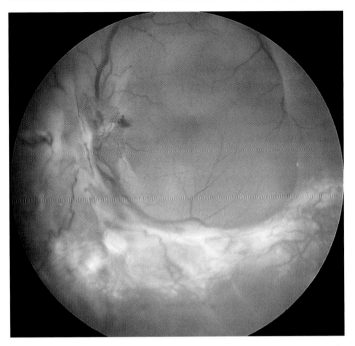

**Figure 6.54** Inferior tractional retinal detachment secondary to advanced proliferative diabetic retinopathy

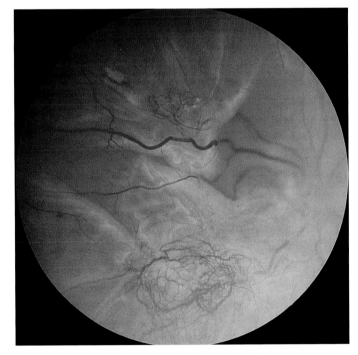

**Figure 6.55** Combined tractional–rhegmatogenous retinal detachment and retinal neovascularisation in advanced proliferative diabetic retinopathy

## Exudative retinal detachment

**Symptoms.** Photopsia is absent because there is no vitreo-retinal traction, although floaters may be present if there is associated vitritis. The visual field defect may develop suddenly and progress rapidly. Depending on the cause, both eyes may be involved simultaneously (e.g. Harada disease).

### Signs

1. **The RD** has a convex configuration, just like a rheg-matogenous RD, but its surface is smooth and not corrugated. It is very mobile and exhibits the phenomenon of *'shifting fluid'* in which SRF responds to the force of gravity and detaches the area of retina under which it accumulates. For example, in the upright position, the SRF collects under the inferior retina, but on assuming the supine position for several minutes, the inferior retina flattens and the SRF shifts posteriorly, detaching the macula and superior retina.

2. **SRF** may be so deep that the RD can be seen with the slit lamp without the aid of a lens, and it may even touch the back of the lens (Fig. 6.56). The cause of the RD, such as a choroidal tumour (Fig. 6.57), may be apparent when the fundus is examined, or the patient may have an associated systemic disease responsible for the RD (rheumatoid arthritis, Harada disease, toxaemia etc.).

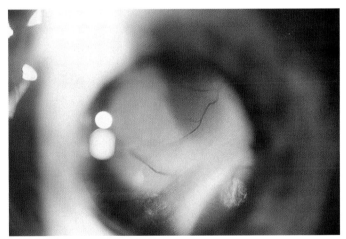

**Figure 6.56** Very deep exudative retinal detachment

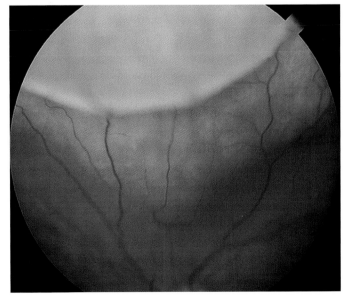

**Figure 6.57** Choroidal tumour associated with overlying exudative retinal detachment (Courtesy of J. Shields and A. Singh)

249

3. **'Leopard spots'** consisting of scattered areas of subretinal clumping may be seen after the detachment has flattened (Fig. 6.58).

## *Differential diagnosis*

### DEGENERATIVE RETINOSCHISIS

*Symptoms.* Photopsia and floaters are absent because there is no vitreoretinal traction. A visual field defect is seldom observed because spread posterior to the equator is rare. If present, it is absolute and not relative as in RD. Occasionally symptoms occur as a result of either vitreous haemorrhage or development of progressive RD.

### *Signs*

1. **Breaks** may be present in one or both layers in eyes with retinoschisis.

2. **The elevation** is convex, smooth, thin and relatively immobile (see Fig. 6.25) unlike the opaque and corrugated appearance of a rhegmatogenous RD. The thin inner leaf of the schisis cavity may be mistaken, on cursory examination, for an atrophic longstanding rhegmatogenous RD, but demarcation lines and secondary cysts in the inner leaf are absent.

### CHOROIDAL DETACHMENT

*Symptoms.* Photopsia and floaters are absent because there is no vitreoretinal traction. A visual field defect may be noticed if the choroidal detachment is extensive.

### *Signs*

1. **Low intraocular pressure** is common as a result of concomitant detachment of the ciliary body.

2. **The anterior chamber** may be shallow in eyes with extensive choroidal detachments.

3. **The elevations** are brown, convex, smooth and relatively immobile (Fig. 6.59). Temporal and nasal bullae tend to be most prominent. Large 'kissing' choroidal detachments may obscure the view of the fundus. Because the detachments are limited anteriorly only by the scleral spur, the peripheral retina and ora serrata can be seen with ease without scleral indentation (Fig. 6.60). The elevations do not extend to the posterior pole because they are limited by the firm adhesion between the suprachoroidal lamellae where the vortex veins enter their scleral canals.

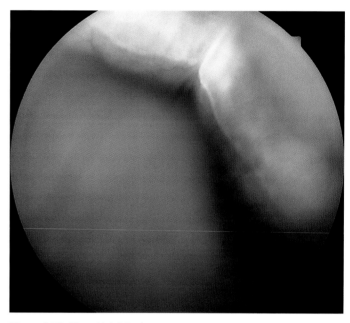

**Figure 6.59** Choroidal detachment

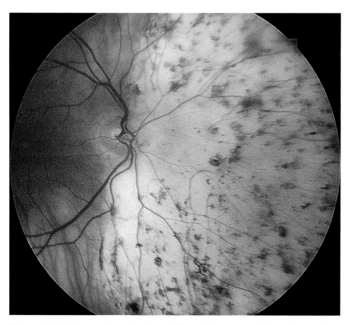

**Figure 6.58** 'Leopard spot' pigmentation following resolution of exudative retinal detachment

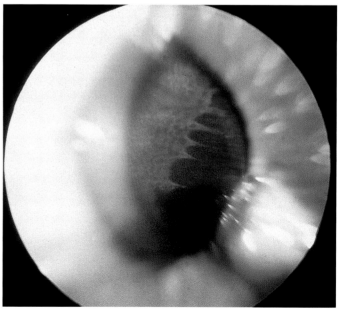

**Figure 6.60** Choroidal detachment with visibility of the pars plana (Courtesy of P. Morse)

## UVEAL EFFUSION SYNDROME

The uveal effusion syndrome is a rare, idiopathic condition which most frequently affects middle-aged hypermetropic men. It is characterised by ciliochoroidal detachment followed by exudative RD (Fig. 6.61) which may be bilateral. Following resolution 'leopard-spot' mottling may be seen. Uveal effusion may be mistaken for RD complicated by choroidal detachment or a ring melanoma of the anterior choroid.

# Prophylaxis of Rhegmatogenous Retinal Detachment

Although, given the right circumstances, most retinal breaks can cause RD, some are more dangerous than others. Important criteria to be considered in the selection of patients for prophylactic treatment can be divided into (a) *characteristics of the break* and (b) *other considerations*.

## CHARACTERISTICS OF BREAK

1. **Type:** a tear is more dangerous than a hole because it is associated with dynamic vitreoretinal traction.

2. **Size:** the larger the break, the more dangerous it is.

3. **Symptomatic** tears associated with acute PVD are more dangerous than those detected on routine examination.

4. **Location** is important for the following reasons:

   - Superior breaks are more dangerous than inferior breaks because, as a result of gravity, SRF is likely to spread more quickly. Superotemporal tears are particularly dangerous because the macula is threatened early in the event of RD.

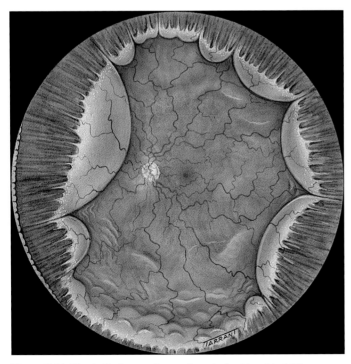

**Figure 6.61** Uveal effusion syndrome characterised by choroidal detachment and exudative retinal detachment

- Equatorial breaks are more dangerous than oral because the latter are usually located within the vitreous base.

5. **'Subclinical RD'** refers to a break surrounded by a small amount of SRF. Because the SRF is usually located anterior to the equator, it does not give rise to a peripheral visual field defect. It is debatable whether incidentally detected subclinical RDs require intervention as they do not invariably progress.

6. **Pigmentation** around a retinal break indicates that it has been present for a long time and the danger of progression to clinical RD is reduced, although chronicity is not a guarantee against future progression.

## OTHER CONSIDERATIONS

1. **Cataract surgery** is known to increase the risk of RD, particularly if associated with vitreous loss.

2. **Myopic** patients are more prone to RD. A retinal break in a myopic eye should be taken more seriously than an identical lesion in a non-myopic eye.

3. **Family history** may occasionally be relevant; any break or predisposing degeneration should be taken seriously if the patient gives a family history of RD.

4. **Systemic diseases** that are associated with an increased risk of RD include Marfan syndrome, Stickler syndrome and Ehlers–Danlos syndrome.

## CLINICAL EXAMPLES

The following clinical examples illustrate the various risk factors just discussed:

1. **Subclinical RD** associated with a large symptomatic U-tear and located in the upper temporal quadrant (Fig. 6.62a) should be treated without delay because the risk of progression to a clinical RD is very high. As the tear is located in the upper temporal quadrant, early macular involvement by SRF is possible. Treatment options include cryotherapy combined with an explant, and pneumatic retinopexy (see below).

> NB: Argon laser photocoagulation alone is less appropriate because the break is surrounded by SRF.

2. **A large U-tear** in the upper temporal quadrant in an eye with symptomatic acute PVD (Fig. 6.62b) should be treated without delay because the risk of progression to clinical RD is high. Although the tear is not associated with SRF yet, it is still dangerous because it is large. Fresh tears such as this, in patients with symptoms of acute PVD, often progress to clinical RD within a few days or weeks unless treated prophylactically. In addition, SRF accumulates more quickly in eyes with PVD because the volume of syneretic fluid is greater than in eyes with atrophic holes or dialyses without PVD. Treatment is by cryotherapy or laser photocoagulation.

> NB: 'No fluid = No explant'.

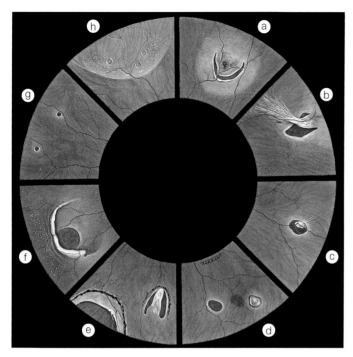

**Figure 6.62** Prophylactic treatment of retinal breaks (see text)

3. **An operculated U-tear** bridged by a patent blood vessel (Fig. 6.62c) should be treated if persistent dynamic vitreoretinal traction on the bridging blood vessel is causing recurrent vitreous haemorrhage. Although eyes with breaks associated with avulsed or bridging blood vessels may be successfully treated by argon laser photocoagulation alone, the possibility of an explant or vitrectomy to reduce traction on the operculum and blood vessel should be considered.

4. **An operculated U-tear** in the lower temporal quadrant detected by chance (Fig. 6.62d) is much safer because there is no vitreoretinal traction. Prophylaxis is therefore not required in the absence of other risk factors.

5. **Pigment demarcation** associated with an inferior U-tear and a dialysis detected by chance are both low-risk lesions (Fig. 6.62e) which have been present for a long time. However, the presence of pigmentation around a large U-tear is not always a guarantee against progression, particularly when associated with other risk factors such as aphakia, myopia or RD in the fellow eye. If necessary, treatment may involve cryotherapy or photocoagulation.

6. **Degenerative retinoschisis** with breaks in both layers (Fig. 6.62f) does not require treatment. Although this lesion represents a full-thickness defect in the sensory retina, the fluid within the schisis cavity is usually viscid and rarely passes into the subretinal space.

7. **Two small asymptomatic holes** near the ora serrata (Fig. 6.62g) do not require treatment because the risk of RD is extremely small as they are probably located within the vitreous base. About 5% of the general population have such lesions.

8. **Small inner layer holes in retinoschisis** (Fig. 6.62h) also carry an extremely low risk of RD as there is no communication between the vitreous cavity and the subretinal space. Treatment is therefore inappropriate.

> **NB:** In the absence of associated retinal breaks, neither lattice nor snailtrack degenerations require prophylactic treatment. However, prophylaxis should be considered if PVD has not yet occurred and the fellow eye has suffered RD in the past.

## CHOICE OF TREATMENT MODALITIES

The three modalities used for prophylaxis are: (a) *cryotherapy*, (b) *laser photocoagulation* using a slit-lamp delivery system, and (c) *laser* using the indirect ophthalmoscopic delivery system combined with scleral indentation. Large areas of cryotherapy may increase the risk of pigment epithelial cell release and subsequent epiretinal membrane formation. Thus, laser is the preferred modality for extensive lesions. For small lesions, there is little evidence to suggest an increased risk with cryotherapy as opposed to laser. In most cases, the treatment modality is based on the surgeon's preference and experience as well as the availability of instrumentation. Other considerations are as follows:

1. **Location of lesion:** an equatorial lesion can be treated by either photocoagulation or cryotherapy. A post-equatorial lesion can be treated only by photocoagulation unless the conjunctiva is incised. Peripheral lesions near the ora serrata can be treated either by cryotherapy or by laser photocoagulation using the indirect ophthalmoscope delivery system combined with indentation. Treatment of very peripheral lesions by laser photocoagulation using a slit-lamp delivery system is difficult because it may be impossible to adequately treat the base of a U-tear.

2. **Clarity of media:** eyes with hazy media are much easier to treat by cryotherapy.

3. **Pupil size:** eyes with small pupils are easier to treat by cryotherapy.

## LASER PHOTOCOAGULATION

### Technique

- Select a spot size of 200 $\mu$m and set the duration to 0.1 or 0.2 seconds.
- Insert the triple-mirror contact lens or one of the wide-field lenses.
- Surround the lesion with two rows of confluent burns of moderate intensity (Fig. 6.63).

### Complications

These are rare, but when they do occur, they are usually associated with excessively heavy treatment to large areas of the retina and may involve both anterior and posterior segments.

1. **Posterior segment**

- Maculopathy: cystoid macular oedema or macular pucker.

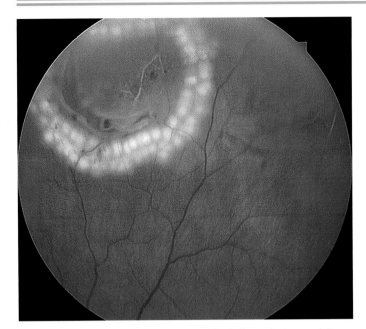

**Figure 6.63** Appearance soon after prophylactic laser photocoagulation of a retinal hole

- Choroidal detachment, which may be associated with secondary angle-closure glaucoma as a result of a forward rotation of the ciliary body.
- Exudative RD, which usually resolves within 1 or 2 weeks.

2. **Anterior segment** problems, which are rare, include:

- Corneal burns.
- Iris burns, which may result in iritis, iris atrophy and sphincter damage.
- Anterior capsular lens opacities.
- Transient myopia.

## CRYOTHERAPY

### Technique

- Instil a topical anaesthetic or inject lidocaine (Xylocaine) subconjunctivally in the same quadrant as the lesion to be treated. For lesions behind the equator, a small conjunctival incision may be necessary to enable the cryoprobe to reach the required location.
- Insert a Barraquer speculum.
- Check the cryoprobe for correct freezing and defrosting and also make sure that the rubber sleeve is not covering the tip.
- While viewing with the indirect ophthalmoscope, gently indent the sclera with the tip of the probe. In order not to mistake the shaft of the probe for the tip, start indenting near the ora serrata and then move the tip posteriorly to the lesion.
- Surround the lesion with a single row of cryo-applications, terminating freezing as soon as the retina whitens. In most cases this can be achieved by one or two applications to the tear itself. Because recently frozen retina soon reverts to its normal colour, it is easier to inadvertently re-treat the same area with cryotherapy than with photocoagulation.

---

> **NB: Do not remove the cryoprobe until it has defrosted completely because premature removal may 'crack' the choroid and give rise to choroidal haemorrhage.**

Pad the eye for about 4 hours to help decrease chemosis and advise the patient to refrain from strenuous physical activity for 7 days. For about 2 days, the treated area appears whitish due to oedema. After about 5 days, pigmentation begins to appear. Initially the pigment is fine and then it becomes coarser and is associated with a variable amount of chorioretinal atrophy (Fig. 6.64).

### Complications

1. **Chemosis and lid oedema** are common.

2. **Transient diplopia** may occur as a result of freezing a rectus muscle.

3. **Vitritis** may occur as a result of excessively heavy treatment.

4. **Maculopathy** is rare, but commoner than with laser treatment.

5. **Choroidal detachment** and **exudative RD** are very rare.

6. **New break formation** (see below).

## CAUSES OF FAILURE

1. **Failure to surround the entire lesion,** particularly the base of a U-tear, is the most common cause of failure. If the most peripheral part of the tear cannot be reached by photocoagulation, then cryotherapy should be used.

2. **Failure to apply contiguous treatment** when treating a large break or a dialysis.

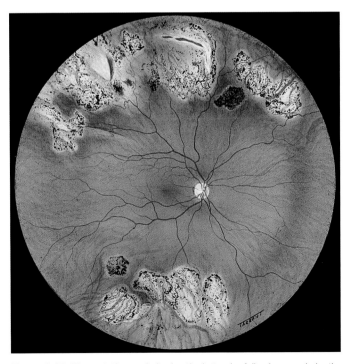

**Figure 6.64** Pigmentation and chorioretinal atrophy following prophylactic cryotherapy

3. **Failure to use an explant or gas tamponade** in an eye with 'subclinical RD'.

4. **New break formation** within or adjacent to the treated area (Fig. 6.65) is usually caused by excessively heavy treatment, particularly of lattice degeneration. New breaks developing away from a treated area are probably not associated with the treatment itself.

## BENIGN PERIPHERAL RETINAL DEGENERATIONS

It is important to recognise the following entirely innocuous peripheral retinal degenerations which do not require prophylaxis (Fig. 6.66).

1. **Microcystoid degeneration** consists of tiny vesicles with indistinct boundaries on a greyish-white background which make the retina appear thickened and less transparent (see Fig. 6.4). The degeneration always starts adjacent to the ora serrata and extends circumferentially and posteriorly with a smooth undulating posterior border. Microcystoid degeneration is present in all adult eyes, increasing in severity with age, and is not in itself causally related to RD, although it may give rise to retinoschisis.

2. **Snowflakes** are minute glistening yellow-white dots which are frequently found scattered diffusely in the peripheral fundus. Occasionally, circumscribed aggregations of snowflakes may be seen near the equator. Foci composed solely of snowflakes are innocuous and require no treatment.

3. **Pavingstone degeneration** is characterised by discrete yellow-white patches of focal chorioretinal atrophy which is present to some extent in 25% of normal eyes (Fig. 6.67).

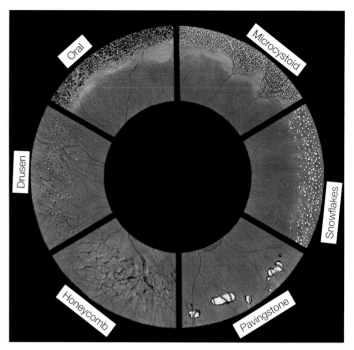

**Figure 6.66** Benign peripheral retinal degenerations (see text)

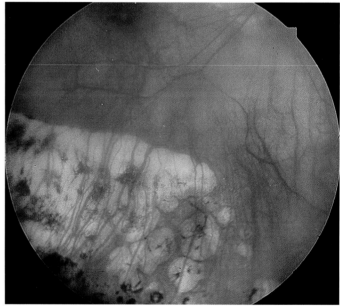

**Figure 6.67** Pavingstone degeneration

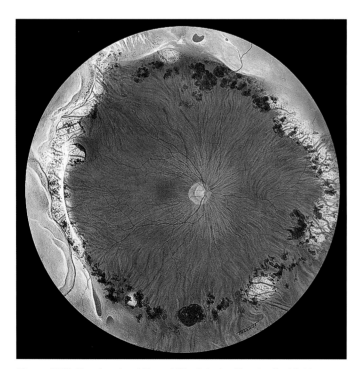

**Figure 6.65** New breaks at 7 and 12 o'clock with subretinal fluid following extensive cryotherapy of lattice degeneration

4. **Honeycomb (reticular) degeneration** is an age-related change characterised by a fine network of perivascular pigmentation which may extend posterior to the equator (Fig. 6.68).

5. **Drusen** are characterised by clusters of small pale lesions which may have hyperpigmented borders (Fig. 6.69). They are similar to drusen at the posterior pole and usually occur in the eyes of elderly individuals.

6. **Oral pigmentary degeneration** is an age-related change consisting of a hyperpigmented band running adjacent to the ora serrata.

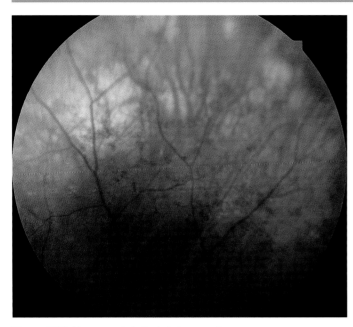

**Figure 6.68** Honeycomb (reticular) degeneration

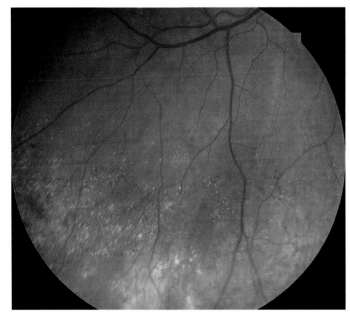

**Figure 6.69** Peripheral drusen

# Surgery

## *Preoperative considerations*

***Prognosis for preservation of central vision.*** The main factors governing visual function following surgical reattachment of the retina are:

1. **Duration of macular involvement.**

- If the macula is uninvolved, most eyes maintain their preoperative visual acuity.
- If the macula is detached for 10 days or less, postoperative visual acuity is excellent.

- If the macula is detached for over 2 months, postoperative visual acuity is usually very poor. However, it must be emphasised that, although visual acuity may be poor, the patient is frequently glad to have restoration of peripheral vision following successful retinal reattachment.

2. **Height of macular detachment,** reflected by preoperative visual acuity, is also important. It appears that photoreceptor cell degeneration is more severe with increasing separation from the RPE.

3. **Age.** Patients 60 years of age or younger obtain better postoperative visual acuity than do older patients.

***Indications for urgent surgery.*** It should be noted that the spread of SRF is governed by three factors:

1. **The position of the primary break:** SRF will spread more quickly from a superior break

2. **The size of the break:** large breaks lead to more rapid accumulation of SRF than do small ones.

3. **State of vitreous gel.** If the vitreous gel is healthy and solid, even giant tears or giant dialyses may not lead to RD. However, if synchysis is advanced as in myopia, progression is usually rapid and the entire retina may become detached within 1 or 2 days.

> **NB:** It is therefore apparent that a patient with a fresh RD involving the superotemporal quadrant but with an intact macula should be operated on as soon as possible. In order to prevent SRF spreading to the macula, the patient should be positioned flat in bed with only one pillow and with the head turned so that the retinal break is in the most dependent position. For example, a patient with a right upper temporal RD should turn his or her head to the right. Preoperative bed rest is also desirable in eyes with bullous RDs because it may lessen the amount of SRF and facilitate surgery. Patients with dense fresh vitreous haemorrhage in whom visualisation of the fundus is impossible should also be operated on as soon as possible if B-scan ultrasonography shows an underlying RD.

***What to tell the patient.*** The function of the retina can be likened to the film in a camera, and an RD can be explained in terms of wallpaper peeling off a wall. Simple diagrams may be helpful in explaining the principles of surgery. Inform the patient that the other eye will also be examined and any weaknesses may be treated. It is also important to emphasise that anatomical success does not equate to visual success and occasionally a second operation is necessary. The patient should be warned that after surgery the eye will be red, tender and slightly painful. There may also be some transient double vision.

***Mydriatics.*** The commonest regimen is dilation with 1% cyclopentolate and 10% phenylephrine drops given at 15-minute intervals for 1 hour preoperatively. One per cent atropine is also usually instilled into the operated eye at the end of the procedure, to maintain good postoperative mydriasis.

NB: If operating under general anaesthesia, it is good practice to carefully examine the fellow eye of patients undergoing RD repair, which should therefore also be dilated as part of the preoperative regimen.

***Prophylactic antibiotics.*** Although postoperative intra-ocular infection is extremely rare following RD surgery, most surgeons use a solution of aqueous 5% povidone–iodine (Betadine) to clean the fornices and operative field immediately prior to surgery. A routine subconjunctival injection of betamethasone and an antibiotic at completion of surgery is also often given.

### Problems with intraocular lens implants

● Lens reflexes and lens edge effects may impede visualisation of the fundus.
● Capsular opacification may impair visualisation of the fundus.
● Intravitreal air injection may displace the lens anteriorly, resulting in subluxation, iris capture and possible corneal damage.

NB: Because of the difficulties with visualisation, and the fact that pseudophakic eyes often have multiple small holes, most surgeons would now adopt a vitrectomy approach to repair this type of detachment

## Pneumatic retinopexy

Pneumatic retinopexy is an outpatient procedure in which an intravitreal expanding gas bubble is used to seal a retinal break and reattach the retina without scleral buckling. The most frequently used gases are sulphur hexafluoride ($SF_6$) and perfluoropropane ($C_3F_8$). Pneumatic retinopexy has the advantage of being a relatively quick, minimally invasive, 'office-based' procedure. However, success rates are usually slightly less than those achievable with conventional scleral buckling surgery.

***Indications.*** The procedure is usually reserved for treatment of uncomplicated RDs with a small retinal break or a cluster of breaks extending over an area of less than two clock hours situated in the upper two-thirds of the peripheral retina.

***Technique*** depends on the amount of SRF as follows:

1. **Shallow SRF** associated with a break which can be easily closed by scleral indentation:

● Treat the retinal breaks with cryotherapy (Fig. 6.70a). Plenty of scleral indentation is helpful in reducing the intraocular pressure and thus facilitating the subsequent intravitreal injection of the gas bubble.
● Inject either 0.5 ml of 100% $SF_6$ or 0.3 ml of 100% $C_3F_8$ into the vitreous cavity (Fig. 6.70b).
● With forceps or a sterile cotton-wool bud, seal the scleral entry site to prevent the escape of gas under the conjunctiva.

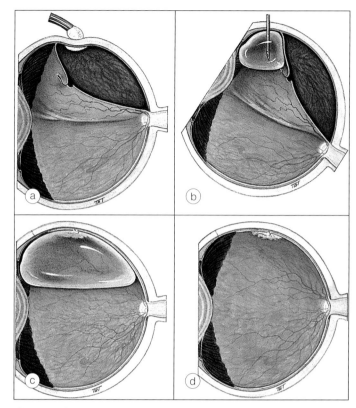

**Figure 6.70** Pneumatic retinopexy (see text)

● If there is no light perception and absence of pulsation of the central retinal artery following the injection, perform an anterior chamber paracentesis to lower the intraocular pressure.
● Postoperatively, position the patient's head so that the break is uppermost and the rising gas bubble is in contact with the tear (Fig. 6.70c and 6.70d), and posturing is maintained for 5–7 days as the gas absorbs.

2. **Moderately bullous RD** associated with a break that cannot be closed by scleral indentation:

● Omit cryotherapy.
● Inject gas.
● As the retina flattens over the next few days, treat the breaks by laser photocoagulation, preferably using the indirect ophthal-moscopic delivery system because it is easier to apply through a gas bubble than is slit-lamp delivery.
● Continue postoperative positioning for 5–7 days until adequate chorioretinal adhesion is established.

## Scleral buckling

### GENERAL CONSIDERATIONS

***Purpose.*** Scleral buckling is a surgical procedure in which material sutured onto the sclera (explant) creates an inward indentation (buckle). Its two main purposes are:

1. **To close retinal breaks** by apposing the RPE to the NR.

2. **To reduce dynamic vitreoretinal traction** at sites of local vitreoretinal adhesion.

### Buckle configurations

1. **Radial** explants are placed at right angles to the limbus (Fig. 6.71a).

2. **Segmental circumferential** explants are placed circumferentially with the limbus to create a segmental buckle (Fig. 6.71b).

3. **Encircling** explants are placed around the entire circumference of the globe to create a 360° buckle and, if necessary, may be augmented by local explants (Fig. 6.71c and 6.71d).

**Materials.** All explants are made from either soft or hard silicone as follows:

1. **Soft silicone (Silastic) sponges** may be round or oval. Round sponges have a diameter of 3 mm, 4 mm or 5 mm. Sponges are most frequently used for local buckling during a non-drainage procedure.

2. **Hard silicone tyres** of various dimensions may be used either to create solitary local buckles, during drain or non-drain surgery, or to supplement an encircling strap.

3. **Hard silicone straps** are used only for 360° buckling.

## EXPLANTS

**General properties.** In order to adequately seal a retinal break, it is essential for the buckle to have adequate length, width and height. The entire break should ideally be surrounded by about 2 mm of buckle. It is also important for the buckle to involve the area of the vitreous base anterior to the tear in order to prevent the possibility of subsequent reopening of the tear and anterior leakage of SRF. The dimensions of the retinal break can be assessed by comparing it with the diameter of the optic disc (1.5 mm) or the end of a scleral indenter.

1. **Width** of a radial buckle depends on the width (distance between anterior horns) of the retinal tear, and its length depends on the length (distance between base and apex) of the tear. In general, the width of the explant should be twice that of the tear.

2. **Height** of a local buckle is determined by the following interrelated factors:

   - The greater the diameter of the explant, the higher the buckle.
   - The greater the separation of suture, the higher the buckle.
   - The tighter the sutures over the explant, the higher the buckle.
   - The lower the intraocular pressure, the higher the buckle. However, if the eye is extremely hard, it will be impossible to create a buckle, irrespective of the diameter of the explant, separation of sutures and tightness of sutures. Conversely, in a very soft eye, a high buckle can be created with a small-diameter sponge.

> NB: Most local buckles lose their effect after about 3 years.

### Indications

1. **Radial buckling**

   - U-tears.
   - Posterior breaks, because of inability to support them on a circumferential buckle.

2. **Segmental circumferential buckling**

   - Multiple breaks located in one or two quadrants and/or at varying distances from the ora serrata.
   - Anterior breaks.
   - Wide breaks such as dialyses.

> NB: A solitary hole can be sealed with either a radial or circumferential buckle.

3. **Encircling explants** are rarely used unless accompanied by a vitrectomy.

## TECHNIQUE

### Preliminary steps

- *Both* pupils should usually be dilated, and, whilst operating on one eye, the eyelids of the fellow eye taped shut to prevent accidental corneal exposure.
- The retinal drawing should be displayed upside-down in a convenient place such as an x-ray viewing box (Fig. 6.72).

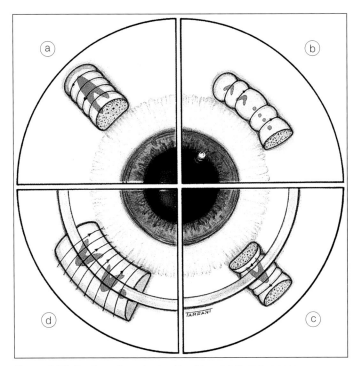

**Figure 6.71** Configuration of scleral buckles. **(a)** Radial sponge; **(b)** circumferential sponge; **(c)** encirclement augmented by a radial sponge; **(d)** encirclement augmented by a solid silicone tyre

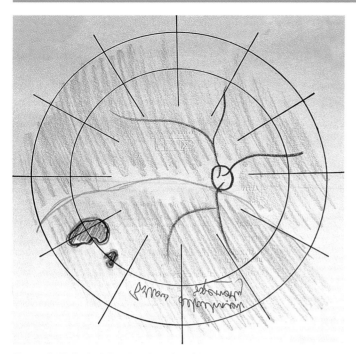

**Figure 6.72** Retinal drawing placed upside down

- One of the key factors in ensuring rapid, stress-free surgery is for the surgeon to plan exactly which technique will be used and inform the theatre staff so that all equipment is available promptly.
- Perform a peritomy appropriate to the extent of scleral exposure required (Fig. 6.73).
- With cellulose sponges, clear the episcleral tissue from the sclera to facilitate subsequent insertion of scleral sutures and drainage of SRF; beginners frequently do not appreciate the importance of this step.

***Bridle sutures*** are used to stabilise the globe and manipulate it into optimal positions during surgery. The technique is as follows:

- Insert a squint hook under a rectus muscle (Fig. 6.74).

> NB: Make sure that you separate the superior rectus from the underlying superior oblique.

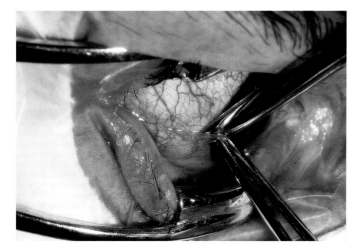

**Figure 6.73** Conjunctival incision

- Pass a reverse mounted needle with a 4/0 black silk suture under (not through) the muscle tendon (Fig. 6.75).
- Secure the suture by twisting it around mosquito forceps (Fig. 6.76) and cut off the excess.
- Repeat the above steps for other tendons as required. Surgery can be carried out with only one or two muscle sutures but is usually easier if three muscles have been slung.

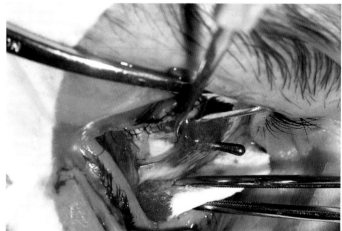

**Figure 6.74** Insertion of squint hook under a rectus muscle

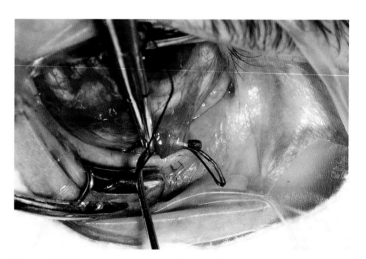

**Figure 6.75** Reverse mounted needle passed under a muscle tendon

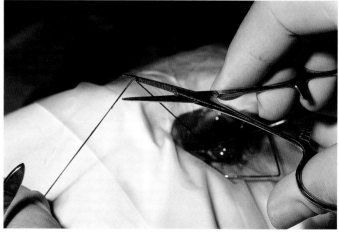

**Figure 6.76** Twisting of suture around mosquito forceps

***Scleral inspection*** must be performed for the following reasons:

1. **To detect anomalous vortex veins** so that they will not be damaged during cryotherapy, scleral buckling or drainage of SRF.

2. **To detect scleral thinning** (Fig. 6.77), which may be associated with the following problems:

   - Penetration of the choroid and retina during insertion of scleral sutures.
   - Cutting out of sutures as they are being tightened over the explant. This is particularly likely to occur when the intraocular pressure is elevated because SRF has not been drained.
   - Scleral rupture during cryotherapy or localisation of breaks.

***Indentation ophthalmoscopy*** should be performed and the findings compared with the fundus drawing. Identification of all retinal breaks is crucial to surgical success.

   - Try to appose the retinal breaks to the RPE by indenting the sclera. If achieved easily, drainage of SRF is not necessary.
   - Assess the dimensions of retinal breaks.

> **NB: Remember that a retinal break in highly elevated retina appears larger and more posterior than one of the same size in a shallow RD.**

***Localisation of all breaks*** is crucial to the correct placement of the scleral buckle.

1. **Technique**

   - Indent the sclera at the site calculated to correspond to the apex of the tear and visualise the indent via the indirect ophthalmoscope. When the indent lies beneath the apex of the tear (Fig. 6.78) press on the sclera to leave a temporary indentation mark. Ask an assistant to dry the area as the indent is released and

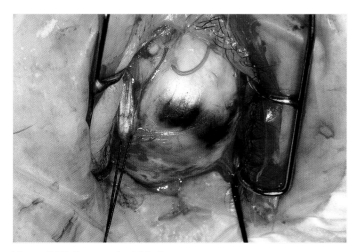

**Figure 6.77** Severe scleral thinning

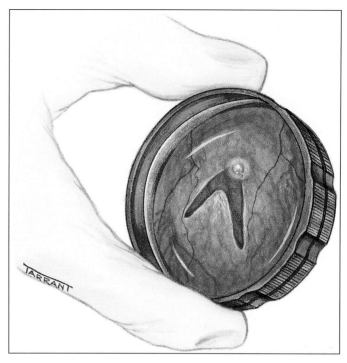

**Figure 6.78** Indentation of the apex of a U-tear

place a spot of surgical ink on the sclera at the site of indent. Re-check the position with indirect ophthalmoscopy.

> **NB: Beware of the tendency to localise breaks too posteriorly in eyes with deep SRF.**

   - If the indentation does not coincide with the break, repeat the procedure until accurate localisation is achieved. In eyes with very large breaks, localise the two ends as well as the midpoint of the posterior flap.

2. **Problems.** Localisation of relatively anterior breaks in eyes with shallow SRF is easy. However, accurate localisation may be very difficult or impossible in eyes with bullous RDs, especially if associated with breaks located behind the equator, in which case a D-ACE (Drain-Air-Cryo-Explant) or vitrectomy procedure would be more appropriate.

***Cryotherapy*** creates an inflammatory chorioretinal lesion which, on scarring, results in a strong bond between the sensory retina and RPE so that retinal breaks are permanently sealed.

1. **Technique**

   - Check that the cryoprobe is able to freeze to -80°C and defrost quickly.
   - Ask for the theatre lights to be turned off.
   - Indent the sclera gently with the tip of the cryoprobe whilst viewing with the indirect ophthalmoscope (Fig. 6.79).

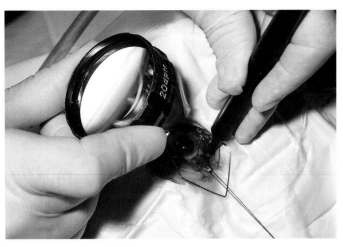

**Figure 6.79** Cryotherapy

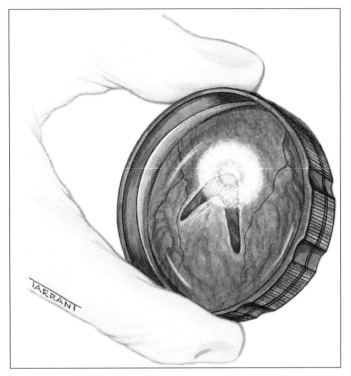

**Figure 6.80** Appearance of the iceball

- Commence freezing by depressing the footswitch and continue until the sensory retina has just turned white (Fig. 6.80).
- Treat any predisposing lesions in attached retina first, as this will soften the globe and may facilitate subsequent treatment of breaks in detached retina. When freezing breaks in detached retina, indent the sclera with the cryoprobe to bring the RPE as close as possible to the break. The break will appear darker as a result of the contrast between the white frozen sensory retina and the underlying RPE and choroid. This phenomenon is useful in differentiating small breaks from areas of retinal thinning.
- Repeat cryotherapy until the entire break has been surrounded by a 2 mm margin. Small holes may require

only one application whereas large tears or long islands of lattice degeneration will require several.

**2. Problems**

a. *Failure of the iceball to appear.* If after about 6 seconds the retinal whitening cannot be visualised, it is very important to ensure that the shaft of the probe has not been mistaken for the tip. If this is the case, the tip itself will be too far posterior and may cause macular damage. It is also important to avoid inadvertent attempts to freeze through the patient's eyelids.

b. *Excessive cryotherapy* is undesirable because it predisposes to pigment fallout, postoperative vitritis and exudative RD. It can be prevented by taking the following precautions:

- Avoid freezing the same area several times. If cryotherapy has to be applied to a large area, refreezing can be avoided by observing normal anatomical landmarks and also noting that recently frozen retina becomes less transparent after about 30 seconds.
- In eyes with very deep SRF it may be impossible to freeze the sensory retina without the formation of a huge iceball within the subretinal space. In these circumstances it may be necessary to perform a D-ACE procedure to ensure that both the RPE and sensory retina are adequately treated or to convert to a vitrectomy procedure.

c. *Premature removal of the cryoprobe* should be resisted because 'cracking' the tip of the probe off the sclera before the iceball has defrosted may cause:

- Choroidal haemorrhage by 'cracking' the frozen choroid.
- Rupture of thin sclera.

d. *Excessive scleral indentation* with the cryoprobe, in vulnerable eyes, may result in the following:

- Penetration through thin sclera.
- Rupture of a cataract incision.
- Closure of the central retinal artery.

### *Insertion of explant*

**1. Technique**

- Select the appropriate-sized explant according to the criteria previously described.
- With callipers, measure the distance separating the sutures (Fig. 6.81) and mark the sclera with indentation by the calliper leg.

---

**NB:** As a general rule, the separation of sutures should be about 1.5 times the diameter of a sponge explant. For example, with a 5 mm explant, separation of sutures should be 7.5 mm (i.e. 5 + 2.5). If a very high buckle is desired, space the sutures even further apart. For solid explants, the suture spacing will depend on the exact explant selected. For example, a 277 explant requires sutures at 9 mm spacing for a 1 mm indent.

---

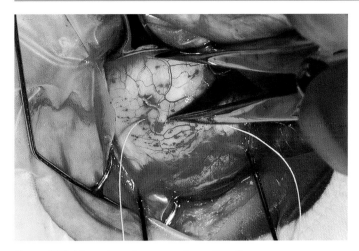

**Figure 6.81** Measuring suture separation with callipers

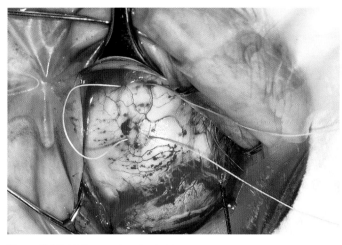

**Figure 6.82** Mattress suture in place

- Insert a mattress-type suture which will straddle the explant using 5/0 Dacron double-ended sutures on a spatulated needle (Fig. 6.82). A quarter-circle needle is best for long anterior placement but a half-circle needle is preferred for relatively posterior placement. The number of sutures will depend upon the length of the explant. Each bite should ideally extend for at least 3 mm and have an even intrascleral course. For radial buckles, the tip of the needle should be pointing posteriorly as it traverses the sclera.
- Pick up one end of the explant with forceps and feed it through the sutures.
- With two Castroviejo needle holders, tie the sutures over the explant (Fig. 6.83).
- After tying the first suture, many surgeons prefer to perform a paracentesis to drop the intraocular pressure and prevent tearing out of the second suture or closure of the retinal circulation.

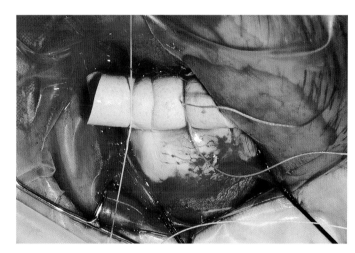

**Figure 6.83** Tying of suture over the sponge

- Check the position of the buckle in relation to the retinal break with the indirect ophthalmoscope (Fig. 6.84). If the break is closed or very nearly closed and there are no other open breaks, the operation can be terminated without drainage of SRF. If the buckle is incorrectly positioned, it should be removed and repositioned.
  - Check the central retinal artery by inspecting the optic disc to ensure flow has not been stopped due to high intraocular pressure. If pulsation is not present or inducible with indentation, then intraocular pressure is above systolic. In this event, massage the globe or repeat the paracentesis. Very rarely it may be necessary to slacken the sutures, massage the globe and then tighten the sutures very slowly.

NB: Examine the fellow eye carefully with scleral indentation, and, if necessary, prophylactically treat with cryotherapy or indirect ophthalmoscopic laser photocoagulation any predisposing lesions.

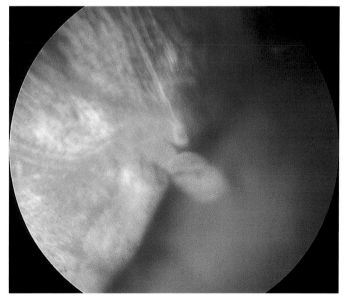

**Figure 6.84** Position of buckle in relation to the tear – in this case the buckle is too anterior

## 2. Problems

a. *Accidental drainage* of SRF may become apparent immediately or when the sutures are being tightened over the sponge, at which point the SRF begins to leak out and the eye becomes soft. Premature drainage of SRF is undesirable because the induced ocular hypotony makes further suture placement difficult and may lead to choroidal haemorrhage. Attempts should be made to remove the suture and either oversew the perforated sclera or adjust the buckle position so that the draining site is tamponaded by the buckle. This may be difficult in very hypotonous eyes which will require an intra-vitreal air injection to restore the intraocular pressure. Very small leaks can often be left as they invariably seal spontaneously.

b. *'Fishmouthing'* is a tendency of certain retinal tears, typically large superior U-tears located at the equator in a bullous RD, to open widely following scleral buck-ing and drainage of SRF (Fig. 6.85a). In some cases the RD may even appear more elevated than before and associated radial folds may make the tear very difficult to close. This problem can be avoided by avoiding fluid drainage unless as part of a D-ACE procedure. Some folds flatten spontaneously during the postoperative period whilst others prevent retinal reattachment by keeping open a communicating retinal break. Manage-ment of this problem involves insertion of an additional radial buckle and injection of air into the vitreous cavity (Fig. 6.85b).

## DRAINAGE OF SUBRETINAL FLUID

**Indications.** Although a large proportion of RDs can be treated successfully with non-drainage techniques, drainage of SRF may be required under the following circumstances:

1. **Deep SRF beneath the retinal break.** In this situation, the application of cryotherapy may be difficult or impos-sible and the RD should be repaired using a **D-ACE** (**D**rain-**A**ir-**C**ryo-**E**xplant) procedure, although such cases are now often repaired via a vitrectomy procedure.

   - **D**rain the SRF to bring the break closer to the RPE.
   - **A**ir injection into the vitreous cavity to counteract the hypotony induced by drainage.
   - **C**ryotherapy to the localised break.
   - **E**xplant insertion.

2. **Immobile retina** is a relative indication for drainage because the non-drainage procedure is successful only if the detached retina is sufficiently mobile to move back against the buckle during the postoperative period. If it is rendered relatively immobile by PVR, a high buckle is required to seal the break, which may only be achieved if the eye is first softened by draining the SRF. However, such eyes are now often treated by vitrectomy.

3. **Longstanding RDs** tend to be associated with viscous SRF which may take a long time (many months) to absorb. Drainage may therefore be necessary to restore macular reattachment quickly, even if the break itself can be closed without drainage.

4. **Danger from raised intraocular pressure.** Eyes in which significant elevation of intraocular pressure may cause problems should be drained or repaired by vitrectomy. This is because with a non-drainage procedure the scleral sutures have to be tightened over the sponge in order to achieve the desired buckling effect. This causes a signifi-cant elevation of intraocular pressure for several hours. The temporary elevation of intraocular pressure is usually harmless although in the following situations it may have detrimental effects:

   - In eyes with advanced glaucomatous field loss it may cause a complete loss of all vision.
   - In eyes with thin sclera the sutures may cut out as they are being tightened.

**Advantages.** Although non-drainage of SRF avoids most of the operative complications, drainage provides immediate contact between the sensory retina and RPE with flattening of the fovea. If this contact is delayed for more than 5 days, a satisfactory adhesion may not develop around the retinal break. This may result in non-attachment of the retina or, in some cases, reopening of the break during the postoperative period. In addition, drainage of SRF allows the use of a large bubble of an internal tamponading agent (air or gas).

**Techniques**

1. **'Prang' technique**

   - Apply digital pressure to the globe until the central retinal artery is occluded and complete blanching of the choroidal vasculature is achieved, in order to prevent haemorrhage from the drainage site.
   - Make a full-thickness perforation with the tip of a 27-gauge hypodermic needle bent 2 mm at the tip in a single, swift but controlled fashion.
   - Following drainage of SRF, inject air to restore ocular pressure either from a syringe and 27-gauge needle or using an air line from a vitrectomy machine attached to a 27-gauge needle. The latter technique has the

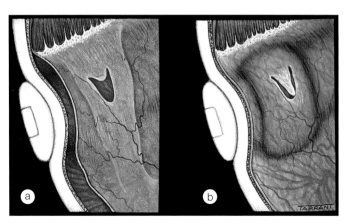

**Figure 6.85** **(a)** 'Fishmouthing' of a U-tear communicating with a radial fold; **(b)** insertion of radial buckle

advantage of a more rapid restoration of intraocular pressure and decreased risk of choroidal haemorrhage.

### 2. 'Cut-down' technique

- Examine the fundus to make sure that the SRF has not shifted.
- Make sure that the intraocular pressure is not elevated by relaxing the traction sutures and lifting the lid speculum from the globe. Drainage of SRF when the intraocular pressure is high may cause retinal incarceration.
- Choose the sclerotomy site beneath the deepest SRF avoiding any vortex veins.
- Perform a radial sclerotomy about 4 mm long and of sufficient depth to allow herniation of a small dark knuckle of choroid into the incision.
- Place a 5/0 Dacron mattress suture across the lips of the sclerotomy (optional).
- Ask the assistant to hold the lips of the sclerotomy apart and inspect the prolapsed knuckle with a +20D lens for the presence of large choroidal vessels. These are usually obvious as they are located most superficially in the choroid. If a large vessel is present, suture the sclerotomy and choose another drainage site.
- If large choroidal vessels are absent, gently apply low-heat cautery to the choroidal knuckle to decrease the risk of choroidal bleeding.
- If this does not result in drainage of SRF, perforate the choroidal knuckle with one of the following:

  - A 25-gauge hypodermic needle on a syringe.
  - A sharp suture needle held by a needle holder (Fig. 6.86).
  - Diathermy pin.
  - Argon endolaser probe.

---

**NB:** (a) A sharp-ended instrument should be introduced tangentially to reduce the risk of retinal damage. (b) It is not always advantageous to drain all the SRF because the eye may become excessively soft. If necessary, partial drainage can be performed by tying the sclerotomy suture into a temporary bow before all the SRF has been drained. The fundus can then be inspected and, if the SRF beneath the tear is sufficiently decreased, the bow can be converted into a permanent knot. This partial drainage of SRF may obviate the necessity to perform an intravitreal injection to prevent excessive ocular hypotony due to drainage of a large volume of SRF.

---

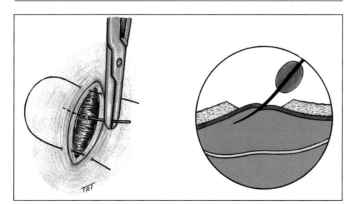

**Figure 6.86** Cut-down technique of drainage of subretinal fluid

### 3. If part of a non-D-ACE type procedure, gradually tighten the sutures over the buckling material to prevent hypotony as the fluid drains. Inspect the fundus to check that the tear is correctly positioned on the buckle (as previously described) and to ensure that the retina is not incarcerated; a normal drainage site is apparent as a small yellow spot.

## *Complications*

1. **Haemorrhage** (Fig. 6.87) is usually caused by damage to a large choroidal vessel.

   a. *Complications.* Although small bleeds may be innocuous because the blood escapes with the SRF, large bleeds may give rise to the following:

   - Postoperative maculopathy and impairment of central vision may occur as a result of gravitation of large amounts of blood in the subretinal space to the fovea.
   - Vitreous haemorrhage as a result of entry of blood into the vitreous cavity through the retinal break.
   - Haemorrhagic choroidal detachment resulting from collection of a large volume of blood in the suprachoroidal space.

   b. *Prevention*

   - Avoid drainage near the vortex ampullae; drainage is usually safe under or just on either side of the vertical recti anterior to the equator as well as just above and below (but not under) the horizontal recti.
   - Avoid drainage through recently frozen sclera because cryotherapy dilates choroidal vessels and increases the risk of bleeding.

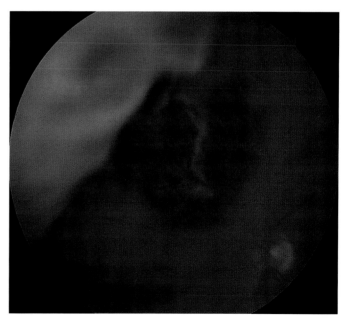

**Figure 6.87** Mild subretinal haemorrhage associated with drainage of subretinal fluid

- Avoid drainage, if possible, in the temporal fundus because in the event of bleeding into the subretinal space the blood may not gravitate towards the fovea.

c. *Management* of significant haemorrhage (Fig. 6.88) is as follows:

- Tighten the sutures over the buckle as quickly as possible in order to increase intraocular pressure and prevent further bleeding.
- Prevent gravitation of blood in the subretinal space to the fovea by rotating the globe and turning the patient's head.

> **NB:** Drainage of suprachoroidal blood by performing a second sclerotomy is unrewarding because the blood has already clotted.

2. **Failure of drainage** of SRF ('dry tap') may be caused by one of the following:

- Failure to perforate the full thickness of the choroid.
- Attempted drainage in an area of flat retina: therefore always check the position of the SRF immediately prior to drainage.
- Incarceration of the retina in the sclerotomy (see later).

3. **Iatrogenic break formation** is caused by perforation of the retina with the needle while draining SRF.

a. *Prevention*

- Do not insert the needle too deeply into the subretinal space.
- Drain where the SRF is deepest – usually near the equator.
- Before draining, check that there is still sufficient SRF to drain and that the SRF has not shifted.

b. *Management*

- If the perforation has occurred within the bed of the buckle, the break should be treated with cryotherapy.

- If the perforation is outside the bed of the buckle and the break is in detached retina, apply cryotherapy to the break and mount it on a small explant. If the break is in flat retina, apply cryotherapy only.

4. **Retinal incarceration** into the sclerotomy is usually due to excessively elevated intraocular pressure at the time of drainage using method 2. As already mentioned, it is one of the causes of a dry tap, although, occasionally, after an initial appearance of SRF, the flow will suddenly cease despite the fact that a large amount of SRF still remains in the eye. Ophthalmoscopy reveals a star-shaped puckering at the drainage site (Fig. 6.89).

a. *Prevention.* Do not drain SRF when intraocular pressure is high.

b. *Management*

- Apply pressure over the sclerotomy site with the tip of a squint hook in an attempt to reposit the incarcerated retina.
- If the incarceration is in the bed of the buckle, no further action is required if it cannot be reposited with the squint hook.
- If the incarceration is away from the bed of the buckle, support the incarcerated area of retina on a local buckle to prevent postoperative traction and possible persistence of SRF.

5. **Vitreous prolapse**

a. *Causes*

- Attempted drainage at the site of flat retina: therefore always check the position of SRF immediately prior to drainage.

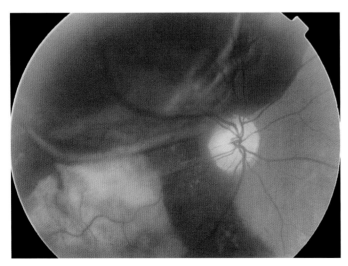

**Figure 6.88** Severe subretinal haemorrhage associated with drainage of subretinal fluid

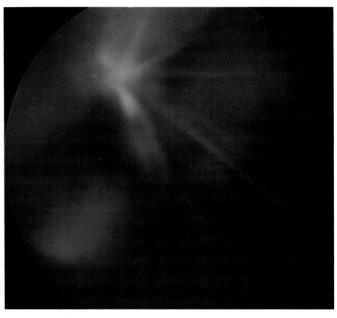

**Figure 6.89** Retinal incarceration into the drainage site

- Drainage near a large break in which retrohyaloid fluid followed by solid vitreous passes through the break and leaks out through the sclerotomy. This fairly rare complication may not always be preventable because it is not always possible to avoid drainage near a large break.

*b. Management*

- Inspect the sclerotomy to make sure that there is no associated retinal incarceration – if incarceration is present, try to reposit the retina with the tip of a squint hook.
- Excise the vitreous prolapse with scissors.
- If the prolapse is in an area of flat retina, apply cryotherapy to the associated iatrogenic retinal tear.
- If the prolapse is in an area of detached retina, take no further action.

## ABSORPTION OF SUBRETINAL FLUID

Following drainage of SRF, the retina should be flat or very nearly flat on the first postoperative day and should remain flat thereafter. Following a non-drainage procedure, the volume of SRF should decrease each day so that the retina is flat by the third or fourth day following most acute RDs.

1. **Reaccumulation of SRF** following drainage or an increase in volume after non-drainage is caused by one of the following:

*a. An open break* which has not been sealed at the time of surgery is by far the most common cause.

*b. Exudative RD* resulting from excessive cryotherapy is very rare. It is important not to re-operate in these cases because the SRF will absorb spontaneously within 1 or 2 weeks.

2. **Slow absorption of SRF.** In some cases the SRF does not increase in volume but either fails to diminish or absorbs very slowly despite the fact that all breaks are closed. This may be caused by one of the following:

*a. Viscid SRF* in eyes with longstanding RD that have not been drained.

*b. Deficient RPE* in eyes with a hypopigmented fundus may be responsible for slow absorption of SRF. The collection of SRF is invariably located inferiorly and eventually absorbs after several weeks. In the meantime, the patient should be advised to sleep with the head elevated in order to prevent spread of SRF to the fovea.

*c. Residual tractional RD* in eyes with fixed folds or severe vitreoretinal traction. In these cases, a localised fold of elevated retina may persist postoperatively for a variable period of time.

## INTRAVITREAL AIR INJECTION

### 1. Indications

- Ocular hypotony after drainage of SRF.
- 'Fishmouthing' of a U-shaped tear.
- Radial retinal folds.

### 2. Technique

- Take a 25-gauge needle on a 5 ml syringe and make sure that both are dry to prevent the formation of small bubbles during injection.
- Fill the syringe with air through a micropore filter.
- With the toothed forceps, grasp a muscle tendon and position the globe so that the injection site is uppermost.
- Steady the globe and insert the needle 4 mm behind the limbus to avoid the vitreous base. Take care not to damage the long posterior ciliary arteries and nerves which run in the suprachoroidal space in line with the horizontal recti. If the eye is very soft following drainage of a large volume of SRF, a preliminary half-thickness scratch incision will facilitate the introduction of the needle without excessively deforming the globe.
- While viewing through the pupil using an indirect ophthalmoscope without a condensing lens, aim the needle at the centre of the vitreous cavity and push it through the pars plana.
- Do not pass the needle into the centre of the vitreous cavity but stop when the tip of the needle is just visible through the pupil. Make sure you have penetrated the non-pigmented epithelium of the pars plana.
- Make a single smooth injection (Fig. 6.90a) and at the same time check the intraocular pressure digitally.
- Quickly withdraw the needle; the incision is self-closing.

### 3. Problems

*a. Loss of fundus visualisation* as a result of the formation of small air bubbles in the vitreous (Fig. 6.90b) is the main disadvantage of air as compared with saline injection. This can be avoided by taking the following precautions:

- Ensure that the syringe and needle are dry.
- Inject with one movement of the plunger
- Do not introduce the needle into the centre of the vitreous cavity.
- The injection site should be uppermost so that the initial few small bubbles collect and remain around the tip of the needle before coalescing into a single large bubble. The small bubbles will usually coalesce after a few minutes. They can also be made to move out of the way by repositioning the globe.

*b. Severe elevation of intraocular pressure* by air injection is undesirable because it may result in corneal oedema, loss of buckle height and anterior displacement of an iris-supported lens with damage to the corneal endothelium. It is therefore better to have an eye that is slightly too soft than too hard. Management is as follows:

- Drain more SRF (if present), bearing in mind the danger of retinal incarceration.
- Aspirate air from the vitreous; this may be difficult if the cornea is oedematous.
- Perform an anterior chamber paracentesis.

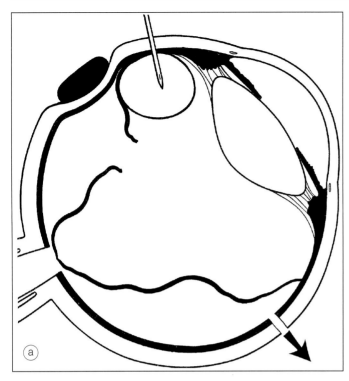

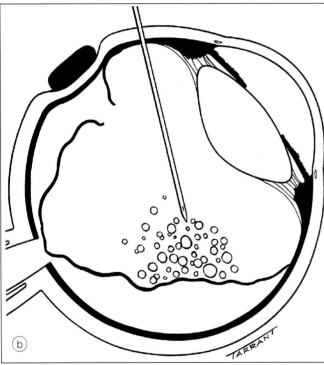

**Figure 6.90** Intravitreal air injection. **(a)** Correct method; **(b)** incorrect method

### 4. Complications

a. *Lens damage* can be avoided by taking into account the tilt of the globe and aiming the needle at the centre of the vitreous cavity and away from the lens.

b. *Retinal damage* may occur if the needle is inserted too posteriorly. Remember that the ora serrata is located 6 mm behind the limbus nasally and 7 mm temporally.

c. *Haemorrhage* is a rare complication resulting from damage to the long posterior ciliary arteries.

d. *Postoperative bacterial endophthalmitis* is very rare.

## CLINICAL EXAMPLES

The following clinical examples will emphasise the most important aspects of management just discussed.

### Fresh retinal detachment

1. **Preoperative considerations.** Examination shows a localised right upper temporal RD due to a U-tear (Fig. 6.91a). The prognosis for central vision is good because the macula is uninvolved. The patient should be operated on as soon as possible because the macula is in great danger for two reasons:

- The break is located in the upper temporal quadrant.
- SRF will spread quickly because the break is large.

2. **Surgical technique of cryotherapy and buckle.** Peritomy should extend from 8.30 to 12.30 o'clock to expose the lateral and superior recti. The tear should close on a 5 mm sponge explant. The sutures should be about 8 mm apart to impart adequate height to the buckle. The sponge should be placed radially (Fig. 6.91b) to prevent 'fishmouthing'. Accurate positioning of the explant is vital in this case. Failure to close the break may be due to an undersized buckle (Fig. 6.91c) or a malposition of the buckle (Fig. 6.91d). Alternatively, a solid 277 or 279 type explant could be used; however, this type of buckle creates less of an indent and is associated with an increased requirement for SRF drainage to ensure hole closure. Drainage of SRF is not otherwise required because:

- The retina is mobile.
- The break can be apposed to the RPE without difficulty.
- The SRF is not very viscous as the RD is fresh.

> **NB: It is also possible to treat this case with a pneumatic retinopexy procedure**

### Longstanding retinal detachment

1. **Preoperative considerations.** Examination shows an extensive right RD with macular involvement associated with a U-tear in the upper temporal quadrant and two small holes in the lower temporal quadrant (Fig. 6.92a). A partially pigmented demarcation line is present at the junction of detached and flat retina, and a secondary intraretinal cyst is present inferiorly. This is therefore a longstanding RD because demarcation marks take about 3 months to develop and secondary retinal cysts usually take about 12 months. The prognosis for restoration of good visual acuity is very poor because the fovea has probably been detached for at least 12 months. There is therefore no urgency for surgery, which can be performed at the patient's and surgeon's convenience.

2. **Surgical technique.** Peritomy should extend from 5.30 to 12.30 o'clock to expose the superior, lateral and inferior

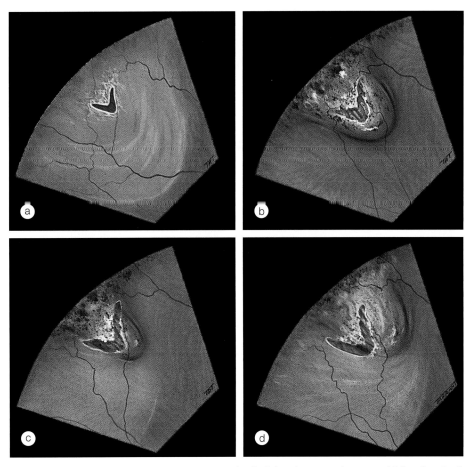

**Figure 6.91** Management of fresh upper temporal retinal detachment and causes of failure (see text)

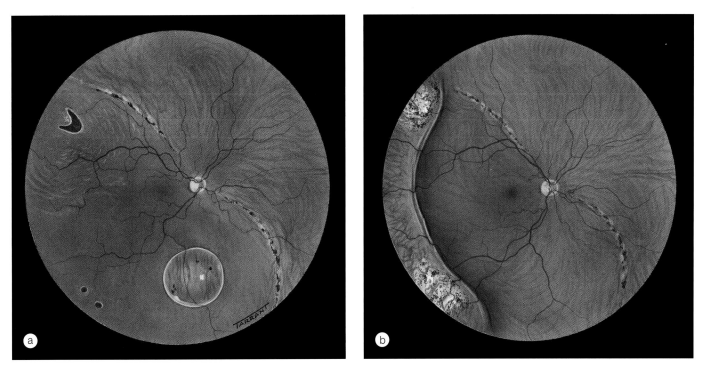

**Figure 6.92** Management of longstanding retinal detachment (see text)

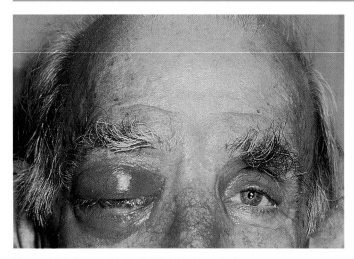

**Figure 6.93** Acute orbital cellulitis following retinal surgery

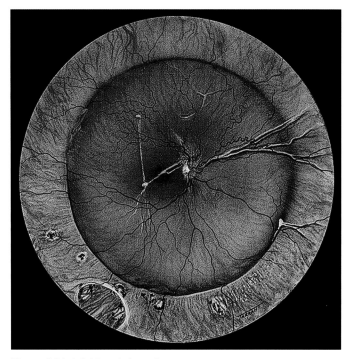

**Figure 6.94** A tight encirclement

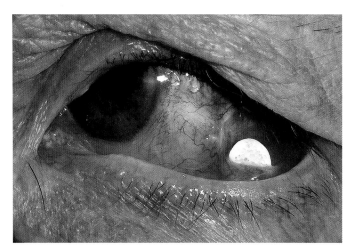

**Figure 6.95** Exposed sponge

recti. The breaks can be sealed with a long 4-mm-wide circumferential sponge explant extending from 7 to 10.30 o'clock or a circumferential solid 277 or 279 type explant (Fig. 6.92b). Drainage of SRF may be required because in longstanding cases SRF is viscous and may take a long time to absorb.

## POST-OPERATIVE COMPLICATIONS

1. **Acute orbital cellulitis** is usually due to infection of explant material (Fig. 6.93).

2. **Sterile vitritis** is rarely seen unless very excessive cryotherapy has been applied.

3. **Choroidal detachment** is caused by transudation of choroidal fluid into the potential space between the sclera and uvea. The two main predisposing factors are:

   - Prolonged severe ocular hypotony.
   - Damage to vortex veins, particularly by large posteriorly placed buckles.

4. **Elevation of intraocular pressure** may be caused by secondary angle-closure as a result of forward displacement of the iris–lens diaphragm and anterior rotation of the ciliary body. This is particularly likely to occur in eyes with pre-existing shallow anterior chambers in which a tight encircling procedure (Fig. 6.94) has obstructed the vortex veins.

5. **Bacterial endophthalmitis** is rare.

6. **Exposure of explant,** usually a sponge, may occur several weeks or months postoperatively (Fig. 6.95).

   a. *Causes*

   - Inadequate coverage of the explant with Tenon's capsule and conjunctiva during closure.
   - Inadequate suturing of the explant to the sclera.
   - Failure to trim the ends of the explant, so a sharp edge erodes through the conjunctiva.
   - Large sponge placed too anteriorly.

   b. *Treatment* involves removal of the sponge (Fig. 6.96), but, if this is performed in the first few postoperative months, it may be associated with redetachment.

7. **Migration of encircling strap**

   - Rarely, a strap may migrate anteriorly and even cut through the tendons of the rectus muscles (Fig. 6.97).
   - Migration into the globe is fortunately extremely rare (Fig. 6.98).

8. **Maculopathy** associated with variable impairment of visual acuity may be seen:

   a. *Macular epiretinal membrane formation* in the form of either cellophane maculopathy or macular pucker.

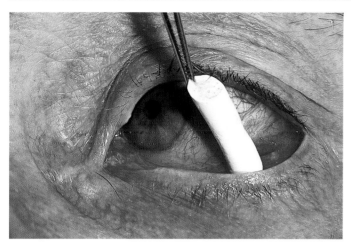

**Figure 6.96** Sponge removal

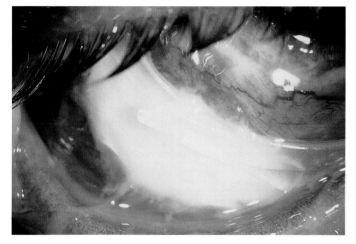

**Figure 6.97** Anterior migration and infection of an encircling strap

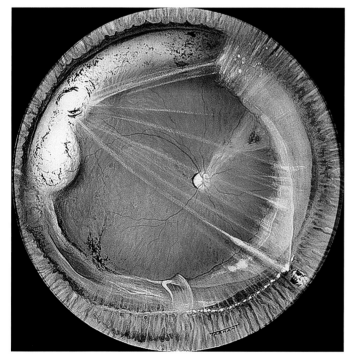

**Figure 6.98** Intraocular migration of an encircling strap

b. *Pigmentary maculopathy* – usually caused by pigment fallout as a result of excessive cryotherapy. Visual acuity, however, is usually unimpaired.

c. *Cystoid macular degeneration* unassociated with leakage of fluorescein from the perifoveal capillaries typically occurs in eyes with longstanding involvement of the macula by SRF. Visual acuity is usually very poor, and, when the cystoid changes resolve, they are replaced by degenerative lesions involving the RPE without any improvement in visual function.

d. *Atrophic maculopathy* is usually caused by the gravitation of blood in the subretinal space due to choroidal haemorrhage at the time of surgery.

e. *Delayed absorption of SRF at the macula,* which may persist for many months and stimulate a detachment of the RPE.

9. **Extraocular muscle imbalance.** Transient diplopia is fairly common during the immediate postoperative period following scleral buckling techniques.

a. *Predisposing factors*

- A large sponge inserted under one of the rectus muscles (Fig. 6.99). In most cases the diplopia resolves spontaneously after a few weeks or months and requires no specific therapy apart from reassurance or the temporary use of prisms. Very rarely the sponge has to be removed.

- Surgical disinsertion of a rectus muscle (usually superior or inferior rectus) in order to place a buckle under the muscle. This is now a rare cause of diplopia as muscle disinsertion is usually unnecessary.

- Rupture of a muscle belly due to excessive traction on the sutures. This may cause a complete and severe palsy unless the cut ends can be approximated. Treatment may be very difficult and requires muscle operations on both eyes.

- Severe conjunctival scarring, usually associated with repeated operations, may cause mechanical restriction of eye movements.

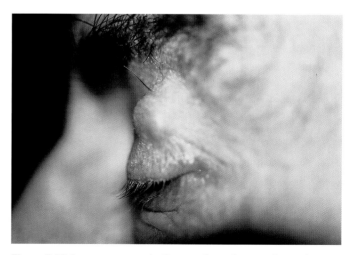

**Figure 6.99** Large sponge under the superior rectus muscle causing vertical diplopia and distortion of the upper eyelid

● Decompensation of a large heterophoria resulting from poor postoperative visual acuity in the operated eye.

b. *Treatment* of persistent diplopia may involve injection of botulinum toxin or surgery.

10. **Changes in refraction.** A local buckle may induce mild astigmatism, while encircling buckles may induce myopia (averages 2.75D) by increasing the axial length of the globe. The induced changes in refraction are usually stable by about the fourth month.

11. **Ptosis** may occur, particularly in elderly patients, due to postoperative stretching of an already attenuated levator aponeurosis by lid oedema.

12. **Cataract,** which is uncommon, may be caused by one of the following:

● Lens injury during intravitreal injections.
● Anterior segment necrosis.
● Progression of pre-existing lens opacities.
● Persistent RD.

## CAUSES OF FAILURE

***Missed breaks.*** It should be emphasised that about 50% of all RDs are associated with more than one break. In most cases the breaks are located within 90° of each other. At surgery, the surgeon should therefore not be satisfied if only one break has been found until a thorough search has been made for the presence of other breaks and the configuration of the RD corresponds to the position of the primary break. In eyes with hazy media or intraocular lens implants, visualisation of the peripheral retina may be difficult and all retinal breaks impossible to detect. As a last resort, the possibility of a hole at or near the posterior pole such as a true macular hole should be considered if no peripheral breaks can be detected.

### Operative causes
The main operative causes of failure to seal all breaks are as follows:

1. **Buckle failure** may be the result of the following:

● Buckle of inadequate size – replace (see Fig. 6.91c).
● Buckle incorrectly positioned – reposition (see Fig. 6.91d).
● Buckle of inadequate height – drain SRF or consider intravitreal gas injection.

2. **'Fishmouthing'** of the retinal tear (Fig. 6.100).

3. **A missed iatrogenic break** caused inadvertently during drainage of SRF.

***Proliferative vitreoretinopathy*** is the most common cause of late failure. The traction forces associated with PVR can occasionally open old breaks and create new ones. Presentation is typically between the fourth and sixth postoperative weeks. After an initial period of visual improvement follow-

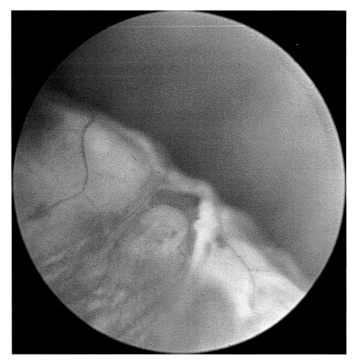

**Figure 6.100** Circumferential buckle with 'fishmouthing' of a U-tear

ing successful retina reattachment, the patient reports a sudden and progressive loss of vision, which may develop within a few hours.

***Reopening of retinal break*** in the absence of PVR may result of one of the following:

1. **Inadequate cryotherapy.** Small round holes do not usually leak postoperatively, even if they have not been adequately treated, provided they are located on the buckle. U-tears of moderate-to-large dimensions may leak postoperatively even though they are initially closed by the buckle, unless they are well surrounded by cryotherapy. This is because persistent traction on the flap of the tear may pull the sensory retina away from the RPE and allow SRF to re-accumulate.

2. **Inadequate buckling** of the vitreous base anterior to the retinal tear may result in reopening of the tear and anterior leakage of SRF.

3. **Late buckle failure** may be due to the following:

● Loosening of the encircling element.
● Spontaneous extrusion of the explant, as previously described.
● Removal of the explant because of infection or exposure, as previously described.

***New break formation*** may occasionally occur in areas subjected to persistent vitreoretinal traction following local buckling. This is less likely to occur following encircling procedures which give a permanent buckle. New inferior retinal breaks can form as a result of upward vitreous traction induced by an expanding intravitreal gas bubble following pneumatic retinopexy.

# Pars plana vitrectomy

## INTRODUCTION

**Main aims.** Pars plana vitrectomy is a microsurgical procedure designed to remove vitreous gel, usually in order to gain access to retinal pathology. The following are the main aims of vitrectomy in the management of RD:

- Removal of vitreous opacities.
- Excision of the posterior hyaloid face up to the posterior border of the vitreous base. Most surgeons believe it important to remove as much gel as possible to decrease the incidence of secondary breaks and other complications. The so-called 'core' vitrectomy which leaves extensive residual gel is usually reserved for cases where it is difficult to achieve good visualisation and gel clearance, such as acute endophthalmitis.
- Release of vitreoretinal traction.
- Retinal manipulation and re-attachment.
- Creation of a space within the vitreous cavity for subsequent internal tamponade.
- Miscellaneous aims, where appropriate, include removal of associated cataract, dislocated lens fragments or intraocular foreign bodies.

**Instrumentation** is complex, and, in addition to the vitreous cutter, many other instruments are available. The diameter of the shafts of most instruments is 0.9 mm (20-gauge) so that they are interchangeable and can be inserted through either sclerotomy.

1. **The cutter** has an inner guillotine blade which oscillates up to 1500 times per minute (Fig. 6.101 bottom), cutting the vitreous gel into tiny pieces and simultaneously removing it by suction into a collecting cassette. Cutter speeds are increasing with improvements in instrument technology, so gel can be removed with minimal transvitreal traction on the retina during surgery.

2. **The intraocular illumination source** is through a 20-gauge fibreoptic probe (Fig. 6.101 top) which delivers light from an 80–150 watt bulb.

3. **The infusion cannula** usually has an intraocular length of 4 mm, although in special circumstances, such as choroidal detachment or eyes with opaque media, a 6 mm cannula may be required.

4. **Accessory instruments**

   a. *Scissors* (Fig. 6.102 right) which can cut either vertically, for retinectomy and segmentation, or horizontally, for delamination of epiretinal membranes.
   b. *Forceps* (Fig. 6.102 left) for grasping epiretinal membranes, internal limiting membranes or foreign bodies.
   c. *Flute needle* and backflush flute needle (Fig. 6.103).
   d. *Endodiathermy* and endolaser delivery systems.

**The wide-angle viewing system** (Fig. 6.104) has revolutionised vitreoretinal surgery, dramatically improving the operative view. Most systems (e.g. BIOM, IBOS) use a combination of an indirect lens hanging beneath the operative microscope combined with a series of prisms to reinvert the image. The systems are non-contact and avoid the need for a skilled assistant to hold the older-style irrigating contact lenses. The field of view is almost out to the ora serrata, and higher magnification lenses are also available for macular work. The systems also provide a good view through poorly dilated pupils. The image quality, however, is very dependent on maintaining a wet cornea with balanced salt solution or hypromellose, and the stereopsis is not quite as good as with a contact lens for very fine macular surgery.

## Tamponading agents

1. **Purposes**

   - To achieve intraoperative retinal flattening by internal drainage of SRF and fluid–gas exchange.
   - To produce internal closure of retinal breaks during the postoperative period.
   - The ideal tamponading agent should have a high surface tension, be optically clear and biologically inert. In the absence of such an ideal substance, the following are in current use.

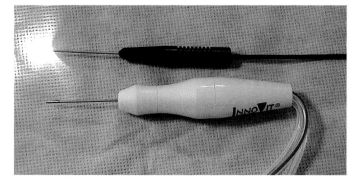

**Figure 6.101** (Top) Illumination pipe; (bottom) cutter

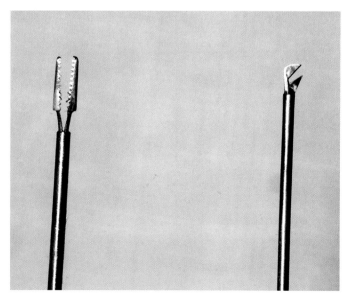

**Figure 6.102** (Left) forceps; (right) scissors

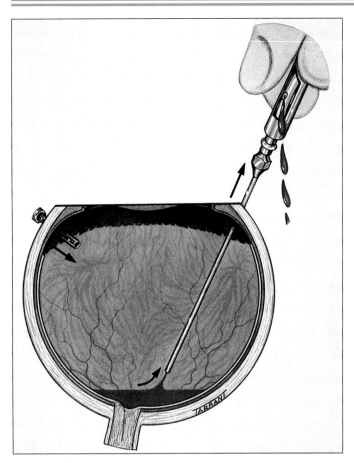

**Figure 6.103** Flute needle in situ

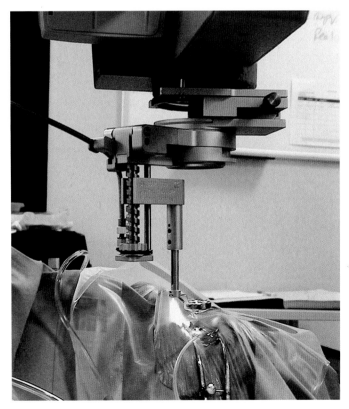

**Figure 6.104** Viewing system for vitreous surgery

2. **Expanding gases.** Although air can be used in certain cases, one of the following expanding gases is usually preferred in order to achieve prolonged intraocular tamponade:

- Sulphur hexafluoride ($SF_6$), which doubles its volume if used at a 100% concentration and lasts 10–14 days.
- Perfluorethane ($C_2F_6$), which triples its volume at 100% and lasts 30–35 days.
- Perfluoropropane ($C_3F_8$), which quadruples its volume at 100% and lasts 55–65 days.

> **NB:** Because the eye is usually left almost entirely gas-filled at the end of the procedure, most tamponading agents are used at an isolumetric concentration (e.g. 20–30% for $SF_6$ and 12–16% for $C_3F_8$).

3. **Heavy liquids** (perfluorocarbons) have a high specific gravity and thus remain in a dependent position when injected into the vitreous cavity. The main indications are as follows:

- To stabilise the posterior retina during epiretinal membrane dissection in eyes with PVR.
- To unfold giant retinal tears.
- To assist in removal of posteriorly dislocated lens fragments or intraocular lens implants.
- To stabilise the retina during retinotomy and macular translocation procedures.
- To aid retinal flattening during surgery of RDs caused by small anterior retinal breaks where aspiration of SRF can be challenging, particularly in phakic eyes. The use of heavy liquids can avoid the requirement for an additional drainage retinotomy. However, it should be emphasised that the vast majority of detachments can be drained directly through the causative break, particularly with the use of wide-angle viewing systems.

4. **Silicone oils** have a low specific gravity and are thus buoyant. They allow for more controlled intraoperative retinal manipulation and may also be used for prolonged postoperative intraocular tamponade. The most commonly used liquid silicones have relatively low viscosity (1000–5000 cs). The 1000 cs silicone is easy to inject and to remove, whilst 5000 cs silicone is less prone to the production of tiny droplets (emulsification). However, variation in viscosity is unrelated to surface tension.

5. **Long-term heavy liquid tamponade.** Although primarily developed for intraoperative use, newer perfluorocarbon compounds are now available for postoperative tamponade of the inferior retina. However, problems have been noted, with potential retinal toxicity and severe postoperative inflammation.

## INDICATIONS

Following the introduction of vitrectomy surgery for RD repair, the indications for vitrectomy surgery have now been expanded to include many other conditions, particularly those affecting the macula. It is impossible in a short textbook to adequately cover a rapidly advancing 'sub-speciality'. Therefore, RD repair will be discussed in some detail, while other indications will be mentioned briefly. Hopefully, this will be sufficient for the general or trainee ophthalmologist, while the specialist vitreoretinal surgeon will consult recent scientific publications for more detailed information.

Although the vast majority of simple rhegmatogenous RDs can be treated successfully by scleral buckling techniques, vitrectomy surgery has greatly improved the prognosis for more complex detachments. As techniques have improved and surgeons' familiarity and confidence have grown, the threshold for vitrectomy surgery has fallen. Many surgeons now feel that morbidity and success rates are better with vitrectomy for all pseudophakic RD, aphakic RD, and those that would otherwise require drainage of SRF. The guidelines below are therefore not absolute but intended to give some insight into the factors influencing the decision-making process.

### Rhegmatogenous RD

1. **In which retinal breaks cannot be visualised** as a result of haemorrhage, vitreous debris, posterior capsular opacity, intraocular lens edge effects. Vitrectomy is crucial to provide an adequate retinal view of all associated breaks. Scleral buckling carries a high risk of failure and PVR in such circumstances, if any retinal breaks are missed.

2. **In which retinal breaks cannot be closed by scleral buckling,** such as:

   - Giant retinal tears (Fig. 6.105).
   - Very posterior tears, particularly if large (Fig. 6.106).
   - Severe vitreoretinal traction as in PVR (Fig. 6.107).

**Tractional RDs,** which are caused by contraction of epiretinal membranes (usually preretinal, only rarely subretinal) rather than retinal breaks – the two main causes are: (a) advanced proliferative diabetic retinopathy and (b) penetrating trauma of the posterior segment. Less common indications for vitrectomy include tractional RD to branch retinal vein occlusion, posterior uveitis, and advanced retinopathy of prematurity.

1. **Indications in diabetic RD**

   a. *Tractional RD threatening or involving the macula* (Fig. 6.108). If necessary, vitrectomy can be combined with internal panretinal photocoagulation (Fig. 6.109). Extramacular tractional RD may be observed because, in many cases, it remains stationary for a long time provided the proliferative retinopathy has been controlled with adequate panretinal photocoagulation.

   b. *Combined tractional–rhegmatogenous RD* should be treated urgently, even if the macula is not involved, because SRF is likely to spread quickly.

2. **Indications in penetrating trauma**

   a. *Prevention of tractional RD.* Unlike diabetic retinopathy where epiretinal membrane proliferation occurs mostly on the posterior retina, fibrocellular proliferation after penetrating trauma tends to develop on the pre-equatorial retina and/or the ciliary body. Treatment is usually aimed at visual rehabilitation and minimising the tractional process.

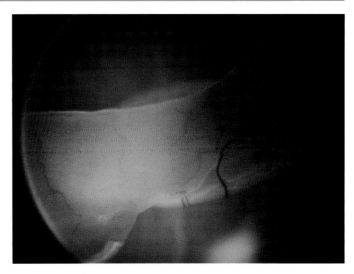

**Figure 6.105** Giant retinal tear

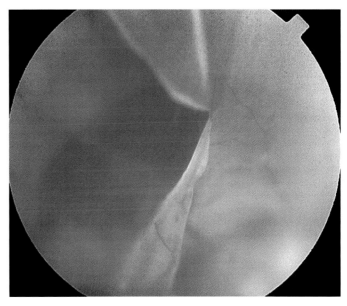

**Figure 6.106** Large posterior tear

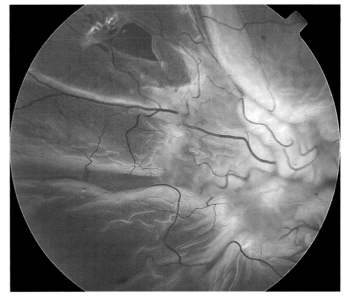

**Figure 6.107** Severe proliferative vitreoretinopathy

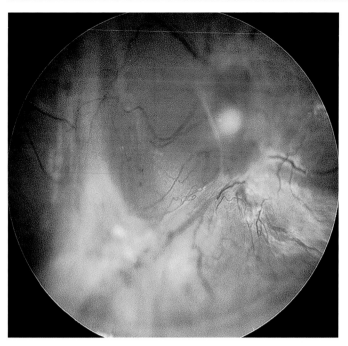

**Figure 6.108** Tractional retinal detachment involving the macula

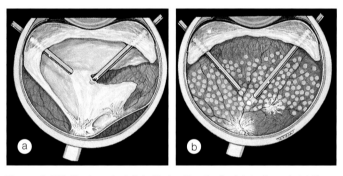

**Figure 6.109** Treatment of diabetic tractional retinal detachment. **(a)** Pars plana vitrectomy; **(b)** laser endophotocoagulation

b. *Late tractional RD,* which is usually associated with an intraocular foreign body, may develop months after otherwise successful removal of the foreign body.

## TECHNIQUE

### Preparation

#### 1. Technique

- Following limbal peritomy, an infusion cannula is secured to the sclera 3.5 mm behind the limbus in pseudophakic or aphakic eyes (4 mm in phakic eyes) at the level of the inferior border of the lateral rectus muscle.
- Two further sclerotomies are made at the 10 and 2 o'clock positions. These can be standard incisions made with an MVR blade or self-sealing sclerotomies.

### 2. Problems

a. *Suprachoroidal or subretinal infusion* can be avoided by ensuring that the infusion port of the cannula has penetrated well into the vitreous cavity and is not covered by uveal tissue or retina. This is more likely to occur in hypotonous eyes with pre-existing choroidal effusions and following penetrating trauma.

b. *Haemorrhage from the entry site* is an uncommon complication which tends to occur at the beginning of the procedure. The bleeding may be controlled by increasing the intraocular pressure via elevation of the infusion bottles but is usually mild and self-limiting.

c. *Incarceration of vitreous and/or retina* into the entry site may occur in eyes with bullous RDs. It can be prevented by plugging the sclerotomies and not starting the intraocular infusion until vitrectomy is about to begin. Any prolapsed vitreous should be abscised without exerting traction flush with the sclera.

d. *Entry-site breaks* may occur immediately behind sclerotomies.

---

**NB: It is important to thoroughly examine entry sites at the end of the procedure and treat any breaks appropriately.**

---

### *Basic vitrectomy*

#### 1. Technique

- Assemble indirect viewing system and insert the vitreous cutter and the fibreoptic light pipe through the upper two sclerotomies (Fig. 6.110).
- Excise the central vitreous gel and posterior capsule thickening if required.
- Identify and excise the posterior hyaloid face as far anteriorly as possible, usually flush with the posterior border of the vitreous base, creating a posterior hyaloid detachment if needed.

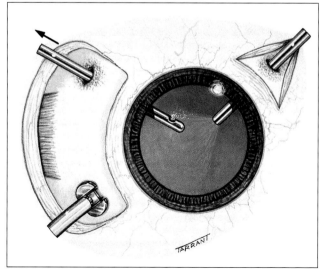

**Figure 6.110** Infusion cannula, light pipe and vitreous cutter in position

## 2. Problems

a. *Miosis* may occur during periods of hypotony or following inadvertent iris manipulation. Mydriasis may be restored either pharmacologically by injecting into the anterior chamber 0.1 ml of a 1:10 000 solution of adrenaline or mechanically by pupil-stretching sutures or retractors.

b. *Corneal epithelial oedema* is more likely to occur following frequent preoperative instillation of dilating drops and if surgery is unduly prolonged. Visualisation of the operating field may be improved by removing the loose epithelium taking care not to damage Bowman's layer and preserving a perilimbal rim of epithelium.

c. *Corneal stromal oedema* with folds in Descemet's membrane occurs more frequently in aphakic eyes and may give rise to annoying distortion and multiple images during fluid–air exchange. Visualisation may be improved by coating the endothelial corneal surface with a viscoelastic substance such as hyaluronic acid.

d. *Lens opacification* may occur as a result of either lens touch by an intraocular instrument or prolonged surgery, especially if fluid–gas exchange is repeated. A phacoemulsification or lensectomy may be required if lens opacification results in significant impairment of the surgical field.

e. *Preretinal haemorrhage* may occur during epiretinal membrane dissection, especially in the presence of proliferative diabetic retinopathy (see later). The risk of bleeding can be minimised by avoiding traction on neovascular tissue. Small bleeding points can be treated by increasing the intraocular pressure via raising the level of the infusion bottle. Larger bleeders may require treatment with unimanual or bimanual bipolar diathermy. Alternatively, careful direct pressure with the tip of an occluded flute needle for a few seconds will often arrest bleeding

f. *Intraretinal haemorrhage* in attached retina usually follows a forcible avulsion of preretinal fibrovascular tissue. The bleeding points can be sealed with the use of unimanual or bipolar diathermy by approximating the tip of the diathermy to the bleeding point and activating the diathermy directly over it.

g. *Expulsive suprachoroidal haemorrhage* is a devastating but fortunately very rare complication which is more likely to occur following periods of hypotony, especially in highly myopic, aphakic eyes. If recognised early, the bleeding may be controlled by the maintenance of a very high intraocular pressure and prompt closure of the entry sites. Drainage of the supra-choroidal blood at the time of surgery is ineffective because clotting occurs immediately.

> **NB: The above basic steps and potential problems apply to all vitrectomies. Subsequent steps depend on the characteristics of the RD.**

### *Large or posterior retinal breaks*

1. **Fluid–air exchange** (Fig. 6.111)
   - Place the tip of the flute needle over or inside the break.
   - The infusion line is turned to air rather than fluid injection.
   - The pressure of the progressively enlarging air bubble will force the SRF into the flute needle and out of the eye (hydraulic retinal re-attachment).

2. **Retinopexy** of the now flat retinal breaks with either trans-scleral cryotherapy or laser endophotocoagulation using minimal energy. Pre-treatment marking of all breaks with bipolar diathermy makes break location easier but is not necessary in all cases.

3. **Prolonged internal tamponade** is achieved by replacing air with a non-expansile concentration of sulphahexafluoride ($SF_6$) or perfluoropropane ($C_3F_8$) gases, or with silicone oil. The non-expansile mixture of gas and air is prepared in a large (50 ml) syringe and the air-filled vitreous cavity is flushed with 20% or 30% $SF_6$–air mixture or 14–16% $C_3F_8$–air mixture.

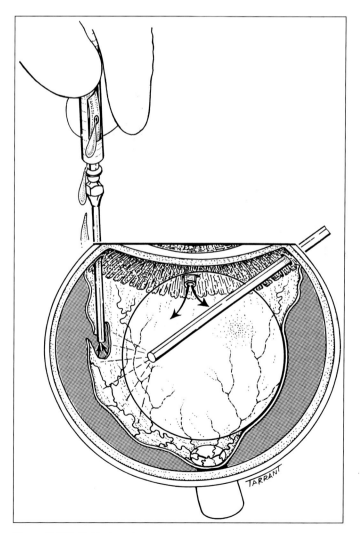

**Figure 6.111** Fluid–air exchange

### Giant retinal tears

1. **Unrolling of the flap** following a complete vitrectomy is achieved using 'heavy' perfluorocarbon liquids. The heavy liquid is slowly injected over the optic disc (Fig. 6.112). The expanding globule will both unfold the retina and expel the SRF through the giant tear into the vitreous cavity and out of the eye via a flute needle.

2. **Subsequent steps**

   ● Laser photocoagulation around the tear is performed directly via endolaser. Cryotherapy or indirect laser is applied to the anterior horns of the tear to avoid lens touch in phakic eyes. Laser photocoagulation is preferable to cryotherapy to treat most of the tear as it is less likely to induce extensive dispersion of the RPE.

   ● Scleral buckling is usually not required because most giant tears tend to involve the superior retina and can be closed by internal tamponade. Occasionally, however, the tear may extend below the horizontal meridian and patients should be asked to posture appropriately during the postoperative period.

   ● Heavy liquid/silicone oil exchange is performed. Some surgeons prefer tamponade with $C_3F_8$ gas, in which case great care must be taken to avoid retinal slippage during heavy liquid/air exchange.

> **NB:** Prophylaxis of the fellow eye is usually recommended because of the high risk of giant tear formation in patients with no obvious trauma as a precipitating factor.

***Proliferative vitreoretinopathy.*** The aims of surgery in PVR are to release transvitreal traction by vitrectomy and tangential (surface) traction by membrane dissection in order to restore retinal mobility and allow closure of retinal breaks.

1. **Membrane dissection.** Localised fixed retinal folds ('starfolds') may be freed by the removal of the central plaque of epiretinal membrane as follows:

   ● Engage the tip of the vertically cutting scissors in the edge of the valley of the membrane between two adjacent retinal folds (Fig. 6.113).
   ● Pull the membrane towards the ora serrata until it peels from the surface of the retina (Fig. 6.114). If the membrane is strongly attached to the retina, or the retina is too mobile, the membrane can be cut with scissors prior to its complete removal. As epiretinal traction is being relieved, the retina will become progres-

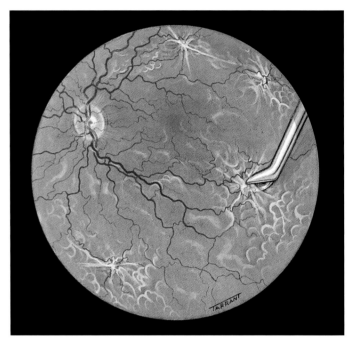

**Figure 6.113** Dissecting of starfolds with vertically cutting scissors in proliferative vitreoretinopathy

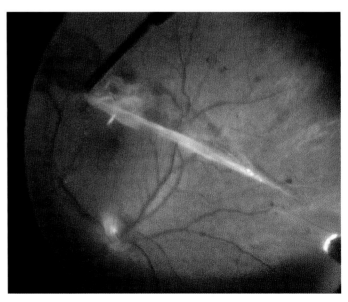

**Figure 6.114** Peeling of an epiretinal membrane

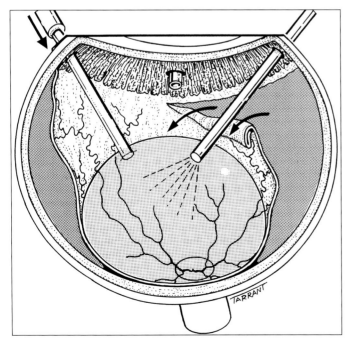

**Figure 6.112** Unrolling of a giant retinal tear using heavy liquid

sively more mobile, so that further attempts at membrane dissection may be hampered. The use of heavy liquids to stabilise the posterior retina greatly improves the ability to continue further dissection towards the vitreous base. In the presence of severe contraction of the vitreous base (anterior PVR), it may be necessary to perform a lensectomy in order to complete the dissection.

- If sufficient traction can be released and there is not significant retinal shortening, a fluid–air exchange can be performed followed by retinopexy; alternatively, retinopexy can be applied under heavy liquid prior to fluid–air exchange.
- The intraocular air is then exchanged for an extended intraocular tamponading agent such as $C_3F_8$ or silicone oil.
- Some surgeons also prefer to insert a local or circumferential scleral explant in such cases, to provide additional relief of any residual traction.

**2. Relieving retinotomy.** The decision to perform a relieving retinotomy is made after epiretinal membrane dissection has been performed as completely as possible but the retinal mobility is deemed insufficient for lasting re-attachment.

- Coagulate the retina and its blood vessels using unimanual diathermy.
- Perform the retinotomy with vertically cutting scissors (Fig. 6.115). To be efficient, the cut must be large and extend through the inferior $180°$.
- Alternatively, the vitreous cutter may be used to perform the retinotomy and remove redundant anterior retina in the same step. Most retinotomies are sited behind the posterior border of the vitreous base and are circumferentially orientated. Occasionally, radial retinotomies are used for rigid posterior margins of long-standing retinal tears.
- Heavy liquid is used to stabilise the retina, allowing laser retinopexy prior to heavy liquid/oil exchange, as for a giant retinal tear.

***Tractional retinal detachments.*** The goal of vitrectomy in tractional RDs is to release anteroposterior and/or circumferential vitreoretinal traction. Because the membranes are vascularised – and the retina often friable – they cannot be

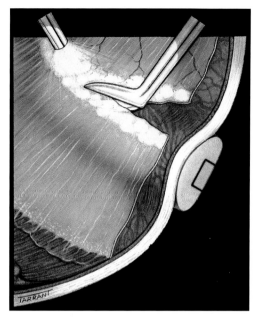

**Figure 6.115** Relieving retinotomy in proliferative vitreoretinopathy

simply peeled from the surface of the retina, as this would result in haemorrhage and tearing of the retina. The two methods of removing fibrovascular membranes in diabetic tractional RDs are the following.

**1. Delamination** involves the horizontal cutting of the individual vascular pegs connecting the membranes to the surface of the retina (Fig. 6.116). This is preferred to segmentation (see below) because it allows the complete removal of fibrovascular tissues from the retinal surface (en-bloc delamination). The technique is as follows:

- Cut a window in the partially detached posterior hyaloid and pass horizontally cutting scissors into the retrohyaloid space.
- Gain access to the cleavage plane between the membrane and the detached retina by elevating a posterior extension of the membrane to which thin atrophic retina is often adherent. Failure to find this plane will cause splitting of the membrane, leading to haemorrhage and inadequate dissection.

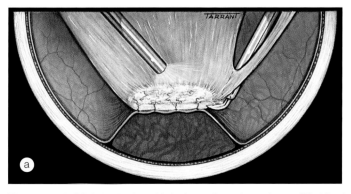 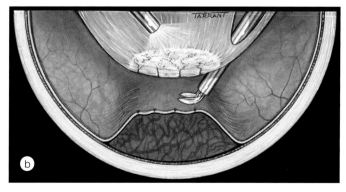

**Figure 6.116 (a)** Delamination with horizontally cutting scissors; **(b)** delamination completed

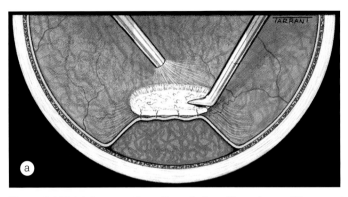 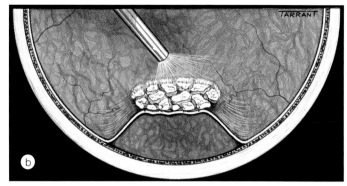

**Figure 6.117 (a)** Segmentation with vertically cutting scissors; **(b)** segmentation completed

- Divide the vascular attachments ('pegs') individually as the remaining posterior hyaloid draws the edges of the freed membrane away from the retinal surface.
- Excise the membrane–posterior hyaloid complex with the cutter.

2. **Segmentation** involves the vertical cutting of epiretinal membranes into small segments (Fig. 6.117). It is used to release circumferential vitreoretinal traction when delamination is difficult or impossible, such as in very mobile combined tractional–rhegmatogenous RD associated with posterior retinal breaks. The technique is as follows:

- Perform a complete vitrectomy and divide the posterior hyaloid attachment to the epiretinal membrane ('truncation' of the posterior hyaloid).
- Engage the lower blade of vertically cutting scissors in the cleavage space between the membrane and the retinal surface.
- Cut the membrane into small segments, usually with the vascular pegs in their centres.
- Seal bleeding points with diathermy.

Provided there are no retinal breaks, internal tamponade is not required in the treatment of tractional RDs ('no tear, no air'). However, in the presence of retinal breaks (pre-existing or iatrogenic) hydraulic re-attachment by fluid–air exchange is performed and the edges of the break are treated with retinopexy. In diabetics, internal tamponade with a long-acting gas is preferred to silicone oil.

## POSTOPERATIVE COMPLICATIONS

***Raised intraocular pressure*** may be caused by the following mechanisms:

1. **Secondary angle-closure glaucoma** may be associated with choroidal swelling and ciliary body rotation. Treatment is with mydriatics and cycloplegics.

2. **Overexpansion of intraocular gas** may cause raised intraocular pressure as a result of complete filling of the vitreous cavity if the concentration of expansile gas used was inadvertently too high. If the intraocular pressure cannot be controlled medically, 0.1–1 ml of the gas should be removed. This may have to be repeated if the remaining gas continues to expand.

3. **Silicone oil-associated glaucoma**

a. *Early glaucoma* is caused by pupil block by silicone oil in the anterior chamber (Fig. 6.118). This occurs particularly in the aphakic eye with an intact iris diaphragm. In aphakic eyes this can be prevented by performing an inferior ('Ando') iridectomy at the time of surgery (Fig. 6.119). The iridectomy allows free passage of aqueous to the anterior chamber so that the silicone remains behind the iris plane and does not block the pupil.

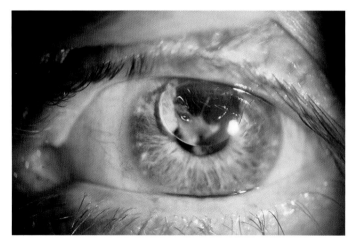

**Figure 6.118** Silicone oil in the anterior chamber

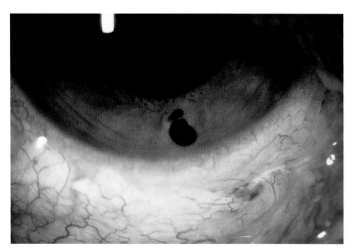

**Figure 6.119** Inferior (Ando) iridotomy

*b.* *Late glaucoma* is caused by emulsified silicone in the anterior chamber (Fig. 6.120) which causes trabecular blockage (Fig. 6.121). This complication may be reduced by an early removal of silicone oil either via the pars plana in phakic eyes or via the limbus in aphakic eyes (Fig. 6.122). Unfortunately, following removal of silicone oil, there is a risk of retinal re-detachment.

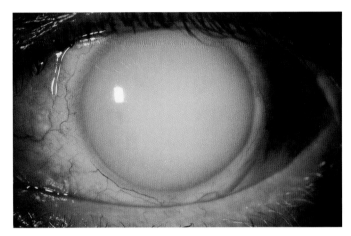

**Figure 6.120** Emulsified silicone oil in the anterior chamber

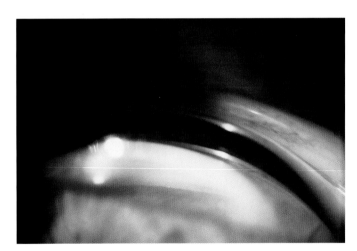

**Figure 6.121** Emulsified silicone oil in the chamber angle which may cause trabecular blockage

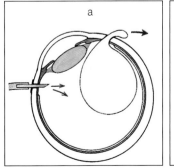
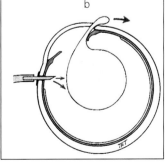

**Figure 6.122** Technique of removal of silicone oil. **(a)** In a phakic eye; **(b)** in an aphakic eye

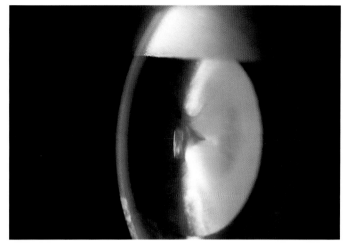

**Figure 6.123** Cataract and emulsified silicone oil (inverted 'pseudo-hypopyon')

4. **Ghost cell glaucoma.** Following a complete vitrectomy in patients with dense vitreous haemorrhage associated with RD, the residual effete red blood cells may enter the anterior chamber and, because their pliability is lost, they mechanically block the trabecular meshwork and impair aqueous outflow. In most cases medical treatment is sufficient to control the pressure, although occasionally an anterior chamber washout may be required.

5. **Steroid-induced glaucoma** may occur due to prolonged postoperative use of strong steroids in susceptible individuals.

*Cataract* may be caused by the following mechanisms:

1. **Gas-induced.** The use of either a large or long-lived intra-vitreal gas bubble almost invariably gives rise to feathering of the posterior subcapsular lens cortex. Fortunately, lens opacification is usually transient in these circumstances.

2. **Silicone-induced.** Almost all phakic eyes with silicone oils eventually develop cataract (Fig. 6.123). The initial hope that the early removal of silicone would prevent lens opacification has not been realised. If a cataract develops, the silicone oil can be removed in conjunction with phaco-emulsification cataract extraction, posterior capsulorhexis and posterior chamber lens implantation.

3. **Delayed cataract formation.** Following successful vitrec-tomy, a large proportion of eyes develop nuclear sclerosis within 1 year if the patient is over 50 years of age.

*Recurrent vitreous haemorrhage.* Most diabetic eyes develop a transient vitreous haemorrhage within the first 2 postoperative days following extensive dissection of fibro-vascular tissue. If the haemorrhage becomes recurrent, or per-sists beyond 1 month, persistent retinal neovascularisation or neovascularisation of the anterior hyaloid should be suspect-ed and treated.

*Retinal re-detachment.* Whilst the initial success rate for retinal re-attachment is generally high, the complex nature of

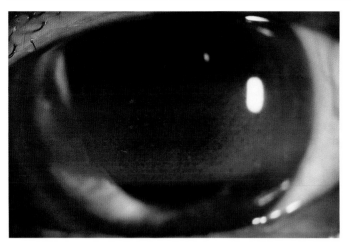

**Figure 6.124** Silicone oil-induced band keratopathy

cases requiring vitrectomy puts such eyes at a higher risk of re-detachment. The commonest time for this to occur is when the intraocular gas bubble has absorbed (usually 3–6 weeks postoperatively) or following removal of silicone oil. Causes include the following:

- Re-opening of the original break may occur because of either inadequate dissection at the time of original surgery in eyes with PVR or the re-proliferation of epiretinal membranes, the latter being more common in eyes with proliferative diabetic retinopathy.
- Failure to detect all breaks present preoperatively and iatrogenic breaks created around pars plana entry sites.

***Band keratopathy*** may occur as a result of prolonged contact between silicone oil and the corneal endothelium (Fig. 6.124).

## FURTHER READING

Asaria RH, Kon CH, Bunce C, et al. How to predict proliferative vitreoretinopathy: a prospective study. *Ophthalmology* 2001;108: 1184–1186.

Asaria RHY, Gregor ZJ. Simple retinal detachments: identifying the at-risk case. *Eye* 2002;16:404–410.

Byer NE. Lattice degeneration of the retina. *Surv Ophthalmol* 1979; 23:213–248.

Byer NE. The long-term natural history of senile retinoschisis with implications for management. *Ophthalmology* 1986;93:1127–1137.

Byer NE. Long-term natural history of lattice degeneration of the retina. *Ophthalmology* 1989;96:1396–1402.

Byer NE. What happens to untreated asymptomatic retinal breaks, and are they affected by posterior vitreous detachment? *Ophthalmology* 1998;105;1045–1049.

Byer NE. Subclinical retinal detachment resulting from asymptomatic retinal breaks. *Ophthalmology* 2001;108:1499–1504.

Byer NE. Perspectives on the management of complications of senile retinoschisis. *Eye* 2002;16:359–364.

Campochiaro PA. Pathogenetic mechanisms in proliferative vitreoretinopathy. *Arch Ophthalmol* 1997;115:237–241.

Charteris DG. Proliferative vitreoretinopathy: pathobiology, surgical management, and adjunctive treatment. *Br J Ophthalmol* 1995; 79:953–960.

Charteris DG, Sethi CS, Lewis GP, et al. Proliferative vitreoretinopathy – developments in adjunctive treatment and retinal pathology. *Eye* 2002;16:369–374.

Cowley M, Conway BP, Campochiaro PA, et al. Clinical risk factors for proliferative vitreoretinopathy. *Arch Ophthalmol* 1989;107: 1147–1151.

Ghazi NG, Green WR. Pathology and pathogenesis of retinal detachment. *Eye* 2002;411–421.

Hassan TS, Sarrafizadeh R, Ruby AJ, et al, The effect of duration of macular detachment on results after scleral buckle repair of primary, macula-off retinal detachments. *Ophthalmology* 2002; 109:146–152.

Hikichi T, Trempe CL. Relationship between floaters, light flashes, or both, and complications of posterior vitreous detachment. *Am J Ophthalmol* 1994;117:593–598.

Kleinmann G, Rechtman E, Pollack A, et al. Pneumatic retinopexy. Results in eyes with classic vs relative indications. *Arch Ophthalmol* 2002;120:1455–1459.

Kon CH, Asaria RH, Occleston NL, et al. Risk factors for proliferative vitreoretinopathy after pars plana vitrectomy: a prospective study. *Br J Ophthalmol* 2000;84:506–511.

Lewis H. Peripheral retinal degenerations and the risk of retinal detachment. *Am J Ophthalmol* 2003;136:155–160.

Minihan M, Tanner V, Williamson TH. Primary rhegmatogenous retinal detachment: 20 years of change. *Br J Ophthalmol* 2001;85: 546–548.

Pastor JC. Proliferative vitreoretinopathy: an overview. *Surv Ophthalmol* 1998;43:3–18.

Ross WH. Visual recovery after macula-off retinal detachment. *Eye* 2002;16:440–446.

Schwartz SG, Kuhl DP, McPherson AR, et al. Twenty-year follow-up for scleral buckling. *Arch Ophthalmol* 2002;120:325–329.

Scott JD. Future perspectives in primary retinal detachment repair. *Eye* 2002;16:349–352.

Sharma T, Challa JK, Ravishankar KV, et al. Scleral buckling for retinal detachment. Predictors for anatomic failure. *Retina* 1994;14: 338–343.

Tanner V, Harle D, Tan J, et al. Acute posterior vitreous detachment: the predictive value of vitreous pigment and symptomatology. *Br J Ophthalmol* 2000;84: 1264–1268.

Tanner V, Minihan M, Williamson TH. Management of inferior retinal breaks during pars plana vitrectomy for retinal detachments. *Br J Ophthalmol* 2001;85:480–482.

Tanner V, Haider A, Rosen P. Phacoemulsification and combined management of intraocular silicone oil. *J Cataract Refract Surg* 1998;24:585–591.

The Eye Disease Case-control Study Group. Risk factors for idiopathic rhegmatogenous retinal detachment. *Am J Ophthalmol* 1993;137:749–757.

The Retina Society Terminology Committee. The classification of retinal detachment with proliferative vitreoretinopathy. *Ophthalmology* 1983;90:121–125.

Wilkinson CP. Evidence-based analysis of prophylactic treatment of asymptomatic retinal breaks and lattice degeneration. *Ophthalmology* 2000;107:12–15.

Wolfensberger TJ, Aylward GW, Leaver PK. Prophylactic 360 degree cryotherapy in fellow eyes of patients with spontaneous giant retinal tears. *Ophthalmology* 2003;110:1175–1177.

# TUMOURS

# TUMOURS OF THE CHOROID

## Choroidal Naevus

Choroidal naevi are present in about 5–10% of Caucasians but are very rare in dark-skinned races. Although they are probably present at birth, growth occurs mainly during the pre-pubertal years and is extremely rare thereafter. For this reason, clinically detectable growth should arouse suspicion of malignancy.

***Histology.*** A naevus is a hamartoma composed of the following four types of naevus cells which are derived from the neural crest.

1. **Spindle cells** with small nuclei and variable pigmentation.

2. **Polyhedral cells** which are deeply pigmented and have small ovoid nuclei ('melanocytoma cells').

3. **Dendritic cells,** with long branching processes, large nuclei, prominent nucleoli and variable pigmentation.

4. **Balloon cells** which are large, non-pigmented, polyhedral and contain foamy cytoplasm.

> **NB:** Choroidal naevi induce secondary changes of the retinal pigment epithelium (RPE), which influence their ophthalmoscopic appearance. These abnormalities include drusen, multilayering of RPE cells, RPE atrophy, accumulation of lipofuscin deposits ('orange pigment'), RPE detachments and choroidal neovascularisation.

### *Diagnosis*

1. **Presentation.** The vast majority of naevi are asymptomatic and detected by routine examination. Rarely, symptoms may be caused by involvement of the fovea by the tumour itself or serous retinal detachment.

2. **Typical naevus**

   - Usually post-equatorial, oval or circular, slate-blue or grey lesion with detectable but not sharp borders (Fig. 7.1).
   - Dimensions are <3 mm in diameter and <1 mm in thickness.

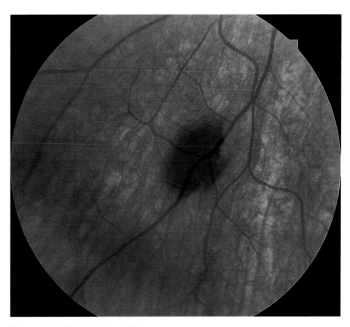

**Figure 7.1** Typical choroidal naevus

- Surface drusen may be present, particularly in the central area of a larger lesion (Fig. 7.2).
- Serous macular detachment is uncommon and may occur either as a direct result of RPE disturbance or secondary to choroidal neovascularisation (Fig. 7.3).

### 3. Atypical naevus

- An amelanotic naevus (Fig. 7.4).
- A 'halo' naevus which is surrounded by a pale zone resembling choroidal atrophy, histologically consisting of balloon-cell degeneration within the tumour cells (Fig. 7.5). This is believed to be associated with a relatively small chance of malignant growth.

### 4. Suspicious tumour

- Symptoms such as blurred vision, metamorphopsia, field loss and photopsia.
- Dimensions are >5 mm in diameter and >1 mm in thickness.
- Traces of surface orange pigment at the level of the RPE, consisting of macrophages containing lipofuscin (Fig. 7.6).
- Absence of surface drusen on a thick lesion.
- Margin of the lesion at or near the optic disc (Fig. 7.7).
- Serous retinal detachment either over the surface of the lesion or inferiorly.

> **NB:** The greater the number of these features, the higher the chance that the lesion is a melanoma.

### 3. Investigations

a. *Fluorescein angiography (FA)* findings depend on the amount of pigmentation within the naevus and associated changes in the overlying RPE. Most naevi are avascular and pigmented, giving rise to hypofluorescence caused by blockage of background choroidal fluorescence. If the lesion is associated with surface drusen, this will result in areas of hyperfluorescence (Fig. 7.8). The latter may also be caused by serous retinal detachment and choroidal neovascularisation.

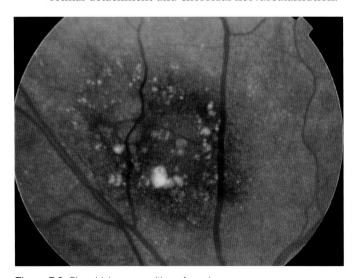

**Figure 7.2** Choroidal naevus with surface drusen

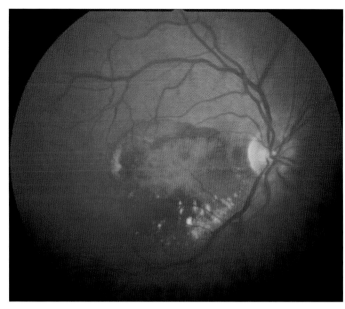

**Figure 7.3** Choroidal naevus with neovascular membrane, haemorrhage and exudates

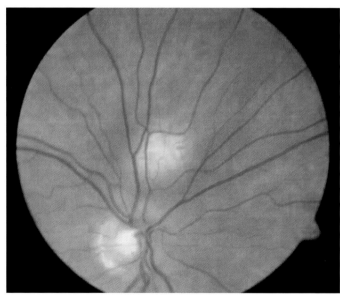

**Figure 7.4** Presumed amelanotic choroidal naevus

> **NB:** FA is usually not helpful in distinguishing a small melanoma from a naevus, although multiple pinpoint areas of hyperfluorescence may predict future growth.

b. *Indocyanine green (ICG) angiography* shows hypofluorescence relative to the surrounding choroid (Fig. 7.9).
c. *Ultrasonography (US)* shows a localised flat or slightly elevated lesion with high internal acoustic reflectivity (Fig. 7.10); a low internal reflectivity is suggestive of malignancy. Although useful in documenting tumour thickness, measurement of basal dimensions is only approximate because tapering margins are difficult to delineate.

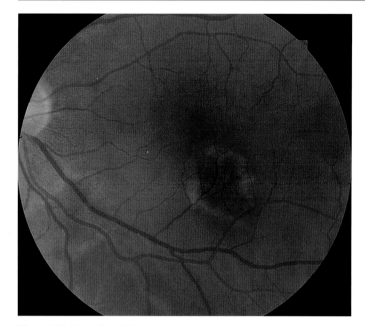

**Figure 7.5** Halo choroidal naevus

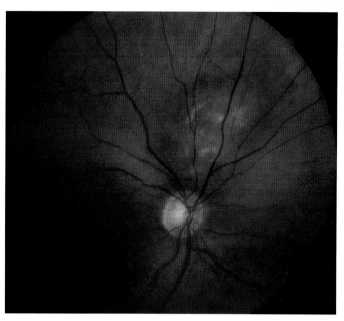

**Figure 7.7** Suspicious juxtapapillary choroidal tumour

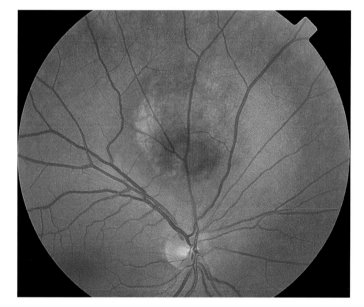

**Figure 7.6** Suspicious choroidal tumour with traces of orange (lipofuscin) pigment

## Management

1. **Typical naevi** do not require special follow-up because the risk of malignant transformation is extremely low, but they should be documented if the patient is reviewed for another condition.

2. **Suspicious tumours** require baseline fundus photography and US, and then indefinite follow-up. It should be sufficient to compare the ophthalmoscopic appearances with a baseline colour photograph, using landmarks such as retinal blood vessels. Fundus photography and US should be repeated if growth is suspected. It is difficult to detect small changes in thickness by US because of measurement variation of ±0.5 mm. Once growth has been documented, the lesion should be reclassified as a melanoma and managed accordingly.

> **NB: It is not known at what stage melanomas begin to metastasise. Lethal systemic spread may start when they are indistinguishable from large, suspicious naevi; consequently, once a definitive clinical diagnosis of malignancy has been made, it may be too late to prevent metastasis. On receiving this information, most patients opt for treatment rather than observation. There is therefore a trend towards earlier treatment, especially if this is unlikely to cause significant visual loss. This approach has been encouraged by the development of transpupillary thermotherapy, which is administered under local anaesthesia on an out-patient basis (see later).**

### Differential diagnosis

1. **Congenital hypertrophy of the RPE** is dark and flat, with a well-defined outline.

2. **Melanocytoma of the choroid** is clinically indistinguishable from a large naevus.

3. **Small melanoma** is usually associated with serous retinal detachment and orange pigment.

## FURTHER READING

Callanan DG, Lewis ML, Byrne SF, et al. Choroidal neovascularization associated with choroidal nevi. *Arch Ophthalmol* 1993;111:789–794.

Shields CL, Cater J, Shields JA, et al. Combination of clinical factors predictive of growth of small choroidal melanocytic tumors. *Arch Ophthalmol* 2000; 118:360–364.

The Collaborative Ocular Melanoma Study Group. Factors predictive of growth and treatment of small choroidal melanoma. COMS report no. 5. *Arch Ophthalmol* 1997;115:1537–1544.

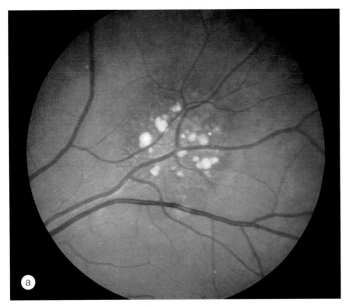

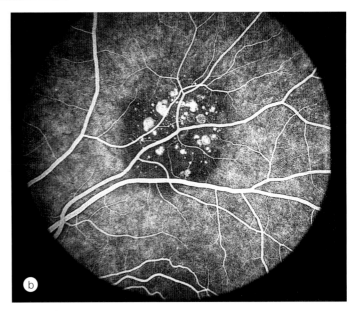

**Figure 7.8 (a)** Typical choroidal naevus with surface drusen; **(b)** FA shows hypofluorescence due to blockage of background choroidal fluorescence and areas of hyperfluorescence corresponding to surface drusen

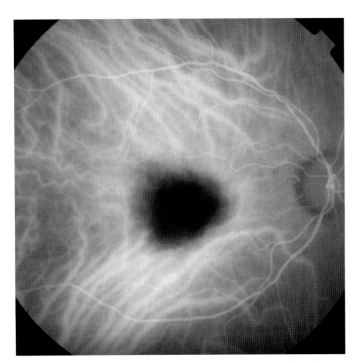

**Figure 7.9** ICG angiogram of a choroidal naevus shows masking of choroidal fluoresecence (Courtesy of B.A. Lafaut)

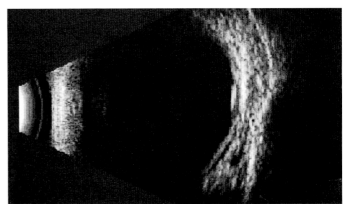

**Figure 7.10** Ultrasonography of a choroidal naevus (Courtesy of Dr. M. Karolczak-Kulesza)

lar melanoma is two to three times more common in blue/grey than brown eyes. Melanoma of the choroid is the most common primary intraocular tumour in adults and accounts for 95% of uveal melanomas (ciliary body, 2%; iris, 3%).

## PREDISPOSITIONS

1. **Congenital ocular melanocytosis** is associated with approximately a 1-in-400 chance of melanoma. It is characterised by an increased population of melanocytes within the uvea and episclera. Clinically, it is manifest by the following:

   ● Multifocal, slate-grey episcleral pigmentation (Fig. 7.11) and hyperpigmentation of the uvea, which gives rise to ipsilateral hyperchromic heterochromia iridis (Fig. 7.12) and hyperpigmentation of the fundus (Fig. 7.13).

   ● Occasional features include iris mammillations (Fig. 7.14) and glaucoma.

## Choroidal Melanoma

### EPIDEMIOLOGY

In general, the overall incidence of uveal melanomas is about five cases per million persons per year, with no significant gender difference. The tumour is extremely rare in children and is much more common in Caucasians than in dark-skinned races. Epidemiological studies suggest that intraocu-

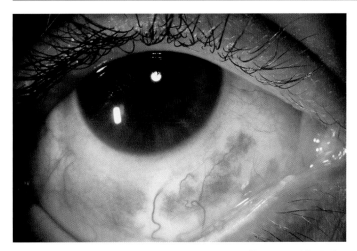

**Figure 7.11** Congenital subepithelial melanocytosis (Courtesy of B. Jay)

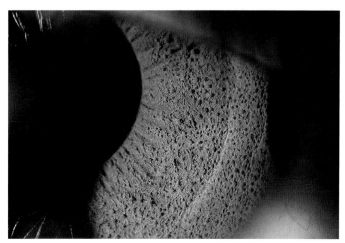

**Figure 7.14** Iris mammilation in naevus of Ota

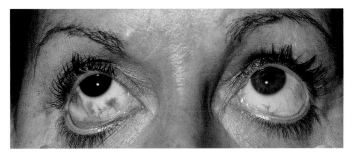

**Figure 7.12** Right iris hyperchromia and subepithelial melanocytosis in naevus of Ota.

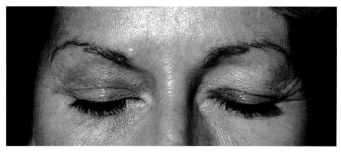

**Figure 7.15** Right cutaneous hyperpigmentation in naevus of Ota.

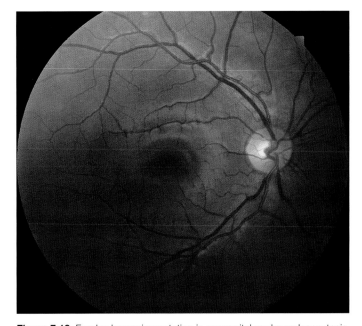

**Figure 7.13** Fundus hyperpigmentation in congenital ocular melanocytosis

- Hyperpigmentation of facial skin, most frequently in the distribution supplied by the first and second divisions of the ipsilateral trigeminal nerve ('oculodermal melanocytosis' or 'naevus of Ota') (Fig. 7.15).

2. **Melanocytoma** is a deeply pigmented naevus which is most commonly recognised at the optic disc but which can occur anywhere in the uveal tract (see later).

3. **Other predispositions**

   - Atypical cutaneous naevi.
   - Familial cutaneous melanoma.
   - Neurofibromatosis-1.

## PATHOLOGY

### Cell type

1. **Spindle B** cells are long and fusiform with an oval nucleus containing a prominent nucleolus.

2. **Epithelioid** cells are large and round with abundant eosinophilic cytoplasm with a large nucleus containing a conspicuous nucleolus.

3. **Intermediate** cells, which have features of both spindle and epithelioid cells.

### Modified Callender classification of uveal melanomas

1. **Spindle cell** melanomas, comprising 45% of tumours, are composed only of spindle cells, with a small percentage described as *fascicular* because of the pallisading or ribbon-like arrangement of cells in parallel rows (Fig. 7.16).

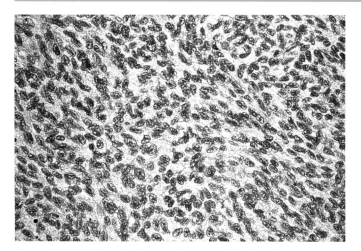

**Figure 7.16** Spindle cell melanoma (Courtesy of A. Garner)

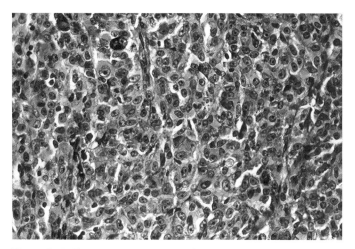

**Figure 7.17** Epithelioid cell melanoma (Courtesy of A. Garner)

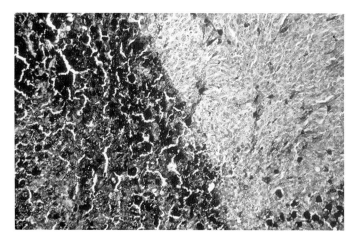

**Figure 7.18** Mixed cell melanoma (Courtesy of A. Garner)

2. **Epithelioid cell** melanomas (5%) consisting only of this cell type (Fig. 7.17).

3. **Mixed cell** melanomas (45%) consisting of the two cell types in variable proportion (Fig. 7.18).

4. **Necrotic** melanomas (5%) in which the predominant cell type is unrecognisable (Fig. 7.19).

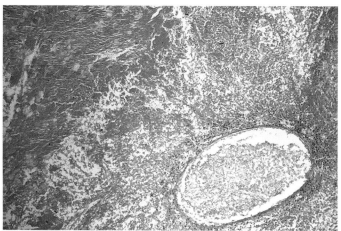

**Figure 7.19** Necrotic melanoma (Courtesy of A. Garner)

## Pattern of tumour spread

- Rupture of Bruch's membrane and RPE, with herniation into the subretinal space, often with the development of a 'collar-stud' shape (Fig. 7.20).
- Perforation of the retina, with vitreous seeding and haemorrhage.
- Invasion of scleral openings for blood vessels and nerves, resulting in orbital spread.
- Invasion of optic nerve is rare, but the tumour may encircle the optic disc.
- Invasion of vortex veins, with metastatic spread. Clinical metastatic disease involves the liver in more than 90% of patients. Other sites such as lung, bone, skin and brain are affected less often and usually in association with liver disease.

> **NB: About 5% of ocular tumours grow diffusely and do not result in a significant increase in choroidal thickness. Extraocular spread is common at the time of diagnosis.**

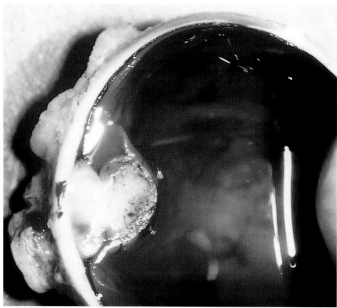

**Figure 7.20** Collar-stud choroidal melanoma

## Prognostic factors for survival

1. **Histological features** implying an adverse prognosis include large numbers of epithelioid cells per high-power field, closed laminin loops within the tumour and lymphocytic infiltration.

2. **Cytogenic abnormalities** within the tumour cells, such as monosomy 3 and gains in chromosome 8, are associated with a 50% death rate at 5 years.

3. **Size:** large tumours have a worse prognosis than small tumours, particularly if the basal diameter exceeds 16 mm.

4. **Extrascleral extension** carries a poor prognosis, because the tumour usually shows aggressive histological and cytological features.

5. **Location:** anterior tumours involving the ciliary body have a worse prognosis.

6. **Local tumour recurrence** after conservative treatment is associated with a poor prognosis for survival. This is probably because the recurrence is an indication that the original tumour was relatively aggressive.

## DIAGNOSIS

**Presentation** peaks at around the age of 60 years and occurs in one of the following ways:

- An asymptomatic tumour detected by chance on fundus examination performed for other reasons.
- A symptomatic tumour causing decreased visual acuity, metamorphopsia, visual field loss, floaters, or photopsia, consisting of a brief 'ball of light' travelling across the visual field two to three times a day, most apparent in subdued lighting.
- Pain due to neovascular glaucoma or uveitis is uncommon.

## Signs

### 1. Common

- An elevated, subretinal, dome-shaped mass, which can be grey (Fig. 7.21), brown, black or amelanotic (Fig. 7.22).
- Surface orange pigment (lipofuscin) is frequently seen (Fig. 7.23).
- If the tumour breaks through Bruch's membrane, it acquires a mushroom-shaped appearance, with visible blood vessels if the tumour is amelanotic (Fig. 7.24).
- Exudative retinal detachment, which is initially confined to the surface of the tumour (Fig. 7.25), and which later shifts inferiorly, becoming bullous and eventually total.
- Dilated and tortuous episcleral ('sentinel') blood vessels if the choroidal tumour involves the ciliary body.

> **NB: Unlike rhegmatogenous retinal detachment, the subretinal fluid shifts with ocular movement and gravity ('shifting fluid'). In addition, the retina does not show the fine, silvery rippling that occurs in rhegmatogenous detachment.**

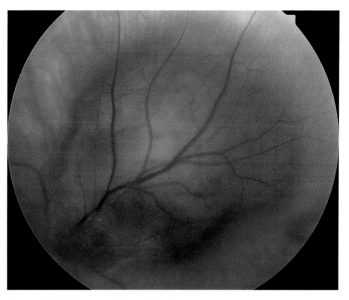

**Figure 7.21** Pigmented choroidal melanoma

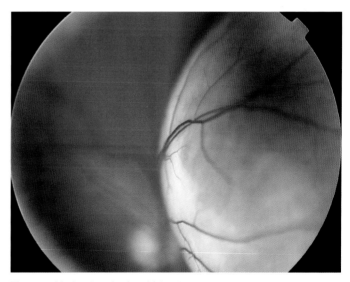

**Figure 7.22** Amelanotic choroidal melanoma

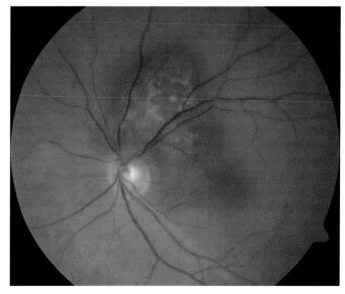

**Figure 7.23** Choroidal melanoma with orange pigment

## 2. Uncommon

- Interference with the choroidal circulation may give rise to a straight line of cobblestone degeneration, pointing outwards from the posterior pole ('comet tail'), often associated with 'bone spicules' (Fig. 7.26).
- Central retinal vein occlusion if the optic nerve is involved.
- An extensive flat, grey or brown, irregular discoloration of the fundus, due to a diffuse tumour (Fig. 7.27).
- Choroidal folds, haemorrhage, rubeosis, secondary glaucoma, cataract and uveitis.

> **NB:** Binocular indirect ophthalmoscopy combined with indirect slit-lamp biomicroscopy is sufficient for diagnosis in the vast majority of cases.

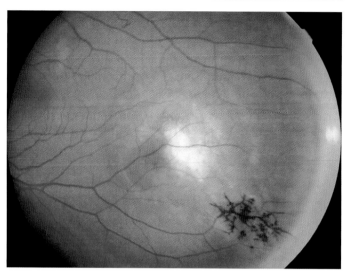

**Figure 7.26** 'Comet's tail' degeneration peripheral to a choroidal melanoma

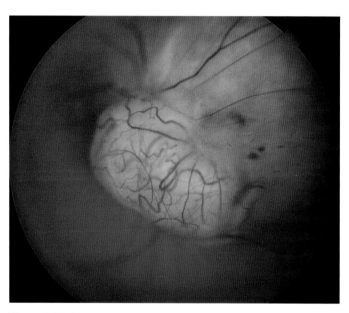

**Figure 7.24** Amelanotic collar-stud choroidal melanoma with visible blood vessels

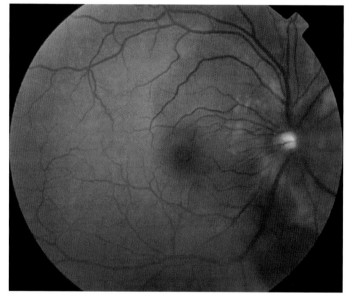

**Figure 7.27** Diffuse choroidal melanoma

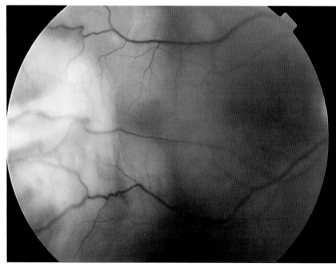

**Figure 7.25** Shallow retinal detachment overlying a choroidal melanoma

***Differential diagnosis.*** Although in the majority of cases the diagnosis is straight-forward, the following conditions should be considered in the differential diagnosis of atypical cases:

### 1. Pigmented lesions

- Large naevus.
- Melanocytoma.
- Congenital hypertrophy of the RPE.
- Haemorrhage in the subretinal space or choroid.
- Metastatic cutaneous melanoma.

### 2. Non-pigmented lesions

- Circumscribed choroidal haemangioma.
- Metastasis.
- Solitary choroidal granulomas associated with sarcoidosis or tuberculosis.

- Posterior scleritis can present with a large elevated lesion, but, unlike melanoma, pain is a common feature.
- Large elevated disciform lesion, particularly if located away from the macula.

### *Investigations*

1. **Visual field examination** does not differentiate a melanoma from a large naevus, although, in the former, visual field loss is more severe.

2. **Transillumination** (Fig. 7.28) gives an approximate indication of tumour extent but has no diagnostic value.

3. **US** is useful in determining tumour size and detecting extraocular extension. B-scan US shows characteristic acoustic hollowness, choroidal excavation and orbital shadowing (Fig. 7.29). A collar-stud configuration is almost pathognomonic (Fig. 7.30). A-scan US provides additional information about internal acoustic reflectivity, which can assist diagnosis.

4. **FA** is of limited diagnostic value because there is no pathognomonic pattern. Collar-stud melanomas show a 'dual circulation'. Most melanomas show a mottled fluorescence during the arteriovenous phase and progressive

leakage and staining (Fig. 7.31). Hypofluorescence may occur if the RPE over a pigmented tumour is either absent or normal.

5. **ICG** provides more information about the extent of the tumour, because there is less interference caused by RPE changes (Fig. 7.32).

6. **MRI,** particularly when combined with surface coils and fat suppression sequences, shows that choroidal melanomas are hyperintense in T1-weighted images (Fig. 7.33) and hypointense in T2-weighted images, but these features are not pathognomonic. Enhancement with gadolinium improves image quality, demonstrating optic nerve and orbital invasion and facilitating differentiation from other tumours.

7. **Colour-coded Doppler imaging** may differentiate pigmented tumours from intraocular haemorrhage, particularly in eyes with opaque media.

8. **Fine needle aspiration biopsy (FNAB)**, aided by immunohistochemistry, is useful when the diagnosis cannot be established by less invasive methods.

9. **Systemic investigation** is aimed at the following:

   a. *Excluding a metastasis to the choroid* if there is uncertainty about whether the ocular tumour is a melanoma or a metastasis. Ocular secondaries arise most frequently from the lung in both sexes and from the breast in women. Occasionally, the primary site is the kidney or gastrointestinal tract. If metastasis is suspected, initial investigations should include chest radiography, rectal examination, serum PSA and CEA, and mammography in females.

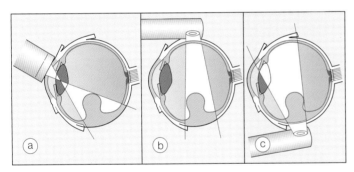

**Figure 7.28** Technique of transillumination. **(a)** Transpupillary; **(b)** transocular; **(c)** trans-scleral (From B. Damato, from *Ocular Tumours*, Butterworth-Heinemann, 2000)

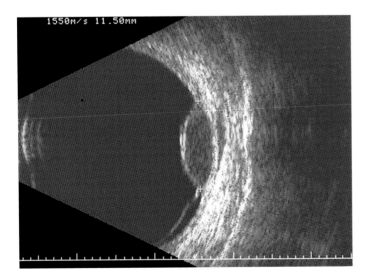

**Figure 7.29** Ultrasonography of a dome-shaped choroidal melanoma showing choroidal excavation

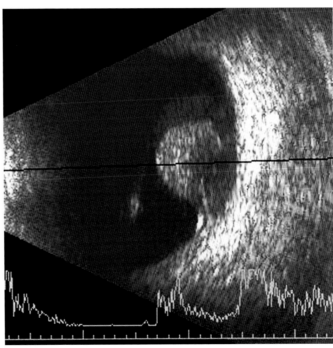

**Figure 7.30** A and B scan ultrasonography of a collar-stud choroidal melanoma

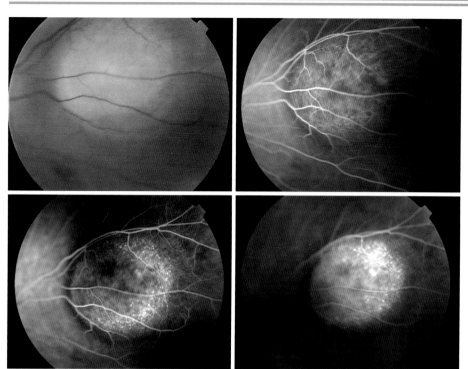

**Figure 7.31** FA of a choroidal melanoma (see text)

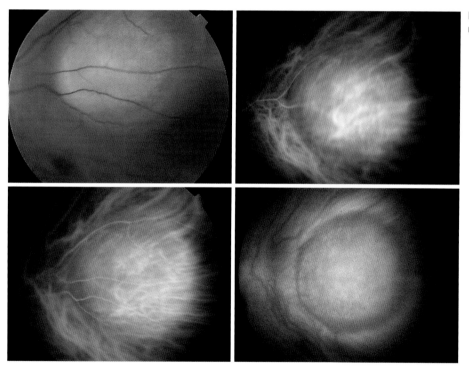

**Figure 7.32** ICG angiogram of a choroidal melanoma (see text)

b. *Detecting metastatic spread from the choroid* if there is an increased suspicion of metastatic disease because of large tumour size (i.e. basal diameter >16 mm), symptoms such as dyspepsia, abdominal pain and weight loss, palpable enlargement of the liver, or abnormal liver function tests. Hepatic involvement can be detected by US, and elevated levels of gamma-glutamyl transpeptidase and alkaline phosphatase.

Chest radiography rarely shows lung secondaries in the absence of liver metastases. Only about 1–2% of patients have detectable metastases at the time of presentation. If screening is undertaken after treatment of the ocular tumour, liver scans and biochemical liver function tests should be performed every 6 months for the first 5–10 years, and then annually.

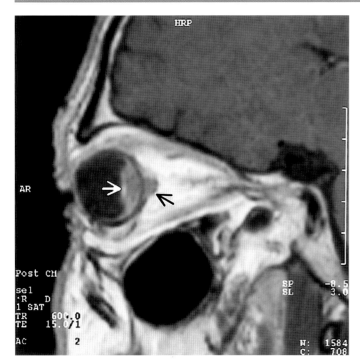

**Figure 7.33** T1-weighted MRI shows a choroidal melanoma (white arrow) and extraocular extension (black arrow) (Courtesy of M. Karolczak-Kulesza)

## MANAGEMENT

Treatment is performed not only to prevent metastatic disease but also to avoid the development of a painful and unsightly eye, preferably conserving as much useful vision as possible. Management should be tailored to the individual patient taking the following factors into consideration:

- Size, location and extent of the tumour, together with effects on vision.
- State of the fellow eye.
- General health and age of the patient.
- The patient's wishes and fears.

***No treatment*** may be appropriate for a slowly growing tumour in the only seeing eye of a very elderly or chronically ill patient. In many centres, if it is not possible to determine clinically whether a tumour is a small melanoma or a large naevus: the lesion is observed and treatment is administered only if growth is documented by sequential US or photography. The risks involved in delaying treatment are uncertain, so it is essential to confirm and document that the patient understands the situation fully. Special measures need to be taken to ensure that the patient is not lost to follow-up.

***Brachytherapy*** with a ruthenium-106 or iodine-125 applicator is usually the treatment of first choice because it is relatively straightforward and effective.

1. **Indications** are tumours less than 20 mm in basal diameter in which there is a reasonable chance of salvaging vision. It is possible to treat tumours up to 5 mm thick with a ruthenium plaque and up to 10 mm thick with an iodine plaque. Supplemental transpupillary thermotherapy may be required to sterilise the tumour or to reduce exudation.

2. **Technique**
   - The tumour is localised by transillumination or binocular indirect ophthalmoscopy.
   - A template consisting of a transparent plastic dummy or metal ring with eyelets is sutured to the sclera with a releasable bow.
   - Once it has been established that the template is correctly positioned, the sutures are loosened and used to secure the radioactive plaque.
   - The plaque is removed once the appropriate dose has been delivered, usually within 3–7 days. At least 80 Gy needs to be delivered to the tumour apex. Tumour regression starts about 1–2 months after treatment and continues for several years.

3. **Tumour response** is usually gradual (Fig. 7.34). Amelanotic tumours tend to become more pigmented as they regress (Fig. 7.35). As long as there is no re-growth or lateral extension of the tumour margins, there should be no cause for concern.

4. **Complications** include retinopathy, papillopathy, vitreous haemorrhage, cataract, neovascular glaucoma, and recurrence of tumour.

5. **Survival** is similar to that following enucleation of comparable tumours.

***Charged particle irradiation*** with protons by means of a cyclotron unit achieves a more homogenous dose of radiation than does brachytherapy. Treatment is fractionated over 4 days, with each dose delivered in less than a minute.

1. **Indications** are tumours unsuitable for brachytherapy because of either large size or posterior location, which might make positioning of a plaque unreliable.

2. **Technique**
   - Radio-opaque tantalum markers are sutured to the sclera and used to locate the tumour radiographically.
   - The patient is seated in a mechanised chair with the head immobilised.
   - The eyes look at an adjustable fixation target.
   - Four fractions of radiotherapy are delivered over 5 days.

3. **Tumour regression** is slower than with brachytherapy, and choroidal atrophy around the base of the tumour takes longer to develop.

4. **Complications** depend on the tumour's size and location and its proximity to the optic disc and fovea. They include loss of lashes, eyelid depigmentation, canaliculitis with epiphora, conjunctival keratinisation, keratitis, maculopathy, optic neuropathy (Fig. 7.36), exudative retinal detachment and neovascular glaucoma. Local tumour recurrence is rare.

5. **Survival results** are similar to those following brachytherapy or enucleation.

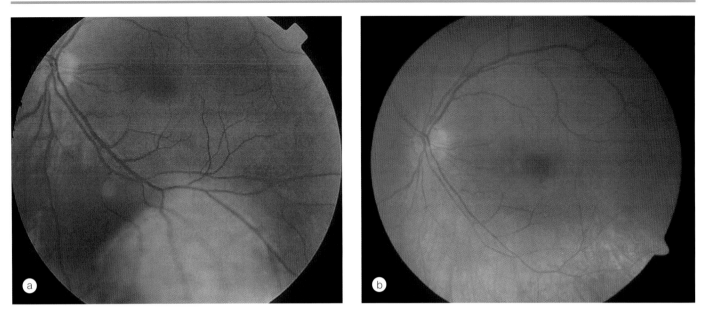

**Figure 7.34** Ruthenium plaque radiotherapy of an inferior choroidal melanoma in the left eye of a 35-year-old female. **(a)** Before brachytherapy when the tumour measured 10 mm by 8 mm by 3.6 mm; **(b)** two years after the brachytherapy, the visual acuity was 6/6 and the tumour was inactive

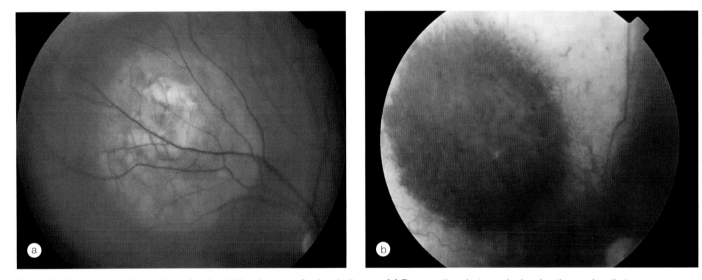

**Figure 7.35** Increased pigmentation of a choroidal melanoma after brachytherapy. **(a)** Preoperative photograph showing the amelanotic tumour; **(b)** 13 years later

**Stereotactic radiotherapy** is still an investigational technique, so the indications, contraindications and outcomes are not yet defined. Radiation is focussed on the tumour by aiming multiple, highly collimated beams from different directions, either concurrently or sequentially, so that only the tumour receives a high dose of radiation.

**Transpupillary thermotherapy (TTT)** uses an infrared laser beam to induce tumour cell death by hyperthermia and not coagulation.

1. **Indications** are selected, small, pigmented tumours, especially those near the optic disc or fovea. The advantages of TTT over radiotherapy include the precision of treatment, immediate tumour necrosis and treatment on an outpatient basis.

2. **Technique**

   ● Overlapping 1-minute applications of a 3 mm diode laser beam are applied all over the tumour surface, adjusting the power so that retinal blanching does not develop before 45 seconds.
   ● A 2 mm rim of surrounding choroid is treated to prevent marginal recurrence.
   ● Adjunctive plaque radiotherapy is administered, if possible, to prevent recurrence from deep intrascleral deposits.
   ● The treatment is repeated after 6 months if there is residual tumour.

3. **Tumour response** is gradual, with the lesion first becoming darker and flatter, eventually disappearing to leave bare sclera (Fig. 7.37).

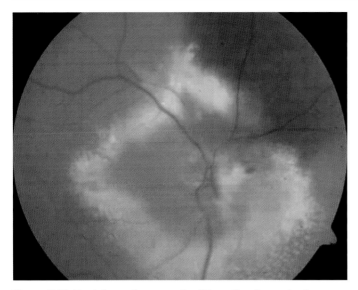

**Figure 7.36** Exudative optic neuropathy 17 months after proton beam radiotherapy of a juxtapapillary choroidal melanoma

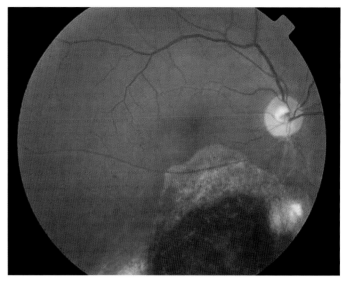

**Figure 7.38** Choroidal melanoma measuring 9 mm by 6 mm by 2.8 mm treated with ruthenium plaque radiotherapy and adjunctive transpupillary thermotherapy. Four years after treatment, the vision was 6/6 and the tumour was inactive, with a thickness of 1.1 mm

4. **Complications** include tumour recurrence, vascular occlusion, neovascularisation and maculopathy.

> **NB: TTT is a useful adjunct to radiotherapy, reducing oedema and preventing local tumour recurrence (Figure 7.38).**

***Trans-scleral choroidectomy*** is a difficult procedure and is therefore not performed widely.

1. **Indications** are carefully selected tumours that are too thick for radiotherapy and usually less than 16 mm in diameter.

2. **Technique**

   - The tumour is localised by transillumination.
   - The eye is decompressed by limited vitrectomy.
   - A partial-thickness scleral flap is created over the tumour (Fig. 7.39a).
   - The tumour is resected together with the deep scleral lamella, if possible leaving retina intact (Fig. 7.39b).
   - After scleral closure (Fig. 7.39c), the eye is filled with balanced salt solution.
   - Adjunctive brachytherapy is administered, either immediately (Fig. 7.39d) or after healing has occurred.

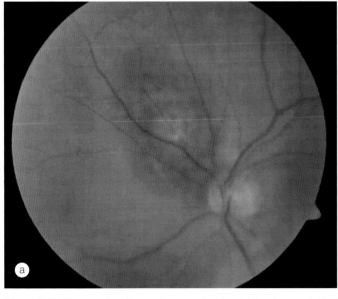

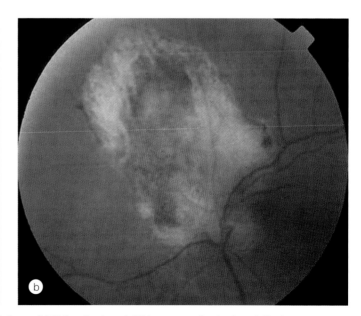

**Figure 7.37** Transpupillary thermotherapy of a choroidal melanoma in the left eye. **(a)** Before treatment, **(b)** two years after treatment, the tumour was inactive and the vision was 6/9

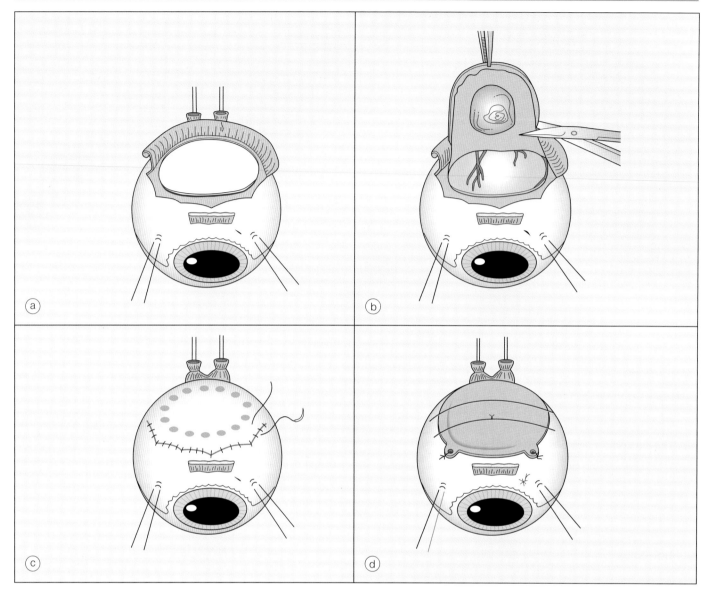

**Figure 7.39** Technique of trans-scleral choroidectomy. **(a)** Scleral flap; **(b)** tumour excision; **(c)** closure of flap; **(d)** plaque insertion (From B. Damato, from *Ocular Tumours*, Butterworth-Heinemann, 2000)

3. **Response** of the RPE may result in hyperpigmentation in and around the coloboma.

4. **Complications** include retinal detachment, if the tumour has invaded retina, and tumour recurrence, particularly if the tumour is more than 16 mm in diameter.

***Trans-retinal choroidectomy*** (Fig. 7.40) is a controversial procedure because of concerns about seeding tumour cells to other parts of the eye and perhaps systemically. It is therefore performed only if it offers the only hope for conserving useful vision, for example, if the tumour extends close to optic disc and if the vision in the fellow eye is poor.

### Enucleation

1. **Indications** for excision of the globe are large tumour size, optic disc invasion, extensive involvement of the ciliary body or angle, irreversible loss of useful vision, and poor motivation to keep the eye.

2. **Technique** is the same as for other conditions, using the surgeon's preferred orbital implant. It is essential to perform ophthalmoscopy and to do this *after* draping the patient, to ensure that the correct eye is treated.

3. **Complications** are the same as with enucleation for other conditions. Orbital recurrence is rare if there is no extra-ocular tumour spread or if any such extension is completely excised.

***Exenteration*** (removal of the globe and orbital contents) is indicated when orbital tumour involvement cannot be controlled by lumpectomy and radiotherapy.

### Treatment of metastatic disease

1. **Systemic** chemotherapy and/or immunotherapy rarely induce responses. Higher rates of remission have been reported with intra-hepatic chemotherapy.

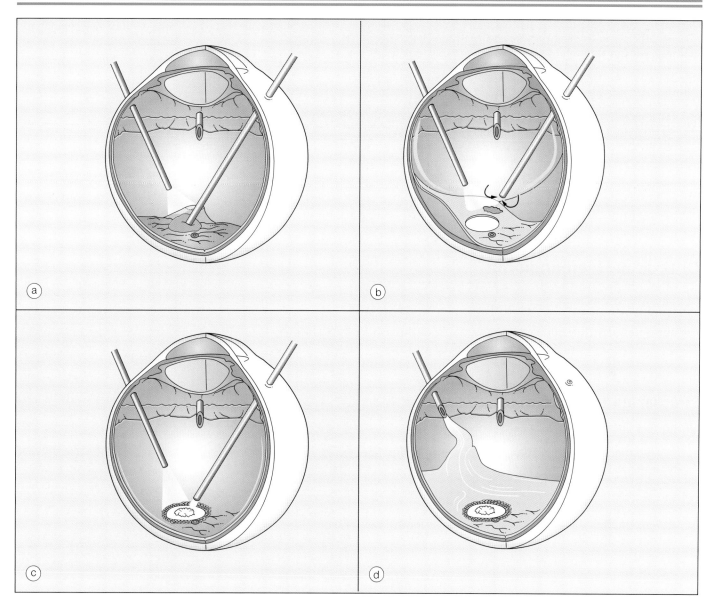

**Figure 7.40** Technique of trans-retinal choroidectomy. **(a)** Retinotomy and tumour excision; **(b)** fluid–air exchange; **(c)** laser endophotocoagulation around the retinotomy; **(d)** air–silicone oil exchange (From B. Damato, *Ocular Tumours*, Butterworth-Heinemann, 2000)

**2. Partial hepatectomy** for removal of small metastatic deposits can significantly prolong life.

## FURTHER READING

Damato BE. An approach to the management of patients with uveal melanomas. *Eye* 1993;7:388–397.

Damato BE, Groenewald C, McGailliard J, et al. Endoresection of choroidal melanoma. *Br J Ophthalmol* 1998;82:213–218.

Damato BE, Paul J, Foulds W. Risk factors for residual and recurrent uveal melanoma after transscleral local resection. *Br J Ophthalmol* 1996;80:102–108.

De Potter P, Jamart J. Adjuvant indocyanine green in transpupillary thermotherapy for choroidal melanoma. *Ophthalmology* 2003; 110:406–414.

Diener-West M, Earle JD, Fine SL, et al. The COMS randomized trial of iodine 125 brachytherapy for choroidal melanoma. *Arch Ophthalmol* 2001;119:969–982.

Finger PT. Radiation therapy for choroidal melanoma. *Surv Ophthalmol* 1997;42:215–232.

Gass JD. Problems in the differential diagnosis of choroidal nevi and malignant melanomas. The XXXIII Edward Jackson Memorial Lecture. *Am J Ophthalmol* 1977;83:299–323.

Gragoudas E, Li W, Goitein M, et al. Evidence-based estimates of outcome in patients irradiated for intraocular melanoma. *Arch Ophthalmol* 2002;120:1665–1671.

Gunduz K, Shields CL, Shields JA, et al. Radiation retinopathy following plaque radiotherapy for posterior uveal melanoma. *Arch Ophthalmol* 1999;117:609–614.

Jampol LM, Moy CS, Murray TG, et al. The COMS randomized trial of iodine 125 brachytherapy for choroidal melanoma. IV. Local treatment failure and enucleation in the first 5 years after brachytherapy. COMS report no. 19. *Ophthalmology* 2002;109: 2197–2206.

Kim JW, Damato BE, Hiscott P. Noncontiguous tumor recurrence of posterior uveal melanoma after local transscleral resection. *Arch Ophthalmol* 2002;120:1659–1664.

Rennie IG. Things that go bump in the light. The differential diagnosis of posterior uveal melanomas. *Eye* 2002;16:325–346.

Robertson DM, Buettner H, Bennett SR. Transpupillary thermotherapy as primary treatment for small choroidal melanomas. *Arch Ophthalmol* 1999;117: 1512–1519.

Shields CL, Cater J, Shields JA, et al. Combined plaque radiotherapy and transpupillary thermotherapy for choroidal melanoma. Tumor control and treatment complications in 270 consecutive patients. *Arch Ophthalmol* 2002;120:933–940.

Shields CL, Shields JA, Cater J, et al. Plaque radiotherapy for uveal melanomas. Long-term visual outcome in 1106 patients. *Arch Ophthalmol* 2000;118:1219–1228.

Shields CL, Shields JA, DePotter P, et al. Transpupillary thermotherapy in the management of choroidal melanomas. *Ophthalmology* 1996;103:1642–1650.

Shields CL, Shields JA, Perez N, et al. Primary transpupillary thermotherapy for small choroidal melanoma in 256 consecutive cases: outcomes and limitations. *Ophthalmology* 2002;109:25–34.

Wilson MW, Hungerford JL. Comparison of episcleral plaque and proton beam radiation therapy for the treatment of choroidal melanoma. *Ophthalmology* 1999;106: 1579–1587.

# Choroidal Haemangioma

Choroidal haemangiomas are rare hamartomas which may be cavernous or mixed cavernous–capillary (Fig. 7.41). The tumour is probably congenital and may lie dormant throughout life or may give rise to symptoms in adulthood. It is almost always solitary and is not usually associated with systemic disease. Most are stationary and a few are slow-growing.

## CIRCUMSCRIBED CHOROIDAL HAEMANGIOMA

### Diagnosis

1. **Presentation** is in the fourth to fifth decades in one of the following ways:

   - Unilateral blurring of central vision, visual field defect or metamorphopsia.
   - Hypermetropia may occur if the retina is elevated by tumour or fluid.
   - Some patients are asymptomatic with normal visual acuity.

2. **Signs**

   - A discrete, smooth, round or oval mass which has the same pink colour as the surrounding choroid. It is located posterior to the equator in the macula or peri-

papillary area (Fig. 7.42). The median base diameter of the lesion is 6 mm and thickness 3 mm.

   - White foci may be present on the surface of the tumour and probably represent fibrous metaplasia of the overlying RPE (Fig. 7.43).

## 3. Complications

- Intraretinal oedema, accumulation of subretinal fluid over the tumour and with cystoid retinal degeneration.
- Exudation may lead to extensive retinal detachment and neovascular glaucoma.
- RPE degeneration, subretinal fibrosis and, rarely, macular atrophy.

## 4. Investigations

a. *US* shows an acoustically solid lesion with a sharp anterior surface and high internal reflectivity, but with

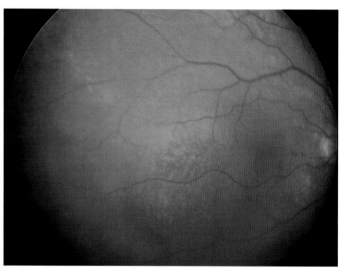

**Figure 7.42** Circumscribed choroidal haemangioma (Courtesy of C. Barry)

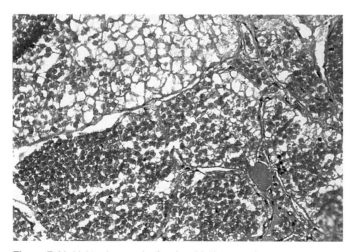

**Figure 7.41** Light micrograph of a choroidal haemangioma

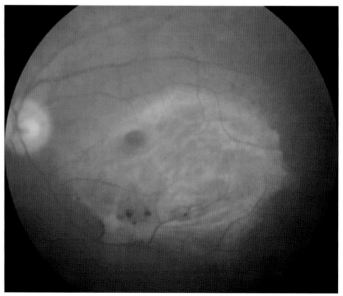

**Figure 7.43** Fibrous metaplasia over a choroidal haemangioma

neither choroidal excavation nor orbital shadowing (Fig. 7.44).

b. *FA* reveals rapid, spotty hyperfluorescence in the pre-arterial or early arterial phase and diffuse intense late hyperfluorescence (Fig. 7.45).

c. *ICG* shows lacy hyperfluorescence in the early frames by 1 minute and hypofluorescence ('washout') at 20 minutes.

d. *MRI* shows that the tumour is iso- or hyperintense to the vitreous in T1-weighted images and isointense in T2-weighted images, with marked enhancement with gadolinium.

***Treatment*** of vision-threatening haemangiomas is as follows:

1. **Photodynamic therapy** using the same method as for choroidal neovascular membranes.

2. **TTT** for lesions not involving the macula, but this causes peripheral visual field loss (Fig. 7.46).

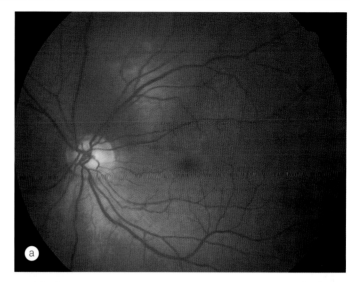

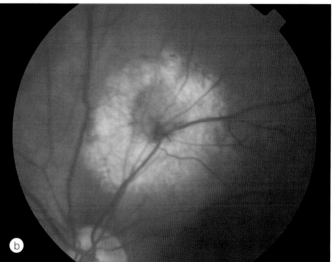

**Figure 7.46** Transpupillary thermotherapy of a juxtapapillary choroidal haemangioma. **(a)** Before treatment, when the tumour measured 10 mm by 7 mm by 1.2 mm and visual acuity 3/60; **(b)** after treatment visual acuity improved to 6/12

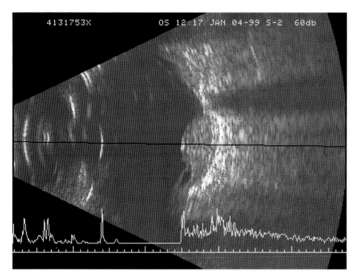

**Figure 7.44** A-scan and B-scan of a choroidal haemangioma

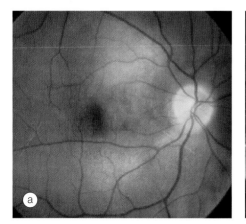
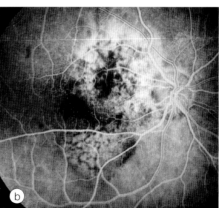
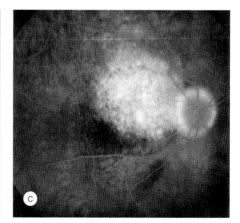

**Figure 7.45 (a)** Circumscribed choroidal haemangioma; **(b)** FA early phase shows spotty hyperfluorescence; **(c)** late phase shows diffuse hyperfluorescence

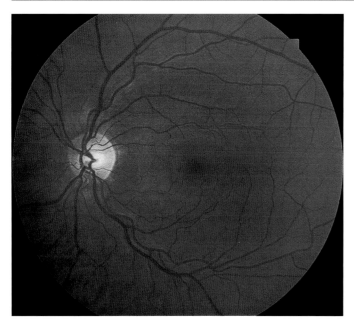

**Figure 7.47** Diffuse choroidal haemangioma.

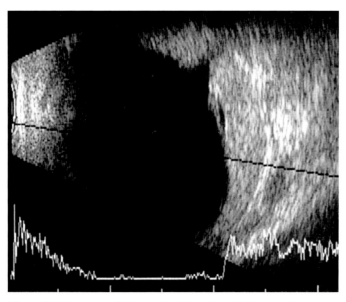

**Figure 7.48** A-scan and B-scan of a diffuse choroidal haemangioma

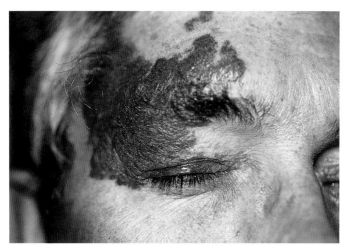

**Figure 7.49** Localised naevus flammeus in Sturge–Weber syndrome

3. **Radiotherapy** involving lens-sparing external beam irradiation, proton beam radiotherapy or plaque brachytherapy. Only a low dose is needed, but even this can cause collateral damage to normal tissues.

### Differential diagnosis

1. **Amelanotic choroidal melanoma** has a yellow-tan colour, often with subtle intrinsic pigment.

2. **Choroidal metastasis** is creamy yellow and may be multifocal. However, metastatic deposits from carcinoid tumour, renal cell carcinoma and thyroid carcinoma may appear orange, similar to a haemangioma.

3. **RPE detachment** is acoustically hollow and shows different features on FA.

## DIFFUSE CHOROIDAL HAEMANGIOMA

Diffuse choroidal haemangioma usually affects over half of the choroid and enlarges very slowly. It occurs almost exclusively in patients with the Sturge–Weber syndrome, ipsilateral to the naevus flammeus.

### Diagnosis

● A deep-red 'tomato ketchup' colour which is most marked at the posterior pole (Fig. 7.47) and diffuse thickening of the choroid, best demonstrated by US (Fig. 7.48).
● Complications include secondary retinal cystoid degeneration and exudative retinal detachment.
● Neovascular glaucoma can result if exudative retinal detachment is not treated.

**Treatment** involves external beam radiotherapy, if troublesome complications arise.

**Sturge–Weber syndrome** (encephalotrigeminal angiomatosis) is a congenital, sporadic phacomatosis.

1. **Classification**

   ● Trisystem disease involves the face, leptomeninges and eyes.
   ● Bisystem disease involves the face and eyes, or the face and leptomeninges.

2. **Signs**

   ● Facial naevus flammeus (port-wine stain), extending over the area corresponding to the distribution of one or more branches of the trigeminal nerve (Fig. 7.49). The lesion is usually unilateral and occasionally bilateral.
   ● Ipsilateral pariental or occipital leptomeningeal haemangioma may cause contralateral or generalised focal or generalised seizures, hemiparesis or hemianopia.
   ● Other features include ipsilateral glaucoma, episcleral haemangioma and iris heterochromia.

## FURTHER READING

Arevalo JF, Shields CL, Shields JA, et al. Circumscribed choroidal hemangioma: characteristic features with indocyanine green videoangiography. *Ophthalmology* 2000;107:344–350.

Garcia-Arumi J, Ramsay LS, Guraya BC. Transpupillary thermotherapy for circumscribed choroidal hemangiomas. *Ophthalmology* 2000;107:351–356.

Jurklies B, Anastassiou G, Ortmans S, et al. Photodynamic therapy using verteporfin in circumscribed choroidal haemangioma. *Br J Ophthalmol* 2003;87:84–89.

Kamal A, Watts AR, Rennie IG. Indocyanine green enhanced trans-pupillary thermotherapy of circumscribed choroidal haemangioma. *Eye* 2000;14:701–705.

Lee V, Hungerford JL. Proton beam therapy for posterior pole circumscribed choroidal haemangioma. *Eye* 1998;12:925–928.

Madreperla SA. Choroidal hemangioma treated with photodynamic therapy using verteporfin. *Arch Ophthalmol* 2001;119:1606–1610.

Porrini G, Giovannini A, Amato G, et al. Photodynamic therapy of circumscribed choroidal hemangioma. *Ophthalmology* 2003;110:674–680.

Rapizzi E, Grizzard WS, Capone A Jr. Transpupillary thermotherapy in the management of circumscribed choroidal hemangioma. *Am J Ophthalmol* 1999;127:481–482.

Robertson DM. Photodynamic therapy for choroidal hemanigioma associated with serous retinal detachment. *Arch Ophthalmol* 2002;120: 1155–1161.

Schmidt-Erfurth UM, Michels S, Kusserow C, et al. Photodynamic therapy for symptomatic choroidal hemangioma. Visual and anatomic results. *Ophthalmology* 2002;109:2284–2294.

Shields CL, Honavar SG, Shields JA, et al. Circumscribed choroidal hemangioma. Clinical manifestations and factors predictive of visual outcome in 200 consecutive cases. *Ophthalmology* 2001; 108:2237–2248.

# Melanocytoma

Melanocytoma is a rare, distinctive, heavily pigmented naevus which is seen most frequently in the optic nerve head but which can arise anywhere in the uvea. In contrast with choroidal melanoma, melanocytomas are relatively more common in dark-skinned individuals. They are slightly more common in females. The tumour consists of deeply pigmented polyhedral or spindle cells with small nuclei (Fig. 7.50).

## *Diagnosis*

1. **Presentation.** Optic nerve head melanocytoma is usually detected by chance but rarely is due to optic nerve dysfunction.

2. **Signs**

   - Optic nerve head melanocytoma is a dark brown or black lesion with feathery edges within the retinal nerve fibre layer, which extends over the edge of the disc (Fig. 7.51).
   - The tumour often occupies the inferior part of the disc, although occasionally it is elevated and occupies the entire disc surface (Fig. 7.52).
   - Melanocytomas of the choroid, ciliary body and iris are extremely rare.
   - Rarely, seeding of the vitreous with pigment particles may occur, and give rise to secondary glaucoma.

3. **Complications,** which are rare, include the following:

   - Malignant transformation to melanoma.
   - Visual field defects which can be either an enlarged blind spot or a scotoma corresponding to a retinal nerve fibre bundle defect.
   - Profound loss of vision is very rare and may be caused by malignant transformation, central retinal vascular obstruction, ischaemic optic neuropathy, neuroretinitis and spontaneous tumour necrosis.

**Treatment** is not required except in the very rare event of malignant transformation.

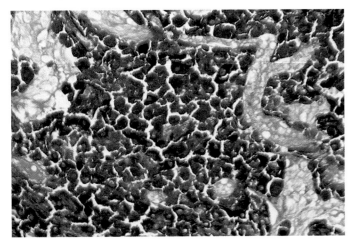

**Figure 7.50** Light micrograph of a melanocytoma showing deeply pigmented, plump cells with small nuclei

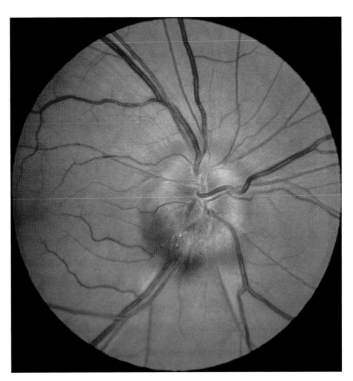

**Figure 7.51** Melanocytoma involving the inferior part of the optic disc and adjacent retina

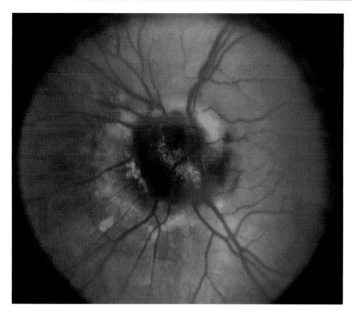

**Figure 7.52** Melanocytoma obscuring most of the optic disc (Courtesy of C. Barry)

## Differential diagnosis

**1. Optic nerve head melanocytoma**

- Choroidal melanoma invading the optic nerve head (Fig. 7.53).
- Other peripapillary pigmented lesions that involve the optic nerve and adjacent retina are adenoma, idiopathic reactive hyperplasia of the RPE, and combined hamartoma of the retina and RPE.

**2. Uveal melanocytoma** is indistinguishable from a naevus or a small melanoma.

# Choroidal Osteoma

Choroidal osteoma (osseous choristoma) is a very rare, benign, slow-growing, ossifying tumour which is more common in women. Both eyes are affected in about 25% of cases but not usually simultaneously. The tumour consists of mature, cancellous bone, which causes overlying RPE atrophy.

## Diagnosis

1. **Presentation** is in the second to third decades with gradual visual impairment if the macula is involved by the tumour itself or by secondary choroidal neovascularisation.

2. **Signs**

- An orange-yellow lesion with well-defined, scalloped borders, most commonly situated at the posterior pole (Fig. 7.54).
- The surface may show pink vascular tufts.
- Overlying RPE changes develop in longstanding cases (Fig. 7.55).
- The thickness is less than 5 mm and the diameter is 3–20 mm.
- Slow growth can occur over several years (Fig. 7.56).

3. **Investigations**

- a. *FA* manifests irregular, diffuse mottled hyperfluorescence during the early and late phases (Fig. 7.57). Choroidal neovascularisation may be evident.
- b. *ICG* shows early hypofluorescence with late staining (Fig. 7.58).
- c. *US* shows a very dense highly reflective lesion (bone) which causes linear orbital shadowing (Fig. 7.59).
- d. *CT* demonstrates bone-like features (Fig. 7.60).

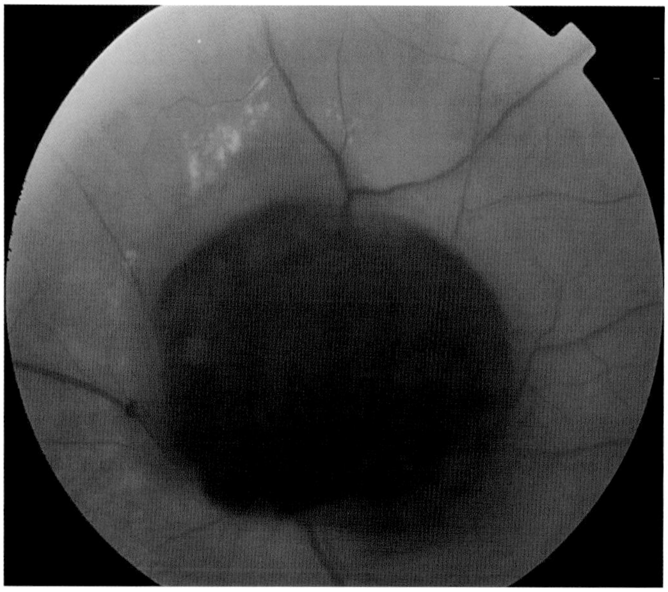

**Figure 7.53** Choroidal melanoma invading the optic disc, mimicking a melanocytoma

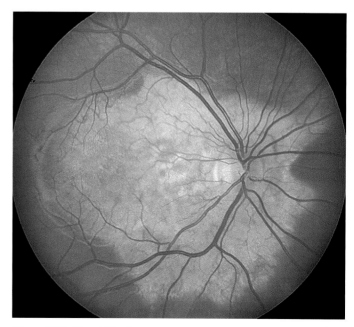

**Figure 7.54** Choroidal osteoma

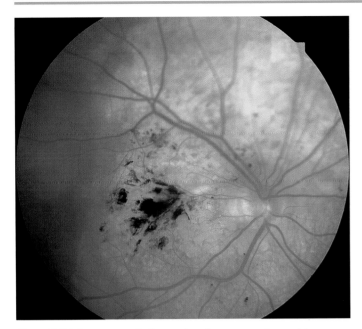

**Figure 7.55** Same eye as in the previous figure, several years later, showing overlying changes in the RPE

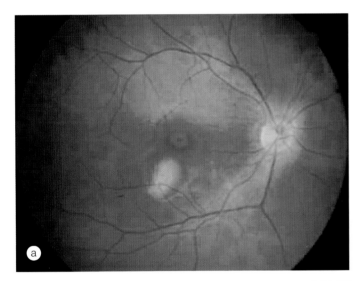

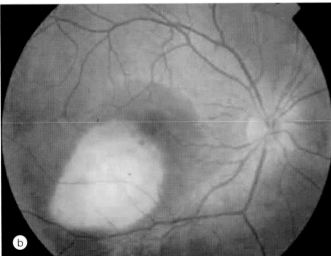

**Figure 7.56** Choroidal osteoma. **(a)** At presentation; **(b)** 7 years later (Courtesy of G. Modarati)

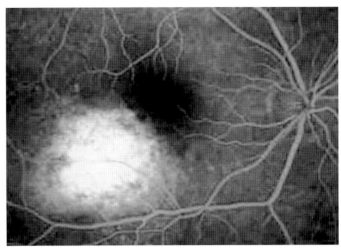

**Figure 7.57** FA of a choroidal osteoma (Courtesy of G. Modarati)

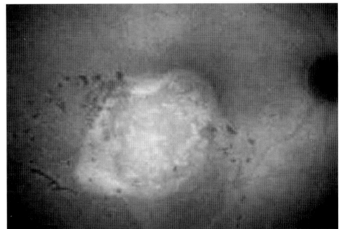

**Figure 7.58** ICG angiogram of a choroidal osteoma (Courtesy of G. Modarati)

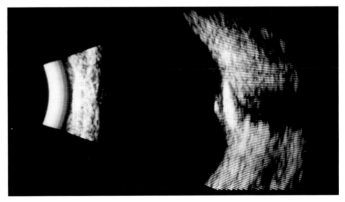

**Figure 7.59** B-scan of a choroidal osteoma

 *e. MRI* shows that relative to vitreous the tumour is hyperintense on T1-weighted images and hypointense on T2-weighted images.

***Treatment*** is usually not appropriate although regression has been reported after photocoagulation and systemic steroid therapy. Secondary choroidal neovascularisation responds poorly to laser therapy.

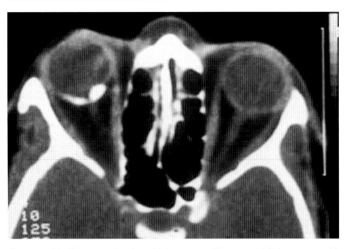

**Figure 7.60** CT scan of a choroidal osteoma (Courtesy of P. Lommatzsch)

### Differential diagnosis

1. **Choroidal metastasis,** which may also be bilateral but typically affects an older age group.

2. **Amelanotic choroidal naevus or melanoma.**

3. **Osseous metaplasia,** which may occur in association with choroidal haemangiomas.

4. **Sclerochoroidal calcification,** which typically develops under the vascular arcades, often bilaterally. It may be idiopathic or associated with hypercalcaemia.

### FURTHER READING

Aylward GW, Chang TS, Pautler SE, et al. A long-term follow-up of a choroidal osteoma. *Arch Ophthalmol* 1998;116:1337–1341.

Browning DJ. Choroidal osteoma: observations from a community setting. *Ophthalmology* 2003;110:1327–1334.

Shields CL, Shields JA, Augsburger JJ. Choroidal osteoma. *Surv Ophthalmol* 1988;33:17–27.

## Metastatic Choroidal Tumours

The choroid is by far the most common site for uveal metastases, accounting for about 90%, followed by the iris and ciliary body. Metastatic tumours to the choroid are more common than primary malignancies but their presence is usually undetected or overshadowed by the patient's general illness. The most frequent primary site is the breast in women and the bronchus in both sexes. A choroidal secondary may be the initial presentation of a bronchial carcinoma, whereas a past history of breast cancer is the rule in patients with breast secondaries. Other less common primary sites include the gastrointestinal tract, kidney and skin melanoma. The prostate is, however, an extremely rare primary site. Patient survival is generally poor, with a median of 8–12 months for all patients; 8–15 months for breast carcinoma and 3–5 months for bronchial carcinoma. In patients with breast carcinoma, risk factors for choroidal metastases include dissemination of disease in more than one organ and the presence of lung and brain metastases.

### Diagnosis

1. **Presentation** is usually with visual impairment, although metastases may be asymptomatic if located away from the macula.

2. **Signs**

   - A fast-growing, creamy-white, placoid or oval lesion most frequently located at the posterior pole (Fig. 7.61).
   - Occasionally, the deposits assume a globular shape and may mimic an amelanotic melanoma (Fig. 7.62).
   - The deposits are multifocal in about 30% of patients and both eyes are involved in 10–30% of cases.
   - Secondary exudative retinal detachment is frequent and may occur in eyes with relatively small deposits.
   - Retinal and optic disc metastases are very rare.

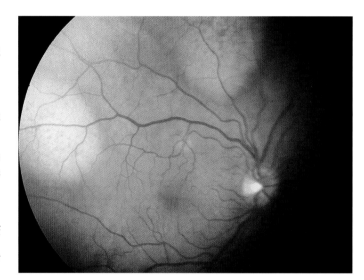

**Figure 7.61** Two choroidal metastases

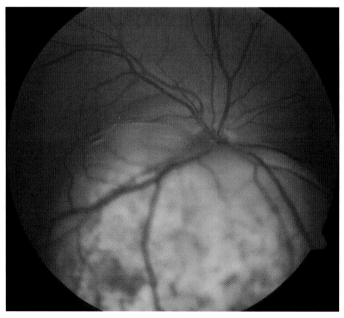

**Figure 7.62** Choroidal metastasis mimicking an amelanotic melanoma

### 3. Ocular investigations

a. *US* shows diffuse choroidal thickening and moderate internal acoustic reflectivity (Fig. 7.63).

b. *FA* shows early hypofluorescence with diffuse late staining (Fig. 7.64) but, in contrast with choroidal melanomas, a 'dual circulation' is not seen.

c. *ICG* shows early hypofluorescence with late isofluorescence (Fig. 7.65) and less evidence of RPE change than with FA.

d. *CT* is not diagnostic but demonstrates the distribution of metastases in the eye and orbit.

e. *MRI*. Compared with the vitreous, metastases tend to be hyperintense on T1-weighted images and hypo- or isointense on T2-weighted images. Gadolinium enhancement is less marked than with melanomas.

f. *Biopsy*, performed by fine needle aspiration, may be appropriate when the primary site is unknown.

### 3. Systemic investigations are aimed at locating the primary tumour, if unknown, and other metastatic sites. These may include the following:

- Full history and physical examination.
- Mammography in females.
- Chest radiography and sputum cytology.

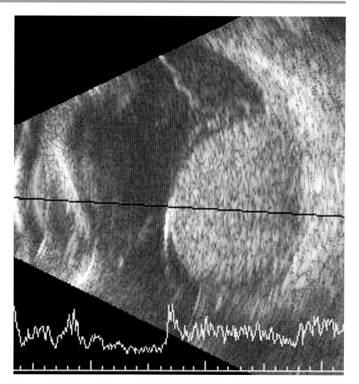

**Figure 7.63** A and B-scan of a choroidal metastasis showing moderate internal acoustic reflectivity

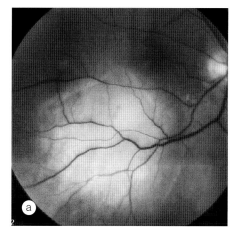 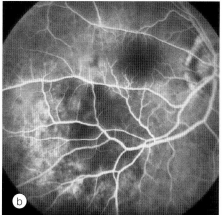 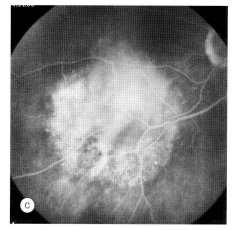

**Figure 7.64** Choroidal metastasis from bronchial carcinoma. **(a)** Red-free image; **(b)** FA shows early hypofluorescence; **(c)** late phase shows diffuse hyperfluorescence due to staining

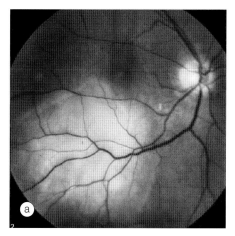 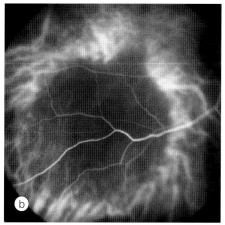 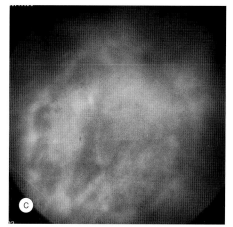

**Figure 7.65** **(a)** Red-free image of the same patient as in the previous figure; **(b)** ICG shows early hypofluorescence; **(c)** late phase isofluorescence

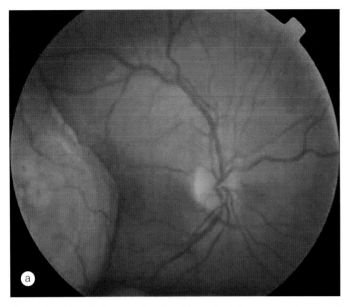
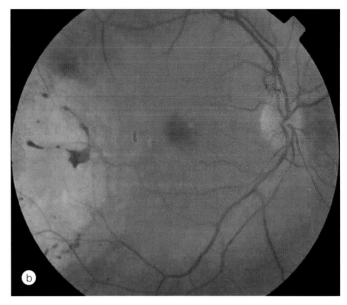

**Figure 7.66** Brachytherapy of a choroidal metastatic adenocarcinoma. **(a)** Before treatment; **(b)** after treatment

- Serum biochemistry, including alkaline phosphatase.
- Abdominal CT.
- Faecal occult blood.
- Urinalysis for red blood cells.

### Treatment

1. **Observation,** if the patient is asymptomatic or receiving systemic chemotherapy.

2. **Radiotherapy,** either external beam or brachytherapy (Fig. 7.66).

3. **TTT** is useful for small tumours with minimal subretinal fluid.

4. **Systemic therapy** for the primary tumour may be beneficial for choroidal metastases.

5. **Enucleation** may be required for a painful blind eye.

### FURTHER READING

Demirci H, Shields CL, Chao AN, et al. Uveal metastasis from breast cancer in 264 patients. *Am J Ophthalmol* 2003;136:264–271.

Kreusel KM, Wiegel T, Stange M, et al. Choroidal metastasis in disseminated lung cancer: frequency and risk factors. *Am J Ophthalmol* 2002;134:445–447.

Shields CL, Shields JA, Gross NE, et al. Survey of 520 eyes with uveal metastases. *Ophthalmology* 1997;104:1265–1276.

## Bilateral Diffuse Uveal Melanocytic Proliferation

Bilateral diffuse uveal melanocytic proliferation (BDUMP) is a very rare paraneoplastic syndrome occurring usually in patients with systemic, often occult, malignancy.

### Diagnosis

#### 1. Signs

- Diffuse thickening of the entire uvea associated with multiple pigmented or non-pigmented, slightly elevated tumours (Fig. 7.67).
- Multiple red-grey patches in the RPE, which may have a reticular pattern.
- Vitreous and anterior chamber cells.
- Anterior uveal cysts and tumours.
- Episcleral nodules.
- Complications include exudative retinal detachment, cataract and raised intraocular pressure.

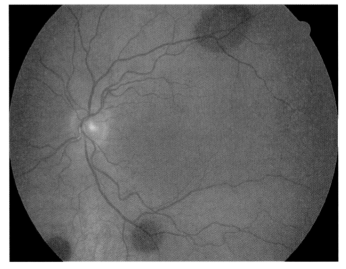

**Figure 7.67** Diffuse uveal melanocytic proliferation (Courtesy of A. M. Leys)

## 2. Investigations

a. *US* shows diffuse choroidal thickening and multiple tumours.

b. *FA* shows masking of background choroidal fluorescence by pigmented tumours and extensive patchy hyperfluorescence in the RPE.

c. *ERG* is often reduced.

**Treatment.** Detection of an occult primary malignancy might enable early treatment to improve survival. There is no effective treatment of the ocular tumours although an anecdotal report suggests that these can regress if the underlying malignancy is successfully treated.

# TUMOURS OF THE RETINA

## Retinoblastoma

Retinoblastoma is the most common primary, intraocular malignancy of childhood. Even so, it is rare, occurring in about 1:20 000 live births. It accounts for about 3% of all childhood cancers.

## PATHOLOGY

### Histology

● The tumour is composed of small basophilic (retinoblastoma) cells with large hyperchromatic nuclei and scanty cytoplasm.

● Flexner–Wintersteiner rosettes represent tumour differentiation and consist of columnar cells around a membrane-bound lumen, into which cytoplasmic processes project (Fig. 7.68a).

● Fleurettes are eosinophilic cells attached at their tip (Fig. 7.68b).

● Homer–Wright rosettes of cells form around a mass of neural fibres (Fig. 7.68c).

● Necrosis is manifest as an area of amorphous material or ghost cells (Fig. 7.68d). It is associated with secondary calcification if mild and uveitis if severe.

● Pseudo-rosettes of retinoblastoma cells form around blood vessels within a necrotic area.

### Patterns of tumour spread

● Endophytic growth into vitreous, with seeding of tumour cells throughout the eye.

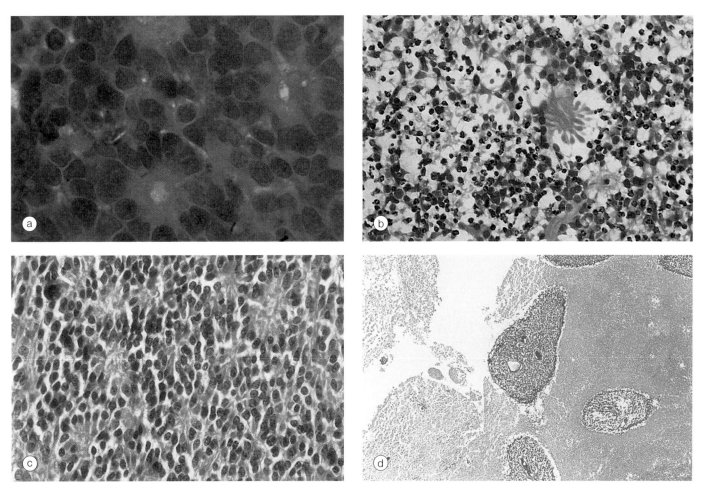

**Figure 7.68** Histology of retinoblastoma: **(a)** Flexner–Wintersteiner rosettes; **(b)** fleurettes; **(c)** Holmer–Wright rosettes; **(d)** necrosis (Courtesy of W. Lee)

- Exophytic growth into subretinal space, causing retinal detachment.
- Optic nerve invasion, with spread of tumour along the subarachnoid space to the brain.
- Choroidal invasion, which if extensive indicates an increased risk of metastasis.
- Diffuse infiltration of the retina, without exophytic or endophytic growth.
- Metastatic spread, which is to regional nodes, lung, brain and bone.

> **NB:** Predictive factors of metastatic disease are large tumour volume (i.e. more than 1 cm³), optic nerve invasion, massive choroidal invasion and orbital spread.

## GENETICS

Retinoblastoma results from malignant transformation of primitive retinal cells before final differentiation. Because these cells disappear within the first few years of life, the tumour is seldom seen after 3 years of age. Retinoblastoma may be hereditable or non-hereditable. The gene predisposing to retinoblastoma (*RB1*) is at 13q14.

1. **Heritable (germline)** retinoblastoma accounts for 40%. In these patients, one allele of the *RB1* (a tumour suppressor gene) has mutated in all body cells. When a further mutagenic event ('second hit') affects the second allele, the cell undergoes malignant transformation. Because all the retinal precursor cells contain the initial mutation, these children develop bilateral and multifocal tumours. Familial cases also carry a predisposition to non-ocular cancers; most notably pinealoblastoma (trilateral retinoblastoma) and osteosarcoma. The risk of second malignancy increases greatly if external beam irradiation has been used to treat the original tumour within the first year of life, and the second tumour tends to arise within the irradiated field.

   - The mutation is transmitted in 50%, but, because of incomplete penetrance, only 40% of offspring will develop the tumour.
   - If a child has heritable retinoblastoma, the chances of any siblings having this disease are 2% if the parents are healthy and 40% if a parent is affected.
   - About 15% of patients with hereditary retinoblastoma manifest unilateral involvement.

2. **Non-heritable (somatic)** retinoblastoma accounts for 60%. The tumour is unilateral, not transmissible, and does not predispose the patient to an increased risk of second non-ocular cancers. If a patient has a solitary retinoblastoma and no positive family history, this is probably, but not definitely, non-heritable, so that the risk in each sibling and in each offspring is about 1%. If examination of the parents reveals a regressed tumour, then these chances increase to 40%.

> **NB:** Siblings at risk of retinoblastoma should be screened for retinoblastoma by US prenatally and by ophthalmoscopy as soon as possible after birth and then regularly until the age of 4 or 5 years.

## DIAGNOSIS

***Presentation*** in the vast majority of cases is within the first 2 years of life. Children with bilateral tumours tend to present earlier (average 12 months) than those with unilateral involvement.

- Leukocoria (white pupillary reflex) is the commonest (60%) and may be first noticed in family photographs (Fig. 7.69).
- Strabismus is the second most common (20%). Fundus examination is therefore mandatory in all cases of childhood strabismus.
- Secondary glaucoma, sometimes associated with buphthalmos, is uncommon.
- Multifocal iris nodules (Fig. 7.70), resembling granulomatous inflammation, or pseudo-hypopyon (masquerade syndrome – Fig. 7.71) can be mistaken for uveitis. This can occur with diffuse retinoblastoma, which tends to present between the age of 5 and 12 years. It is therefore important to consider retinoblastoma in the differential diagnosis of unusual chronic uveitis in children.
- Orbital inflammation (Fig. 7.72) mimicking orbital or preseptal cellulitis may occur with necrotic tumours. It does not necessarily imply extraocular extension and the exact mechanism is not known.
- Orbital invasion with proptosis and bone invasion may occur in neglected cases (Fig. 7.73).

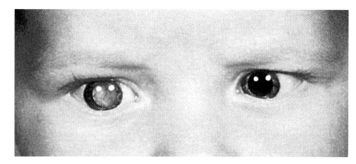

**Figure 7.69** Retinoblastoma causing leukocoria (Courtesy of J. Dudgeon)

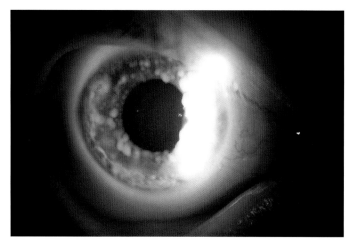

**Figure 7.70** Iris nodule due to iris invasion by retinoblastoma

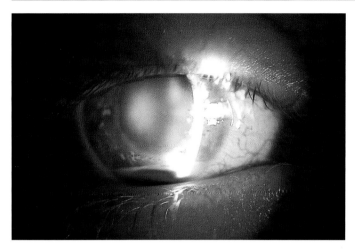

**Figure 7.71** Pseudo-hypopyon due to anterior segment invasion by retinoblastoma

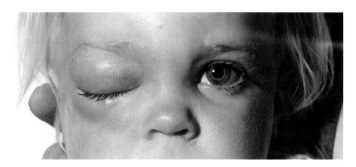

**Figure 7.72** Orbital inflammation associated with retinoblastoma mimicking preseptal cellulitis

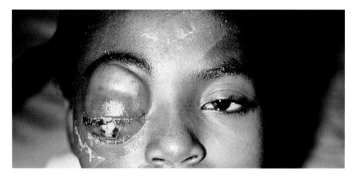

**Figure 7.73** Orbital invasion by neglected retinoblastoma

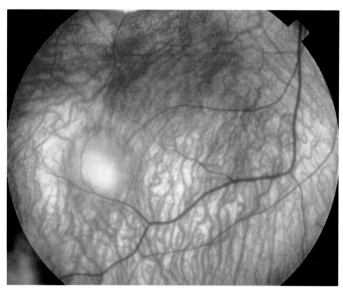

**Figure 7.74** Small intraretinal retinoblastoma

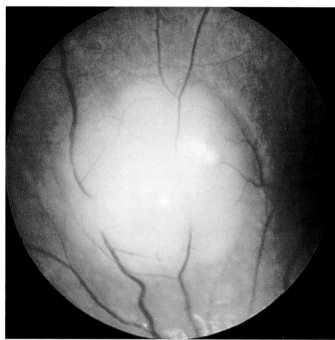

**Figure 7.75** Larger intraretinal retinoblastoma

- Metastatic disease involving regional lymph nodes and brain before the detection of ocular involvement is rare.
- Raised intracranial pressure due to 'trilateral retinoblastoma' before the diagnosis of ocular involvement is a very rare.
- Routine examination of a patient known to be at risk.

***Signs.*** Indirect ophthalmoscopy with scleral indentation must be performed on both eyes after full mydriasis. This is because without indentation pre-equatorial tumours may be missed and one eye may harbour multiple tumours. The clinical signs depend on tumour size and growth pattern.

- An intraretinal tumour is a placoid white lesion (Figs. 7.74 and 7.75).

- An endophytic tumour projects into the vitreous as a white mass (Figs. 7.76 and 7.77).
- An exophytic tumour forms subretinal, multilobulated white masses, with retinal detachment. The tumours may be difficult to visualise if the subretinal fluid is deep (Fig. 7.78).
- Extensive retinoblastoma is characterised by rubeosis iridis, hyphaema, secondary glaucoma and vitreous haemorrhage.
- Spontaneous regression is rare and may either manifest as severe uveitis resulting in phthisis or it may be asymptomatic, resulting in an inactive scar with residual calcium (Fig. 7.79), resembling an irradiated tumour.

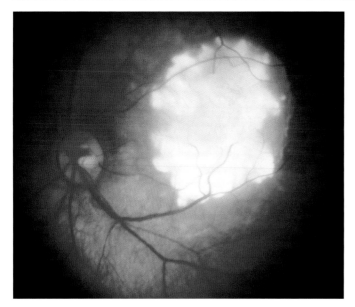

**Figure 7.76** Endophytic retinoblastoma (Courtesy of C. Barry)

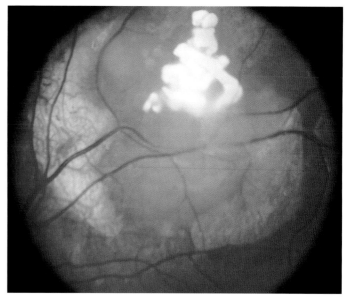

**Figure 7.79** Regressed retinoblastoma with calcific residue

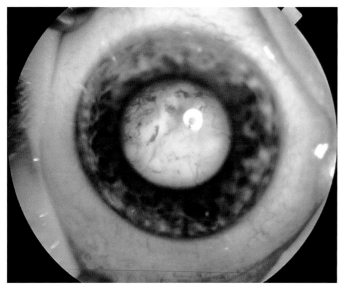

**Figure 7.77** Large endophytic retinoblastoma with surface new blood vessels

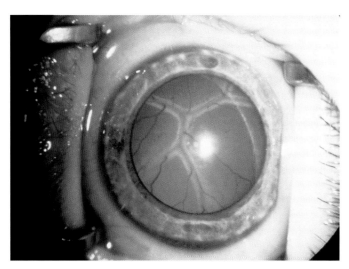

**Figure 7.78** Retinal detachment due to exophytic retinoblastoma

### *Differential diagnosis*

1. **Persistent hyperplastic primary vitreous** is an important cause of congenital leukocoria (see Fig. 9.35). It typically occurs in a microphthalmic eye and is almost always unilateral. It is characterised by a retrolental mass. With time, the mass contracts and pulls the ciliary processes centrally so that they become elongated and visible through the pupil. An associated dehiscence involving the posterior capsule may lead to subsequent cataract formation.

2. **Coats disease** is almost always unilateral, is more common in boys and tends to present later than retinoblastoma. It is characterised by telangiectatic retinal blood vessels, extensive intra- and subretinal yellow exudation, and exudative retinal detachment. The diagnosis is assisted by US or other imaging, which would demonstrate the absence of tumours.

3. **Retinopathy of prematurity,** if advanced, may cause retinal detachment and leukocoria. Diagnosis is usually straightforward because of the history of prematurity and low birth weight.

4. **Toxocariasis**

   - Chronic toxocara endophthalmitis may cause a cyclitic membrane and a white pupil (see Fig. 4.50).
   - Toxocara granuloma at the posterior pole may resemble an endophytic retinoblastoma.

5. **Intermediate uveitis** may mimic the diffuse infiltrating type of retinoblastoma seen in older children.

6. **Retinal dysplasia** is characterised by a congenital pink or white retrolental membrane (see Fig. 9.38) in a microphthalmic eye, with a shallow anterior chamber and elongated ciliary processes.

7. **Incontinentia pigmenti** (Bloch–Sulzberger syndrome) is a rare X-linked dominant disorder affecting girls. It is charac-

terised by vesiculobullous dermatitis on the trunk and extremities (see Fig. 9.40). Malformations of teeth, hair, nails, bones and central nervous system (CNS) may also be present. About one-third of children develop cicatricial retinal detachment in the first year of life, which may cause leukocoria.

8. **Retinocytoma** (retinoma) is thought to be a benign variant of retinoblastoma. It is characterised by calcified mass associated with RPE alteration and chorioretinal atrophy. The appearance is remarkably similar to that of a retinoblastoma following irradiation.

9. **Retinal astrocytoma,** which may be multifocal and bilateral (see Fig. 7.92).

### Investigations

1. **US** is used mainly to assess tumour size. It also detects calcification within the tumour (Fig. 7.80) and is helpful in the diagnosis of simulating lesions.

2. **CT** demonstrates gross involvement of the optic nerve, orbital and CNS extension, and the presence of calcification (Fig. 7.81). However, it entails a significant dose of radiation, which may be dangerous in patients with germinal mutations.

3. **MRI** cannot detect calcification, but is superior to CT for optic nerve evaluation and for detection of a pinealoblastoma, especially when contrast is used (Fig. 7.82). MRI may also be useful to differentiate retinoblastoma from simulating conditions.

4. **Systemic** investigations such as bone marrow aspiration and lumbar puncture are performed only in patients with optic nerve involvement or evidence of extraocular extension.

5. **Genetic** studies require fresh tumour tissue from the enucleated eye and a blood sample for DNA analysis. Blood samples from the patient's relatives and a sperm sample from the father may also be useful.

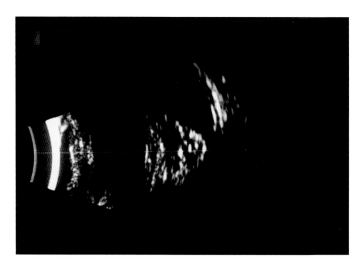

**Figure 7.80** Ultrasonography with low gain of a retinoblastoma showing echoes from calcification (Courtesy of H. Atta)

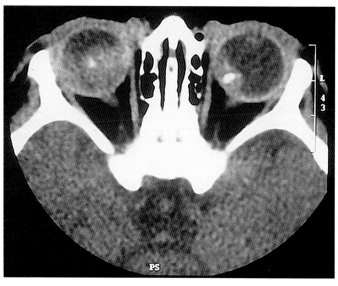

**Figure 7.81** Axial CT shows bilateral advanced retinoblastomas (Courtesy of K. Nischal)

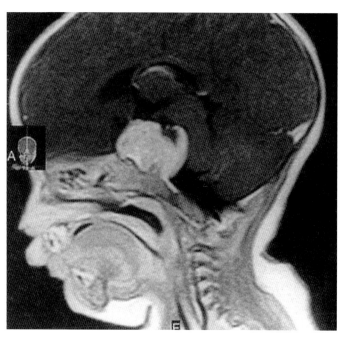

**Figure 7.82** Sagittal MRI shows pinealoblastoma (Courtesy of J. Pe'er)

### TREATMENT

This is related to tumour size; location and associated findings such as retinal detachment, subretinal and vitreous tumour seeds; and the state of the fellow eye.

**Small tumours,** no more than 4 mm diameter and 2 mm thickness may be treated by:

1. **TTT** is indicated for posterior tumours.

2. **Cryotherapy** using the triple freeze-thaw technique is useful for pre-equatorial tumours.

3. **Chemotherapy** without other treatment can be attempted for a macular tumour, to conserve as much vision as possible.

**Medium-size tumours,** up to 12 mm wide and 6 mm thick may be treated by:

1. **Brachytherapy** is indicated if there is no vitreous seeding. Following treatment, the tumour regresses, leaving a calcific residue (Fig. 7.83).

2. **Chemotherapy** with carboplatin, vincristine and etoposide, which may be combined with cyclosporine. The drugs are given intravenously in 3-week cycles over a 4–9-month period, depending on disease severity. This may be followed by local treatment with cryotherapy or thermotherapy to consolidate tumour control.

3. **External beam radiotherapy** should be avoided, if possible, due to the high risk of complications such as cataract formation, radiation retinopathy and cosmetic deformities. In patients with germinal mutations, there is also a risk of inducing a second malignancy such as sarcoma of bone or connective tissue.

**Large tumours** may be treated by:

1. **Chemotherapy** to shrink the tumour (chemoreduction), facilitating subsequent local treatment, thereby avoiding enucleation or external beam radiotherapy. Chemotherapy also will have a beneficial effect if a smaller tumour is present in the fellow eye or if there is a pinealoblastoma.

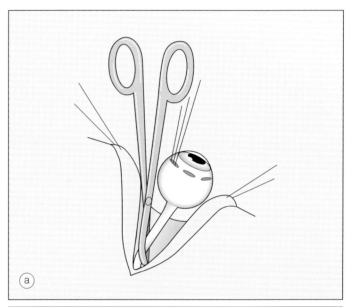

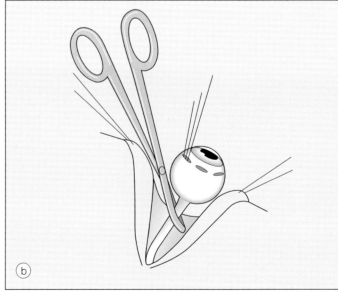

**Figure 7.83** Brachytherapy of retinoblastoma. **(a)** Before treatment; **(b)** after treatment, showing typical 'cottage cheese' appearance (Courtesy of N. Bornfeld)

**Figure 7.84** Enucleation. **(a)** Correct technique involving a long optic nerve segment; **(b)** incorrect (From B. Damato, from *Ocular Tumours*, Butterworth-Heinemann, 2000)

2. **Enucleation** if there is rubeosis, vitreous haemorrhage or optic nerve invasion. Enucleation is also indicated if chemoreduction fails or a normal fellow eye makes aggressive chemotherapy inappropriate. It is also useful for diffuse retinoblastoma because of poor visual prognosis and high risk of recurrence with other therapeutic modalities. Post-enucleation adjuvant therapy in high-risk cases significantly reduces the occurrence of metastatic disease. Enucleation should be performed with minimal manipulation and it is imperative to obtain a long piece of optic nerve (8–12 mm) (Fig. 7.84a). There is no contraindication to the insertion of an orbital implant. Unfortunately, subsequent shortening of the fornices and retraction of the implant (post-enucleation socket syndrome) may require further surgical intervention.

***Extraocular extension*** beyond the lamina cribrosa is treated with chemotherapy after enucleation. Extension to the cut end of the optic nerve or extension through the sclera is treated with chemotherapy and irradiation of the affected orbit.

***Metastatic disease*** is treated with high-dose chemotherapy, total body irradiation and bone marrow rescue. Patients with malignant cells in the cerebrospinal fluid may require intrathecal methotrexate.

> **NB:** If any eye with retinoblastoma has been conserved, follow-up is necessary every 1–3 months for the first year, then every 3–4 months for the next year or two, then 6-monthly until the age of about 5 years, then annually until the age of about 10 year. Orbital scans are indicated in high-risk cases. Patients with heritable retinoblastoma also need brain scans for pinealoblastoma and appropriate advice or management regarding second malignant neoplasms in later life.

## FURTHER READING

Benz MS, Scott UI, Murray TG, et al. Complications of systemic chemotherapy as treatment of retinoblastoma. *Arch Ophthalmol* 2000;118:577–578.

Gombos DS, Kelly A, Coen P, et al. Retinoblastoma treated with primary chemotherapy alone: the significance of tumour size, location, and age. *Br J Ophthalmol* 2002;86:80–83.

Hungerford J. Factors influencing metastasis in retinoblastoma. *Br J Ophthalmol* 1993;77:541.

Karcioglu ZA, Al-Mesfer SA, Abboud E, et al. Workup for metastatic retinoblastoma: a review of 261 patients. *Ophthalmology* 1997; 104:307–312.

Kingston JE, Hungerford JL, Madreperla SA, et al. Results of combined chemotherapy and radiotherapy for advanced intraocular retinoblastoma. *Arch Ophthalmol* 1996;114:1339–1343.

O'Brien JM. Alternative treatment in retinoblastoma. *Ophthalmology* 1998;105:571–572.

Shields CL, De Potter P, Himelstein BP, et al. Chemoreduction in the initial management of intraocular retinoblastoma. *Arch Ophthalmol* 1996;114:1330–1338.

Shields CL, Honavar SG, Meadows AT, et al. Chemoreduction plus focal therapy for retinoblastoma: factors predictive of need for treatment with external beam radiotherapy or enucleation. *Am J Ophthalmol* 2002;133:657–664.

Shields CL, Honavar SG, Shields JA, et al. Factors predictive of recurrence of retinal tumors, vitreous seeds, and subretinal seeds following chemoreduction for retinoblastoma. *Arch Ophthalmol* 2002;120:460–464.

Shields CL, Santos MC, Diniz W, et al. Thermotherapy for retinoblastoma. *Arch Ophthalmol* 1999;117:885–893.

Shields CL, Shields JA, Cater J, et al. Plaque radiotherapy for retinoblastoma. Long-term tumor control and treatment complications in 208 tumors. *Ophthalmology* 2001;108:2116–2121.

Shields CL, Shields JA, Needle M, et al. Combined chemotherapy and adjuvant treatment for intraocular retinoblastoma. *Ophthalmology* 1997;104:2101–2111.

Singh AD. Visual results in children treated for retinoblastoma [Editorial]. *Eye* 2002;16:115–116.

Watts P, Westall C, Colpa L, et al. Visual results in children treated for macular retinoblastoma. *Eye* 2002;16:75–80.

Wilson MW, Rodriguez-Galindo C, Haik BG, et al. Multiagent chemotherapy as neoadjuvant treatment for multifocal retinoblastoma. *Ophthalmology* 2001; 108:2106–2115.

# Astrocytoma

Astrocytoma of the retina or optic nerve head is a rare benign tumour which does not usually threaten vision. The tumour is composed of large fibrillary astrocytes, calcospherites and blood vessels, which may be abundant (Fig. 7.85). Astrocytomas may be encountered as an incidental solitary lesion in normal individuals and, rarely, in patients with neurofibromatosis, but most notably occur in association with tuberous sclerosis. About 50% of patients with tuberous sclerosis have fundus astrocytomas, which may be multiple and bilateral.

## DIAGNOSIS

- A semi-translucent nodule (Fig. 7.86a and 7.86b) which stains but does not leak fluorescein (Fig. 7.86c and 7.86d) or a white, well-circumscribed plaque, usually in the fundus periphery (Fig. 7.87).
- A peripapillary, calcific, nodular, mulberry-like lesion (Fig. 7.88).
- An intermediate type of lesion with features of both types may also be encountered.
- Most tumours are static in size and appearance, although a minority may grow and become more calcified (Fig. 7.89).
- Secondary cystic degeneration may occur (Fig. 7.90).
- Rare complications include subretinal exudation and vitreous haemorrhage.

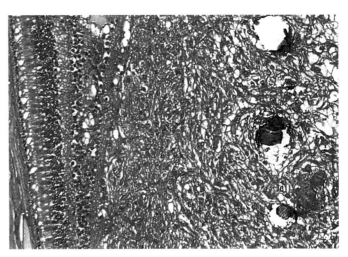

**Figure 7.85** Light micrograph of a retinal astrocytoma showing fibrillary astrocytes and calcospherites (Courtesy of P. Hiscott)

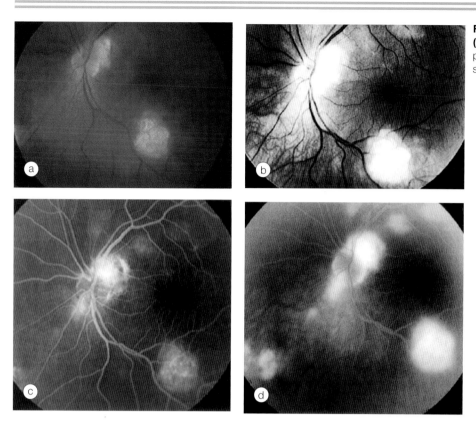

**Figure 7.86** Optic nerve and retinal astrocytomas. **(a)** Colour image; **(b)** red-free image; **(c)** FA venous phase shows hyperfluorescence; **(d)** late phase shows staining

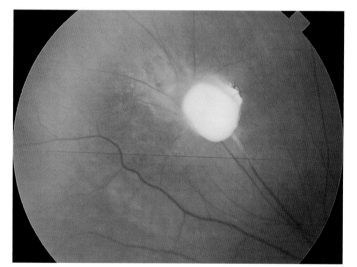

**Figure 7.87** Retinal astrocytoma

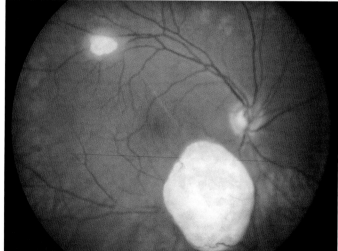

**Figure 7.88** Longstanding retinal astrocytomas

### Differential diagnosis

1. **Optic disc drusen,** if large and exposed.

2. **Myelinated nerve fibres** may resemble a small, flat astrocytoma.

3. **Retinoblastoma,** endophytic or regressed, may mimic a mulberry astrocytoma.

***Tuberous sclerosis*** (Bourneville disease) is an autosomal dominant phacomatosis characterised by the development of hamartomas in multiple organ systems from all primary germ layers. The classic triad of (a) *epilepsy,* (b) *mental retardation* and (c) *adenoma sebaceum* occurs in only a minority of patients, but is diagnostic when present.

### 1. Cutaneous signs

- Adenoma sebaceum, consisting of fibroangiomatous red papules with a butterfly distribution around the nose and cheeks, is universal (Fig. 7.91).

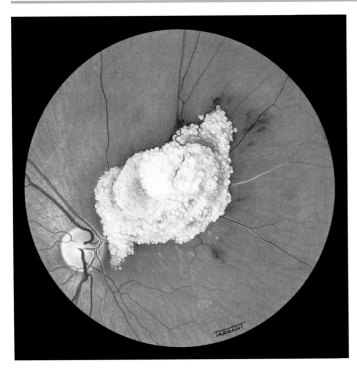

**Figure 7.89** Calcified mulberry-like retinal astrocytoma

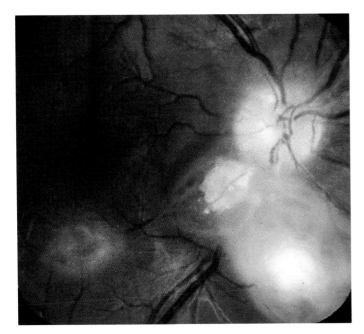

**Figure 7.90** Retinal astrocytoma with cystic degeneration

- Ashleaf spots are hypopigmented macules on the trunk, limbs and scalp. In infants with sparse skin pigmentation, they are best detected using ultra-violet light, under which they fluoresce (Wood's lamp).
- Confetti skin lesions.
- Shagreen patches consist of diffuse thickening over the lumbar region (Fig. 7.92).
- Fibrous plaques on the forehead.
- Skin tags (molluscum fibrosa pendulum).
- Café-au-lait spots.
- Subungual hamartomas.

### 2. Neurological features

- Scattered cerebral astrocytic hamartomas are universal (Fig. 7.93).
- Mental retardation.
- Seizures.

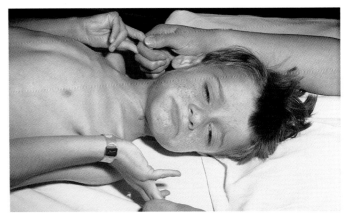

**Figure 7.91** Adenoma sebaceum in a patient with tuberous sclerosis during an epileptic fit

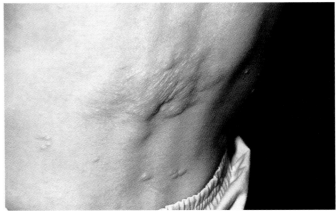

**Figure 7.92** Shagreen patches in tuberous sclerosis

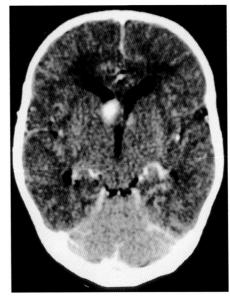

**Figure 7.93** CT shows scattered cerebral astrocytic hamartomas in tuberous sclerosis

313

### 3. Visceral tumours

- Renal angiomyolipomas and cysts.
- Cardiac rhabdomyomas.
- Pulmonary lymphangiomatosis.

## FURTHER READING

Zimmer-Galler IE, Robertson DM. Long-term observation of retinal lesions in tuberous sclerosis. *Am J Ophthalmol* 1995;119: 318–324.

# Capillary Haemangioma

Capillary haemangioma of the retina or optic nerve head is a rare, sight-threatening vascular hamartoma which can occur in isolation. However, about 50% of patients with solitary capillary haemangiomas and virtually all patients with multiple lesions have von Hippel–Lindau disease (vH-L). The prevalence of retinal capillary haemangiomas in patients with vH-L is approximately 60%.

## ENDOPHYTIC HAEMANGIOMA

### Diagnosis

1. **Presentation.** The median age at diagnosis in patients with vH-L is earlier (18 years) than in those without vH-L (36 years). The tumour may be detected by screening of those at risk or because of symptoms due to macular exudates or retinal detachment.

2. **Signs,** in chronological order:

   - A tiny red lesion located within the capillary bed between an arteriole and a venule (Fig. 7.94).
   - A small, well-defined nodule (Fig. 7.95).
   - A round orange-red mass associated with dilatation and tortuosity of the supplying artery and draining vein due to arteriovenous shunting, so that both vessels appear similar (Fig. 7.96).
   - Fibrotic angiomas are white and without feeder vessels.

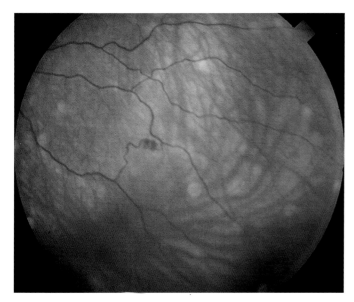

**Figure 7.94** Very early retinal capillary haemangioma

### Complications

- Hard exudate formation in the area surrounding the tumour and/or at the macula (Fig. 7.97).
- Macular oedema and cellophane maculopathy.
- Epiretinal membrane formation.
- Retinal detachment, which may be tractional (Fig. 7.98), rhegmatogenous or exudative.
- Vitreous haemorrhage.
- Secondary glaucoma and phthisis.

### OTHER TYPES

1. **Exophytic haemangioma** is less common and arises from the outer retina in the juxtapapillary region and

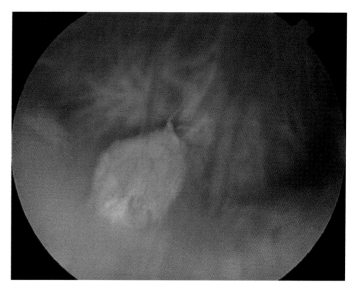

**Figure 7.95** Retinal capillary haemangioma

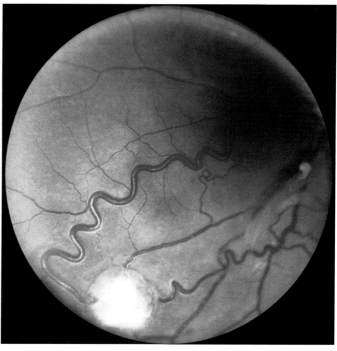

**Figure 7.96** Retinal capillary haemangioma with vascular dilatation

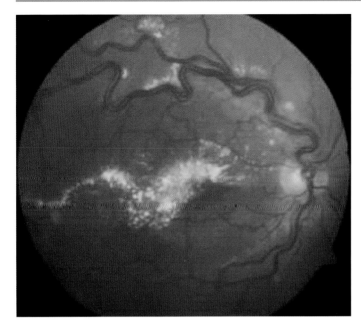

**Figure 7.97** Macular hard exudates associated with retinal capillary haemangioma

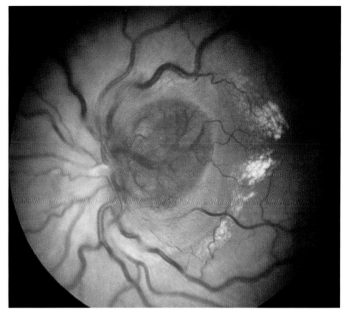

**Figure 7.100** Capillary haemangioma of the optic disc with macular exudates (Courtesy of K. Nischal)

presents with visual loss. It is characterised by a sessile, ill-defined lesion with dilated blood vessels, which may be associated with retinal oedema and haemorrhage (Fig. 7.99), and exudative retinal detachment.

2. **Optic nerve head haemangioma** develops at the optic disc, causing visual loss from exudation (Fig. 7.100).

## INVESTIGATIONS

FA shows early hyperfluorescence and late leakage (Fig. 7.101).

## TREATMENT

1. **Argon laser photocoagulation** for small peripheral lesions. Following successful treatment, the calibre of the feeding blood vessels returns to normal (Fig. 7.102).

2. **Cryotherapy** for larger peripheral lesions (Fig. 7.103) or those with exudative retinal detachment. Vigorous treatment of a large lesion may cause a temporary but extensive exudative retinal detachment.

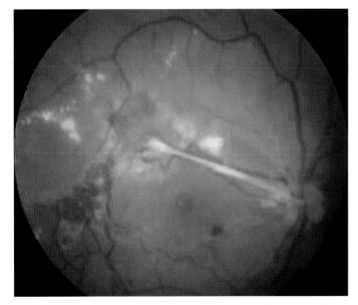

**Figure 7.98** Tractional retinal detachment associated with retinal capillary haemangioma

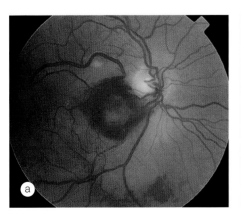
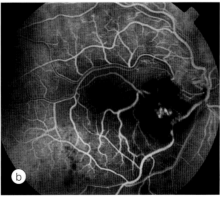
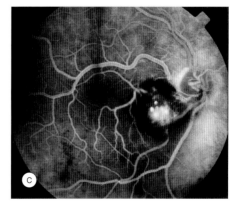

**Figure 7.99** **(a)** Juxtapapillary exophytic retinal capillary haemangioma with subretinal haemorrhage; **(b)** and **(c)** FA shows progressive central hyperfluorescence of the tumour with surrounding hypofluorescence due to blockage by blood

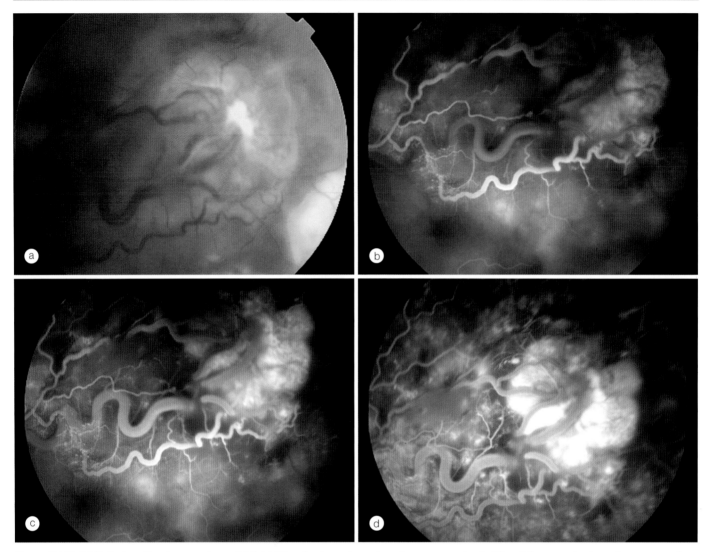

**Figure 7.101** **(a)** Retinal capillary haemangioma; **(b)** & **(c)** FA early phase shows hyperfluorescence due to filling; **(d)** progressive hyperfluorescence due to leakage

3. **Brachytherapy** for lesions too large for cryotherapy.

4. **Vitreoretinal surgery** may be required for non-absorbing vitreous haemorrhage, epiretinal fibrosis or tractional retinal detachment. If appropriate, the tumour may be destroyed by endolaser photocoagulation.

## VON HIPPEL–LINDAU DISEASE

vH-L is caused by a mutation on the short arm of chromosome 3 and inherited in an autosomal dominant fashion.

### Clinical features

- CNS haemangioma involving the cerebellum (Fig. 7.104), spinal cord, medulla or pons affects about 25% of patients with retinal tumours.
- Phaeochromocytoma.
- Renal cell carcinoma and pancreatic islet cell carcinoma.
- Cysts of the testis, kidneys, ovaries, lungs, liver and pancreas.
- Polycythaemia, which may be the result of factors released by a cerebellar or renal tumour.

***Screening*** is vital because it is impossible to predict which patients with retinal haemangiomas will harbour systemic lesions. The ophthalmologist must therefore refer all such patients for systemic and neurological evaluation. Relatives should also be screened, because of the dominant inheritance pattern of the disease. Apart from physical examination, the following screening protocol should be regularly performed in patients with established vH-L and relatives at risk.

1. **Annual screening**

   - Physical examination.
   - Ophthalmoscopy from age 5 years, increased to 6-monthly from 10 to 30 years.
   - Renal ultrasonography from age 16 years.
   - Twenty-four hour urine collection for estimation of vanillyl mandelic acid and catecholamine levels from age 10 years to detect phaeochromocytoma.

2. **Screening every 2 years** involves abdominal and brain MRI scans from age 15 years.

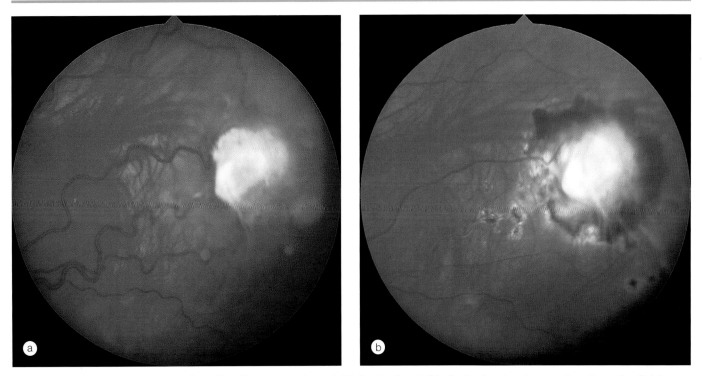

**Figure 7.102** Laser photocoagulation of retinal capillary haemangioma. **(a)** Before treatment; **(b)** after treatment; note regression of vascular dilatation

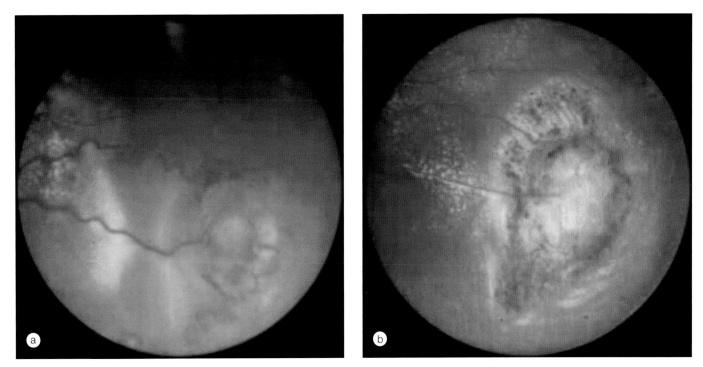

**Figure 7.103** Cryotherapy of retinal haemangioma. **(a)** Before treatment; **(b)** after treatment (Courtesy of W.S. Foulds)

***Genetic tests*** are indicated in all patients with suspected disease and in first- and second-degree relatives. With modern techniques, the sensitivity is almost 100%.

## FURTHER READING

Atebara NH. Retinal capillary hemangioma treated with verteporfin photodynamic therapy. *Am J Ophthalmol* 2002;134:788–790.

Garcia-Arumi J, Sararols LH, Cavero L, et al. Therapeureputic options for capillary papillary hemangiomas. *Ophthalmology* 2000;107: 48–54.

Girmens JF, Erginay A, Massin P, et al. Treatment of von Hippel-Lindau retinal hemangioblastoma by the vascular endothelial growth factor receptor inhibitor SU5416 is more effective for associated macular edema than for the hemangioblastoma. *Am J Ophthalmol* 2003;136:194–196.

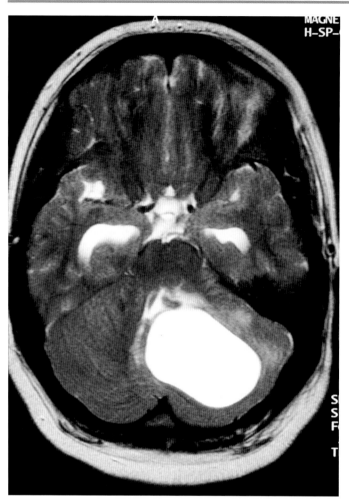

**Figure 7.104** Cystic cerebellar haemangioma (Courtesy of A. Singh)

- Because of sluggish flow of blood, the red cells may sediment and separate from plasma, giving rise to 'menisci', or fluid levels within the lesion, best seen on FA (Fig. 7.107).
- Complications, which are uncommon, include haemorrhage and epiretinal membrane formation.

**Treatment** involving photocoagulation should be avoided as it may result in haemorrhage or tumour enlargement. Rarely, vitrectomy may be necessary for non-absorbing vitreous haemorrhage.

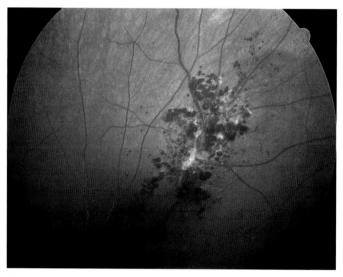

**Figure 7.105** Retinal cavernous haemangioma (Courtesy of C. Barry)

Singh AD, Nouri M, Shields CL, et al. Retinal capillary hemangioma. A comparison of sporadic cases and cases associated with von Hippel-Lindau disease. *Ophthalmology* 2001;108:1907–1911.

Singh AD, Shields JA, Shields CL. Solitary retinal capillary hemangioma: hereditary (von Hippel-Lindau disease) or non-hereditary? *Arch Ophthalmol* 2001;119:232–234.

Webster AR, Maher ER, Moore AT. Clinical characteristics of ocular angiomatosis in von Hippel-Lindau disease and correlation with germline mutation. *Arch Ophthalmol* 1999;117:371–378.

# Cavernous Haemangioma

Cavernous haemangioma of the retina or optic nerve head is a rare, congenital, unilateral, vascular hamartoma. It can be inherited in an autosomal dominant fashion in combination with lesions of the skin and CNS ('neuro-oculo-cutaneous phacomatosis' or 'cavernoma multiplex').

## Diagnosis

1. **Presentation** may be in the second to third decades with vitreous haemorrhage or, more frequently, as a chance finding.

2. **Signs**

   - Sessile clusters of saccular aneurysms resembling a 'bunch of grapes' on the retina (Fig. 7.105) or optic nerve head (Fig. 7.106).

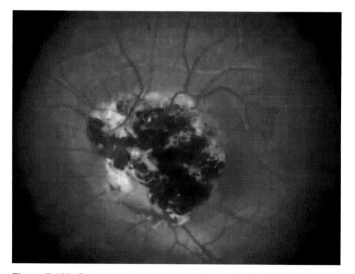

**Figure 7.106** Cavernous haemangioma at the optic disc (Courtesy of P. Lommatzsch)

# Racemose Haemangioma

Racemose haemangioma (also known as arteriovenous malformation) of the retina and optic nerve head is a rare, usually unilateral, congenital malformation involving direct commu-

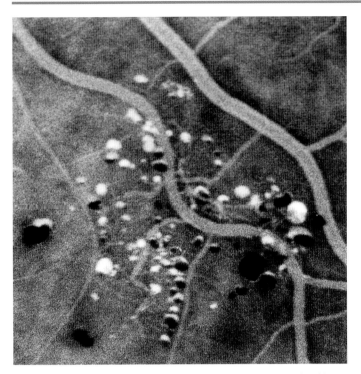

Figure 7.107 FA of a cavernous haemangioma shows fluid levels with hypofluorescence corresponding to red blood cells and hyperfluorescence corresponding to plasma

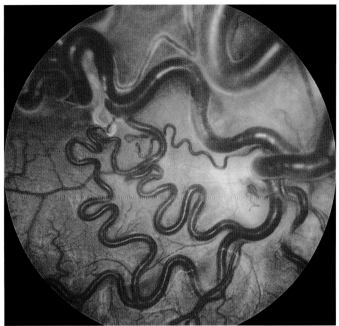

**Figure 7.108** Racemose haemangioma

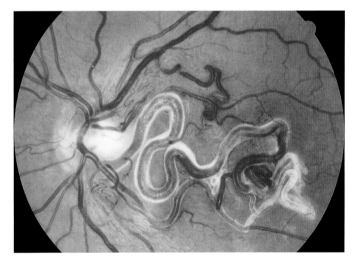

**Figure 7.109** Racemose haemangioma with sclerotic blood vessel

nication between the arteries and veins without an intervening capillary bed. Some patients have similar ipsilateral lesions involving the midbrain, baso-frontal region and posterior fossa (an association referred to as the Wyburn–Mason syndrome). Brain involvement may lead to spontaneous haemorrhage or epilepsy. Occasionally, malformations may involve the maxilla, mandible and orbit. Facial skin lesions have also been reported.

## Diagnosis

1. **Presentation** may be with visual impairment or, more commonly, as a chance finding.

2. **Signs**

   - Enlarged, tortuous blood vessels which are often more numerous than in a normal fundus, with the vein and artery appearing similar (Fig. 7.108).
   - With time, the vessels become more dilated and tortuous, and may become sclerotic (Fig. 7.109).
   - Rare complications of very large lesions include exudation and vitreous haemorrhage.

3. **FA** usually shows increasing vascular hyperfluorescence but absence of leakage (Fig. 7.110a and b).

**Treatment** is not required.

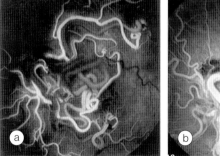
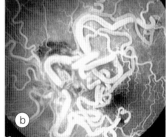

**Figure 7.110** FA of a cavernous haemangioma shows progressive hyperfluorescence of blood vessels but absence of leakage

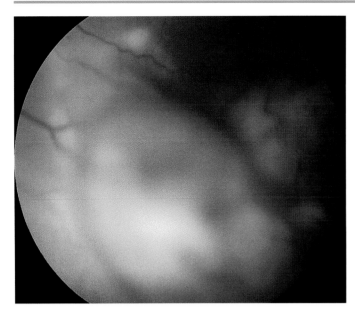

**Figure 7.111** Vasoproliferative tumour

# Vasoproliferative Tumour

Retinal vasoproliferative tumour is a rare gliovascular lesion which occurs in healthy individuals.

### Diagnosis

1. **Presentation** is in the fifth to sixth decades with blurring of vision due to macular exudation.

2. **Signs**

   - A solitary, highly vascularised, yellow, retinal or subretinal mass usually located in the retinal periphery (Fig. 7.111).
   - Complications include haemorrhage, exudation, cystoid macular oedema, epiretinal fibrosis and exudative retinal detachment.

**Treatment** involving cryotherapy, laser photocoagulation or brachytherapy may be beneficial but the visual prognosis is guarded.

### FURTHER READING

Heimann H, Bornfeld N, Vij O, et al. Vasoproliferative tumours of the retina. *Br J Ophthalmol* 2000;84:1162–1169.

Jain K, Berger AR, Yucil YH, et al. Vasoproliferative tumours of the retina. *Eye* 2003;17:364–368.

Sarraf D, Payne AM, Kitchen ND, et al. Familial cavernous hemangioma: an expanding ocular spectrum. *Arch Ophthalmol* 2000; 118:969–973.

Shields CL, Shields JA, Barrett J, et al. Vasoproliferative tumors of the ocular fundus. Classification and clinical manifestations in 103 patients. *Arch Ophthalmol* 1995;113:615–623.

# Primary Intraocular Lymphoma

Primary intraocular–CNS lymphoma is an uncommon, diffuse, highly malignant, large B-cell (non-Hodgkin) lymphoma.

It arises within the brain, spinal cord, leptomeninges and/or the eye and has a poor prognosis, with a 5-year survival rate of less than 33%.

## DIAGNOSIS

### CNS lymphoma

1. **At presentation,** the following four profiles are seen:

   - Solitary or multiple intracranial nodules.
   - Diffuse meningeal or periventricular lesions.
   - Localised intradural spinal masses.
   - Intraocular involvement.

2. **The diagnosis** is usually made by identifying malignant lymphocytes in the brain, cerebrospinal fluid or vitreous.

***Intraocular lymphoma*** involves the vitreous and retina and frequently represents a diagnostic challenge, masquerading as uveitis. Both eyes are eventually affected in 80% of cases, but often asymmetrically.

1. **'Chronic anterior uveitis'** unresponsive to steroids.

2. **'Intermediate uveitis'** in an elderly patient may initially be responsive to steroids but subsequently becomes unresponsive. The vitreous typically shows large clumps or sheets composed of malignant cells.

3. **Posterior segment**

   - Multifocal, large, yellowish, sub-RPE infiltrates (Fig. 7.112).
   - Occasionally, coalescence of the lesions may form a ring encircling the equator, which is pathognomonic for lymphoma (Fig. 7.113).
   - Less frequent manifestations include diffuse retinal infiltrates (Fig. 7.114) resembling viral retinitis, vascular sheathing and occlusion, and multifocal tiny deep white lesions which can be misdiagnosed as inflammatory.

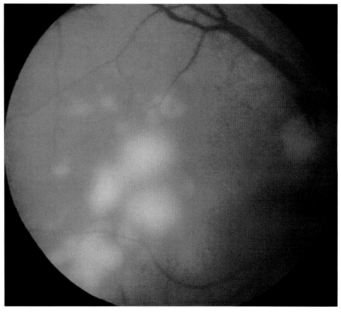

**Figure 7.112** Multiple sub-RPE infiltrates in primary intraocular lymphoma (Courtesy of A. Cruess)

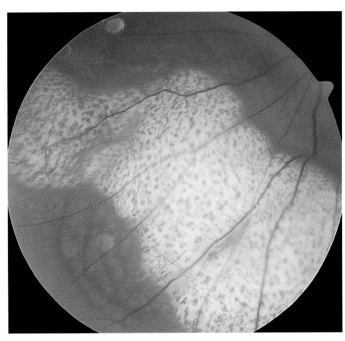

**Figure 7.113** Coalescent infiltration in primary intraocular lymphoma

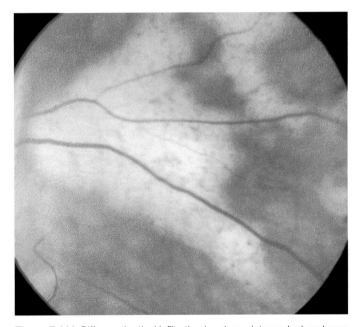

**Figure 7.114** Diffuse subretinal infiltration in primary intraocular lymphoma

---

**NB: Most patients presenting with primary intraocular lymphoma develop CNS lymphoma within 2 or 3 years.**

---

### Investigations

1. **Intraocular biopsy** by pars plana vitrectomy, 20-gauge needle vitreous biopsy or FNAB of subretinal nodules. The lymphoma cells (Fig. 7.115) are fragile, and, to prevent a false-negative result, it is important to examine the sample without delay. Any steroid therapy should be stopped a few days before this investigation.

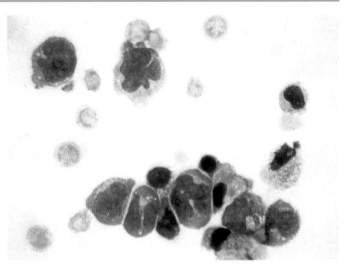

**Figure 7.115** Vitreous biopsy in primary intraocular lymphoma showing lymphoma cells with large irregular nuclei (Courtesy of P. Smith)

2. **Clinical neurological examination** for signs of CNS disease.

3. **MRI brain scan** – should be performed repeatedly with contrast enhancement.

4. **Lumbar puncture** – to detect lymphoma cells in cerebrospinal fluid.

### Treatment

1. **Systemic treatment** involves external beam radiotherapy to the eyes, sometimes in conjunction with whole brain radiotherapy, and/or systemic or intrathecal chemotherapy.

2. **Intravitreal** methotrexate may be used as primary treatment and for recurrences following systemic therapy.

### FURTHER READING

Char DH, Ljung BM, Miller T, et al. Primary intraocular lymphoma (ocular reticulum cell sarcoma) diagnosis and management. *Ophthalmology* 1988;95:625–630.

de Smet MD, Vancs VS, Kohler D, et al. Intravitreal chemotherapy for the treatment of recurrent intraocular lymphoma. *Br J Ophthalmol* 1999;83:448–451.

Hoffman PM, McKelvie P, Hall AJ, et al. Intraocular lymphoma: a series of 14 patients with clinicopathological features and treatment outcomes. *Eye* 2003;17:513–521.

Ridley ME, McDonald HR, Sternberg P Jr, et al. Retinal manifestations of ocular lymphoma (reticulum cell sarcoma). *Ophthalmology* 1992;99:1153–1160.

Smith JR, Rosenbaum JT, Wilson DJ. Role of intravitreal methotrexate in the management of primary central nervous system lymphoma with ocular involvement. *Ophthalmology* 2002;109:1709–1716.

# TUMOURS OF THE RETINAL PIGMENT EPITHELIUM

## Congenital Hypertrophy of the Retinal Pigment Epithelium

Congenital hypertrophy of the retinal pigment epithelium (CHRPE) is a common benign lesion which may be (a) *typical*, either solitary or grouped, or (b) *atypical*. It is important to differentiate the two types because the latter may have important systemic implications.

## TYPICAL CHRPE

### 1. Solitary

- A unilateral, flat, dark-grey or black, well-demarcated, round or oval lesion one to three disc diameters in size (Figs. 7.116 and 7.117).
- Depigmented lacunae, which often enlarge or coalesce, may be present, particularly in older patients (Fig. 7.118).

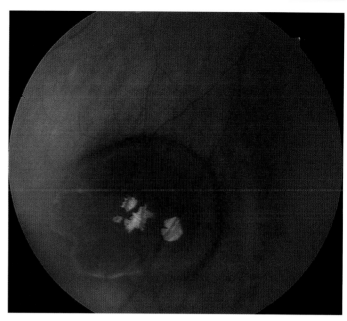

**Figure 7.118** Typical congenital hypertrophy of the RPE with hypopigmented lacunae

- Some lesions may become depigmented with only a thin rim of residual pigment remaining at their margin (Fig. 7.119).
- Occasionally CHRPE is juxtapapillary (Fig. 7.120).

### 2. Grouped

- Usually unilateral, variably sized, sharply circumscribed, round or oval, dark-grey or black lesions, often organised in a pattern simulating animal footprints (bear-track pigmentation) (Fig. 7.121). The lesions are often confined to one sector or quadrant of the fundus, with the smaller spots usually located more centrally.

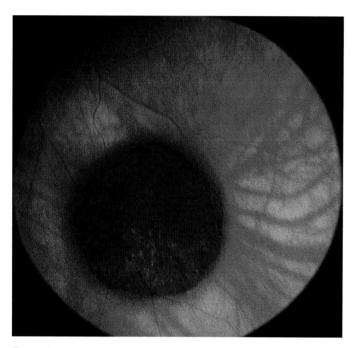

**Figure 7.116** Typical congenital hypertrophy of the RPE

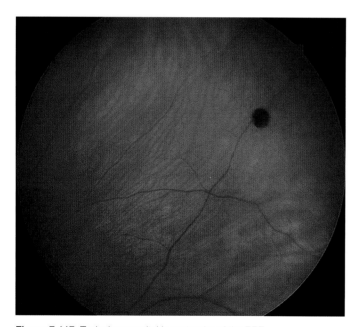

**Figure 7.117** Typical congenital hypertrophy of the RPE

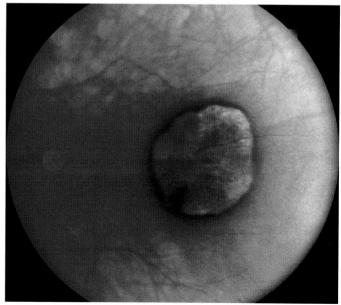

**Figure 7.119** Typical congenital hypertrophy of the RPE, which is nearly completely hypopigmented except for a peripheral ring

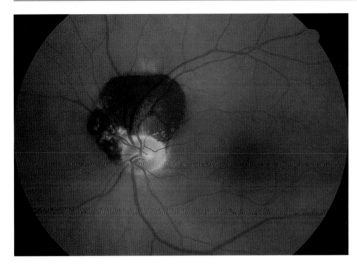

**Figure 7.120** Juxtapapillary congenital hypertrophy of the RPE

develop in adolescence (Fig. 7.124). If untreated, virtually all patients with FAP develop carcinoma of the colorectal region by the age of 50 years. From the age of 10 years, persons at risk should undergo regular endoscopic examinations, and a prophylactic total colectomy should be performed early in adult life in all affected persons. As a result of the dominant inheritance pattern, intensive survey of family members is imperative. The FAP gene has been identified on 5q21–q22. Thus, molecular genetic analysis may identify carriers of the disease in selected cases. Over 80% of patients with FAP have atypical CHRPE which is present at birth. A positive criterion for FAP is the presence of at least four lesions whatever their size, or at least two lesions, one of which must be large. Such fundus lesions in a family member should therefore arouse suspicion of FAP.

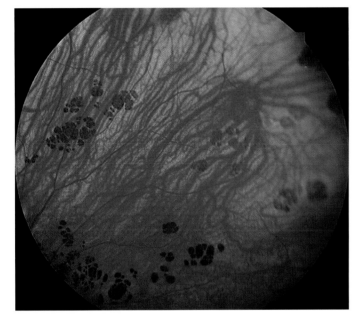

**Figure 7.121** Grouped ('bear-track') congenital hypertrophy of the RPE

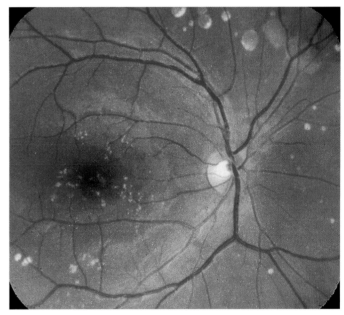

**Figure 7.122** Depigmented grouped ('polar-bear-track') congenital hypertrophy of the retinal pigment epithelium (Courtesy of J.D.M. Gass, from *Stereoscopic Atlas of Macular Diseases*, Mosby, 1997)

- Occasionally the lesions may be depigmented ('polar-bear tracks') (Fig. 7.122).

## ATYPICAL CHRPE

### Signs

- Multiple, bilateral, widely separated, frequently oval or spindle-shaped lesions of variable size associated with hypopigmentation at one margin (Fig. 7.123).
- The lesions have a haphazard distribution and may be pigmented, depigmented or heterogeneous.

### Systemic implications

1. **Familial adenomatous polyposis (FAP)** is a dominantly inherited condition characterised by adenomatous polyps throughout the rectum and colon which usually start to

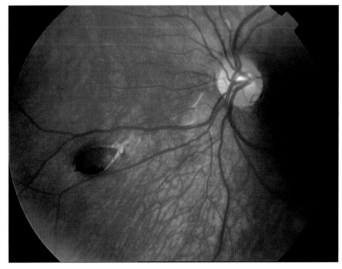

**Figure 7.123** Atypical congenital hypertrophy of the RPE

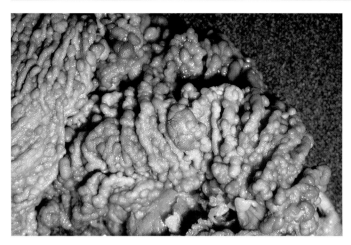

**Figure 7.124** Intestinal adenomatous polyposis

2. **Gardner syndrome** is characterised by FAP, osteomas of the skull and mandible, and cutaneous soft tissue tumours such as epidermoid cysts, lipomas and fibromas.

3. **Turcot syndrome** is characterised by FAP and tumours of the CNS, particularly medulloblastoma and glioma.

## Combined Hamartoma of the Retina and Retinal Pigment Epithelium

Combined hamartoma of the retina and RPE is a rare, usually unilateral malformation which may be juxtapapillary or peripheral. It predominantly affects males and usually occurs sporadically in normal patients, as well as in individuals with neurofibromatosis types 1 and 2, tuberous sclerosis, Gorlin syndrome and incontinentia pigmenti.

### JUXTAPAPILLARY

1. **Presentation** is in late childhood or early adulthood with blurred vision and metamorphopsia.

2. **Signs.** Deep, slightly elevated, greyish-brown pigmentation associated with variable intra- and epiretinal gliosis, a fine network of dilated capillaries and vascular tortuosity (Fig. 7.125).

### *Peripheral*

1. **Presentation** is in early childhood with strabismus.

2. **Signs**

   - A linear ridge associated with retinal distortion and vascular stretching (Fig. 7.126).
   - Complications of both types include retinal and/or optic nerve head distortion, macular oedema, choroidal neovascularisation and, rarely, retinoschisis and retinal detachment.

3. **Treatment** involving removal of epiretinal membranes by vitreoretinal surgery may be attempted but the visual results are often disappointing.

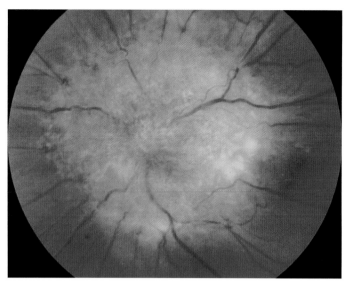

**Figure 7.125** Juxtapapillary combined hamartoma of the retina and RPE

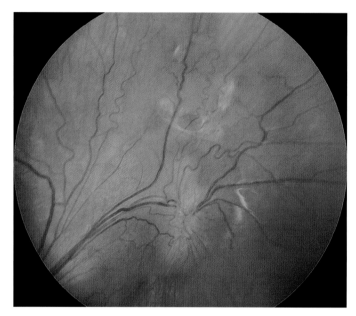

**Figure 7.126** Retinal distortion associated with combined hamartoma of the retina and RPE

## Congenital Hamartoma of the Retinal Pigment Epithelium

1. **Signs**

   - This is a rare, small, jet-black, nodular RPE lesion, with well-defined margins, which involves the overlying retina. Common associated features include minimally dilated retinal feeding vessels and surrounding retinal traction.
   - The lesion is typically located immediately adjacent to the foveola and is 1.5 mm or less in base diameter (Fig. 7.127).

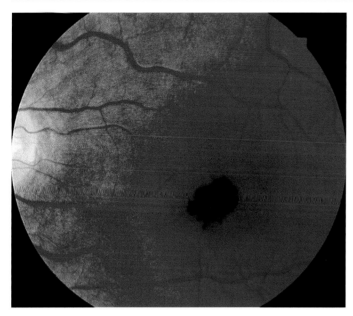

**Figure 7.127** Congenital hamartoma of the RPE

- Visual acuity is usually normal, but may occasionally be impaired as a result of surrounding foveal traction or central foveal involvement.
- The lesion does not appear to enlarge and many patients are asymptomatic in the absence of foveal traction.

**2. Treatment** is not appropriate.

## FURTHER READING

Gass JD. Focal congenital anomalies of the retinal pigment epithelium. *Eye* 1989;3:1–18.

Shields CL, Shields JA, Marr BP, et al. Congenital simple hamartoma of the retinal pigment epithelium. A study of five cases. *Ophthalmology* 2003;110.1005–1011.

Shields JA, Shields CL, Gunduz K, et al. Neoplasms of the retinal pigment epithelium. The 1998 Albert Ruedeman, Sr, Memorial Lecture. Part 2. *Arch Ophthalmol* 1999;117:601–608.

# Chapter **8**

# ACQUIRED OPTIC NERVE DISORDERS

## Applied Anatomy

### GENERAL STRUCTURE

1. **Afferent fibres.** The optic nerve carries about 1.2 million afferent nerve fibres which originate in the retinal ganglion cells. Most of these synapse in the lateral geniculate body, although some reach other centres, notably the pre-tectal nuclei in the midbrain. Nearly one-third of the fibres subserve the central 5° of the visual field. Within the optic nerve itself, the nerve fibres are divided into about 600 bundles (each containing 2000 fibres) by fibrous septae derived from the pia mater (Fig. 8.1).

2. **Oligodendrocytes** provide axonal myelination. Congenital myelination of retinal nerve fibres is the result of anomalous intraocular extension of these cells.

3. **Microglia** are immunocompetent phagocytic cells which probably modulate apoptosis (programmed death) of retinal ganglion cells.

4. **Astrocytes** line the spaces between axons and other structures. When axons are lost in optic atrophy, astrocytes fill in the empty spaces.

5. **Surrounding sheaths**

   a. *The pia mater* is the delicate innermost sheath containing blood vessels.

   b. *The subarachnoid space* is continuous with the cerebral subarachnoid space and contains cerebrospinal fluid (CSF).

   c. *The outer sheath* comprises the arachnoid mater and the tougher dura mater. The latter is continuous with the sclera. Optic nerve fenestration involves incision of the outer sheath.

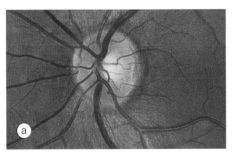
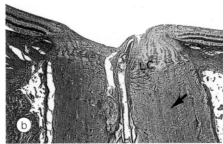
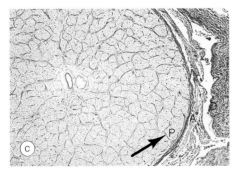
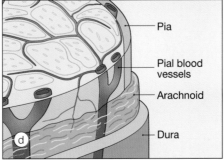

**Figure 8.1** Structure of the optic nerve.
**(a)** Clinical appearance; **(b)** longitudinal section, LC = lamina cribrosa, arrow points to a fibrous septum; **(c)** transverse section, P = pia, A = arachnoid, D = dura; **(d)** surrounding sheaths and pial blood vessels (Courtesy of Wilmer Institute)

## RETINAL NERVE FIBRES

An understanding of the distribution of the 1.2 million ganglion cell axons as they pass across the retina to enter the scleral canal to form the optic nerve head (optic disc) is the key to the interpretation of visual field loss in relation to optic nerve cupping in glaucoma.

1. **Within the retina** the arrangement is as follows (Fig. 8.2):

   - Fibres arising from the macula follow a straight course to the optic nerve head, forming a spindle-shaped area (papillomacular bundle).
   - Fibres arising from the nasal retina also follow a relatively straight course to the optic nerve.
   - Fibres arising temporal to the macula follow an arcuate path around the papillomacular bundle to reach the optic nerve head. They do not cross the horizontal raphé that extends from the foveola to the temporal retinal periphery, demarcating the superior and inferior halves of the retina.

   > **NB:** The arcuate fibres reaching the superotemporal and inferotemporal aspects of the optic nerve head are most vulnerable to glaucomatous damage; the fibres in the papillomacular bundle are the most resistant.

2. **Within the optic nerve head** the retinal fibres are arranged as follows (Fig. 8.3):

   - Fibres from the peripheral fundus lie deep within the retinal nerve fibre layer (i.e. nearer the pigment epithelium) but occupy the most peripheral (superficial) portion of the optic nerve.
   - Fibres arising near to the optic nerve lie superficially within the nerve fibre layer (i.e. nearer the vitreous) but they occupy the central (deep) portion of the optic nerve.

## ANATOMICAL SUBDIVISIONS

The optic nerve is approximately 50 mm long from globe to chiasm and can be subdivided into four segments.

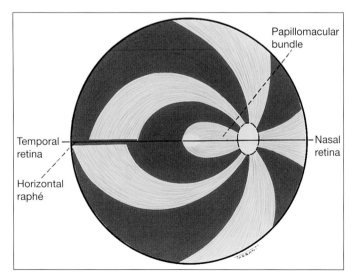

**Figure 8.2** Anatomy of retinal nerve fibres

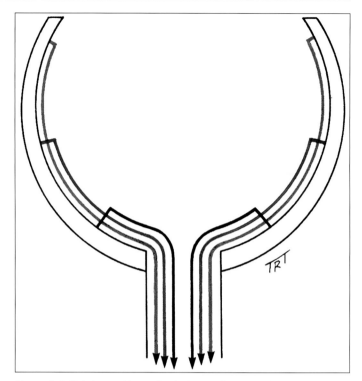

**Figure 8.3** Relative positions of retinal nerve fibres. (Red) peripheral; (blue) equatorial; (black) central

1. **Intraocular** segment (optic disc, nerve head) is the shortest, being 1 mm deep and 1.5 mm in vertical diameter. Disorders affecting this part of the optic nerve include inflammation (papillitis), oedema, abnormal deposits (drusen) and glaucoma.

2. **Intraorbital** segment is 25–30 mm long and extends from the globe to the optic foramen at the orbital apex. Its diameter is 3–4 mm because of the addition of the myelin sheaths to the nerve fibres. At the orbital apex, the nerve is surrounded by the tough fibrous annulus of Zinn, from which originate the four rectus muscles. Because the superior and medial rectus muscles partly originate from the nerve sheath itself, inflammatory optic neuropathy (e.g. retrobulbar neuritis) may be associated with pain on ocular movement. Within the orbit the optic nerve is slack and S-shaped, allowing for eye movements without stretching.

   > **NB:** Because of this redundancy, the optic nerve does not become unduly stretched until proptosis is severe.

3. **Intracanalicular** segment traverses the optic canal and measures about 6 mm. Unlike the intraorbital portion, it is fixed to the canal, since the dura mater fuses with the periosteum.

4. **Intracranial** segment joins the chiasm and varies in length from 5 to 16 mm (average 10 mm). Long intracranial segments are particularly vulnerable to damage by adjacent lesions such as pituitary adenomas and aneurysms.

# AXOPLASMIC TRANSPORT

This is the movement of cytoplasmic organelles within a neurone, between the cell body and the terminal synapse (Fig. 8.4a and b). Orthograde transport involves movement from the cell body to synapse, and retrograde transport is characterised by the converse. Rapid axoplasmic transport is an active mechanism requiring oxygen and is energised by ATP. Axoplasmic flow may be interrupted by a variety of insults, including hypoxia and toxins that interfere with ATP production. Retinal cotton-wool spots are the result of accumulation of organelles due to interruption of axoplasmic flow between the retinal ganglion cells and their terminal synapses. Papilloedema is similarly caused by hold up of axoplasmic flow at the lamina cribrosa (Fig. 8.4c and d).

# OPTIC NERVE HEAD

1. **The posterior scleral foramen** (scleral canal) is the conduit for the retinal nerve fibres leaving the eye. It is usually oval in its vertical axis and has an average vertical diameter of 1.75 mm, which is, however, related to the size of the optic disc and the globe itself. Eyes with small canals therefore have small optic discs (e.g. hypermetropia) and those with large canals have large discs (e.g. myopia). Variations in the mode of scleral entry of the optic nerve give rise to anomalous congenital optic disc appearances, particularly tilted discs.

2. **The lamina cribrosa** consists of a series of plates of collagenous connective tissue which stretch across the posterior scleral foramen. It is perforated by 200–400 openings (pores) containing bundles of retinal nerve fibres. The largest pores are arranged in a vertical hourglass distribution at the superior and inferior poles, have thin connective tissue supports, and contain large nerve fibres which are most vulnerable to glaucomatous damage. The superficial openings of the pores appear as grey dots deep within the optic cup. The appearance of the pores correlates with the severity of glaucomatous damage. If the damage is slight, the pores are small and round; in moderately damaged eyes, they are oval; and in severe damage, they are slit-like.

3. **The optic cup** is a pale depression in the centre of the optic nerve head which is not occupied by neural tissue. On direct ophthalmoscopy, it is best evaluated by observing the bending of the small blood vessels as they cross the disc, although on slit-lamp indirect ophthalmoscopy, the actual borders of the cup may be appreciated three dimensionally. The pallor of the cup results from exposure of the lamina cribrosa and lack of glial tissue in the centre of the disc. The size of the cup is related to the diameter of the disc. A small disc will have a small cup because the nerve fibres are crowded as they leave the eye, while a large disc will have a larger cup because the retinal nerve fibres are less crowded.

4. **Blood supply.** The superficial nerve fibre layer (Fig. 8.5) and the prelaminar layer are supplied by the central retinal artery and the pial plexus derived from collateral branches of the ophthalmic artery. The laminar and postlaminar layers are supplied by the rich capillary network derived from the circle of Zinn-Haller, which receives blood from three sources: (a) choroidal feeder vessels, (b) short posterior ciliary vessels and (c) pial vessels derived from distal branches of the ophthalmic artery.

**Figure 8.4 (a)** & **(b)** Normal axoplasmic transport; **(c)** & **(d)** interruption of axoplasmic transport in papilloedema (Courtesy of Wilmer Institute)

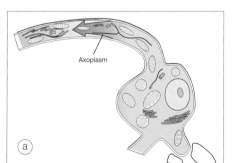
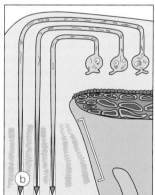
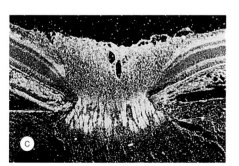
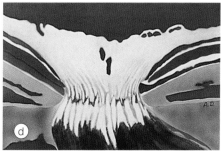

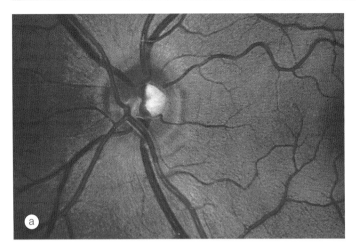

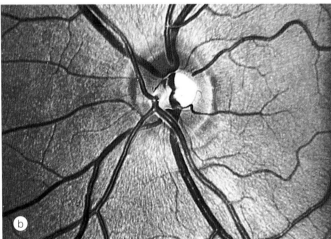

**Figure 8.5** Retinal nerve fibre striations. **(a)** Colour image; **(b)** red-free image (Courtesy of Wilmer Institute)

# The Optic Disc

## NORMAL APPEARANCE

1. **The optic cup** may have one of three main appearances:

   - A small dimple-like central cup (Fig. 8.6).
   - A punched-out deep central cup (Fig. 8.7).
   - A cup with a sloping temporal wall (Fig. 8.8).

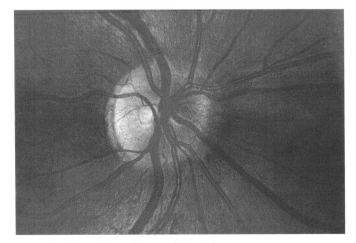

**Figure 8.6** Normal disc with a small (dimple) cup

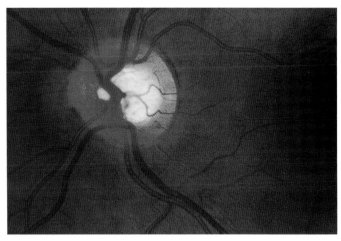

**Figure 8.7** Normal disc with a punched-out deep central cup

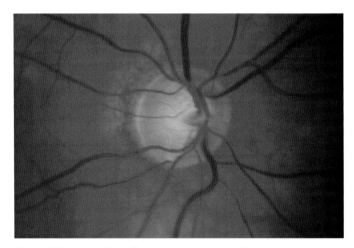

**Figure 8.8** Normal disc with a sloping temporal wall

2. **The cup–disc ratio** indicates the diameter of the cup expressed as a fraction of the diameter of the disc and should be measured in both vertical (Fig. 8.9) and horizontal meridia. This ratio is genetically determined and is also dependent on the area of the disc. The neuroretinal rim occupies a relatively similar area in different eyes; large discs therefore have large cups with high cup–disc ratios (Fig. 8.10). Most normal eyes have a vertical cup–disc ratio of 0.3 or less; only 2% have a ratio greater than 0.7. A ratio greater than 0.7 is suspicious, although it may not be pathological. In any individual, asymmetry of 0.2 or more between the eyes should also be regarded with suspicion until glaucoma has been excluded.

3. **The neuroretinal rim** is the tissue between the outer edge of the cup and the disc margin. The normal healthy rim has an orange or pink colour and shows a characteristic configuration. The inferior rim is the broadest, followed by the superior, nasal and temporal ('ISNT'). A large physiological cup is due to a mismatch between the size of the scleral canal and the number of traversing nerve fibres, which, in health, remains constant. Pathological cupping is caused by an irreversible decrease in the number of nerve fibres, glial cells and blood vessels.

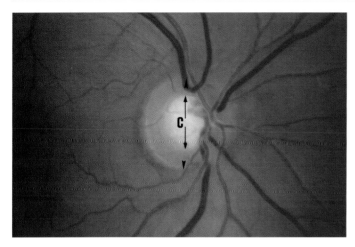

**Figure 8.9** Vertical cup–disc ratio (C = cup; arrows = edge of the optic disc)

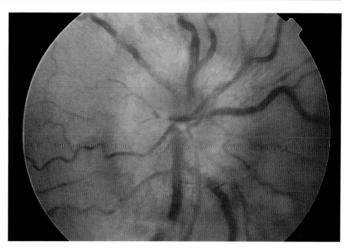

**Figure 8.11** Swollen optic disc

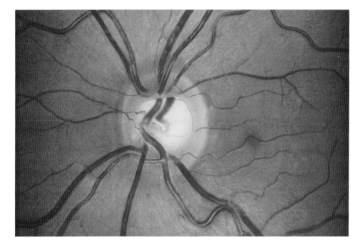

**Figure 8.10** Normal disc with a large physiological cup

4. **The blood vessels** from within the optic nerve enter the disc centrally and then course nasally, following the edge of the cup. The central retinal artery is usually nasal to the vein.

## DISC APPEARANCE IN OPTIC NEUROPATHIES

### Classification

There is no direct correlation between the appearance of the optic disc and visual function. The main appearances in acquired optic nerve disorders are the following:

1. **Normal disc** is classically associated with retrobulbar neuritis, although the disc may initially appear normal in Leber optic neuropathy and compressive lesions.

2. **Disc swelling** (Fig. 8.11) is a feature of papilloedema, anterior ischaemic optic neuropathy, papillitis and the acute stage of Leber optic neuropathy. It may also occur with compressive lesions before the development of optic atrophy.

3. **Optociliary shunts** (Fig. 8.12) represent retinochoroidal venous collaterals at the optic disc and develop as a compensatory mechanism for chronic venous compression, most frequently caused by optic nerve sheath meningioma and, occasionally, optic nerve glioma.

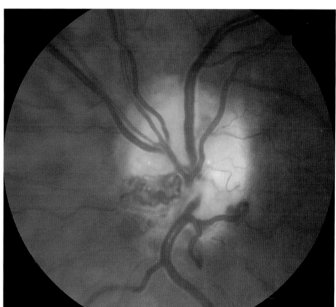

**Figure 8.12** Optociliary shunts

4. **Optic atrophy,** which represents the end result of almost any of the aforementioned clinical conditions and may be primary or secondary (see below).

5. **Glaucomatous** damage is characterised by cupping (Fig. 8.13).

***Primary optic atrophy*** occurs without antecedent swelling of the optic nerve head. It may be caused by lesions affecting the visual pathways from the retrolaminar portion of the optic nerve to the lateral geniculate body. Lesions anterior to the optic chiasm result in unilateral optic atrophy, whereas those involving the chiasm and optic tract will cause bilateral atrophy.

1. **Signs**

   - Pale, flat disc with clearly delineated margins, reduction in number of small blood vessels on the disc surface

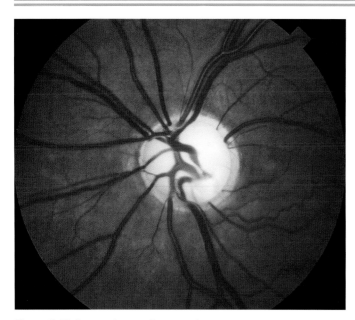

**Figure 8.13** Severe glaucomatous cupping

(Kestenbaum sign) and attenuation of peripapillary blood vessels, and thinning of the retinal nerve fibre layer (Fig. 8.14).

- The atrophy may be diffuse or sectoral depending on the cause and level of the lesion. Temporal pallor may indicate atrophy of fibres from the papillomacular bundle, which enters the optic nerve head on the temporal side.

2. **Causes**

- Following retrobulbar neuritis.
- Compressive lesions such as tumours and aneurysms.
- Hereditary optic neuropathies.
- Toxic and nutritional optic neuropathies.

***Secondary optic atrophy*** is preceded by swelling of the optic nerve head.

1. **Signs** vary according to the cause. The main features are (Fig. 8.15):

- White or dirty grey, slightly raised disc with poorly delineated margins due to gliosis.
- Reduction in number of small blood vessels on the disc surface.

2. **Causes** include chronic papilloedema, anterior ischaemic optic neuropathy and papillitis.

# Optic Neuritis

## CLASSIFICATION

Optic neuritis is an inflammatory, infective or demyelinating process affecting the optic nerve. It can be classified both ophthalmoscopically and aetiologically as follows.

### *Ophthalmoscopic*

1. **Retrobulbar neuritis,** in which the optic disc appearance is normal, at least initially, because the optic nerve head is not involved. It is the most frequent type in adults and is frequently associated with multiple sclerosis (MS).

2. **Papillitis,** in which the pathological process affects the optic nerve head primarily, or is secondary to contiguous retinal inflammation. It is characterised by variable hyperaemia and oedema of the optic disc, which may be associated with peripapillary flame-shaped haemorrhages (Fig. 8.16). Cells in the posterior vitreous may be seen. Papillitis is the most common type of optic neuritis in children, although it can also affect adults.

3. **Neuroretinitis** is characterised by papillitis in association with inflammation of the retinal nerve fibre layer and a macular star fig. (Fig. 8.17). It is the least common type of optic neuritis and is almost never a manifestation of demyelination.

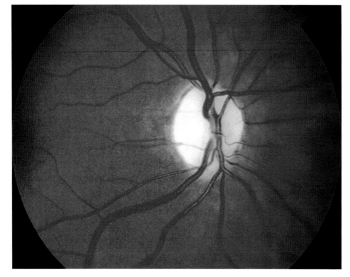

**Figure 8.14** Primary optic atrophy

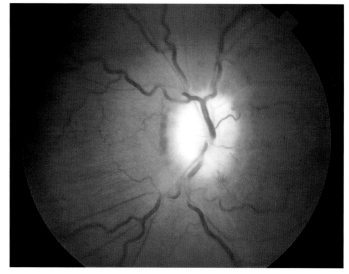

**Figure 8.15** Secondary optic atrophy

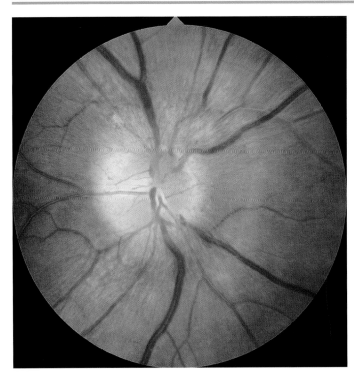

**Figure 8.16** Papillitis

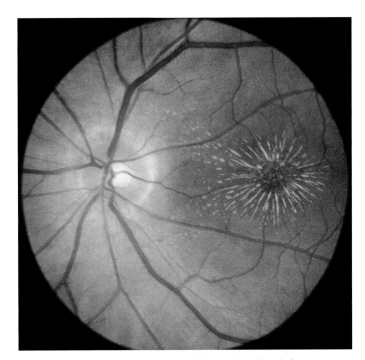

**Figure 8.17** Neuroretinitis (Courtesy of Western Eye Hospital)

### *Aetiological*

1. **Demyelinating,** which is by far the most common cause.

2. **Parainfectious,** which may follow a viral infection or immunisation.

3. **Infectious,** which may be sinus-related, or associated with cat-scratch fever, syphilis, Lyme disease, cryptococcal meningitis in patients with AIDS, or herpes zoster.

4. **Non-infectious** causes include sarcoidosis and systemic autoimmune diseases such as systemic lupus erythematosus, polyarteritis nodosa and other vasculitides.

## DEMYELINATING OPTIC NEURITIS

*Demyelination* is a pathological process by which normally myelinated nerve fibres lose their insulating myelin layer. The myelin is phagocytosed by microglia and macrophages, subsequent to which astrocytes lay down fibrous tissue (the plaque). A demyelinating disease disrupts nervous conduction within the white matter tracts within the brain, brain stem and spinal cord; peripheral nerves are not involved.

1. **Demyelinating diseases** which may cause ocular problems are the following:

   a. *Isolated optic neuritis,* with no clinical evidence of generalised demyelination, although in a high proportion of cases this subsequently develops.
   b. *MS,* which is by far the most common.
   c. *Devic disease* (neuromyelitis optica), which is a rare disease that may occur at any age. It is characterised by bilateral optic neuritis and subsequent development of transverse myelitis (demyelination of the spinal cord) within days or weeks.
   d. *Schilder disease,* which is a very rare, relentlessly progressive, generalised disease with an onset prior to the age of 10 years and death within 1 to 2 years. Bilateral optic neuritis without subsequent improvement may occur.

2. **Ocular features**

   a. *Visual pathway* lesions most frequently involve the optic nerves and cause optic neuritis. Demyelination may occasionally involve the optic chiasm, and rarely the optic tracts or radiations.
   b. *Brain-stem* lesions may result in internuclear ophthalmoplegia (Fig. 8.18) and other gaze palsies, ocular motor cranial nerve palsies, trigeminal and facial nerve palsies and nystagmus.

3. **Association of optic neuritis with MS.** Although some patients with optic neuritis have no clinically demonstrable associated systemic disease, the following close association exists between optic neuritis and MS.

   - Patients who develop optic neuritis but have normal brain MRI have a 16% probability of developing MS within 5 years.
   - At the first episode of optic neuritis, approximately 50% of patients with no other clinical signs of MS will show demyelinating lesions on MRI (Figs. 8.19 and 8.20). These patients carry a high risk of developing clinical MS within 5–10 years.
   - Optic neuritis occurs in 70% of patients with established MS.
   - In a patient with optic neuritis, the subsequent risk of MS is increased with winter onset, HLA-DR2 positivity and Uhtoff phenomenon (worsening of symptoms on elevation of body temperature, such as with exercise or a hot bath).

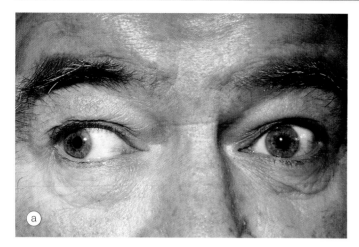

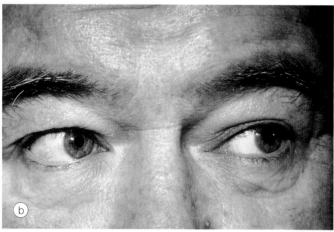

**Figure 8.18** Left internuclear ophthalmoplegia. **(a)** Defective left adduction on right gaze; **(b)** normal left gaze

### Diagnosis of optic neuritis

1. **Presentation** is usually between the ages of 20 and 50 years (mean around 30 years) with subacute monocular visual impairment. Some patients experience positive

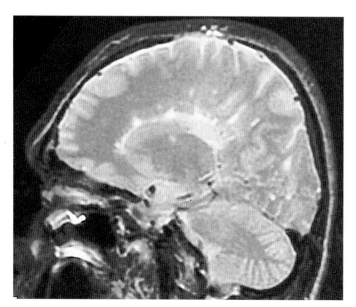

**Figure 8.19** Sagittal T1-weighted MRI showing periventricular plaques of demyelination

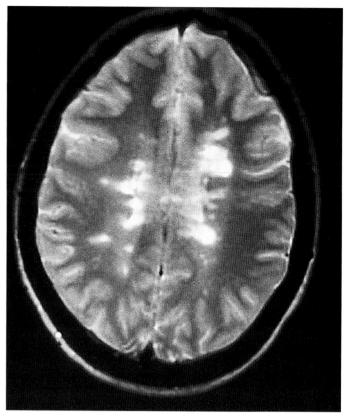

**Figure 8.20** Axial T2-weighted MRI showing periventricular plaques of demyelination

visual phenomena (phosphenes) characterised by tiny white or coloured flashes or sparkles. Discomfort or pain in or around the eye is common and frequently exacerbated by ocular movements. This may precede or accompany the visual loss and usually lasts a few days. Frontal headache and tenderness of the globe may also be present.

2. **Signs**

   - Visual acuity is usually between 6/18 and 6/60 although rarely it may be reduced to no light perception.
   - Other signs of optic nerve dysfunction (i.e. afferent pupillary defect [APD], dyschromatopsia, diminished light-brightness appreciation and impairment of contrast sensitivity).
   - The optic disc is normal in the majority of cases (retrobulbar neuritis); the remainder show papillitis.
   - Temporal disc pallor may be seen in the fellow eye, indicative of previous optic neuritis.

3. **Visual field defects**

   - The most common is diffuse depression of sensitivity in the entire central 30°. This is followed in frequency by altitudinal/arcuate defects and then by focal central/centrocaecal scotomas (Fig. 8.21).
   - Focal defects are frequently accompanied by an element of superimposed generalised depression.
   - The asymptomatic fellow eye may also manifest visual field loss at presentation.

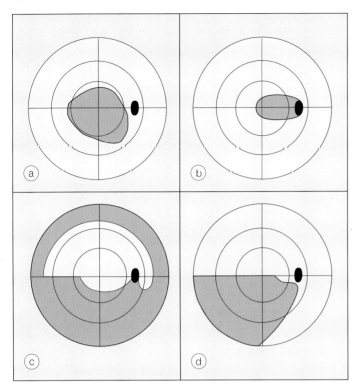

**Figure 8.21** Visual field defects in optic neuritis. **(a)** Central scotoma; **(b)** centrocaecal scotoma; **(c)** nerve fibre bundle defect; **(d)** altitudinal defect

4. **Course.** Vision worsens over several days to 2 weeks and then begins to recover within 2 to 4 weeks. Initial recovery is fairly rapid and then levels off but continues over 6 to 12 months.

***Prognosis of optic neuritis.*** Approximately 75% of patients recover visual acuity to 6/9 or better; 85% recover to 6/12 or better, even if visual acuity was reduced to no light perception during the attack. However, despite return of visual acuity, other parameters of visual function, such as colour vision, contrast sensitivity and light-brightness appreciation, often remain abnormal. A mild APD may persist and optic atrophy may ensue, particularly following recurrent attacks. About 10% of patients develop chronic optic neuritis characterised by slowly progressive or stepwise visual loss, unassociated with periods of recovery.

***Treatment of optic neuritis***

1. **Indications.** When visual acuity within the first week of onset is worse than 6/12, treatment may speed up recovery by 2 to 3 weeks. This is relevant in the patients with poor vision in the fellow eye or those with occupational requirements. Treatment, however, does not influence the eventual visual outcome.

2. **Regimen**

   a. *Intravenous methylprednisolone sodium succinate* (1 g daily) for 3 days, followed by oral prednisolone (1 mg/kg daily) for 11 days and then tapered for 3 days.

   b. *Intramuscular interferon beta-1a* at the first episode of optic neuritis is beneficial in reducing the development of clinical demyelination over the following 3 years in patients at high risk of MS based on the presence of subclinical brain MRI lesions.

## PARAINFECTIOUS OPTIC NEURITIS

Optic neuritis may be associated with various viral infections such as measles, mumps, chickenpox, rubella, whooping cough and glandular fever. It may also occur following immunisation. Children are affected much more frequently than adults.

### Diagnosis

1. **Presentation** is usually 1–3 weeks following a viral infection, with acute severe visual loss, which may involve both eyes. This may be associated with other neurological features such as headache, seizures or ataxia (meningoencephalitis).

2. **Signs.** The optic discs most frequently manifest bilateral papillitis, although occasionally there may be a neuroretinitis or the discs may be normal.

***Treatment*** is not required in the vast majority of patients because the prognosis for spontaneous visual recovery is very good. However, when visual loss is severe and bilateral or involves an only seeing eye, intravenous steroids should be considered.

## INFECTIOUS OPTIC NEURITIS

1. **Sinus-related** optic neuritis is an infrequent condition characterised by recurrent attacks of unilateral visual loss associated with severe headache and spheno-ethmoidal sinusitis. Possible mechanisms of optic neuropathy include direct spread of infection, occlusive vasculitis and bony defects in the wall of the sinus. Treatment is with systemic antibiotics and, if appropriate, surgical drainage.

2. **Cat-scratch fever** (benign lymphoreticulosis) is caused by *Bartonella henselae* or, less commonly, *Bartonella quintana*, which is inoculated by a cat scratch or bite. Numerous ophthalmological features have been described, most notably neuroretinitis (see below).

3. **Syphilis** may cause acute papillitis or neuroretinitis during the primary or secondary stages. Involvement may be unilateral or bilateral and is frequently associated with a mild vitritis.

4. **Lyme disease** (borreliosis) is a spirochaetal infection caused by *Borrelia burgdorferi* which is transmitted by a tick bite. It may cause neuroretinitis and, occasionally, acute retrobulbar neuritis, which may be associated with other neurological manifestations and may mimic MS. Treatment of neurological involvement is with intravenous ceftriaxone 2 g daily for 14 days.

5. **Cryptococcal meningitis** in patients with AIDS may be associated with acute optic neuritis, which may be bilateral.

6. **Varicella zoster virus** most frequently causes papillitis by spread from contiguous retinitis (i.e. acute retinal

necrosis, progressive outer retinal necrosis). Primary optic neuritis is uncommon but may occur in patients with herpes zoster ophthalmicus.

## NON-INFECTIOUS OPTIC NEURITIS

***Sarcoid-associated*** optic neuritis affects 1–5% of patients with neurosarcoid. It may develop during the course of the disease or be its presenting manifestation. Optic nerve involvement may be indistinguishable from that in demyelination, although the optic nerve head may exhibit a characteristic lumpy appearance suggestive of granulomatous infiltration and there may be an inflammatory reaction in the vitreous. The response to steroid therapy is often rapid although vision may decline if treatment is tapered or stopped prematurely and some patients require long-term low-dose therapy. Methotrexate may also be used as an adjunct to steroids or as monotherapy in steroid-intolerant patients.

***Autoimmune*** optic nerve involvement may be in the form of retrobulbar neuritis or anterior ischaemic optic neuropathy (see below). Some patients may also experience slowly progressive visual loss suggestive of optic nerve compression. Treatment is with systemic steroids.

### Neuroretinitis

1. **Presentation** is with unilateral, painless, visual impairment which starts gradually and then becomes most marked after about a week.

2. **Signs**

   - Visual acuity is impaired to a variable degree.
   - Signs of optic nerve involvement are usually mild or absent because visual loss is largely due to macular oedema rather than optic nerve dysfunction.
   - Papillitis associated with peripapillary and macular oedema; venous engorgement and splinter-shaped haemorrhages may be present in severe cases.
   - A macular star figure composed of hard exudates subsequently ensues (Fig. 8.22).
   - Central or centrocaecal scotoma.

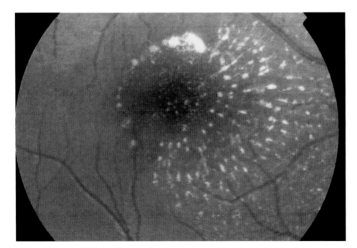

**Figure 8.22** Macular star

3. **Course** in most cases lasts between 6 and 12 months, with return to normal or near-normal visual acuity in the majority of patients, with resolution of the papillitis and then of the macular hard exudates. Initially, however, the hard exudates tend to become more prominent as the optic disc swelling is resolving. Some patients may subsequently develop an involvement of the fellow eye. Although recurrent disease is uncommon, it has a different clinical profile, characterised by signs of optic nerve dysfunction, and carries a poor visual prognosis.

4. **Fluorescein angiography** (FA) shows diffuse leakage from superficial disc vessels.

5. **Systemic associations.** About 25% of cases are idiopathic (Leber idiopathic stellate neuroretinitis). Cat-scratch fever is responsible for 60% of cases. Other notable causes include syphilis, Lyme disease, mumps and leptospirosis.

6. **Treatment** varies according to the underlying cause. Recurrent idiopathic cases may require steroids and/or azathioprine.

## FURTHER READING

Bar S, Segal M, Shapira R, et al. Neuroretinitis associated with cat scratch disease. *Am J Ophthalmol* 1990;110:703–705.

Beck RW, Arrington J, Murtagh FR, et al. Optic Neuritis Study Group. Brain magnetic resonance imaging in acute optic neuritis. *Arch Neurol* 1993;50:841–846.

Champs Study Group. Inteferon beta-1 for optic neuritis patients at high risk of multiple sclerosis. *Am J Ophthalmol* 2001;132:463–471.

Cunningham ET, Koehler JE. Ocular bartonellosis. *Am J Ophthalmol* 2000;300:340–348.

Hull TP, Bates JH. Optic neuritis after influenza vaccination. *Am J Ophthalmol* 1997;124:703–704.

Optic Neuritis Study Group. The clinical profile of acute optic neuritis. Experience of the Optic Neuritis Treatment Trial. *Arch Ophthalmol* 1991;109:1673–1678.

Optic Neuritis Study Group. The 5-year risk of MS after optic neuritis: experience of the Optic Neuritis Treatment Trial. *Neurology* 1997;49:1404–1413.

Optic Neuritis Study Group. Visual function five years after optic neuritis: experience of the Optic Neuritis Treatment Trial. *Arch Ophthalmol* 1997;115:1545–1552.

Reed BJ, Scales DK, Wong MT, et al. *Bartonella henselae* neuroretinitis in cat scratch disease; diagnosis, management and sequelae. *Ophthalmology* 1998; 105:459–466.

Sellebjerg F, Nielsen HS, Frederiksen JL, et al. A randomized, controlled trial of oral high-dose methylprednisolone in acute optic neuritis. *Neurology* 1999; 52:1479–1484.

Suhler EB, Lauer AK, Rosenbaum JT. Prevalence of serologic evidence of cat scratch disease in patients with neuroretinitis. *Ophthalmology* 2000;107:871–876.

Totan Y, Cekic O. Bilateral retrobulbar neuritis following measles in an adult. *Eye* 1999;13:383–384.

# Ischaemic Optic Neuropathy

## NON-ARTERITIC ANTERIOR ISCHAEMIC OPTIC NEUROPATHY

Non-arteritic anterior ischaemic optic neuropathy (NAION) is the most common optic neuropathy in the elderly. It is the result of a partial or total infarction of the optic nerve head caused by occlusion of the short posterior ciliary arteries. It typically occurs as an isolated event in patients between the ages of 55 and 70 years with structural crowding of the optic nerve head so that the physiological cup is either very small or absent. Predisposing systemic conditions include hypertension, diabetes mellitus, hypercholesterolaemia, collagen vascular disease, antiphospholipid antibody syndrome, hyperhomocysteinaemia, sudden hypotensive events, cataract surgery and administration of sildenafil citrate (Viagra).

### Diagnosis

1. **Presentation** is with sudden, painless, monocular visual loss which is not associated with premonitory visual obscurations. Visual loss is frequently discovered on awakening, suggesting that nocturnal hypotension may play an important role.

2. **Signs**

   - Visual acuity, in about 30% of patients, is normal or only slightly reduced. The remainder have moderate-to-severe impairment.
   - Visual field defects are typically inferior altitudinal, but central, paracentral, quadrantic and arcuate defects may be seen.
   - Dyschromatopsia is proportional to the level of visual impairment, in contrast with optic neuritis, in which colour vision may be severely impaired when visual acuity is reasonably good.
   - Disc pallor associated with diffuse or sectoral oedema, which may be surrounded by a few splinter-shaped haemorrhages (Fig. 8.23a). The oedema gradually resolves and pallor ensues (see Fig. 8.24a).

3. **FA** during the acute stage shows localised disc hyperfluorescence (Fig. 8.23b) which becomes more intense and then eventually involves the entire disc (Fig. 8.23c and 8.23d). Once optic atrophy develops, FA shows unequal choroidal filling during the arterial phase (Fig. 8.24b); the late stages show increasing disc hyperfluorescence (Fig. 8.24c and 8.24d).

4. **Special investigations** include serological studies, fasting lipid profile and blood glucose. It is also very important to exclude occult giant-cell arteritis (GCA) and other autoimmune diseases.

**Treatment.** There is no definitive treatment, although any underlying systemic predispositions should be corrected. Aspirin is effective in reducing systemic vascular events and is frequently prescribed in patients with NAION; however, it does not appear to reduce the risk of involvement of the fellow eye.

**Prognosis.** In most patients there is no further loss of vision, although, in a small percentage, visual loss continues for 6 weeks. Recurrences in the same eye occur in about 6% of patients. Involvement of the fellow eye occurs in about 10% of patients after 2 years and 15% after 5 years, an incidence lower than previously assumed. When the second eye becomes involved, optic atrophy in one eye and disc oedema in the other gives rise to the 'pseudo-Foster Kennedy syndrome' (Fig. 8.25). Two important risk factors for fellow eye involvement are poor visual acuity in the first eye and diabetes mellitus.

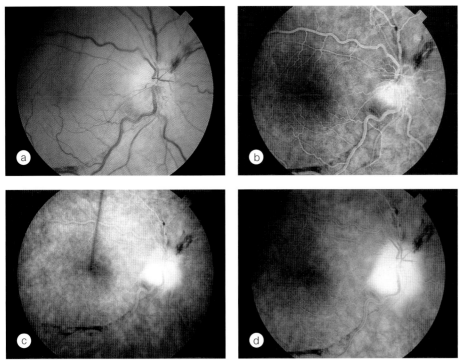

**Figure 8.23** Acute non-arteritic anterior ischaemic optic neuropathy (see text)

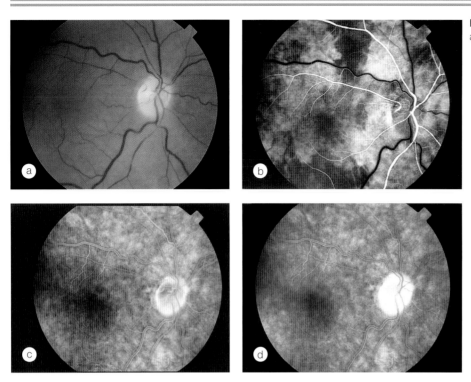

## ARTERITIC ANTERIOR ISCHAEMIC OPTIC NEUROPATHY

***Giant-cell arteritis*** (GCA) is a granulomatous necrotising arteritis (Fig. 8.26) with a predilection for large and medium-size arteries, particularly the superficial temporal, ophthalmic, posterior ciliary and proximal vertebral. The severity and extent of involvement are associated with the quantity of elastic tissue in the media and adventitia. Intracranial arteries, which possess little elastic tissue, are usually spared.

1. **Presentation** is usually in the seventh to eighth decades with the following:

- Scalp tenderness, first noticed when combing the hair, is a frequent presenting complaint.
- Headache, sometimes severe, may be localised to the frontal, occipital or temporal areas or more generalised.
- Jaw claudication is virtually pathognomonic. It is caused by ischaemia of the masseter and causes pain on speaking and chewing.
- Polymyalgia rheumatica is characterised by pain and stiffness in proximal muscle groups (typically the shoulders). It is characteristically worse in the morning and after exertion and may precede cranial symptoms by many months.

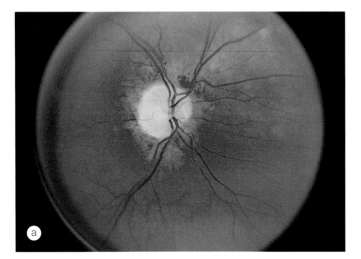

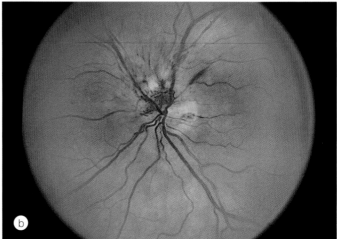

**Figure 8.25** Pseudo-Foster Kennedy syndrome associated with non-arteritic anterior ischaemic optic neuropathy. **(a)** Optic atrophy; **(b)** disc swelling (Courtesy of Wilmer Institute)

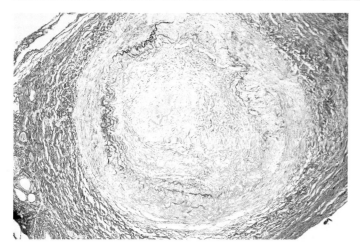

**Figure 8.26** Histology of giant-cell arteritis, showing granulomatous infiltration, disruption of the internal elastic lamina, proliferation of the intima and complete occlusion of the lumen (Courtesy of A. Garner)

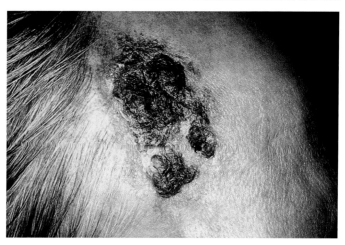

**Figure 8.28** Scalp necrosis in giant-cell arteritis

- Non-specific symptoms such as neck pain, weight loss, fever, night sweats, malaise and depression are common.
- Blindness of sudden onset with minimal systemic upset (occult arteritis) is uncommon.

## 2. Other features

- Superficial temporal arteritis is characterised by thickened, tender, inflamed and nodular arteries (Fig. 8.27), which cannot be flattened against the skull. Pulsation is initially present, but later ceases, a sign strongly suggestive of GCA, since a non-pulsatile superficial temporal artery is highly unusual in a normal individual. In very severe cases, scalp gangrene may ensue (Fig. 8.28).

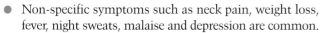

NB: The best location to examine pulsation is directly in front of the tragus of the ear.

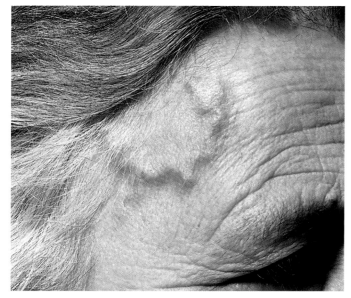

**Figure 8.27** Dilatation and tortuosity of the superficial temporal artery in giant-cell arteritis

- Complications include dissecting aneurysms, aortic incompetence, myocardial infarction, renal failure and brain-stem stroke.

## 3. Diagnostic tests

a. *Erythrocyte sedimentation rate* (ESR) is often very high, with levels of >60 mm/h. In interpreting the ESR, the following should be borne in mind.

- The normal ESR equals roughly half the age in men; and is 5 mm higher in women.
- ESR levels of 40 mm/h may be 'normal' in diabetics and in the elderly.
- Approximately 20% of patients with GCA have a normal ESR.

b. *C-reactive protein* (CRP) is invariably raised and may be helpful when ESR is equivocal.

c. *Temporal artery biopsy* (TAB) should be performed if GCA is suspected.

- Steroids should never be withheld pending biopsy, which should ideally be performed within 3 days of commencing steroids.
- Systemic steroids for more than 7 days may suppress histological evidence of active arteritis; however, this is not invariable and biopsy should still be performed even if steroid therapy has been commenced considerably earlier. This is for two reasons: firstly, if positive, it justifies long-term administration of steroids in a population highly prone to their adverse effects; secondly, if negative, it provides some justification for tailing off and stopping steroid therapy.
- In patients with ocular involvement, it is advisable to take the biopsy from the ipsilateral side. The ideal location is the temple, because it avoids damage to a major branch of the auriculotemporal nerve.
- At least 2.5 cm of the artery should be taken and serial sections examined, because of the phenome-

non of 'skip lesions' – segments of histologically normal arterial wall may alternate with segments of granulomatous inflammation.

● Lack of pulsation may render TAB difficult, especially in inexperienced hands; not uncommonly, a segment of nerve is excised and sent for histological examination.

4. **Treatment** involves the administration of systemic steroids.

5. **Ophthalmic features**

a. *Arteritic anterior ischaemic optic neuropathy* (AAION) is the most common (Fig. 8.29). In untreated patients, the incidence is 30–50%, of which one-third develop bilateral involvement. Posterior ischaemic optic neuropathy is much less common (see below).

b. *Transient ischaemic attacks* (amaurosis fugax) may precede infarction of the optic nerve head.

c. *Cotton-wool spots* are uncommon. They are probably caused by platelet microembolisation from the partially thrombosed ophthalmic or central retinal artery. Because GCA is a disease of medium-sized or large arteries, it cannot involve terminal arterioles to produce cotton-wool spots.

d. *Cilioretinal artery occlusion* may be combined with AAION (see Fig. 2.92).

e. *Central retinal artery occlusion* is usually combined with occlusion of a posterior ciliary artery. This is because the central retinal artery often arises from the ophthalmic artery by a common trunk with one or more of the posterior ciliary arteries. However, ophthalmoscopy shows occlusion of only the central retinal artery; the associated ciliary occlusion can be detected only by FA.

f. *Ocular ischaemic syndrome* due to involvement of the ophthalmic artery is rare.

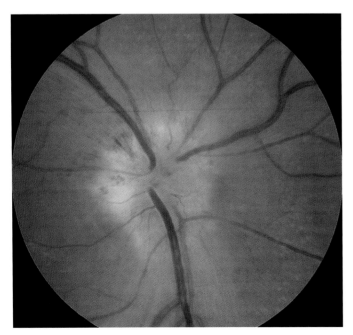

**Figure 8.29** Arteritic anterior ischaemic optic neuropathy

g. *Diplopia*, transient or constant, may be caused by ischaemia of the ocular motor nerves or extraocular muscles.

### Diagnosis of AAION

1. **Presentation** is with sudden, profound unilateral visual loss which may be accompanied by periocular pain and preceded by transient visual obscurations and flashing lights. Bilateral simultaneous involvement is rare. Most cases occur within a few weeks of the onset of GCA, although at presentation about 20% of patients do not have systemic symptoms (i.e. occult GCA).

2. **Signs,** in chronological order:

● Pale and swollen optic disc with small splinter-shaped haemorrhages on its margin (Fig. 8.30a).

> **NB: A strikingly pale ('chalky white') oedematous disc is particularly suggestive of GCA.**

● Over 1–2 months, the swelling gradually resolves and severe optic atrophy (Fig. 8.30b) and blindness ensues.

3. **FA** shows severe hypoperfusion of the choroid.

### Treatment of AAION is aimed at preventing blindness of the fellow eye, although occasionally the second eye may become involved despite early and adequate steroid administration, usually within 5 days after starting treatment.

1. **Regimen**

a. *Intravenous methylprednisolone sodium succinate* 1 g/day for 3 days together with oral prednisolone 80 mg daily. After 3 days the oral dose is reduced to 60 mg/day and then 50 mg/day for 1 week each. The daily dose is then reduced by 5 mg weekly – headache, ESR and CRP permitting – until l0 mg is reached. Maintenance daily therapy is ideally 10 mg/day, although higher doses may be required to control headache.

b. *Oral prednisolone* (80–120mg daily) alone may be administered if intravenous therapy is inappropriate.

2. **Duration** of treatment is governed by the patient's symptoms and the level of the ESR or CRP. Symptoms may, however, recur without a corresponding rise in ESR or CPR, and vice versa. Most patients need treatment for 1–2 years, although some may require indefinite maintenance therapy.

> **NB: Injudicious use of steroids may cause greater harm than the disease itself. Steroid-induced complications may necessitate the use of steroid-sparing agents such as azathioprine.**

### Prognosis of AAION is very poor because visual loss is usually permanent, although, very rarely, prompt administration of systemic steroids may be associated with partial visual recovery.

# POSTERIOR ISCHAEMIC OPTIC NEUROPATHY

Posterior ischaemic optic neuropathy (PION), also termed retrobulbar optic neuropathy, is much less common than the anterior variety. It is caused by ischaemia to the retrolaminar portion of the optic nerve which is supplied by the surrounding pial capillary plexus; only a small number of capillaries actually penetrate the nerve and extend to its central portion among the pial septae. The diagnosis PION is made after other causes of retrobulbar optic neuropathy, such as compression or inflammation, have been excluded. PION occurs in the following three settings.

1. **Operative** develops following a variety of surgical procedures, most notably involving the spine. The major risk factors appear to be anaemia and hypovolaemic hypotension. Bilateral involvement is common and the visual prognosis is poor.

2. **Arteritic** is associated with GCA and carries very poor visual prognosis.

3. **Non-arteritic** is associated with the same systemic risk factors as anterior ischaemic optic neuropathy, but is not associated with small optic discs. The visual prognosis is similar to that with NAION.

# DIABETIC PAPILLOPATHY

Diabetic papillopathy is an uncommon condition characterised by transient visual dysfunction associated with optic disc swelling which may occur in both type 1 and type 2 diabetics. The underlying pathogenesis is unclear but may be the result of small-vessel disease.

## Diagnosis

1. **Presentation** is usually with milder optic nerve dysfunction and slower progression than in NAION or optic neuritis.

2. **Signs**
   - Visual acuity is usually 6/12 or better.
   - Unilateral or bilateral, mild disc swelling and hyperaemia (Fig. 8.31). Disc surface telangiectasia is common, and, when severe, may be mistaken for neovascularisation on cursory examination.
   - Visual field defects in the form of generalised constriction or central scotomas.

*Prognosis* is relatively good despite the lack of definitive treatment. Systemic steroids are of questionable benefit and tend to compromise diabetic control. In most cases, spontaneous resolution occurs within several months, with stabilisation or improvement of visual acuity, although mild optic atrophy may ensue.

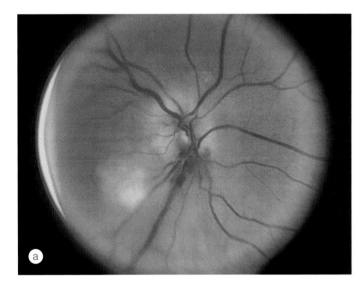

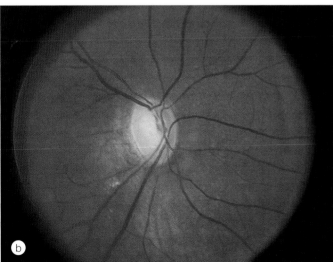

**Figure 8.30 (a)** Arteritic anterior ischaemic optic neuropathy; **(b)** optic atrophy 3 months later (Courtesy of Wilmer Institute)

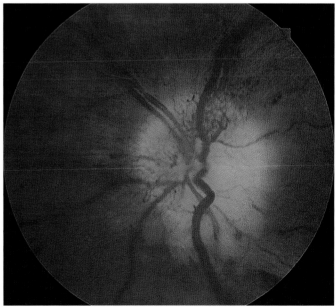

**Figure 8.31** Diabetic papillopathy

## FURTHER READING

Aiello PD, Trautmann JC, McPhee TJ, et al. Visual prognosis in giant cell arteritis. *Ophthalmology* 1993;100:550–555.

Alexandrakis G, Lam BL. Bilateral posterior ischemic optic neuropathy after spinal surgery. *Am J Ophthalmol* 1999;127:354–355.

Boone MI, Massry GG, Frankel RA, et al. Visual outcome in bilateral nonarteritic anterior ischemic optic neuropathy. *Ophthalmology* 1996;103:1223–1228.

Chan CCK, Paine M, O'Day J. Steroid management in giant cell arteritis. *Br J Ophthalmol* 2001;85:1061–1064.

Hattenhauer MG, Leavitt JA, Hodge DO, et al. Incidence of non-arteritic anterior ischemic optic neuropathy. *Am J Ophthalmol* 1997;123:103–107.

Hayreh SS, Podhajsky PA, Raman R, et al. Giant cell arteritis: validity and reliability of various diagnostic criteria. *Am J Ophthalmol* 1997;123:285–296.

Hayreh SS, Podhajsky PA, Zimmerman B. Nonarteritic anterior ischemic optic neuropathy – time of onset of visual loss. *Am J Ophthalmol* 1997;124:641–647.

Hayreh SS, Podhajsky PA, Zimmerman B. Ocular manifestations of giant cell arteritis. *Am J Ophthalmol* 1998;125:509–520.

Hayreh SS, Podhajsky PA, Zimmerman B. Ipsilateral recurrence of nonarteritic anterior ischemic optic neuropathy. *Am J Ophthalmol* 2001;132:734–742.

Hayreh SS, Zimmerman B. Visual deterioration in giant cell arteritis patients while on high dose corticosteroid therapy. *Ophthalmology* 2003;110:1204–1215.

Liu GT, Glaser JS, Schatz NJ, et al. Visual morbidity in giant cell arteritis. Clinical characteristics and prognosis of vision. *Ophthalmology* 1994;101:1779–1785.

Newman NJ, Scherer R, Langenberg P, et al, for the Ischemic Optic Neuropathy Decompression Trial Research Group. The fellow eye in NAION: report from the Ischemic Optic Neuropathy Decompression Trial follow-up. *Am J Ophthalmol* 2002;134:317–328.

Sadda S, Nee M, Miller NR, et al. Clinical spectrum of posterior ischemic optic neuropathy. *Am J Ophthalmol* 2001;132:743–750.

Salomon O, Huna-Baron R, Kurtz S, et al. Analysis of prothrombic and vascular risk factors in patients with nonarteritic anterior ischemic optic neuropathy. *Ophthalmology* 1999;106:739–742.

# Hereditary Optic Neuropathy

## LEBER HEREDITARY OPTIC NEUROPATHY

Leber hereditary optic neuropathy (LHON) is a rare disease which is the result of maternal mitochondrial DNA mutations, most notably 11778. The condition typically affects young adult males, although in atypical cases the condition may affect females and present at any age between 10 and 60 years. The diagnosis of LHON should therefore be considered in any patient with bilateral optic neuritis, irrespective of age.

### Diagnosis

1. **Presentation** is typically with unilateral, acute or sub-acute, severe, painless visual loss. The fellow eye becomes similarly affected within days or weeks (but no longer than 2 months) after the first.

2. **Signs** during the acute stage are often subtle and easily overlooked; in some patients the disc may be entirely normal.

- In typical cases there are dilated capillaries on the disc surface which may extend onto adjacent retina (telangiectatic microangiopathy), vascular tortuosity and swelling of the peripapillary nerve fibre layer (Fig. 8.32). Telangiectatic microangiopathy may be present in asymptomatic female relatives.

- Subsequently, the telangiectatic vessels regress and severe optic atrophy ensues.

> **NB:** Surprisingly, the pupillary light reactions may remain fairly brisk.

3. **FA** shows absence of dye leakage.

4. **Visual field** defects usually consist of centrocaecal scotomas.

***Treatment*** is generally ineffective although many modalities, including steroids, hydroxocobalamin and surgical intervention, have been tried. Smoking and excessive consumption of alcohol should be discouraged, to minimise potential stress on mitochondrial energy production.

***Prognosis*** is poor, although some visual recovery may occur in a minority of cases even years later. Most patients suffer severe, bilateral and permanent visual loss, with a final visual acuity of 6/60 or less. The 11778 mutation carries the worst prognosis.

## HEREDITARY OPTIC ATROPHY

The hereditary optic atrophies (neuropathies) are a very rare heterogeneous group of disorders that are primarily characterised by bilateral optic atrophy.

### Kjer syndrome

1. **Inheritance** is autosomal dominant.

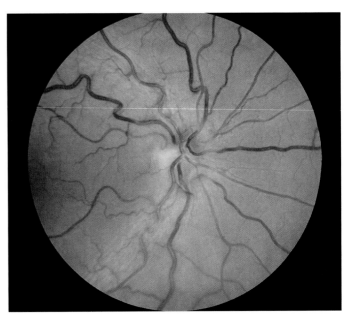

**Figure 8.32** Acute stage of Leber optic neuropathy

2. **Presentation** is usually in the first decade with insidious visual loss.

3. **Signs** – mild temporal pallor or diffuse optic atrophy.

4. **Prognosis** is variable (final visual acuity 6/12–6/60), with considerable differences within and between families.

5. **Systemic abnormalities** are absent.

### Behr syndrome

1. **Inheritance** is autosomal recessive.

2. **Presentation** is in the first decade with visual loss which stabilises after a variable period of progression.

3. **Signs** – diffuse optic atrophy.

4. **Prognosis** is variable, with moderate-to-severe visual loss and nystagmus.

5. **Systemic abnormalities** include spastic gait, ataxia and mental handicap.

**Wolfram syndrome** is also referred to as DIDMOAD (Diabetes Insipidus, Diabetes Mellitus, Optic Atrophy and Deafness).

1. **Inheritance** is autosomal recessive.

2. **Presentation** is between the ages of 5 and 21 years.

3. **Signs** – diffuse optic atrophy.

4. **Prognosis** is very poor (final visual acuity is <6/60).

5. **Systemic abnormalities** (apart from DIDMOAD) include anosmia, ataxia, seizures, mental handicap, short stature, endocrine abnormalities and elevated CSF protein.

# Toxic Optic Neuropathy

## NUTRITIONAL OPTIC NEUROPATHY

Nutritional optic neuropathy (tobacco–alcohol amblyopia) typically affects heavy drinkers and cigar and pipe smokers who are deficient in protein and the B vitamins. Most patients have neglected their diet, obtaining their calories from alcohol instead. Some of those affected also have defective vitamin B12 absorption and may develop pernicious anaemia.

### Diagnosis

1. **Presentation** is with insidious-onset, progressive, bilateral, usually symmetrical visual impairment associated with dyschromatopsia.

2. **Signs.** The optic dics at presentation are normal in most cases. Some patients show subtle temporal pallor, splinter-shaped haemorrhages on or around the disc, or minimal disc oedema.

3. **Visual field defects** are bilateral, relatively symmetrical, centrocaecal scotomas. The margins of the defects are difficult to define with a white target but are easier to plot and larger when using a red target.

**Treatment** involves weekly injections of 1000 units of hydroxocobalamin for 10 weeks. Multivitamins are also administered and patients should be advised to eat a well-balanced diet and abstain from drinking and smoking.

**Prognosis** is good in early cases provided patients comply with treatment, although visual recovery may be slow. In advanced and unresponsive cases, there is permanent visual loss as a result of optic atrophy.

## DRUG-INDUCED OPTIC NEUROPATHY

**Ethambutol** (Myambutol, Mynah) is used in combination with isoniazid and rifampicin in the treatment of tuberculosis. Toxicity is dose- and duration-dependent, the incidence being 6% at a daily dose of 25 mg/kg; rarely, 15 mg/kg may be toxic. Toxicity is unusual and may occur after at least 2 months of therapy (average is 7 months).

> **NB:** Isoniazid may also rarely cause toxic optic neuropathy, particularly in combination with ethambutol.

1. **Presentation** is with symmetrical insidious visual impairment associated with dyschromatopsia.

2. **Signs** include normal or slightly swollen optic discs with splinter-shaped haemorrhages.

3. **Visual field defects** usually consist of central or centro-caecal scotomas, although bitemporal or peripheral constriction may occur.

4. **Prognosis** is good following cessation of treatment, although recovery may take up to 12 months. A minority of patients develop permanent visual impairment as a result of optic atrophy.

5. **Screening** should be at about 3-monthly intervals if the daily dose exceeds 15 mg/kg. The drug should be stopped immediately if symptoms develop.

**Amiodarone** is an anti-arrhythmia drug used in the treatment of ventricular tachycardia and fibrillation, and in restoration of sinus rhythm in atrial fibrillation. Common systemic side effects include thyroid dysfunction, pulmonary toxicity, peripheral neuropathy and gastrointestinal problems. Vortex keratopathy (Fig. 8.33), which is innocuous, is virtually universal. Other uncommon ocular side effects include anterior subcapsular lens opacities, multiple chalazia, dry eyes and optic neuropathy. The last-mentioned affects only 1–2% of patients and is not dose-related.

1. **Presentation** is with insidious unilateral or bilateral visual impairment.

2. **Signs** are bilateral optic disc swelling that may persist for a few months after medication is stopped.

3. **Visual field defects** may be mild and reversible, or severe and permanent.

4. **Prognosis** is variable because cessation of the drug may not inevitably bring about improvement.

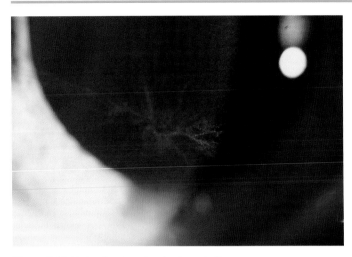

**Figure 8.33** Vortex keratopathy due to amiodarone

5. **Screening** is not appropriate because there is no way to identify those at risk. Patients should, however, be warned of the small risk of toxicity and to report any suggestive symptoms.

6. **Differential diagnosis** includes NAION, which also affects patients with systemic vascular disease. However, amiodarone optic neuropathy typically has a more insidious onset, milder visual loss, a longer duration of disc oedema and is more commonly bilateral than NAION.

***Vigabatrin*** is an antiepileptic drug, used mainly as second-line therapy. A significant percentage of patients develop dyschromatopsia and constricted visual fields when the total dose is 1500 g or more. The defects develop between 1 month to several years of starting therapy and are often permanent despite discontinuation of the drug. Product literature advises visual field testing at 6-monthly intervals.

### FURTHER READING
Macaluso DC, Shults WT, Fraunfelder FT. Features of amiodarone-induced optic neuropathy. *Am J Ophthalmol* 1999;127:610–612.
Mantyjarvi M, Tuppurainen K, Ikaheimo K. Ocular side effects of amiodarone. *Surv Ophthalmol* 1998;42:360–366.
Nagra PK, Foroozan R, Savino PJ, et al. Amiodarone induced optic neuropathy. *Br J Ophthalmol* 2003;87:420–422.

## Glaucomatous Optic Neuropathy

Glaucomatous damage results in characteristic signs involving (a) *retinal nerve fibre layer*, (b) *parapapillary area* and (c) *optic disc*.

### RETINAL NERVE FIBRE CHANGES
In normal eyes, the retinal nerve fibre layer is best seen on slit-lamp biomicroscopy using a green filter (Fig. 8.34). In glaucoma, subtle retinal nerve fibre layer defects precede the development of detectable optic disc and visual field changes. Retinal nerve fibre dropout may be diffuse or localised. Early localised damage is characterised by slit defects in the retinal nerve fibre layer (Fig. 8.35). As glaucomatous damage pro-

gresses, the defects become larger. The atrophic area becomes darker due to enhanced visualisation of the retinal pigment epithelium (RPE) and the retinal blood vessels become prominent (Fig. 8.36).

## PARAPAPILLARY CHANGES
Chorioretinal atrophy surrounding the optic nerve head is conceptualised as consisting of two zones – an inner 'beta' zone, bordering the disc margin, which in turn is concentrically surrounded by an outer 'alpha' zone (Fig. 8.37).

1. **Zone beta** exhibits chorioretinal atrophy with visibility of the sclera and large choroidal blood vessels.

2. **Zone alpha** displays variable irregular hyper and hypopigmentation of the RPE.

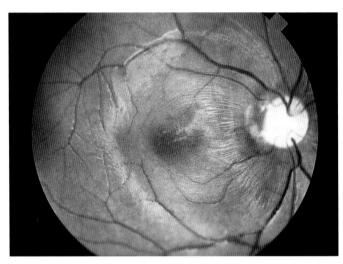

**Figure 8.34** Normal retinal nerve fibre layer; best seen with a green filter (Courtesy of J. Salmon)

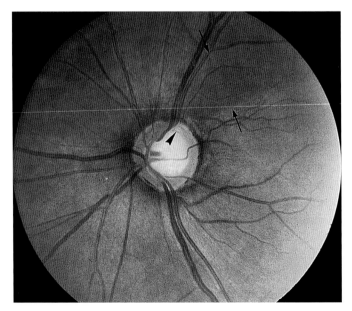

**Figure 8.35** Broad wedge-shaped superior retinal nerve fibre layer defect (arrows) associated with thinning of the neuroretinal rim (Courtesy of J. Salmon)

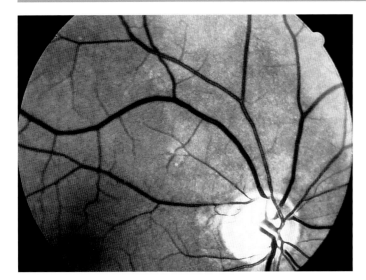

**Figure 8.36** Diffuse retinal nerve fibre layer atrophy in advanced glaucoma; no striations are visible and the retinal blood vessels appear dark and sharply defined (Courtesy of J. Salmon)

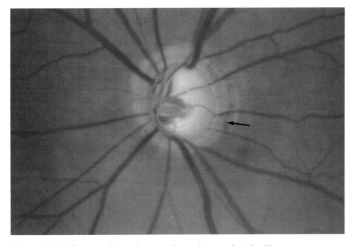

**Figure 8.37** Parapapillary changes (arrow) associated with gross glaucomatous damage (Courtesy of J. Salmon)

Although the alpha zone is larger in patients with primary open-angle glaucoma (POAG), its frequency is similar in glaucomatous and normal subjects. However, the beta zone is not only larger but also occurs more frequently in patients with POAG than in normal individuals. In unilateral POAG, the changes are more advanced in the affected eye. In ocular hypertension, the presence and size of parapapillary changes correlates with the subsequent development of optic disc and visual field damage. Approximately half of all ocular hypertensive eyes that convert to POAG exhibit progression of parapapillary atrophic changes.

## OPTIC DISC CHANGES

Optic disc damage is superimposed upon physiological cupping present prior to the onset of raised intraocular pressure (IOP). If an eye with a small cup develops glaucoma, the cup will increase in size, but during the early stages, its dimensions may still be smaller than that of a large physiological cup (Fig. 8.38). An estimation of cup size alone is therefore of limited value in the diagnosis of early glaucoma, unless it is found to be increasing. Glaucomatous cups are usually larger than physiological cups, although a large cup is not necessarily pathological. Assessment of the thickness, symmetry and colour of the neuroretinal rim is, however, more important. The spectrum of disc damage in glaucoma ranges from highly localised tissue loss with notching of the neuroretinal rim to diffuse concentric enlargement of the cup as well as vascular changes.

1. **Subtypes of glaucomatous damage.** The appearance and pattern of disc damage may correlate with sub-types of glaucoma and provide clues as to the pathogenic mechanisms involved as follows:

   a. *Type 1* (focal ischaemic) disc is characterised by focal tissue loss at the superior and/or inferior poles (polar notching) and an otherwise relatively intact neuroretinal rim (Fig. 8.39). The notch may be associated with localised field defects with early threat to fixation. Paradoxically, a large reduction in IOP may be bene-

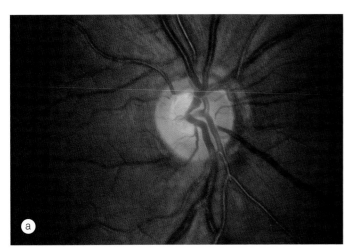

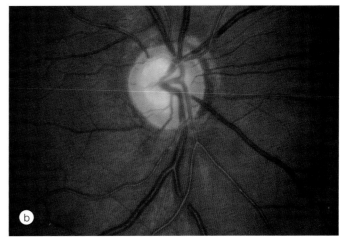

**Figure 8.38 (a)** Normal optic disc with a small cup; **(b)** 2 years later the disc shows concentric glaucomatous enlargement (Courtesy of J. Salmon)

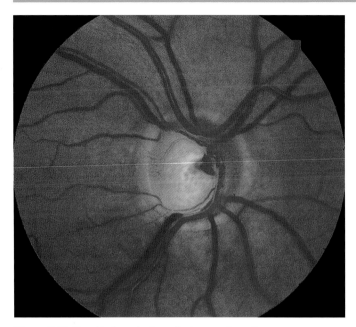

**Figure 8.39** Focal ischaemic (type 1) glaucomatous disc

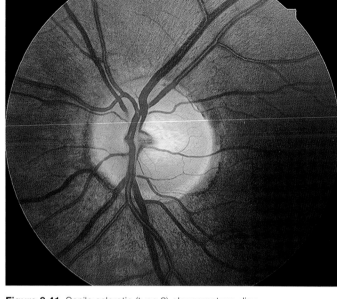

**Figure 8.41** Senile sclerotic (type 3) glaucomatous disc

ficial. Type 1 discs tend to occur in females who may have vasospasm and migraine.

b. *Type 2* (myopic glaucomatous) disc is characterised by polar notching and a temporal crescent in the absence of degenerative myopia (Fig. 8.40). It is associated with dense superior or inferior scotomas, which threaten fixation in 50% of cases. Progression of damage is frequent and may be rapid. Type 2 discs tend to occur in younger patients, particularly males.

c. *Type 3* (senile sclerotic) disc is characterised by a shallow, saucerised cup and a gently sloping neuroretinal rim, a 'moth-eaten' appearance, parapapillary atrophy and peripheral visual field loss (Fig. 8.41). It tends to affect

older patients (both genders equally), and is associated with ischaemic heart disease and hypertension. Circulatory abnormalities have also been demonstrated in the retrobulbar vessels.

d. *Type 4* (concentrically enlarging) disc is caused by diffuse loss of nerve fibres involving the entire cross-section of the optic nerve head. It is characterised by thinning of the entire neuroretinal rim without notching (Fig. 8.42) and is frequently associated with diffuse visual field loss. At presentation, the IOP is often significantly elevated. Type 4 discs tend to occur in younger patients and affect both genders equally.

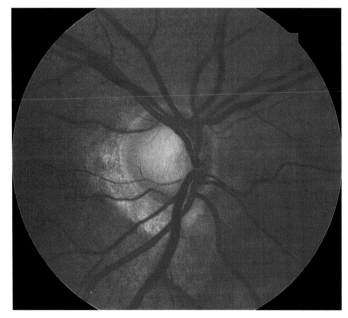

**Figure 8.40** Myopic (type 2) glaucomatous disc

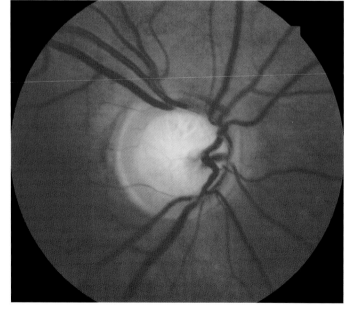

**Figure 8.42** Concentrically enlarging (type 4) glaucomatous disc

*e. Mixed.* At least two-thirds of eyes have a mixed appearance, potentially the result of multiple pathogenic mechanisms.

## 2. Non-specific signs of glaucomatous damage

*a. Baring of circumlinear blood vessels* is a sign of early thinning of the superior or inferior neuroretinal rim. It is characterised by a space between a superficial blood vessel which runs from the superior or inferior aspects of the disc towards the macula and the disc margin (Fig. 8.43).

*b. Nasal cupping* is a sign of severe thinning of the nasal neuroretinal rim in which there is a space between the rim and the central disc vasculature (Fig. 8.44).

*c. Bayoneting* is characterised by double angulation of a blood vessel as it dives sharply backwards and then turns along the steep wall of the excavation before angling again onto the floor of the disc (Fig. 8.45).

*d. The laminar dot sign* is caused by exposure of the lamina cribrosa due to loss of neuroretinal tissue. It is often seen in eyes with advanced glaucomatous damage (Fig. 8.46) but is not specific for glaucoma.

*e. Disc haemorrhages* are flame-shaped and extend onto the nerve fibre layer most frequently inferotemporally (Fig. 8.47). Their significance is as follows:

- About 25% of individuals over the age of 50 years with a disc haemorrhage have established glaucoma. The presence of disc haemorrhages may also be a sign of uncontrolled glaucoma.
- Disc haemorrhages tend to come and go, but often precede a defect in the retinal nerve fibre layer or visual field loss by up to 18 months.
- Disc haemorrhages may occur in non-glaucomatous eyes of patients with systemic hypertension or anaemia.

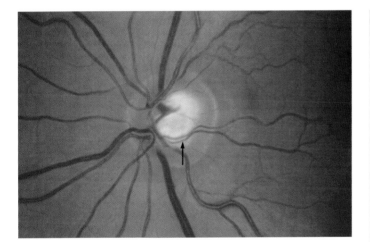

**Figure 8.43** Baring of an inferior circumlinear blood vessel (arrow) (Courtesy of J. Salmon)

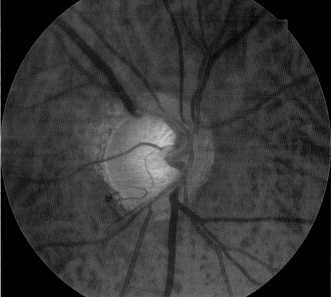

**Figure 8.45** Bayoneting of the superotemporal vein

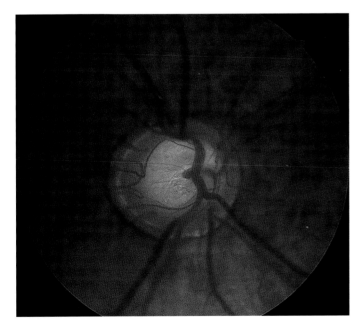

**Figure 8.44** Nasal cupping

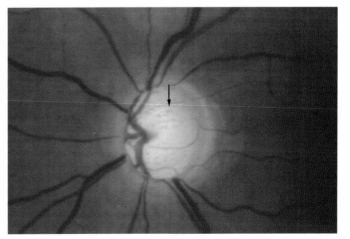

**Figure 8.46** Laminar dot sign due to exposure of the lamina cribrosa (Courtesy of J. Salmon)

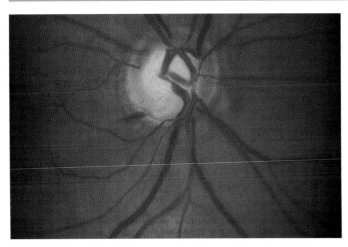

**Figure 8.47** Flame-shaped disc haemorrhage associated with inferior notching

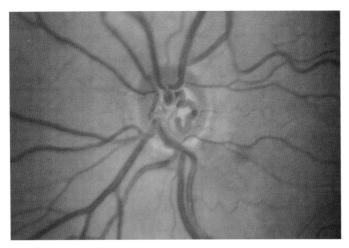

**Figure 8.48** Disc shunts (Courtesy of J. Salmon)

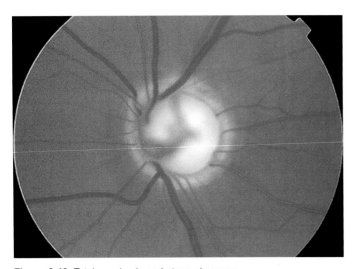

**Figure 8.49** Total cupping in end-stage glaucoma

f. *Disc shunts* between the central retinal and parapapillary veins or between two retinal veins are seen in a small minority of cases (Fig. 8.48).

g. *End-stage damage* is characterised by deep excavation and loss of all neuroretinal tissue (Fig. 8.49).

## FURTHER READING

Broadway DC, Nicolela MT, Drance SM. Optic disc appearance in primary open-angle glaucoma. *Surv Ophthalmol* 1999;43:223–243.

Jonas JB, Budde WM, Panda-Jonas S. Ophthalmoscopic evaluation of the optic nerve head. *Surv Ophthalmol* 1999;43:293–320.

Nicolela MT, Drance SM. Various glaucomatous optic nerve appearances: clinical correlations. *Ophthalmology* 1996;103:640–649.

Nicolela MT, Drance SM, Broadway DC, et al. Agreement among clinicians in the recognition of patterns of optic disk damage in glaucoma. *Am J Ophthalmol* 2001;132:836–844.

Spaeth GL. A new classification of glaucoma including focal glaucoma. *Surv Ophthalmol* 1994;38:9–17.

Sturmer J. Pattern of glaucomatous neuroretinal rim loss. *Ophthalmology* 1993; 100:63–68.

Van Buskirk M, Cioffi GA. Glaucomatous optic neuropathy. *Am J Ophthalmol* 1992;113:447–452.

# Papilloedema

Papilloedema is swelling of the optic nerve head secondary to raised intracranial pressure. It is nearly always bilateral, although it may be asymmetrical. All other causes of disc oedema in the absence of raised intracranial pressure are referred to as 'disc swelling' and usually produce visual impairment. All patients with papilloedema should be suspected of having an intracranial mass unless proved otherwise. However, not all patients with raised intracranial pressure will necessarily develop papilloedema. Tumours of the cerebral hemispheres tend to produce papilloedema later than those in the posterior fossa. Patients with a history of previous papilloedema may develop a substantial increase in intracranial pressure but fail to redevelop papilloedema because of glial scarring of the optic nerve head.

### Cerebrospinal fluid

1. **Circulation** (Fig. 8.50a)

   - CSF is formed by the choroid plexus in the ventricles of the brain.
   - It leaves the lateral ventricles to enter the third ventricle through the foramina of Munro.
   - From the third ventricle, it flows through the sylvian aqueduct to the fourth ventricle.
   - From the fourth ventricle, the CSF passes through the foramina of Luschka and Magendie to enter the subarachnoid space, some flowing around the spinal cord and the rest bathing the cerebral hemispheres.
   - Absorption is into the cerebral venous drainage system through the arachnoid villi.

2. **Normal opening pressure** of CSF on lumbar puncture is <80 mmH$_2$O in infants, <90 mmH$_2$O in children and <210 mmH$_2$O in adults.

### Causes of raised intracranial pressure (Fig. 8.50b)

- Obstruction of the ventricular system by congenital or acquired lesions.
- Space-occupying intracranial lesions, including haemorrhage.
- Impairment of CSF absorption via arachnoid villi, which may be damaged by meningitis, subarachnoid haemorrhage or cerebral trauma.

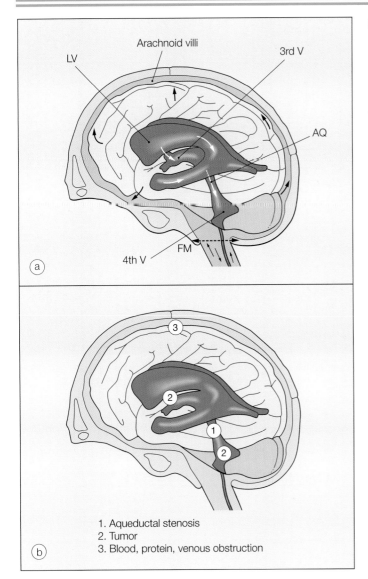

(a)

(b)

1. Aqueductal stenosis
2. Tumor
3. Blood, protein, venous obstruction

**Figure 8.50 (a)** Circulation of cerebrospinal fluid; **(b)** causes of raised intracranial pressure (Courtesy of Wilmer Institute)

- Idiopathic intracranial hypertension (pseudotumour cerebri).
- Diffuse cerebral oedema from blunt head trauma.
- Severe systemic hypertension.
- Hypersecretion of CSF by choroid plexus tumour, which is very rare.

## Clinical features of raised intracranial pressure

1. **Headaches** may come on at any time of day but characteristically occur early in the morning and may wake the patient from sleep. They tend to get progressively worse and patients usually present to hospital within 6 weeks. The headaches may be generalised or localised, and may intensify with head movement, bending or coughing. Patients with lifelong headaches often report a change in character of the headache. Very rarely, headache may be absent.

2. **Sudden nausea and vomiting,** often projectile, may partially relieve the headache. Vomiting may occur as an isolated feature or may precede the onset of headaches by months, particularly in patients with fourth ventricular tumours.

3. **Deterioration of consciousness** may be slight, with drowsiness and somnolence. Dramatic deterioration of consciousness is indicative of brain-stem distortion and tentorial or tonsillar herniation, and requires prompt attention.

4. **Visual**

   a. *Transient obscurations* lasting a few seconds are frequent in patients with papilloedma.

   b. *Horizontal diplopia* due to sixth-nerve palsy caused by stretching of one or both sixth nerves over the petrous tip. It is therefore a false localising sign.

   c. *Visual failure* occurs late in patients with secondary optic atrophy due to longstanding papilloedema (see below).

### Stages of papilloedema

1. **Early** (Fig. 8.51)

   - Visual symptoms are absent and visual acuity normal.
   - Optic discs show hyperaemia and mild elevation. The disc margins (initially nasal, later superior, inferior and temporal) appear indistinct, and swelling of the peripapillary retinal nerve fibre layer develops.
   - There is loss of previous spontaneous venous pulsation. However, as about 20% of normal individuals do not manifest spontaneous venous pulsation, its absence does not necessarily imply raised intracranial pressure. Preserved venous pulsation renders the diagnosis of papilloedema unlikely.

2. **Established** (Fig. 8.52)

   - Transient visual obscurations may occur in one or both eyes, lasting a few seconds, often on standing.
   - Visual acuity is normal or reduced.
   - Optic discs show severe hyperaemia and moderate elevation with indistinct margins, which may initially be asymmetrical. The optic cup and the small vessels

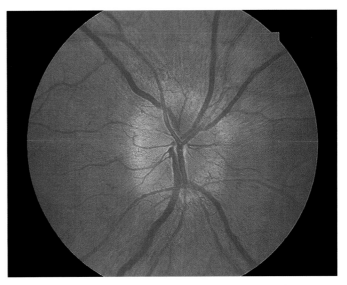

**Figure 8.51** Early papilloedema

on the disc are obscured. Venous engorgement, peri-papillary flame-shaped haemorrhages and frequently also cotton-wool spots may be seen. As the swelling increases, the optic nerve head appears enlarged; circumferential retinal folds may develop on its temporal side. Hard exudates may radiate from the centre of the fovea in the form of a 'macular fan' – an incomplete star with the temporal part missing.

- The blind spot is enlarged.

### 3. Longstanding (vintage) (Fig. 8.53)

- Visual acuity is variable and the visual fields begin to constrict.
- Optic discs are markedly elevated with a 'champagne cork' appearance. Cotton-wool spots and haemorrhages are absent. Optociliary shunts and drusen-like crystalline deposits (corpora amylacea) may be present on the disc surface.

### 4. Atrophic (secondary optic atrophy) (Fig. 8.54)

- Visual acuity is severely impaired.
- The optic discs are a dirty grey colour, slightly elevated, with few crossing blood vessels and indistinct margins.

## *Differential diagnosis of papilloedema*

### 1. Bilateral disc elevation

- High hypermetropia.
- Buried disc drusen (see Chapter 9).

### 2. Bilateral disc swelling may be caused by:

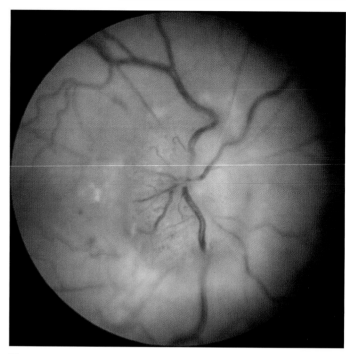

**Figure 8.53** Longstanding papilloedema

- Malignant hypertension.
- Bilateral papillitis.
- Bilateral compressive thyroid ophthalmopathy.
- Bilateral simultaneous anterior ischaemic optic neuropathy.
- Bilaterally compromised venous drainage in central retinal vein occlusion or carotid–cavernous fistula.

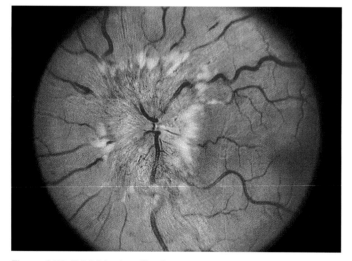

**Figure 8.52** Established papilloedema

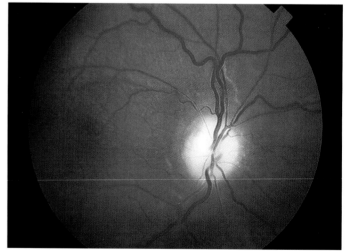

**Figure 8.54** Atrophic papilloedema

# Chapter 9

# CONGENITAL ANOMALIES

## Retina and Choroid

### CHOROIDAL COLOBOMA

In the fully developed eye, the embryonic fissure is inferior and slightly nasal, and extends from the optic nerve to the margin of the pupil (anterior part of the optic cup). A coloboma is the absence of part of an ocular structure as a result of incomplete closure of the embryonic fissure. It may involve the entire length of the fissure (complete coloboma) or only part (i.e. iris, ciliary body, retina and choroid, or the optic disc). A chorioretinal coloboma may be unilateral or bilateral and usually occurs sporadically in otherwise normal individuals.

1. **Signs**

   - Sharply circumscribed, white area devoid of blood vessels, of variable size, in the inferior fundus, associated with a corresponding visual field defect (Figs. 9.1 and 9.2).
   - Colobomas of the optic disc and iris may be present.

2. **Complications.** Retinal detachment may occur either due to a break outside and unrelated to the coloboma or within the coloboma. The latter break is difficult to visualise because of lack of contrast between the break and retina due to absence of choroidal background.

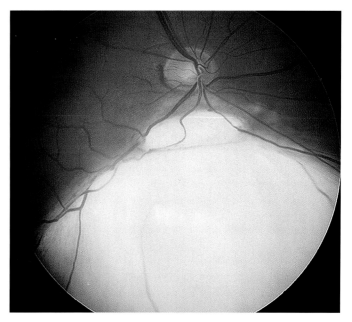

**Figure 9.2** Large chorioretinal coloboma

### MYELINATED NERVE FIBRES

Normally, optic nerve myelination stops at the cribriform plate, but in a minority of cases the ganglion cells retain a myelin sheath.

1. **Signs.** White feathery streaks running within the retinal nerve fibre layer towards the disc (Figs. 9.3–9.5).

2. **Associations** of very extensive nerve fibre myelination (Fig. 9.6) are high myopia and amblyopia.

### RETINAL MACROVESSEL

1. **Signs.** A unilateral, large, aberrant retinal vessel, usually a vein, is present in the posterior pole and may cross the foveal region and horizontal raphe (Fig. 9.7). Because arteriovenous anastamoses are often present, the condition may be considered to be a variant of racemose angiomatosis. The visual prognosis is excellent.

2. **Fluorescein angiography (FA)** may show early filling and delayed emptying of the vessel, and a dilated capillary bed surrounding the macrovessel is often present. Areas of capillary non-perfusion and foveal cysts may also be seen.

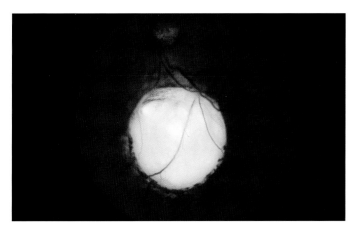

**Figure 9.1** Circumscribed chorioretinal coloboma

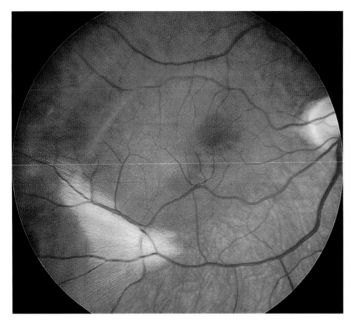

**Figure 9.3** Peripheral myelinated retinal nerve fibres

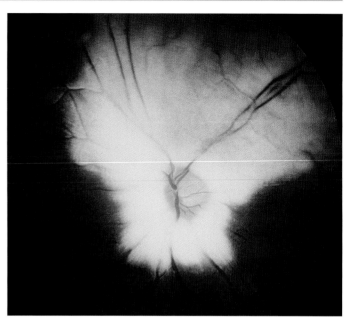

**Figure 9.5** Extensive retinal nerve fibre myelination

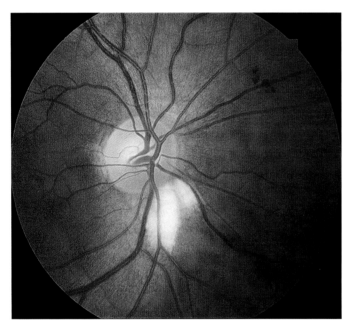

**Figure 9.4** Peripapillary myelinated nerve fibres

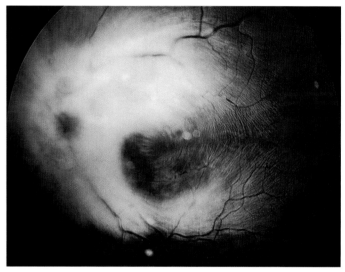

**Figure 9.6** Very extensive retinal nerve fibre myelination

## FAMILIAL RETINAL ARTERIOLAR TORTUOSITY

1. **Inheritance** is autosomal dominant.

2. **Signs.** Tortuous small retinal arterioles, normal venules (Fig. 9.8) and the frequent occurrence of intermittent superficial intraretinal haemorrhages.

3. **FA** shows vascular competence.

4. **Differential diagnosis**

   ● Coarctation of the aorta may also be associated with arteriolar tortuosity alone, without venous involvement.

● Causes of combined arteriolar and venous tortuosity (Fig. 9.9) include Fabry disease, Maroteaux–Lamy syndrome, macroglobulinaemia, cryoglobulinaemia, leukaemia and polycythaemia rubra vera.

## AICARDI SYNDROME

1. **Inheritance** is X-linked dominant. The condition is lethal in utero for males.

2. **Signs**

   ● Bilateral, multiple depigmented 'chorioretinal lacunae' clustered around the disc are pathognomonic (Fig. 9.10).
   ● Optic disc coloboma, hypoplasia and pigmentation.

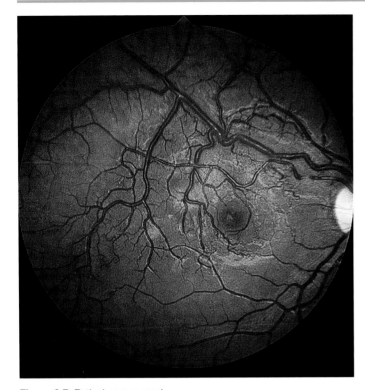

**Figure 9.7** Retinal macrovessel

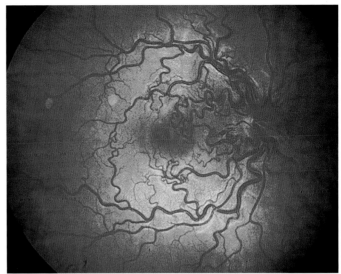

**Figure 9.9** Combined arterial and venous tortuosity

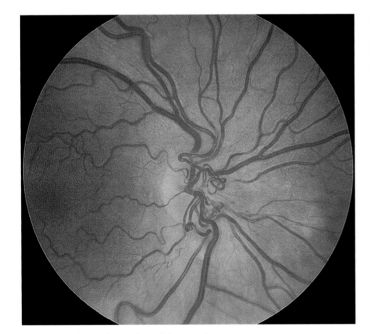

**Figure 9.8** Familial retinal arterial tortuosity

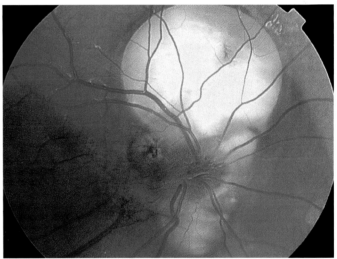

**Figure 9.10** Chorioretinal lacunae and optic disc anomaly in Aicardi syndrome

- Microphthalmos and iris colobomas (Fig. 9.11), as well as persistent pupillary membranes and cataract (Fig. 9.12).

3. **Systemic features** include infantile spasms, agenesis of the corpus callosum (Fig. 9.13), skeletal malformations and psychomotor retardation. Other serious central nervous system (CNS) malformations may also be present and death usually occurs within the first few years of life.

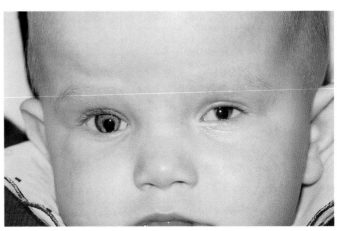

**Figure 9.11** Bilateral iris colobomas and left microphthalmos

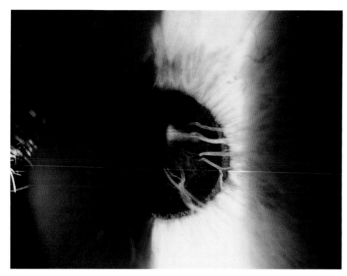

**Figure 9.12** Persistent pupillary membrane and anterior capsular lens opacities

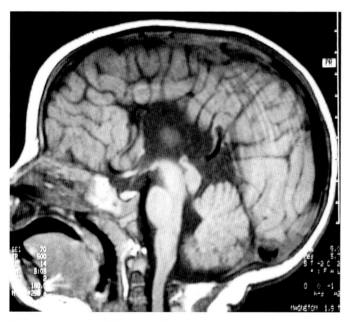

**Figure 9.13** Sagittal MRI shows absence of the corpus callosum (Courtesy of K. Nischal)

# Optic Disc

## PRE-PAPILLARY LOOP

1. **Signs.** A unilateral, vascular loop extending from the disc into the vitreous cavity and then back (Fig. 9.14).

2. **Complications**

   • Obstruction in the distribution of the retinal artery supplying the loop occurs in 10% of cases.
   • Vitreous haemorrhage is rare.

## BERGMEISTER PAPILLA

This is an uncommon unilateral anomaly that is derived from avascular remnants of the hyaloid system and is characterised by raised glial tissue on the disc surface (Fig. 9.15).

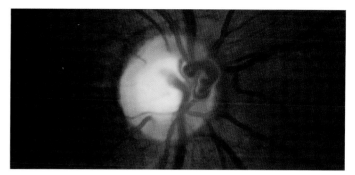

**Figure 9.14** Pre-papillary loop

## TILTED DISC

A tilted optic disc is a common, usually bilateral, anomaly caused by an oblique entry of the optic nerve into the globe. This results in pseudo-rotation of the superior pole of the disc, angulation of the optic cup axis and elevation of the neuroretinal rim.

1. **Signs** (Fig. 9.16 and 9.17a and b)

   • Small, oval or D-shaped disc in which the axis is most frequently directed inferonasally but may be horizontally or nearly vertically. The disc margin is indistinct where the retinal nerve fibres are elevated.
   • Inferonasal chorioretinal thinning.
   • Situs inversus in which the temporal vessels deviate nasally before turning temporally.
   • Associated changes include peripapillary chorioretinal atrophy, variable myopic astigmatic refractive error and posterior staphyloma.

2. **Perimetry** may show superotemporal defects that do not obey the vertical midline (Fig. 9.17c).

3. **Complications,** which are uncommon, include choroidal neovascularisation and sensory macular detachment.

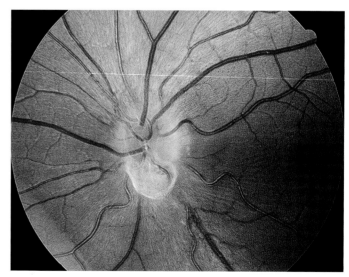

**Figure 9.15** Bergmeister papilla

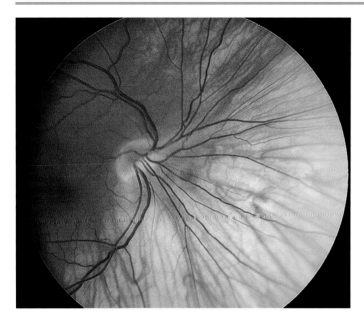

**Figure 9.16** Tilted disc

NB: On cursory examination, the visual field defects may be mistaken for those due to chiasmal compression and lead to unnecessary neuroradiological investigations. In eyes with tilted discs, the field defects are relative in nature, non-progressive and may resolve when a larger test stimulus is used or after optic correction. In addition, the defects are usually surrounded by a normal peripheral visual field and frequently cross the vertical meridia.

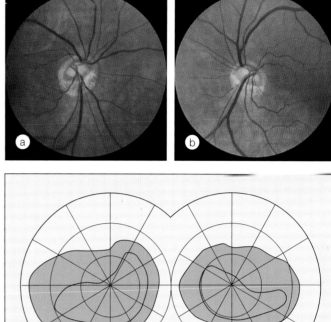

**Figure 9.17** **(a)** & **(b)** Tilted optic discs; **(c)** associated superotemporal visual field defects that do not obey the vertical midline (Courtesy of Wilmer Institute)

## OPTIC DISC PIT

### *Diagnosis*

### 1. Signs

- Visual acuity is normal in the absence of complications.
- The disc is larger than normal and contains a round or oval pit of variable size.
- The pit is usually located in the temporal aspect of the disc (Fig. 9.18a) but may occasionally be central.
- Visual field defects are common and may mimic those due to glaucoma.

2. **FA** of the pit shows early hypofluorescence (Fig. 9.18b) and late hyperfluorescence (Fig. 9.18c).

3. **Maculopathy** in the form of serous detachment (Fig. 9.19a) develops in about 45% of eyes with non-central disc pits, most frequently at about puberty. The subretinal fluid is thought to be derived from the vitreous; less likely sources are the subarachnoid space and leakage from abnormal vessels within the base of the pit (Fig. 9.19b).

4. **Evolution of macular involvement**

- Initially, there is a schisis-like separation of the inner layers of the retina which communicates with the pit.

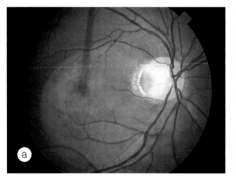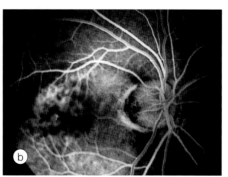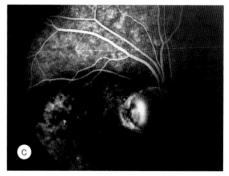

**Figure 9.18** **(a)** Optic disc pit; **(b)** FA early venous phase shows hypofluorescence of the pit; **(c)** later phase shows hyperfluorescence of the pit. Also note mottled hyperfluorescence at the posterior pole due to RPE atrophy secondary to previous serous macular detachment

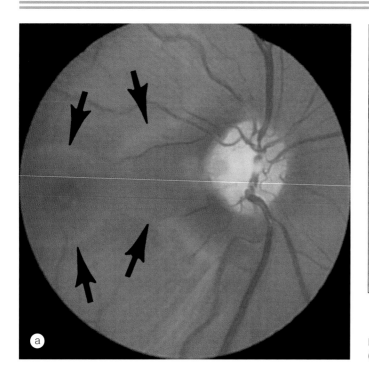

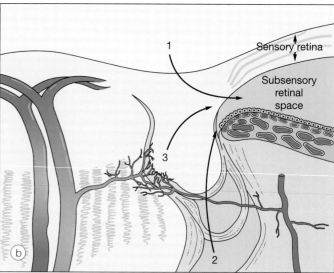

**Figure 9.19 (a)** Optic disc pit and serous macular detachment; **(b)** possible sources of subretinal fluid

● This is followed by serous detachment of the outer retinal layers, which may be associated with subretinal deposits (Fig. 9.20). This appearance may be mistaken for central serous retinopathy.

> **NB: It is important to examine the optic disc carefully in all patients with suspected central serous retinopathy.**

### Treatment options

1. **Observation** at 3-monthly intervals for evidence of spontaneous resolution of the detachment, which occurs in up to 25% of cases.

2. **Laser photocoagulation** may be considered if visual acuity is deteriorating. The burns are applied along the temporal aspect of the disc. The success rate is 25–35%.

3. **Vitrectomy** with air–fluid exchange, postoperative prone positioning and subsequent laser photocoagulation may be considered if laser alone is unsuccessful. The success rare is 50–70%.

## OPTIC DISC DRUSEN

Optic disc drusen (hyaline bodies) are composed of hyaline-like calcific material within the substance of the optic nerve head (Fig. 9.21). Clinically, they are present in about 0.3% of the population and are often bilateral. Although only a minority of relatives manifest disc drusen, nearly half have anomalous disc vessels and absence of the optic cup.

### Signs

1. **Buried drusen.** In early childhood, drusen may be difficult to detect because they lie deep beneath the surface

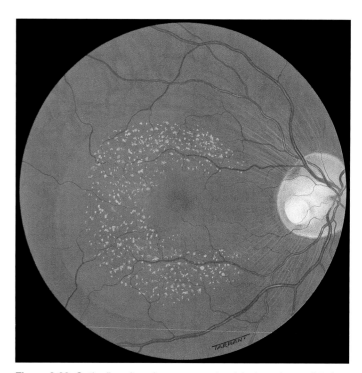

**Figure 9.20** Optic disc pit and serous macular detachment associated with subretinal deposits

of the disc (Fig. 9.22c and d). In this setting, the appearance may mimic chronic papilloedema (Fig. 9.22a and b). Signs suggestive of disc drusen are:

● Elevated disc with a scalloped margin without a physiological cup.

● Hyperaemia is absent and the surface vessels are not obscured, despite the disc elevation.

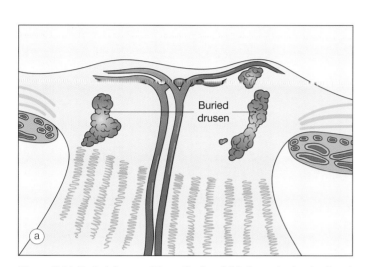

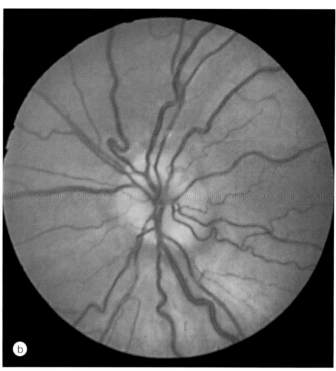

**Figure 9.21** Buried drusen of the optic disc. **(a)** Schematic showing location; **(b)** clinical appearance

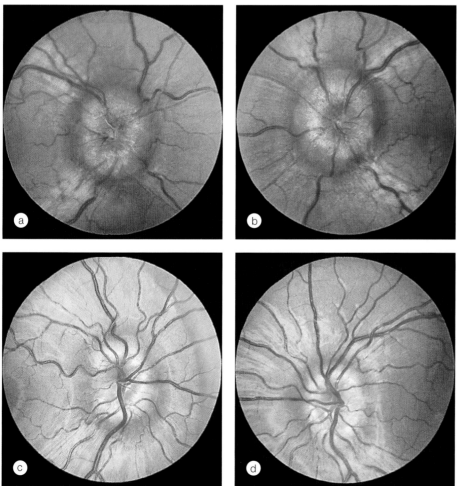

**Figure 9.22 (a)** & **(b)** Chronic papilloedema; **(c)** & **(d)** buried optic disc drusen (Courtesy of Wilmer Institute)

- Anomalous vascular patterns, including early branching, increased number of major retinal vessels and vascular tortuosity.
- Spontaneous venous pulsation may be present in 80% of cases.

2. **Exposed drusen.** During the early teens, drusen usually emerge at the surface of the disc as waxy pearl-like irregularities (Fig. 9.23).

### Complications

- Juxtapapillary choroidal neovascularisation is uncommon (Fig. 9.24) and may require laser photocoagulation.
- Occasionally, a progressive but limited loss of visual field with a nerve fibre bundle pattern may occur.

*Associations* include retinitis pigmentosa, angioid streaks and Alagille syndrome.

*Special investigations* may be necessary for the definitive diagnosis of disc drusen, particularly when buried.

1. **Ultrasonography** (Fig. 9.25) is the most readily available and reliable method because of its ability to detectcalcific deposits. With the grain turned down, drusen can still be recognised by their high acoustic reflectivity.

2. **CT** (Fig. 9.26) is less sensitive than ultrasonography and may miss small drusen. Drusen may, however, be detected incidentally on CT, when performed in the course of investigation of other pathology.

3. **FA** shows the phenomenon of autofluorescence prior to dye injection (Fig. 9.27a) and then progressive hyperfluorescence but no leakage of dye (Fig. 9.27b and 9.27c). Buried drusen show more subtle findings because of attenuation from the overlying tissue.

## OPTIC DISC COLOBOMA

Disc colobomas are usually sporadic, although autosomal dominant inheritance has been described. They may be unilateral or bilateral.

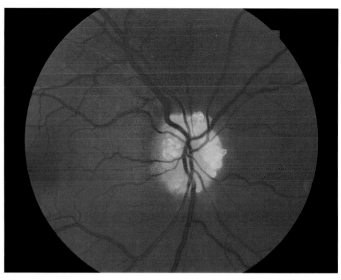

**Figure 9.23** Exposed optic disc drusen

### Diagnosis

1. **Signs**

   - Visual acuity is often decreased.
   - The disc shows a discrete, focal, glistening, white, bowl-shaped excavation, decentred inferiorly so that the inferior neuroretinal rim is thin or absent and normal disc tissue is confined to a small superior wedge (Fig. 9.28a).
   - The optic disc itself may be enlarged but the retinal vasculature is normal.

2. **Visual fields** show a superior defect (Fig. 9.28b) which, in conjunction with the disc appearance, may be mistaken for normal-tension glaucoma.

3. **Ocular associations** include microphthalmos and colobomas of the iris and fundus.

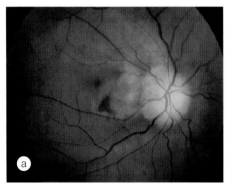
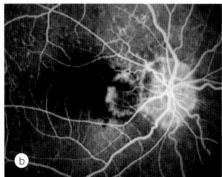
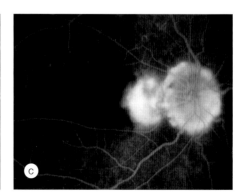

**Figure 9.24** Juxtapapillary choroidal neovascularisation associated with optic disc drusen. **(a)** Macular oedema and haemorrhage; **(b)** FA early venous phase showing lacy hyperfluorescence; **(c)** late phase showing more intense and diffuse hyperfluorescence due to leakage as well as hyperfluorescence of the optic disc

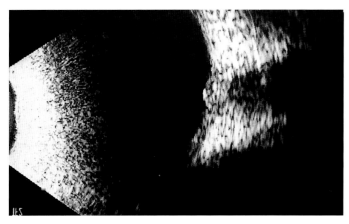

**Figure 9.25** B-scan of optic disc drusen

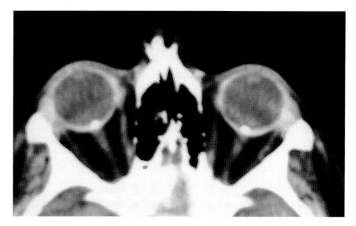

**Figure 9.26** Axial CT shows bilateral optic disc drusen

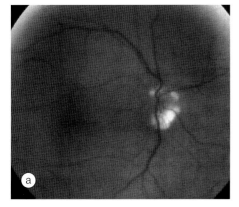

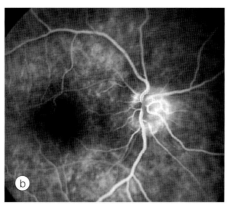

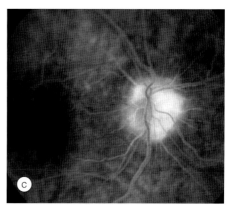

**Figure 9.27** Optic disc drusen. **(a)** Autofluorescence; **(b)** & **(c)** FA shows increasing hyperfluorescence but no leakage

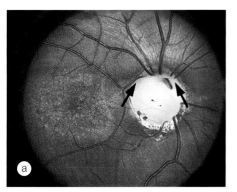

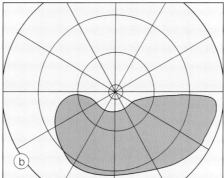

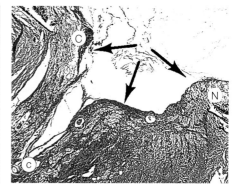

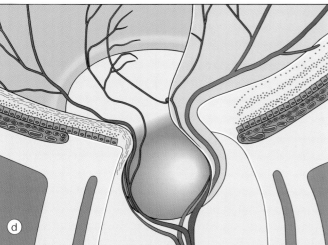

**Figure 9.28** **(a)** Optic disc coloboma with a residual superior wedge of normal disc tissue (arrow) associated with normal retinal nerve fibres; RPE changes at the macula are the result of previous serous detachment; **(b)** corresponding inferior island of visual field; **(c)** longitudinal histological section shows a crater-like defect (arrows), one side of which consists only of collagenous connective tissue (C) and the other is normal (N); **(d)** schematic shows the coloboma (Courtesy of Wilmer Institute)

## Complications

- Serous retinal detachment at the macula may occur (see Fig. 9.28a).
- Progressive enlargement of the excavation and neural rim thinning despite normal intraocular pressure has been described.
- Rhegmatogenous retinal detachment may occur in eyes with associated chorioretinal colobomas.

**Systemic associations** are numerous. The most notable are as follows:

1. **Chromosomal anomalies** include Patau syndrome (trisomy 13), Edward syndrome (trisomy 18) and cat-eye syndrome (trisomy 22).

2. **'CHARGE'** association comprises *C*oloboma, *H*eart defects, choanal *A*tresia, *R*etarded growth and development, *G*enital and *E*ar anomalies.

3. **Other syndromes** include Meckel–Gruber, Goltz, Lenz microphthalmos, Walker–Warburg, Goldenhar, Dandy–Walker cyst and Rubinstein–Taybi.

## MORNING GLORY ANOMALY

Morning glory anomaly is a very rare, usually unilateral sporadic condition. Bilateral cases, which are rarer still, may be hereditary.

### Signs

- Visual acuity is usually very poor.
- A large disc with a funnel-shaped excavation (Fig. 9.29). A central core of whitish glial tissue, representing persistent hyaloid remnants, lies at the base of the excavation.
- The disc is surrounded by an elevated annulus of chorioretinal pigmentary disturbance.
- The blood vessels emerge from the rim of the excavation in a radial pattern like the spokes of a wheel. They are increased in number and it is difficult to distinguish arteries from veins.

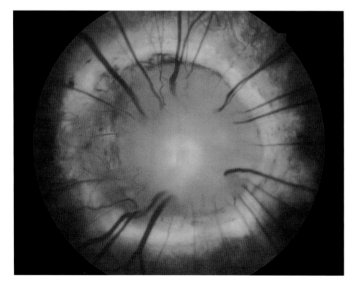

**Figure 9.29** Morning glory anomaly

- Serous retinal detachment develops in about 30% of cases.

**Systemic associations,** which are uncommon, include the following:

1. **Frontonasal dysplasia,** the most important, is characterised by a malformation complex comprising: (a) mid-facial anomalies consisting of hypertelorism, depressed nasal bridge, hare lip and cleft palate; (b) basal encephalocele, absent corpus callosum (see Fig. 9.13) and pituitary deficiency.

2. **Neurofibromatosis type 2** is much less common.

## OPTIC NERVE HYPOPLASIA

The hypoplastic optic nerve, unilateral or bilateral, is characterised by a diminished number of nerve fibres. It may occur as an isolated anomaly in an otherwise normal eye, in a grossly malformed eye or in association with a heterogeneous group of disorders most commonly involving the midline structures of the brain.

**Predispositions** include specific agents used by the mother during gestation, including excess alcohol, LSD, quinine, protamine zinc insulin, steroids, diuretics, cold remedies and anticonvulsants. Superior segmental optic nerve hypoplasia may be associated with maternal diabetes.

### Diagnosis

1. **Signs**

   - Visual acuity can vary from normal to no light perception.
   - Small grey disc surrounded by a yellow halo of hypopigmentation caused by concentric chorioretinal atrophy (double-ring sign) (Fig. 9.30). The outer ring represents what would have been the normal disc margin.
   - The distance from the fovea to the temporal border of the optic disc often equals or exceeds three times the disc diameter – this strongly suggests disc hypoplasia.
   - Despite the small size of the disc, the retinal blood vessels are of normal calibre, although they may be tortuous.
   - Superior segmental hypoplasia ('topless optic disc') is characterised by relative superior entry of the central retinal artery, superior retinal nerve fibre bundle deficiency, superior yellow halo and superior disc pallor associated with inferior altitudinal or sector-like visual field defects. Visual acuity is usually good. There is an association with maternal type 1 diabetes mellitus.

2. **Other features** vary considerably, depending on the severity. They include visual field defects, dyschromatopsia, afferent pupillary defect, foveal hypoplasia, aniridia, microphthalmos, strabismus and nystagmus in severe bilateral cases. Mild cases may be overlooked and the slight reduction of visual acuity mistaken for amblyopia and treated by occlusion.

### Systemic associations

1. **de Morsier syndrome** (septo-optic dysplasia) is present in about 10% of cases. In addition to bilateral optic nerve hypoplasia, this involves a spectrum of midline develop-

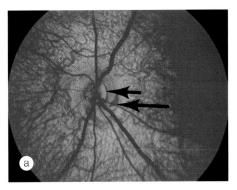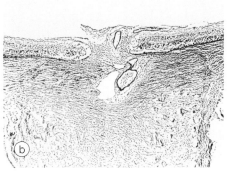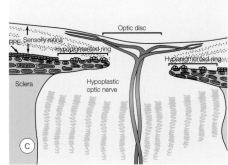

**Figure 9.30** Optic nerve hypoplasia. **(a)** Optic disc hypoplasia; disc outline (short arrow), hypopigmented ring (long arrow); **(b)** longitudinal histological section shows hypoplasia of the disc and retrolaminar optic nerve; **(c)** schematic shows absence of peripapillary retinal pigment epithelium (Courtesy of Wilmer Institute)

mental brain defects which may or may not be associated with endocrine abnormalities. These defects include absence or dysgenesis of the septum pellucidum, thinning or agenesis of the corpus callosum (see Fig. 9.15) and dysplasia of the anterior third ventricle. Hypopituitarism with low growth hormone levels is common; if recognised early, the hormone deficiency can be corrected and normal growth resumed. It has been suggested that retinal venous tortuosity in patients with bilateral optic nerve hypoplasia may be a marker for potential endocrine dysfunction.

2. **Frontonasal dysplasia** is an occasional association.

## MISCELLANEOUS ANOMALIES

1. **Megalopapilla,** in which the horizontal and vertical disc diameters are 2.1 mm or more (Fig. 9.31).

2. **Peripapillary staphyloma** is a usually unilateral condition in which a relatively normal disc sits at the base of a deep excavation whose walls, as well as the surrounding choroid and retinal pigment epithelium show atrophic changes (Fig. 9.32). Visual acuity is markedly reduced, and

local retinal detachment may be present. Frontonasal dysplasia is an occasional association.

3. **Optic disc dysplasia** is a descriptive term for a markedly deformed disc that does not conform to any recognisable category (Fig. 9.33).

4. **Papillorenal syndrome** is an autosomal dominant condition characterised by hypoplastic kidneys, renal failure and optic disc anomalies. The discs appear 'vacant', with replacement of the central retinal vasculature by vessels of cilioretinal origin.

5. **Optic nerve aplasia** is an extremely rare condition characterised by absence of the optic nerve, the ganglion cell layer and the retinal vasculature.

# Vitreous

## PERSISTENT HYALOID ARTERY

Persistent hyaloid artery is a unilateral condition seen in 95% of premature infants and rarely in adults.

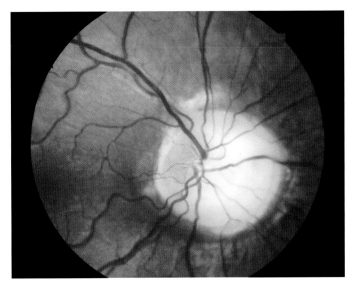

**Figure 9.31** Megalopapilla

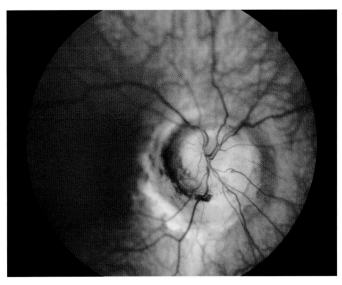

**Figure 9.32** Peripapillary staphyloma

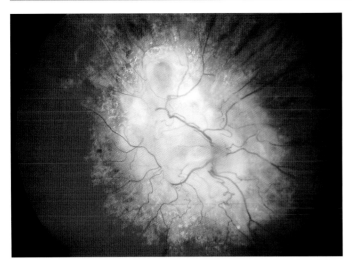

**Figure 9.33** Dysplastic disc (Courtesy of C. Barry)

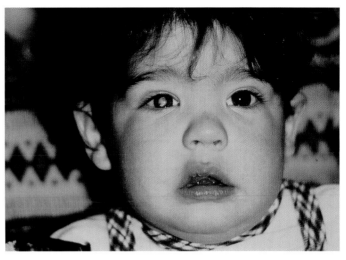

**Figure 9.35** Right leukocoria due to persistent hyperplastic primary vitreous

1. **Signs.** Glial remnants extending from the disc to the lens (Cloquet canal). The artery may contain blood at its point of attachment to the posterior lens capsule (Mittendorf spot) (Fig. 9.34).

2. **Complications.** Vitreous haemorrhage is rare.

3. **Ocular associations** include posterior vitreous cyst, optic disc coloboma and optic nerve hypoplasia.

## PERSISTENT HYPERPLASTIC PRIMARY VITREOUS

Persistent hyperplastic primary vitreous (PHPV) is an important cause of leukocoria. It typically occurs in a microphthalmic eye and is almost always unilateral (Fig. 9.35).

1. **Signs**

   • Retrolental mass into which elongated ciliary processes are inserted (Fig. 9.36).

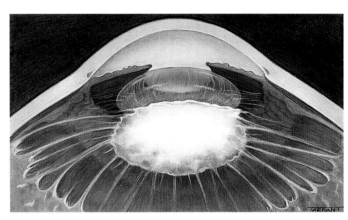

**Figure 9.36** Persistent hyperplastic primary vitreous with elongated ciliary processes

   • With time, the mass contracts and pulls the ciliary processes centrally so that they become visible through the pupil.

2. **Complications** include cataract formation due to a capsular dehiscence.

3. **Treatment** involving vitreoretinal surgery may be successful in salvaging some vision in selected early cases.

## POSTERIOR PERSISTENT HYPERPLASTIC PRIMARY VITREOUS

This is a very rare unilateral anomaly characterised by a dense white membrane or a prominent retinal fold extending from the optic disc to the peripheral retina or retrolental space (Fig. 9.37).

## RETINAL DYSPLASIA

Retinal dysplasia is caused by failure of retinal and vitreous development. It may be unilateral or bilateral.

1. **Signs**

   • Congenital blindness with roving eye movements in bilateral cases.

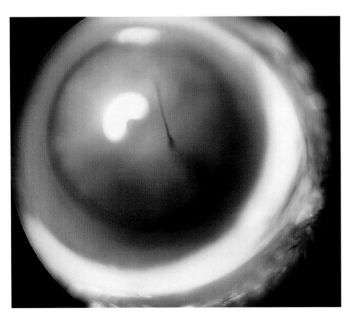

**Figure 9.34** Persistent hyaloid artery

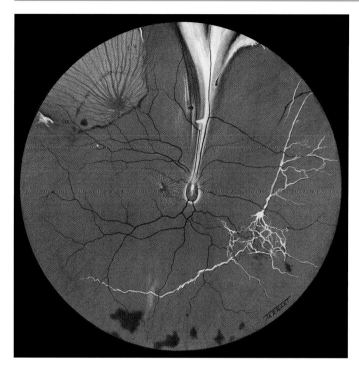

**Figure 9.37** Posterior hyperplastic primary vitreous

- Pink or white retrolental masses resulting in leukocoria (Fig. 9.38).
- Microphthalmos, shallow anterior chamber and elongated ciliary processes.

2. **Systemic associations,** which are usually associated with bilateral involvement, include Norrie disease, incontinentia pigmenti (see below), Warburg syndrome, Patau syndrome, Edward syndrome and osteoporosis–pseudoglioma– mental retardation syndrome.

## INCONTINENTIA PIGMENTI (BLOCH–SULZBERGER SYNDROME)

1. **Inheritance** is X-linked dominant with the gene locus on Xq28. The condition is lethal in utero for males.

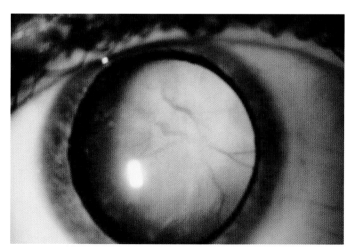

**Figure 9.38** Retinal dysplasia

2. **Presentation** is with vesiculobullous rash on the trunk and extremities (Fig. 9.39) which is later replaced by linear pigmentation (Fig. 9.40).

3. **Ocular signs**

- Retinal dysplasia or neovascularisation resulting in cicatricial retinal detachment in the first year of life, which may cause leukocoria, occurs in one-third of cases.
- Cataract, optic atrophy and strabismus may be present.

4. **Systemic features** include malformations of teeth, hair, nails, bones and CNS.

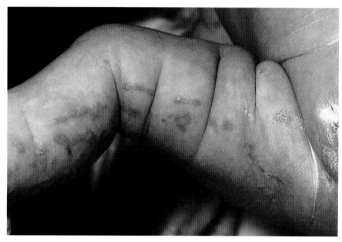

**Figure 9.39** Vesiculobullous skin lesions in incontinentia pigmenti

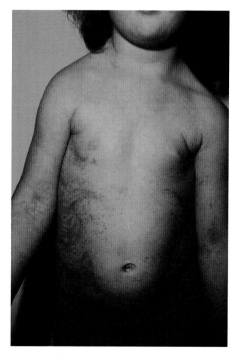

**Figure 9.40** Linear skin hyperpigmentation in incontinentia pigmenti

## FURTHER READING

Brodsky MC. Congenital optic disc anomalies. *Surv Ophthalmol* 1994;39;89–112.

Brown GC, Brown MM. Treatment of retinal detachment associated with congenital excavation defects of the optic disc. *Ophthalmic Surg* 1995;26:11–15.

Cohen SY, Quentel G, Guiberteau B, et al. Macular serous retinal detachment caused by subretinal leakage in tilted disc syndrome. *Ophthalmology* 1998;105:1831–1834.

Lincoff H, Kreissig I. Optical coherence tomography of pneumatic displacement of optic disc pit maculopathy. *Br J Ophthalmol* 1998;82:367–372.

Parsa CF, Silva ED, Sundin OH, et al. Redefining papillorenal syndrome: an under-diagnosed cause of ocular and renal morbidity. *Ophthalmology* 2001;108:738–749.

Sobol WM, Blodi CF, Folk JC, et al. Long-term visual outcome in patients with optic nerve pits and serous retinal detachment of the macula. *Ophthalmology* 1990; 97:1539–1542.

Vongphanit J, Mitchell P, Wang JJ. Population prevalence of tilted optic discs and the relationship of this sign to refractive error. *Am J Ophthalmol* 2002;133:679–685.

# INDEX